# THE DEVELOPMENT OF EMOTIONAL COMPETENCE IN YOUNG CHILDREN

# The Development of Emotional Competence in Young Children

Susanne A. Denham

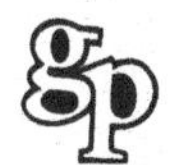


THE GUILFORD PRESS
New York London

A Division of Guilford Publications, Inc.
370 Seventh Avenue, Suite 1200, New York, NY 10001
www.guilford.com



Printed in the United States of America

This book is printed on acid-free paper.

Last digit is print number: 9 8 7 6 5 4 3 2 1

**Library of Congress Cataloging-in-Publication Data**

Names: Denham, Susanne A., author.
Title: The development of emotional competence in young children / Susanne A. Denham.
Description: New York : The Guilford Press, 2023. | Includes bibliographical references and index.
Identifiers: LCCN 2022053677 | ISBN 9781462551743 (paperback) | ISBN 9781462551750 (hardcover)
Subjects: LCSH: Emotions in children. | Developmental psychology. | BISAC: PSYCHOLOGY / Developmental / Child | SOCIAL SCIENCE / Social Work
Classification: LCC BF723.E6 D36 2023 | DDC 155.4/124—dc23/eng/20221212
LC record available at *https://lccn.loc.gov/2022053677*

# Preface

## WHY THIS BOOK IS NEEDED AND THE APPROACH TAKEN

Emotions are omnipresent in all our lives. Young children are no exception, and an explosion of knowledge about their feelings has occurred in the last 30 years. And, although preschoolers' emotions are fascinating and important in their own right, they are absolutely pivotal in how young children learn to engage in relationships and interactions with other people and are able to attain important aspects of school readiness. In short, young children's emotions are central to everything they do—how do they express emotions and regulate them when they are either too muted or too strong? How do they understand their own and others' emotions? These aspects of emotional competence develop enormously during the preschool years and are vital supports for social and school success.

Thus, this book is needed to afford a clear picture of the elements and importance of preschoolers' emotional competence. The amazing abilities preschoolers acquire in this area, as well as their relative weaknesses, are important to describe. Parents, early childhood educators, students, researchers, and other interested individuals can find this book useful in its thick description of how emotional competence evolves during this period.

Further, young children's emotional lives, as important as they are, do not unfold in a vacuum. Adults in their lives play crucial roles in how preschoolers come to be emotionally competent—they show emotions, react to children's emotions, and can even teach about emotions. So another clear need for this book emerges in its take-home messages about how early childhood emotional competence may be fostered—or, unfortunately, hindered—by parents, individual teachers, and an educational system.

In covering these topics, I take the following approaches: In discussing the elements of emotional competence—emotional expressiveness, emotion knowledge, and emotion regulation—I present what I consider to be a reasonable theoretical approach that outlines the key aspects of each element. I then describe, where knowledge is available, how young children change over time but also show stable individual differences, their own uniqueness, for each aspect. I take a similar approach in describing the theory supporting the components of how parents and teachers socialize emotional competence, and then in addressing each of its components in turn, along with issues in these adults' own emotional lives that may impact their socialization. In describing how young children's emotional competence contributes to their social and academic competence, I define each of these constructs and then look at the contribution made by each separate element of emotional competence. Finally, I felt the need to introduce the boundary conditions in which the development of emotional competence may be difficult for young children and to end with considering how we can educate for preschoolers' emotional competence.

## WHAT'S NEW IN THIS VOLUME

There have been many developments since the publication of my earlier volume, *Emotional Development in Young Children*, in 1998. First, I have tried to keep up with definitional issues about emotions themselves and emotional competence in particular. Views of emotion regulation have become clearer, and the study of the topic has proliferated. Further, research methods have expanded and improved to paint a detailed picture of how emotional competence helps young children become better social partners and more focused learners in school. These new developments are reflected in Chapters 10 and 11.

Given the expanding view that researchers have taken about emotional competence in the ensuing years, I am now able to comment upon the ways in which varying cultures are similar and different, especially in terms of how young children's emotional competence is socialized and how it contributes to social competence. Moreover, much more can be said about the biological bases of, and their contributions to, emotional competence during the preschool period. Finally, the role of education in promoting young children's emotional competence also has blossomed. Thus, material on teachers' contributions is given in an entirely new chapter, Chapter 9. Then the progress made in assessing emotional competence and in the programming that promotes young children's emotional competence is outlined in Chapter 13.

Nonetheless, the "bones" of both books remain quite similar—the expression, regulation, and understanding of emotions form the ingredients of emotional competence. There are developmental trajectories for each of these components, and they are affected by both intra- and interpersonal factors. Individual differences in each of the components occur and are important to both social and academic outcomes. Some children have more difficulty attaining emotional competence. This much remains clear.

## TOPIC COVERAGE UNIQUE TO THIS BOOK

No other book to my knowledge goes into as much depth and breadth about the development of each element of emotional competence during the preschool period. In particular, there is comprehensive coverage of the expression of empathy and self-conscious emotions, as well as a comparative look at emotion regulation as both product and process. In terms of emotion knowledge, the coverage extends through many personalized aspects that are difficult for young children.

Finding out and pulling together the specifics of how such emotional competence affords "a leg up" on other important developments are another important focus. Regarding the contribution of emotional competence, I believe this material to be uniquely wide ranging, especially in reference to the way emotional competence can facilitate young children's preacademic learning.

My emphasis on adult emotion socialization is not new, but including that of teachers is, as is a glimpse of how both internal and external forces can influence the development of preschoolers' emotional competence. Finally, stepping back and looking at assessment and programming as part of a whole educational system for preschool emotional competence development is, I feel, an important contribution.

## AUDIENCE AND RATIONALE FOR ORGANIZING THIS BOOK: HOW TO READ OR TEACH FROM IT

My plan has been to make this volume useful to several audiences: researchers, students at both undergraduate and graduate levels, early childhood educators, and others who care about the emotional development of children. Thus, I see it as a valuable tool for use in both courses and self-study.

Given such flexibility in terms of audience, I believe the chapters in this book could be approached in multiple ways. Of course, I think all the chapters integrate well in telling the full story of preschool emotional competence development as I think it should be told. And, as already noted, I have tried to organize the book by first describing the three elements of emotional competence in detail, then explaining how emotional competence facilitates development in other domains, and finally discussing how individual adults and even the educational system, as well as exacerbating conditions, affect such development.

As such, the book reads well as a whole. If it is used in the university or college classroom, a chapter per week could be assigned. For researchers, early childhood educators, and other interested persons, which chapters to read certainly could be dictated by interest (e.g., perhaps just the chapters describing the elements of emotional competence), although, again, it seems that the chapters fit together as a whole.

## PEDAGOGICAL FEATURES

Throughout the chapters I have tried to envision the emotional life of the preschooler. This perspective gives me a lot of joy, and I hope to convey that to the reader; we need to peer into the hearts of our children to know how to help them develop emotionally. In this light, I use many examples to illustrate points and concepts. Further, I often expand these examples into vignettes—so you can follow many of the children I have known or conjured—Joey, Mike, Rodney, Jimmy, Benjie, Carrie, Colin, Layne, and Leah, for example—throughout the book. In a more serious vein, perhaps, I also give section and chapter summaries to aid the reader in following along in what can be a rather complex narrative.

## ACKNOWLEDGING SUPPORT AND DIRECTION

I have felt very supported in taking on this challenging endeavor during a pandemic (although the task may have actually promoted sanity!). First and foremost, I thank my editor, C. Deborah Laughton, who has encouraged me and helped me course-correct when needed, as well as shared the joys of grandparenting with me.

Second, I'm truly indebted to a stellar group of reviewers, all already known to me to be astutely involved in the study of young children's emotional competence, as well as supportive colleagues. More even than this, their ability to assist me in fine-tuning the volume was enormous. So, thank you, Linda Camras, Susan Campbell, Deborah Laible, Jeff Liew, Susan Rivers, and Kate Zinsser. You all form a cadre of incredibly helpful partners in this venture.

Finally, I thank those whose emotions are of utmost importance to me—my daughters, Sarah and Jessie, and grandchildren, Maddie and Andrew. I couldn't do this, or much of anything else, without you.

# Brief Contents

# Extended Contents

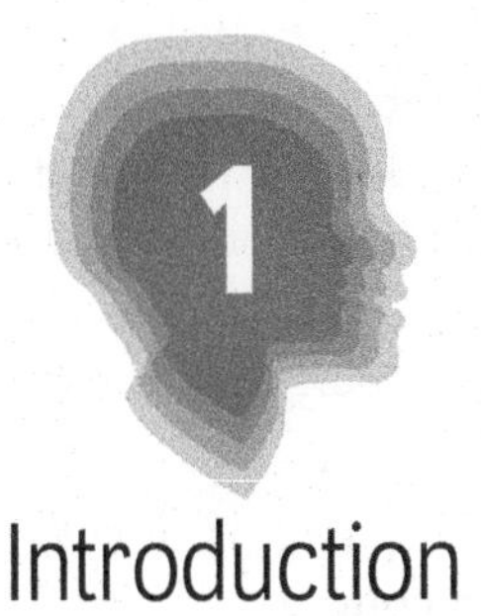

# 1 Introduction

## INTRODUCTION

The social–emotional skills that preschoolers normally develop are quite impressive. Consider the following example:

> Four-year-olds Joey and Mike are pretending to be pirates. They have rubber swords, cocked hats, "gold" coins, and even a stuffed parrot. They are having a lot of fun. Joey finds the buried treasure—hurray! But then things get complicated, changing fast and furiously, as interaction often does. Mike suddenly decides to be the Queen's Navy, and Joey must "sword-fight" him. Then Jimmy, who has been hovering nearby, tries to join in. No way! Joey wants Jimmy to leave. At almost the same minute, Mike steps on a Lego and starts to cry. And Rodney, the class bully, approaches, laughing at Joey and Mike for making believe and at Mike for crying. Joey deals with all of them: He comforts Mike appropriately, manages to tell Jimmy to stay out of the game without alienating him, and does his best to ignore Rodney's teasing. When their teacher calls them to have a snack, everybody is satisfied with the morning.

This is much more than a simple playtime; a lot of emotional transactions are occurring. Joey's clear, convincing, and appropriate expressions of emotions aid him in getting what he wants socially:

- When Joey finds the buried treasure, his face shows absolute joy.
- When challenged by Mike as the Queen's Navy, he roars with rage and acts very brave.

- He displays just the right intensity of anger to tell Jimmy to "keep out." Not too strongly, though—Joey doesn't want Jimmy to shout back, "I'm not your friend!" Joey's understanding of emotions also allows him to respond quickly but accurately—helping him in the tough job of regulating his own emotions and responding to those of others—during rapidly shifting, highly charged play experiences.
- Joey responds to Mike's crying by first quietly giving his friend a chance to pull himself together, and then comforting him. Misinterpreting Mike's grimace as anger could have led Joey to act angry himself, hurting his friend's feelings and endangering their relationship.
- When Rodney comes over, Joey appears noncommittal, masking his anger and fear.

So, within a 5-minute play period, several different elements of emotional competence are called for if the social interaction is to proceed successfully. Taken together, the expression, understanding, and regulation of emotions are vital for determining how Joey gets along with others, how he understands himself, and whether he feels good in his world, within himself, and with other people. Joey is one "emotionally smart" little guy; he is developing "emotional competence."

## THE NATURE OF EMOTION

But what *are* emotions, anyway? Before we delve further into toddlers' and preschoolers' emotional competence, it is important to consider the nature of emotions and their experience. Thus I briefly review the history of the study of emotions. Given this foundation, I consolidate my own view, specifying what I mean by *emotion* and its experience, the interplay between emotion and cognition, and how emotions are regulators of, and are regulated by, the behavior of the self and others. Throughout I posit what I consider to be useful theoretical viewpoints.

At first glance, the need to define as common a human phenomenon as emotion may seem a bit strange, but the scientific study of emotion has a disjointed history. In initial studies of adult emotion, psychologists carefully pondered their own internal processes. After repeated self-observations, they described their conscious experiences of emotion. So early in the history of psychology, subjective qualities such as feelings were respectable topics for study (Buss, Cole, & Zhou, 2019).

However, it admittedly was difficult to observe internal states objectively (Izard, 2010). With behaviorism gaining ascendance in psychology, introspection was no longer considered an acceptable means of study. Only behaviors were investigated, nothing intrapsychic. Phenomena requiring any inferences—such as motivation, thoughts, and feelings—were rejected as unobservable, reducible to overt behavior, and unworthy of scientific scrutiny. So unsurprisingly, emotions were largely ignored for several decades. They were relegated to the status of afterthoughts—nuisances to be examined when they got in the way of "harder" behavioral science.

Then, with a swing of the scientific pendulum, unobservable psychological internal states were not only deemed acceptable, but seen as central to an understanding of human functioning. Still, however, emotions were overlooked: This revolution in psychology was strictly cognitive, and emotions still took a back seat. In their zeal, cognitive psychologists at first considered emotions mere by-products of cognitive appraisal, and thus still not worthy of focused, unitary study. Clearly a more balanced view of emotion was still necessary. It also turns out that this issue of how cognition impacts emotion continues as a longstanding issue.

Perspectives about emotional development that gained ascendance after the cognitive revolution included efforts to situate emotion's relation to cognition in a more balanced manner. The discrete emotions framework is a prominent, early, and continuing example of such perspectives. It holds that emotions can be grouped into a set of very specific, largely facial, responses, which are biologically based responses to specific stimuli, are evolutionarily "old," and are recognizable throughout cultures (e.g., Izard, 1991, 1993a, 1993b, 2007). Such "basic" emotions invoke specific cognitions, behaviors, and regulatory efforts. More important, they are rapid, automatic, and nonconscious, requiring minimal or only rudimentary appraisal. Each basic emotion includes a unique feeling component as part of its neurobiological activation, which may be invariant over the lifespan (Izard, 2007).

Within discrete emotions theory, cognition is considered an important part of "emotion schemas"—for example, emotions such as shame and guilt, where self-evaluation is particularly relevant, require the support of, or are activated by, cognition (Ackerman, Abe, & Izard, 1998). More broadly, emotions interact with cognitive appraisals of ongoing events and higher-order cognitions like the aforesaid self-evaluations to become emotion schemas, going beyond basic emotions to incorporate individual- and culture-specific unions of feelings, motivational and regulatory processes, learned labels, and concepts. Memories, already-constructed concepts, and thoughts connected to a child's self-evaluation, beliefs, and values, strongly supported by language and other social cognitive development, help to create such emotion schemas. According to Izard (2007), the ability to form such schemas may be built into the neurobiological systems that underlie emotions and perceptual/cognitive action.

Thus, Rodney's developing emotion schemas are likely to differ substantially from Jimmy's. When Rodney's teacher tells him he must clean up when he isn't ready to (i.e., he can't get his way), memories of his father punishing him for merely having his toys on the living room floor (that wasn't fair!!), along with the somewhat contradictory admonishment to "stick up for yourself" form the cognitive substrate of an emotion schema. Predicting that his teacher will yell if he doesn't clean up, but that he needs to defend himself, he gets MAD!! He experiences emotion befitting his own individualized schema, supported by cognitions about his experiences with his father and the language to describe them.

In contrast, when Jimmy hears the teacher's request, he appraises the situation as one of obligation because of his Chinese mother's teaching about complying with adults, but his biologically based fearful temperament also engenders stress hormone output (Izard, 2007). So he feels a little scared as he quickly puts away toys. His schema for the same event was very different from Rodney's.

Despite the apparent heuristic power of the emotion schema construct, developmental researchers continue to struggle regarding when and how cognition interfaces with emotions. Thus, although Izard and others who developed theories after the cognitive revolution clearly did not ignore the influence of cognition, some newer theoretical frameworks give more prominence to the action of cognition and language within emotional experience and expression (e.g., Hoemann, Xu, & Barrett, 2019; Holodynski & Seeger, 2019). My stance would be that Izard's notion of emotion schemas allows for many aspects of these more recent theorists' contributions.

Despite competing theoretical frameworks, it is most likely that these two important systems, emotion and cognition, work in concert. It seems to me that, after infancy, sometimes emotional experience *precedes* cognition, sometimes it is *preceded by* cognition, and often it *co-occurs with* cognition, as in emotion schemas. In my view, then, although these newer perspectives give us many useful ideas that will be subsequently discussed, emotion and cognition often work together in the creation of emotional experience—although at times one or the other "takes the lead," neither takes precedence over the other (Lewis & Michalson, 1983).

Although cognition was not integrated into all parts of discrete emotions theory, and some of the theory's tenets have not entirely held up in empirical scrutiny (e.g., Walle & Dahl, 2020), this stance allowed developmental researchers to make predictions about emotional development and the methodologies with which to test them. Given this theory and several others (e.g., functionalism, to which I adhere and which is discussed later; Barrett, 2020; Buss et al., 2019), emotion development research blossomed. In fact, the number of peer-reviewed citations for preschoolers and emotions rose from a low of 140 from 1960 to 1980, to over 1,100 in next two decades, exploding to over 4,400 from 2001 to 2020. This exponential increase has fueled developmental scientists' thinking about emotion itself. In what follows, I outline my own somewhat eclectic conception of emotion, and its nature, process, functions, and position within social relationships and culture.

## Emotional Experience: Emotion and Cognition Together

There is little disagreement that emotional experience originates with autonomic nervous system arousal, but what happens next, and how and why, continue to be the subject of much debate (see Buss et al., 2019; Fischer, Shaver, & Carnochan, 1989; Flores-Kanter & Medrano, 2020; Izard, 1993a; Lazarus, 1991; LoBue, Pérez-Edgar, & Buss, 2019; Stein, Trabasso, & Liwag, 1993). My view of how emotional experiences occur can be seen in Figure 1.1.

First, there is arousal. The autonomic nervous system is aroused by a notable change in the person's world. This change can be caused by an environmental event, by the actions of the individual, by the actions of others, or even by memories. Sometimes the response to this arousal is limited to lower, more primitive brain systems, such as the amygdala and medial prefrontal cortex (Diamond, Stuss, & Knight, 2002; Flores-Kanter et al., 2020; Izard, 2007). When the "bottom drops out" on the "kiddie" roller coaster ride, this accident is certainly a sudden and intense environmental change for a 5-year-old girl. And when a 4-year-old boy's mother blocks access to the cookies on the table, her actions are noteworthy. In both instances emotions ensue quickly and

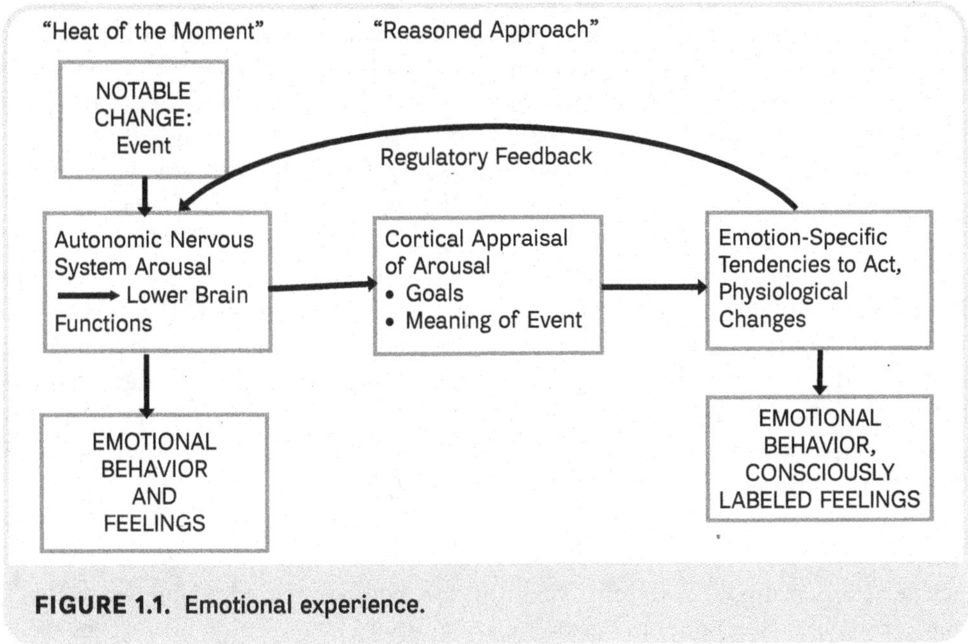


**FIGURE 1.1.** Emotional experience.

automatically, along with their attendant behaviors: The 5-year-old hides her eyes and screams; the 4-year-old glares at his mother and stomps his foot. This "bottom-up" process of emotional experience is portrayed in the leftmost column of Figure 1.1. Quick and relatively effortless, it involves perception more than cognition.

Individuals experience these lower-level emotional experiences across the lifespan, but during early childhood much brain development takes place (e.g., the ventromedial and dorsolateral prefrontal cortex; Diamond et al., 2002; LeDoux, 1996; Tsujimoto, 2008), such that "top-down" functioning becomes increasingly important to the nature of emotional experience (Cole, Lougheed, & Ram, 2018). Moreover, the anterior cingulate cortex develops and functions as a bridge between the limbic system and neocortex, facilitating the constant, dynamic interaction between emotion and cognition. These developments in the brain from toddlerhood onward allow emotion, motivation, and cognition to work together strongly, influencing emotional experience by creating an increasingly complicated network of desired outcomes, or goals, and emotion concepts (i.e., emotion schemas). The creation and utilization of emotion schemas are effortful, although not necessarily conscious.

Hence the need for cortical brain involvement in much of emotional experience is clear: Notable changes and attendant arousal give children important information about their ongoing goals and their ability to cope with events, but this information needs to be held in mind and *understood,* not just automatically reacted to. A child (or an adult, for that matter) needs to *represent* the notable change, the new thing that has happened. Interpretations of the emotion-eliciting circumstance are necessary, and implicate cognitive processes like attention, language, memory, reasoning, and planning. How does the event affect ongoing goals, if at all? Can the child deal with these consequences? These cognitive aspects of an emotional experience are portrayed in the middle column of Figure 1.1.

As 2½-year-old Jessica is playing on the floor, she suddenly sees a large toy action figure, black and rather menacing—certainly unique in her experience—moving into the room on its own. This is a new thing! (Arousal takes place here.) This object must have some sort of effect on her world. But what? (What does this arousal mean? Interpretation is required.) She continues to watch Darth Vader as he comes closer. Slowly she understands that this guy is totally unpredictable. He may interfere with her goal of staying safe. Darth Vader is scary!

Cognition plays an important role in the emotion Jessica finally experiences—in this sense the appraisal theoretical perspective is fully integrated here (Lazarus, 1991). Before any specific emotional reaction is felt by her, or discerned by others, she must attend to the notable event, comprehend it, and interpret it. These interpretations and construals of events' relations to ongoing goals lead not only to felt emotions, but also to actions associated with each specific emotion and to physiological changes in arousal, as portrayed in the rightmost column of Figure 1.1.

In the version of Jessica's experience given here, she feels afraid because of her interpretation of Darth Vader's approach (felt emotion). She turns and runs toward her mother, screaming, "I scared" (goal-directed, emotion-related action; labeled feelings). If she finds her mom, her physiological arousal lessens. But if she realizes she is alone, she feels increased arousal instead. So the results of Jessica's emotion-related actions also influence her arousal and may feed back into new construals and changing emotional experience. As the child matures, self-monitoring of these emotion-related actions and of concomitant changes in arousal comes into play (e.g., an older child's arousal may change as he holds his ground, Darth Vader comes closer, and the child sees he's not a threat). This pathway is portrayed at the top of Figure 1.1.

Sometimes the precise experience of emotional arousal depends on *which* of several goals the child focuses on. For instance, Jessica may have two goals—having fun and remaining safe. The approach of Darth Vader may affect either goal or both. If she cannot remain safe, Jessica will feel afraid. If Darth Vader looks like an interesting toy, she may feel happiness.

In these ways, the argument of whether emotion is predominant over cognition in emotional experiences, or vice versa, can be resolved based on what we are learning about brain development (Diamond et al., 2002). Some emotional experiences do not involve cognition; they are mostly automatic. But because the cortical path to emotion predominates after about the middle of the first year, this intimate union of cognition and emotion is usually what is referred to when emotions are discussed (Izard, 1991; LeDoux, 1996; Stein et al., 1993). The conceptions of emotion put forward in Figure 1.1 thus inform the rest of this volume.

## Emotions as Regulators of the Behavior of Self and Others

### *The Functionalist Perspective*

An important way of looking at emotions, upon which the just-described viewpoint largely rests, focuses on a child's goals, accenting the *functions* of various emotions. What do emotions *do* for children and the people with whom they interact? The functionalist perspective notes that children's emotions provide both children and others with information (see Buss et al., 2019; Campos & Barrett, 1984; Saarni, Campos, Camras, & Witherington, 2006). The information inherent in the experience and expression of emotion is important to a child because it can shape behavior during and after the vent, in accordance with the child's goals.

Thus each emotion has a unique function serving a person's goals for achieving, maintaining, or regaining well-being, both social and cognitive (Cole et al., 2018; Saarni et al., 2006). For example, Jessica in the previous example appraised Darth Vader's arrival as a threat to the goal of safety and is ready to flee. An angry child has had a goal blocked and will work to overcome the obstacle, such as when Mike and Joey literally cross swords over their differing plans for play. In contrast, sadness is marked by an appraisal that an important goal will not be attained and must be abandoned; Jimmy was sad when denied entry to the playtime.

Thus differing emotions affect children's thinking, behavior, and feelings in unique ways and benefit from different regulatory strategies (Barrett, 2020; Dennis & Kelemen, 2009); they also have different consequences, especially in the differing behaviors they elicit from others, because emotional expressions can help others to describe and predict the child's behavior (Walle & Campos, 2012; Widen & Russell, 2010b).

In this functionalist view, then, emotional experience and expressiveness not only are important information for oneself *but also* for others—others' behaviors often constitute antecedent conditions for a child's emotions, but the child's emotions' effects on others are equally important. The experience and expression of emotion signal whether the child or other people need to modify or continue their own goal-directed behavior (Saarni, 2001; Walle & Campos, 2012). For example, if a girl experiences anger while playing at the puzzle activity table with another child, she may tell her mother "I don't want *her* to come to my birthday party." The experience of anger gave her information that affects her subsequent behavior. But her anger also gives information to others that affects their behavior—the play partner who witnessed her anger may seek to avoid her until she is calm, and maybe even until the next day. The information inherent in emotions is crucial to self *and* others. Take another example:

> Eighteen-month-old Amy expresses anger when her parents curtail her freedom to run around the room. She does not want to get into her high chair; in fact, her goal is to continue to dash from the window to the door and back again. Because she experiences this anger, she is likely to engage in specific behaviors, such as kicking and yelling, in service of the goal of freedom. As for her parents, Amy's kicking and yelling lets them know that she does not like the restriction of the high chair. The parents react to this behavior with distractions such as singing, or, in contrast, by yelling at her to sit still. Peers and siblings too benefit from witnessing Amy's expression of emotion. When Amy's 3-year-old brother witnesses her social signal of anger, he may know from experience that his most profitable response is to retreat.

Another example is fear:

> If Marco experiences fear when Billy arrives at day care, the experience of fear gives him important signals that affect his subsequent behavior. He gives Billy a wide berth, seeks the lap of a caregiver, and remains vigilant during his day. Marco's expression of fear gives

important signals to other people that affect their subsequent behavior too. His caregivers are watchful because they wish to know what is bothering him so that they can help him, and Billy also studies him, ready to take advantage by grabbing a toy.

Joey's "pirate" play, described earlier, is likewise replete with evidence of emotions' links to his ongoing goals. When he is happy about finding the buried treasure, his experience of happiness makes him want to continue this enjoyable activity. At the same time, Joey's expression of joy tells his friend Mike that it is an opportune time to join him in flinging "gold doubloons" in the air.

In sum, the experience and expression of emotion signal that the goal-directed behavior of the child or other people needs to be modified or continued. So emotions are important both interpersonally and intrapersonally, and intimately *include* (but are not limited to) cognition, in terms of children's appraisals of how events impact their goals (Walle & Dahl, 2020). As noted by Barrett (2020), the development of emotional competence *can* include the conceptual foundation suggested by Hoemann et al. (2019) and the symbolic representation upon which Holodynski and Seeger (2019) rest portions of their notion of internalized experience and expression of emotion. These viewpoints require careful study and inclusion in our evolving thinking about emotional competence. At the same time, the development of emotional competence is not just the orderly, progressive development implied in those perspectives—it is dynamic, with expressions, feelings, brain development, and aspects of physiological arousal all changing across micro- and macro-level time spans (Barrett, 2020; Cole et al., 2018). Given this level of complexity, the functional perspective offers a fruitful, advantageous lens with which to examine such development. And its inclusion of emotion's influence on others as well as the self leads to another important perspective to consider.

### *The Social Constructivist Perspective*

As already noted, there is no doubt that emotional expressiveness is a powerful interpersonal regulator and that this social side of emotion is important. Some prominent researchers and theorists go even further to assert that this interpersonal function of emotion is central to the very nature of emotional expression and experience (Gergen, 1985; Russell, 1989). This social constructivist approach thus focuses on emotions as social products. According to Saarni and Crowley (1990), emotions and social relations are inseparable. Saarni (1987) states that "emotion's meaningfulness is grounded in human relationships . . . transactions among people [are] the primary focus for feelings to be experienced, observed or inferred, talked about, and elaborated into expectancies for guiding one through future interpersonal interactions" (p. 535–536; see also Boiger & Mesquita, 2012). Interpersonal communication is crucial not only to emotional experience and expression, but also to emotion knowledge and regulation.

According to Saarni (2001), children *make sense of emotions*, as in the functionalist view already described, especially within social interactions. Even very young children learn the "feeling rules" of their community from their own experiences and the socialization of adults—what to feel in differing situations, how to interpret and manage these feelings, and how to react to the feelings of others (Hochschild, 1979).

That is, emotions and emotional competence skills are affected strongly by socialization according to cultural values and norms; for example, how two culture's value and respond to anger and shame may differ markedly (Cole, Tamang, & Shrestha, 2006). Cultural transmission of beliefs and practices regarding emotional competence is a theme I return to frequently in this book. What is adaptive in one cultural group may not be in another (Raval & Walker, 2019).

Thus, to summarize this perspective, emotion-relevant expectations, beliefs, and values are transmitted by social partners during emotional events. As much as emotional competence skills affect interpersonal relations, interpersonal interactions and their contexts guide the development and articulation of these skills (Halberstadt, Denham, & Dunsmore, 2001). The experience, expression, regulation, and interpretation of emotions all depend on one's sociocultural environment and interactions within relationships. Therefore, children's emotional worlds develop with input from socializers, the first of whom are parents. The general tenets, developmental progressions, and outcomes for emotional competence and its socialization may have universal aspects, but we must consider cultural variations as well (Saarni & Crowley, 1990).

## WHAT IS EMOTIONAL COMPETENCE?

Given my theoretical view consolidating a way of describing emotional experience and its function and position within social and cultural milieus, it is time to turn to a definition of *emotional competence*, the focus of the volume. Emotional competence can be defined as *emotional effectiveness*, by which a child can reach short- and long-term goals during or after emotion-eliciting encounters (Saarni, 1999). As exemplified in Joey's play, emotionally competent young children begin to (1) experience and purposefully express a broad variety of emotions, without incapacitating intensity or duration; (2) understand their own and others' emotions; and (3) regulate their emotion whenever its experience is "too much" or "too little" for their own comfort or others' needs and expectations.

It is important to view this development within the context of young children's key developmental tasks. During the early childhood years, emotional competence skills are organized around the developmental tasks of maintaining positive emotional engagement with the physical and social world, making and maintaining relationships with other children and adults, and managing emotional arousal in the context of social interaction and new cognitive demands (Parker & Gottman, 1989; Waters & Sroufe, 1983). These skills are not easy ones for young children, especially because they are just entering the peer arena. As well, the new classroom context that so many young children experience can be very taxing; they are being asked to sit still, pay attention, follow directions, approach group play, complete preacademic tasks, and get along with others in ways that challenge their emerging abilities. The emotional competence skills that develop dramatically during early childhood can assist with these hurdles, and help preschoolers succeed at developmental tasks.

These abilities continue to develop throughout the lifespan, but as Joey shows us, preschool-age children are surprisingly adept at several components of emotional competence. A preview of the exemplary types of competencies mastered by preschoolers includes the following (Camras & Halberstadt, 2017; Halberstadt et al., 2001; Saarni, 1990).

## Emotion Expressiveness

- Using gestures to express nonverbal emotional messages about a social situation or relationship (e.g., Joey hugged Mike when he stepped on the Lego).
- Demonstrating empathic involvement in others' emotions (e.g., Jimmy kissed his baby sister when she fell and hurt her knee).
- Displaying complex social and self-conscious emotions, such as guilt, pride, shame, and contempt, in appropriate contexts (e.g., Mike hung his head when his mother discovered forbidden chocolate all over his face).
- Realizing that one may feel a certain way "on the inside," but show a different demeanor "on the outside"—especially showing that an overt expression of socially disapproved feelings can be controlled, while expressing more socially appropriate emotions (e.g., Jimmy was somewhat fearful of an adult classroom visitor, but showed no emotion or even a slight smile).

## Emotion Knowledge

- Discerning one's own emotional states (e.g., Rodney realized that he mostly feels sad, but also a little bit angry, when getting time-out from his preschool teacher).
- Discerning others' emotional states (e.g., Jimmy knew that Daddy's smile as he comes into the house meant that his workday was satisfactory and he probably won't yell tonight).
- Using the vocabulary of emotion (e.g., Rodney reminisced with his mother about family sadness when a pet died).

## Emotion Regulation

It is important to note that emotions are regulators of behavior within oneself (intrapersonal, as when Joey reins in his annoyance with Mike) and in interactions with others (interpersonal, as when Joey retreated in the face of Rodney's contempt) (Cole, Martin, & Dennis, 2004).

- Coping with aversive or distressing emotions or the situations that elicit them (e.g., even though he was very upset, Joey used his mother's assistance instead of hitting when his younger brother grabbed all the toys, and his mother knew he needed help because of his distress).
- Coping with pleasurable emotions or the situations that elicit them (e.g., when his toddler sister loudly belched, Mike took a deep breath and downplayed his laughter when it began to feel uncontrollable, but even so, his sister looked offended).
- Strategically "up-regulating" the experience and expression of emotions at appropriate

times (e.g., Joey grimaced in anger to make Rodney retreat; he sang out loud to share his happiness at play with Mike).

Although these components of emotional competence are often viewed as individual differences, and often are discussed as such throughout this book, I also emphasize their social roots, informed by both the functionalist and social constructivist perspectives. Preschoolers' unique developmental and social histories and exposure to specific contexts all influence how they experience and interpret emotional transactions. But although children's emotional competence is grounded in their own personal goals and is intimately connected to their own sociocultural context, it also develops in concert with their individual abilities and vulnerabilities related to cognitive skills and influenced by temperament-related emotional dispositions (Saarni, 2001).

Thus, in the next sections of this introductory chapter, I address developmental change and stability, as well as individual differences, in young children's emotional competence, and devote special attention to these contributors: (1) intrapersonal (i.e., cognition, language, and temperament); and (2) interpersonal (i.e., socialization, with an expanded emphasis on culture). Then I briefly introduce topics as they appear in the following chapters of this volume: the outcomes of emotional competence during early childhood for both social competence and preacademic school success. Having introduced these matters, I propose an overarching model of emotional competence during early childhood. Then I turn to the consideration of children who have difficulties in their emotional competence development, along with the need to accurately assess early childhood emotional competence and offer programming to promote its development. Next I describe where I think the field of emotional competence is headed, both theoretically and methodologically, along with an outline of subsequent chapters. Finally, I offer a call for action.

## DEVELOPMENTAL CHANGE IN TODDLERS' AND PRESCHOOLERS' EMOTIONAL COMPETENCE

With this introduction to the nature and importance of emotional competence in early childhood, and some delineation of the nature of emotion itself, it is time to consider developmental change in emotional competence across early childhood. The age period from 2 to 5 years is a time of change for children and caregivers alike. Progress in all areas of children's development—talking, thinking, running, jumping, and playing together—seems to occur daily. Adults are often delighted with these new abilities, especially with children's growing deftness in interacting with both grownups and peers.

As amply described earlier, these new proficiencies are not limited to isolated language, cognitive, social, and motor skills. Children from 2 to 5 years of age are more emotionally sophisticated than we ever previously imagined. The many changes in emotional competence during this age period have prompted developmental psychologists to try to describe them more fully, to search for the contributions of socialization and maturation to such change, and to find ways to examine and promote this development. This focus is particularly auspicious because it signifies an increasing ability to describe specific children, and to predict their behavior, in terms of physical, social, cognitive, *and* emotional attributes.

Accounts of any child's behavior are arid and incomplete unless they include information on emotions. The important developmental question "What changes over time?" cannot be answered fully without knowing the details about children's emotional lives. Children obviously reason in a more abstract way and become more motorically adept as development proceeds. But knowing about developmental change in emotional competence—that 2-year-olds' negativity generally wanes considerably, or that kindergartners are at the threshold of understanding finer complexities of emotional experience—is invaluable to filling out a more complete picture of children at these ages.

These age-related changes have important implications. Different levels of emotional competence in children who differ in age should be expected, often because of advances in language, perspective taking, and other cognitive abilities. In a group of young children, older preschoolers' expression and understanding of emotions differ from toddlers' and even from younger preschoolers'. A 4-year-old at the playground with her mother, upon seeing another child crying, is no longer so likely to freeze, or even to cry herself, as she was at 18 months. Instead, she is likely to look concerned and ask, "Why is he crying?"

The upper limit of this age range—around the transition to kindergarten—is often a time when children experience growth in their understanding of the causes and consequences of emotions and of their complexity. For example, during a busy day in kindergarten, two boys may discuss who is sitting at and who is missing from their snack table. They may commiserate over their shared emotions: "John is here. That's the happy thing." "But Darryl is not, and that's the sad thing. We need to see if we can find him on the playground." Another 5-year-old may assert, "Only our moms know what we really feel on the inside." Still another may smile wanly when offered an unfamiliar food by her favorite aunt, instead of refusing it with an ill-tempered retort. Because of these myriad changes in emotional competence, preschoolers' lives with parents, siblings, peers, and teachers change as well, and their attainment of social and preacademic skills can increase.

In this book, I examine all the component skills of emotional competence—experience and expression, knowledge, and regulation—from the organizing perspective of developmental change across the toddler and preschool periods. Another important organizing perspective focuses on what may stay relatively the same—individual differences in emotional competence.

## INDIVIDUAL DIFFERENCES IN EMOTIONAL COMPETENCE

Normative change in emotional competence, although important, does not tell the whole story. Caregivers often focus on critical individual differences in children's emotional competence: "She gets upset so easily. I wish I could help her calm down." Or "He drew a smile on his picture of himself on the potty. Isn't that super? I love it that he feels proud about what he's done!" Hence, as noted earlier, the important developmental question "What stays relatively the same over time?" also cannot be answered fully without knowing more about children's emotional lives. We may know that a 3-year-old girl can alternate feet while climbing stairs. However, this is not the same as knowing that she sings gaily as she does so, or stomps in anger over an insult incurred an hour ago, or must be coaxed to come upstairs because the "bogeyman" might be there—and that we see similar propensities, perhaps expressed somewhat differently—when she is 5 years old.

Where could preschoolers' budding emotional skills possibly come from? What fuels the development milestones they successfully meet (what is changing?) and their unique individual profiles of emotional competence (what stays relatively the same?)? No doubt, both intrapersonal and interpersonal contributors, along with brain development, are critical for both developmental change and individual stability. How do other areas of children's development, such as cognition, fuel emotional competence? How do parents, other caregivers, siblings, and peers contribute to preschoolers' growing emotional competencies and to individual differences among them? I now consider these questions.

## Intrapersonal Contributions to Individual Differences in Emotional Competence

Children's specific abilities and attributes can promote or hinder emotional competence. Some children are blessed with cognitive and language skills that allow them to better understand their social–emotional world and better communicate their feelings, wishes, desires, and goals for social interactions and relationships (Cutting & Dunn, 1999). Differences in these abilities contribute to differences in emotion expressiveness, knowledge, and regulation. As an example of cognition influencing emotion knowledge, a preschooler who can reason flexibly may more readily perceive how another person's emotional reactions might differ from her own in a specific situation—though they delight *me*, others may fear swimming pools.

> Jenny knows that her friend is afraid of climbing to the top of the jungle gym, even though it is Jenny's favorite activity on the playground. This knowledge of her friend's feelings moderates Jenny's behavior during play with her. The direction of this moderation is governed by other factors: If Jenny is kind, she avoids this activity when playing with her friend; if she is a bit more self-concerned, she teases and goads her.

Thus, preschoolers differ in their age-appropriate abilities to categorize complex elements, such as other people, and to take the perspective of these other persons. These cognitive abilities may support their emotional competence skills—expressiveness, knowledge, and regulation. In fact, in the new theory of constructed emotion (e.g., Hoemann et al., 2019), *all* of emotion development solely consists of the development of linguistic emotion concepts. The strong version of this theory asserts that children only experience and perceive emotions after sufficient brain development to assemble "embodied" emotion concepts that give meaning to arousal and guide behavior, using similar prior experiences. After taking in information from their bodies and the world, children (and others) linguistically *categorize* the information to experience emotion (Hoemann et al., 2019).

The cognitive constructivist view is useful in that conceptualizing emotions and their attendant arousal may help children to know when, and perhaps how, to regulate emotion and behavior based on prior behavior. However, as Barrett (2020) points out, children's emotions are not just concepts—as I've noted, emotions are *functional*—they are organized around the need to motivate and mobilize action tendencies that may include our social interaction partners. In short, and to reiterate earlier conclusions, emotion concepts are important ways in which brain development and cognition influence emotional competence, but they are not its sole determinants. What may be some other intrapersonal attributes that influence the meeting of developmental milestones and contribute to individual differences in preschoolers' emotional competence?

In a less-strict view focusing on language, language skill clearly supports emotional competence in young children, allowing them to represent experience and communicate with others about feelings (Pons, Lawson, Harris, & DeRosnay, 2003). It may especially serve emotion regulation, helping children codify a menu of goal-related emotion regulation strategies, and allowing them to internalize the expression of emotion for regulation that is more efficient and socially satisfactory (Holodynski & Seeger, 2019). Language also allows children to ask for help with their feelings; for example, children with better language skills as toddlers expressed less-intense anger as 4-year-olds (Roben, Cole, & Armstrong, 2013).

Young children's growth in emotion knowledge also benefits from their language skills (Martin, Williamson, Kurtz-Nelson, & Boekamp, 2015; Martins, Osório, Veríssimo, & Martins, 2016; Seidenfeld, Johnson, Cavadel, & Izard, 2014). More verbal children can ask better questions about their own and others' emotions, discussing emotions and the means of dealing with them in conversations with parents and peers. Understanding the answers given by parents and peers may present an advantage in dealing with emotions (Pons et al., 2003). Such conversations also may motivate parents especially to talk more with their children about emotions and their regulation; exposure to discussions about emotions promotes emotional competence (Ogren & Johnson, 2020).

Temperament also is an important intrapersonal element that can guide the development of emotional competence. Children with different emotional dispositions (i.e., temperaments) may demonstrate specific patterns of expressiveness. Further, they may be well- or ill-equipped to develop certain components of emotional competence, especially emotion regulation (Calkins & Mackler, 2011). For example, an especially negative child may find that she or he has a greater need for emotion regulation, even though this may be difficult. Moreover, negativity may be related to difficulties in understanding emotions (e.g., shyer children had less-developed emotion knowledge in DeRosnay, Fink, Begeer, Slaughter, & Peterson, 2014). In contrast, a child whose temperament allows him to shift attention from a distressing situation to focus on comforting actions, objects, or thoughts is better able to regulate his emotions—Benny hums to himself when working on writing letters and focusing on that helps him feel a bit calmer during this challenging task.

## Interpersonal Contributions to Individual Differences in Emotional Competence

Although each child brings a particular set of abilities and propensities to his or her emotional life, other persons clearly play a role in the development of emotional competence, as already noted in the discussion of the social constructivist perspective. That is, interpersonal socialization factors also contribute in a major way to the development of individual differences in emotional competence. Children learn much from various socializing agents about the appropriate expression of emotions, the nature of emotional expressions and situations, means of coping with emotions, and even potential reactions to others' positive and negative emotions.

During this point in the lifespan, the foremost socializers are parents. Most preschoolers enjoy continued close contact with their parents and teachers during this period, even as they move into peer relationships. Parental modeling, contingent reactions to children's emotions, and coaching (i.e., teaching and discussing) contribute to the children's own patterns of expressiveness, emotion knowledge, and emotion regulation (Eisenberg, Cumberland, & Spinrad, 1998).

Parents' own patterns of expressiveness are reflected in their children's expressiveness. Even preschoolers themselves are aware of these associations. When asked to articulate how she feels when her mother is happy, a preschooler may assert, "I give Mommy a big hug!" Another child reflects on his angry father: "I hide from him, I go outside; I don't like him when he's mad." Furthermore, parents who talk about emotions and foster this ability in their children enable their children to express certain optimal patterns of emotions.

> Ranjit's mother calmly discusses her son's anger over not being allowed to sample grapes freely from the produce aisle as they stroll through the grocery store. A few shoppers eye her skeptically. But as Ranjit grudgingly grumbles about his desires, he is learning to use words to communicate emotional needs, rather than launching into a full-blown tantrum.

And parents' specific reactions to their children's emotions encourage or discourage certain patterns of expressiveness. In this example, the mother's calm response fosters not only Ranjit's acceptance of his own anger, but also his modulation of its intensity.

These aspects of socialization also contribute to young children's emotion knowledge. Parents' talking about emotion-laden experiences in daily life, accepting and encouraging children's emotional expressiveness, and expressing predominantly positive emotions all promote children's emotion knowledge.

> When Joanna's father discusses her feelings about the end of the preschool year—the joy of an upcoming trip to the beach, and the accompanying sadness about missing friends—the guidance is quite direct. If Joanna's parents accompany their emotion teaching with positive expressiveness and a readiness to cultivate her emotional life by reacting to her emotions in a helpful, accepting way, then she is even more motivated to tackle the thorny issues centering around emotion knowledge.

Last, it is likely that parents' own emotions, teaching, and reactions to children's emotions influence children's means of emotion regulation.

> Watching his mother break out in tears for the third time that day, Larry witnesses one way to deal with situations that require emotion regulation—just vent them! But he does not get to talk to his mother much about feelings, because she is too busy "letting out her anger." Perhaps the only message he does get is when his mother justifies her outbursts. The mother's scathing reactions to Larry's own emotions lead him to suppress his expressiveness, at least when she is present.

Other socializers' contributions to emotional competence also are important. Especially in the last decades, there is a new spotlight on how early childhood caregivers and educators contribute to preschoolers' emotional competence. Although the same mechanisms can be seen in their emotion socialization, their effects on emotional competence may differ in the larger group environment of the classroom (Denham, Ferrier, & Bassett, 2020).

Peers and siblings also can be very effective socializers of emotion. Their socialization is likely to differ substantially from that of parents, however: If a younger sibling becomes angry in a grocery store, the older sibling is not likely to be as patient and accepting as Ranjit's mother in the earlier example—anger, ridicule, or even desertion is far more probable! Obviously, the preschooler in question could deduce from these reactions that some people do *not* tolerate his anger—an equally important lesson.

### *More on Culture*

Cultural, historical, and socially embedded contexts influence the creation and interpretation of the beliefs and practices in which emotions are experienced, expressed, understood, regulated, and socialized (De Leersnyder, Boiger, & Mesquita, 2015; Saarni, 1987, 1998, 2001; Saarni & Crowley, 1990). In this view, emotions are ongoing, dynamic, and *interactive* (Boiger & Mesquita, 2012). Within the aforementioned socialization framework, parents convey culturally specific patterns of expressiveness and different reactions to children's emotions, and directly teach children cultural information on the ways to express, regulate, and understand emotions. Parental behavior lets children know *what matters* in the world of emotions.

It is crucial to remember that emotional competence and its socialization occur in both collectivistic/relational and individualistic cultural contexts, and it is best to understand both emotional competence and its socialization in terms of the balance of both these continua in the specific setting (Friedlmeier, Çorapçı, & Cole, 2011). Thus, for example, in more collectivistic/relational cultural contexts, the view of the self is more interdependent, whereas independence is accentuated in more individualistic contexts; moreover, emotional goals differ across these continua. That is, in individualistic cultures, the emotional goal is to enhance self-esteem via promoting positivity and allowing expression of negativity, whereas more collectivistic/relational cultures focus on the welfare of the group and its harmony. What these varying goals mean for emotional competence can be exemplified by the emphasis on empathy and shame in collectivistic/relational cultures, and by the opposing accent on pride and anger in individualistic ones, for example. How then might young children's emotional experience and expression, knowledge, and regulation, as well as the socialization mechanisms of modeling, teaching, and responding to children's emotions, be similar or different across cultural contexts? In the ensuing chapters, I attempt to answer these questions.

## THE COMPLEX LINKAGE BETWEEN EMOTIONAL COMPETENCE AND SOCIAL AND SCHOOL SUCCESS

It is one thing to understand that children show differing patterns of emotional competence across ages and individuals. It is quite another matter to realize that these differences have a very real impact on how children work and play together and even on how they master preacademic skills like learning letters and numbers. Not only must parents, educators, and psychologists know what to look for in terms of young children's emotional development, they must know why such development is so crucial, and what aspects of it need fostering.

All the component abilities of emotional competence are important in their own right but also buttress broader aspects of development. Much more detail is given in subsequent chapters, but it is important to note several points here. First, the components of emotional competence help to ensure effective social interactions and young children's overall social competence—their listening, cooperating, appropriate help seeking, joining interactions, and negotiating (Denham & Weissberg, 2004). Second, young children also utilize emotional competence to facilitate learning alongside and in collaboration with teachers and peers (Denham, Brown, & Domitrovich, 2010). Thus emotional competence supports not only social competence, but also early school success (generally defined in this volume as positive attitudes toward learning, persistence, adjustment to classroom routines, and the growth of preacademic competence; Denham, Bassett, Mincic, et al., 2012; Romano, Babchishin, Pagani, & Kohen, 2010).

More specifically, preschoolers who understand and regulate emotions, and are more emotionally positive when they enter school, are at a double advantage throughout their primary years. They can more easily develop positive and supportive relationships with peers and teachers, as well as more easily participate in school and achieve at higher levels (Garner & Waajid, 2008; Graziano, Reavis, Keane, & Calkins, 2007; Izard et al., 2001; Leerkes, Paradise, O'Brien, Calkins, & Lange, 2008). Conversely, children who enter school with fewer emotional competence skills are more often rejected by peers, develop less-supportive relationships with teachers, participate less in class, enjoy school less, achieve at lower levels, and are at risk for later behavior problems (Denham, Bassett, Mincic, et al., 2012; Denham, Bassett, Thayer, et al., 2012; Herndon, Bailey, Shewark, Denham, & Bassett, 2013). Aspects of these skills are even uniquely associated with adult experiences of education, employment, mental health, and avoidance of crime and substance use (Jones, Greenberg, & Crowley, 2015). In short, emotional competence greases the cogs of a successful early social and school experiences, with potentially long-lasting effects. In later chapters I go into greater detail on these advantages of emotional competence.

More specifically, regarding emotional expressiveness, a child who is sad or angry—either sitting on the sidelines of the group or querulously huffing around the room—is less likely to be able to understand, let alone tend to, the emotional needs of others, rendering him a rather poor playmate. Furthermore, this child also probably is too upset, too often, to develop positive attitudes about school, follow class schedules reliably, or focus on preacademic tasks.

Young children who understand emotion better also have more positive peer relations. The youngster who understands the emotions of others should interact more successfully when a friend gets angry with him or her, and the preschooler who can talk about his or her own emotions also is better able to negotiate disputes with friends.

> If Matthew really wants the toy Jesse is holding, and is becoming increasingly frustrated, he may call to his teacher, "Jesse is making me mad. Put on the timer so we'll know when it's my turn." Matthew probably also has more friends than he would if he progressed through his day grabbing and hitting when angry. Matthew also might be able to ask the teacher to help him when he's frustrated doing a hard number task with manipulatives.

Or if a preschooler sees a peer bickering with another friend and correctly deduces the peer's sadness, she comforts her friend rather than retreating or even entering the fray. These accurate perceptions of emotion help children to react appropriately, thus bolstering their relationships. Additionally, knowing readily how to deal with peers' emotions—because they are accurately comprehended—allows preschoolers to give more "space" to preacademic tasks.

Learning to get along in groups of age-mates also presses the preschool child toward regulating emotional expressiveness. A preschooler who begins to regulate his or her own emotions gets along more successfully with peers. In the previous example, Matthew regulates his anger, and Jesse is glad that he does!

In sum, Joey, our "pirate" friend, uses emotion understanding, expressiveness, and regulation at full capacity during his play with peers, and this skill makes him a super playmate—he is more able to behave prosocially, and thus is often part of his peers' plans and is better liked, with more friends than other children. At the same time, because of his emotional competence skills, he has the personal resources that allow him to be better ready to sit still, follow rules and directions, pay attention, and focus on preacademic tasks. So to maximize social competence and early school success, researchers and others must scrutinize how emotional competence allows a child to mobilize personal and environmental resources within peer interactions. This inquiry benefits from a consideration of how components of emotional competence work together.

## Interrelations among Components of Emotional Competence

As important as relations are between each component of emotional competence and social competence or preacademic success, it also is important to note that these components also are likely to support one another as an interrelated network (Eisenberg, Sadovsky, & Spinrad, 2005); when functioning optimally, they work together in an integrated way. In fact, all aspects of emotional competence work together to promote children's social and preacademic success (Denham, Bassett, Mincic, et al., 2012). So, although in subsequent chapters I describe the expression, understanding, and regulation of emotions separately, it is my hope that the complex interrelations of these components of emotional competence will become obvious.

All components of emotional competence are intricately interdependent (Denham, 1986; Giesbrecht, Miller, & Müller, 2010; Hudson & Jacques, 2014; Lindsey, 2017). In particular, as Cole, Martin, et al. (2004) theorized and Denham, Bassett, Mincic, et al. (2012) demonstrated, emotion regulation and expressiveness often operate in concert. Children who experience intense negative emotions and are unable to regulate their expressions of such emotion, are especially likely to suffer difficulties in social relationships (Contreras, Kerns, Weimer, Gentzler, & Tomich, 2000). A crybaby does not fare well on the playground, and a grouch is not welcome during make-believe. In contrast, however, even children who are high in negative emotionality are buffered from peer status problems by good emotion regulation skills, which parents and caregivers can teach them (e.g., Eisenberg, Fabes, Shepard, et al., 1997).

Jenny, who is angry and sullen day after day, and just can't seem to regulate her feelings, is unlikely to learn much about her playmates' emotions, at least partially because they avoid her. If Rodney develops successful strategies for regulating anger during a conflict, he may better recognize and understand both his own emotions and his friend's and may experience guilt over causing distress.

The emotion regulation that facilitates social interactions rests upon a foundation of other aspects of emotional competence. Specifically, emotion knowledge also may support positive, regulated emotional expressiveness, especially in predicting social competence and school success (Denham, Bassett, Thayer, et al., 2012; Denham, Caverly, et al., 2002; Di Maggio, Zappulla, & Pace, 2016).

Five-year-old Joey can "read" the emotions of his friends. He smiles easily at his friend Allen to cheer him up after a teacher's reprimand but sneers a bit at the outcast whose sickly smile indicates a bid for play. Joey can also understand his own emotional signals and fine-tune them so he can continue to be the undisputed leader of his group. When he realizes that he feels a little jittery during small-group time, he tries to still his tapping feet and dancing pencil, because other people (including his teacher) don't like him to behave this way. Besides, he really can do his alphabet work—there's no need to be tense!

In this vignette, we can see that the development of emotion regulation is necessary because of preschoolers' increasingly complex emotionality and the demands of their social world to maintain an even keel. It also is clearly supported by their increased comprehension of their own and others' emotionality. Preschoolers' emotional experience also becomes more and more complicated as they begin to feel blends of emotions and finely nuanced emotions (e.g., guilt or shame), and to better comprehend the emotional messages of parents and peers. So, with so much going on emotionally, some organized emotional gatekeeper—emotion regulation—must be cultivated.

Preschoolers' attention is becoming more riveted on success with friends, and this developmental focus also demands emotion regulation. In short, emotional expressiveness, knowledge, and regulation are working together, inextricably linked.

All these assertions about the interconnectedness of early emotional competence abilities have been corroborated: 4-year-olds with more positive profiles of emotional expressiveness, emotion regulation, *and* emotion knowledge did indeed show greater social and preacademic success as evaluated later that school year and in kindergarten (Denham, Bassett, Mincic, et al., 2012). Emotional competencies worked together to ensure the preschoolers' positive outcomes.

Further, it can be important to demonstrate relations among the aspects of emotional competence as outcomes in their own right. In a study of tantrums, preschoolers' self-reports of general sadness/distress and their lack of emotion knowledge, as well as parents' reports of their dysregulated sadness, use of venting to regulate emotions, anger reactivity, and anger and distress in tantrums, were all intricately related (Giesbrecht et al., 2010). Thus expressivity, emotion knowledge, and emotion regulation all showed associations. As another example, Lindsey (2017) noted the relation between young children's mutual positive affect and emotion knowledge. Finally, Hudson and Jacques (2014) showed that understanding emotions in general, and display rules in particular, contributed to 5- to 7-year-olds' ability to regulate emotion during a disappointing gift task.

In sum, emotional competence components do not operate in isolation. They support or weaken one another and promote or make difficult social and preacademic competence. Peers and adults experience children's emotional competence skills working together during interaction and as supports for learning. In forthcoming chapters, I expand on these interrelations where evidence is available. At this point, though, the ways we understand the nature of emotion and of the components of emotional competence and their potential interrelations and outcomes during early childhood have been discussed. I can now present a model to pull together these important ideas.

## A MODEL OF EMOTIONAL COMPETENCE

Both intra- and interpersonal contributions to the interrelated dimensions of emotional competence and the contributions of emotional competence to social and preacademic competence form the foundation of a developmental model. I argue that both intrapersonal factors (e.g., temperament, cognitive ability, and language) and interpersonal socialization of emotion (i.e., modeling, coaching or teaching about emotions, and reactions to children's emotions) within the preschool period contribute to the young child's expression, knowledge, and regulation of emotions, and that these elements of emotional competence contribute to indices of social and preacademic competence (see Figure 1.2). I use this model as a guiding framework throughout the book. I focus on the elements of emotional competence, the contributory pathways from the children themselves and the people around them, and the outcomes that are important in their world. This model helps conceptualize the explanations I expand upon in the coming chapters. It serves as a road map that describes typical development and suggests a template from which to evaluate less typical development.

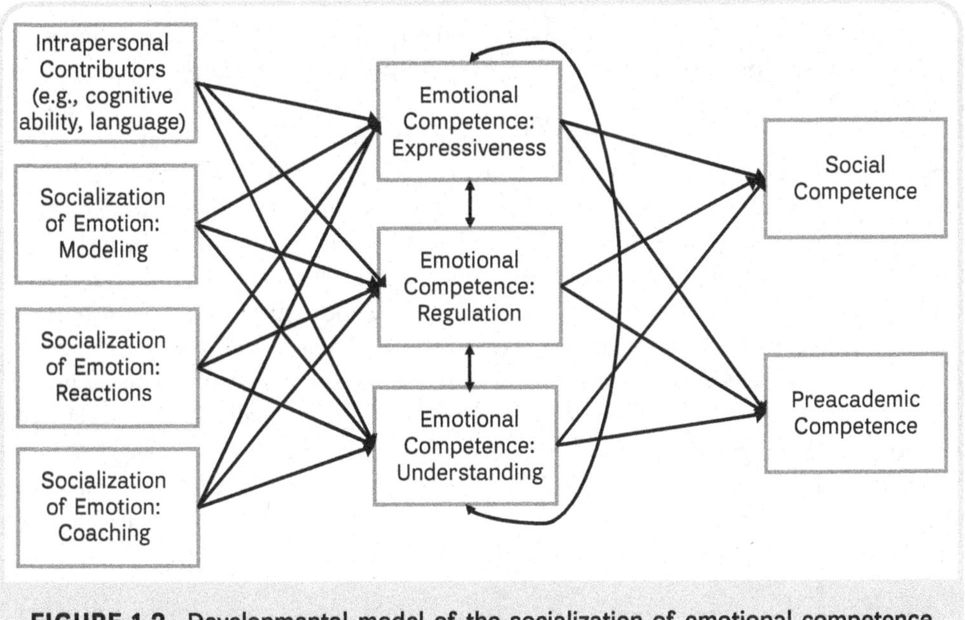


**FIGURE 1.2.** Developmental model of the socialization of emotional competence leading to social competence.

## DIFFICULTIES IN THE DEVELOPMENT OF EMOTIONAL COMPETENCE

Thus the model in Figure 1.2 helps to illustrate what I consider to be theoretically universal transitions to and from young children's emotional competence. But what happens when the development of emotional competence goes awry? It is well and good to study the emotional development of young children, as fascinating as it is, but what use can we make of this knowledge? An applied focus is an important foundation for this book.

Many broad societal problems with which communities struggle have strong emotional undercurrents. Often mental health difficulties are centered on deficits or unusual patterns of emotional expressiveness, knowledge, and regulation. At the core of marital difficulties and child abuse lie anger, contempt, and shame. The experience of debilitating depression and anxiety is primarily emotional. On our highways and in our cities, images of anger predominate and too often explode into violence.

To focus more specifically on childhood development, the lack of emotional competence is obviously central to intractable difficulties. Even a cursory review of the literature on behavior disorders reveals repeated mentions of emotional factors. Anger and other negative affects, as well as lack of positive affect or emotional support, are consistently described as characteristics of both children with behavior problems and their parents (Dadds, Sanders, Morrison, & Rebetz, 1992; Gardner, 1989; Mullin & Hinshaw, 2007; Rubin, Burgess, & Hastings, 2002). Moreover, such emotion-related behavioral characteristics often predict continuity in both externalizing and internalizing psychopathy (Werner, 1989). Thus, when developmental milestones of emotional competence are not negotiated successfully, preschoolers are at risk for psychopathology, both during preschool and later in life (Zahn-Waxler, Iannotti, Cummings, & Denham, 1990).

Of course, the direction of effect also can be the reverse of emotional competence deficits contributing to difficulties in optimal development and psychological health. Intrapersonal issues, such as cognitive impairment, autism spectrum disorder, or other psychopathology like oppositional defiant disorder or attention deficit disorder, can contribute to deficits in emotional competence. Similarly, interpersonal issues, such as child abuse and interparental violence, and other poor emotion socialization practices can hinder the development of emotional competence. Living in conditions of demographic risk (e.g., low income, chaos, systemic racism) also can negatively impact young children's emotional competence. In this book, I discuss all the issues related to emotional competence difficulties, organizing them according to intrapersonal, interpersonal, and mixed contributors to difficulties in emotional development. Knowing how emotional competence develops both typically and atypically points to the need for assessment and programming in this area.

## ASSESSMENT AND PROGRAMMING TO PROMOTE EARLY CHILDHOOD EMOTIONAL COMPETENCE

To solve these pressing problems, emotional competence and the means for strengthening it must be addressed. Realizing when and how young children are at risk for delays and learning to recognize disturbances in the expected milestones of emotional competence are equally necessary. Recognizing the importance of emotional competence in young children and finding the means for cultivating it are essential tasks for caregivers. A knowledge of risk factors and of how to identify delays in the development of emotional competence as well as how to intervene are vital if the centrality of developing emotional competence is to be taken seriously (Knitzer, 1993). Thus the burgeoning literature on how to assess emotional competence during early childhood and on how to create efficacious programming, both targeted and universal, will be delineated within a framework showing how these components contribute to a model of early childhood education.

## STUDYING THE YOUNG CHILD'S EMOTIONAL LIFE: THIS VOLUME AND BEYOND

If emotional competence is so very important, it behooves researchers, educators, and parents to understand what is really going on in the young child's emotional world. Ecologically valid measurement systems that require an investigator to enter a child's world, rather than vice versa, best allow researchers to discern young children's emotional competence. Thus I argue forcefully—and attempt to illustrate amply throughout this book—that studies should be conducted during children's typical play and family activities, either by directly assessing children or by observing them in the social contexts in which they typically live. Ambiguous data or negative results may emanate from less-sensitive modes of study. Since the publication of *Emotional Development in Young Children* in 1998, many investigators have taken up his challenge.

How can we study emotional expressiveness and regulation—two important components of emotional competence? Fortunately, better operational definitions and other methodological advances have enabled successful examinations of children's emotional expressiveness patterns, whether these studies focus on microanalytic facial expressions of emotions or on more comprehensive, global indicators. In addition, new paradigms that challenge preschoolers' emotion regulation, as well as dynamic ways to view such emotion regulation in real time, are emerging with good effect.

And how can we learn more about how preschoolers understand emotions? Asking young children to verbalize about issues of emotional competence leads directly to a quagmire of demands: A preschooler might think, "What does this person want me to do or say? How should I be feeling and acting in this setting?" Even more important, such means of questioning exist in a social vacuum (Saarni, 1987, 1990). A preschooler might query, "What is this lady talking about? Can I answer her at all? Why can't I just go play?" Fortunately, ecologically valid means of examining understanding of emotion are available in response to these concerns.

Thus the stage has been set for a more fruitful inquiry into developmental change and individual differences in preschoolers' emotional competence. I attempt in this volume to give a picture of an exciting time—the unfolding of a vital set of emotional skills that sustain children's well-being, relationships, and even school success. I intend to explore the evidence of these indispensable early capacities to express, understand, and deal with one's own emotions and those of others. It is my hope to convey some of the energy inherent in this field of inquiry and to inspire continued research into these engaging capabilities.

Then, in subsequent chapters I explore these important aspects of the changing emotional competencies of toddlers and preschoolers (see the middle column of Figure 1.2). First, in Chapter 2, I describe patterns and developments in children's emotional expressiveness—their consistent manner of showing emotions in various situations. I survey children's changing expression of the simplest, most basic emotions, which are separable according to facial, vocal, and behavioral indices; they include happiness, sadness, anger, and fear. I also consider the beginnings of empathy in Chapter 2. Next, in Chapter 3, I examine the emergence of more complicated emotions, which involve other people and self-consciousness and/or other cognitive abilities, either implicitly or explicitly; they include shame, guilt, shyness, embarrassment, and pride. I also discuss children's increasing display of blended emotions, as well as their expanding demonstration of emotional display rules.

In Chapters 4 and 5, examining toddlers' and preschoolers' understanding of emotion, I take the view that young children are developing an impressive body of knowledge about both internal states and the causes of behavior. Consequently, in Chapter 4, I explore their growing awareness of emotions in general and of specific discrete emotions, working from a model that melds my own approach to the skills involved in emotion knowledge (Bassett, Denham, Mincic, & Graling, 2012) and that of Pons and colleagues (e.g., Pons, Harris, & de Rosnay, 2004). I describe toddlers' and preschoolers' abilities to use emotion labels, to recognize emotion situations, and to demonstrate knowledge of emotions' causes and consequences. Young children's use of emotion language within their families also is addressed. In addition, in Chapter 5, I describe the development of more complex aspects of understanding of emotion, such as knowledge of equivocal situations, conflicting expressive and situational cues, personalized experience of emotion, ways of regulating both positive and negative emotions, display rules, and simultaneity and ambivalence.

Developmentalists are making big strides in operationalizing fascinating aspects of emotion regulation—to investigate its emotional, cognitive, and behavioral components; I outline how I and others have come to understand emotion regulation in Chapter 6, what we know about developmental change and about individual differences in emotion regulation and in children's use of regulatory strategies. I also explore new views of young children's ability to regulate their emotional expressiveness, including a consideration of the fluid, dynamic, contextually bound in-the-moment emergence of emotions in real time, as well as their reorganization over developmental time. In Chapters 2 through 6, I also describe intrapersonal elements that are likely to contribute to individual differences in emotional competence during the preschool period. Adults need to know what to expect in terms of preschoolers' emotional expressiveness and regulation, as well as their understanding of their own and others' emotions. If they do, they not only help children, but also create a more positive emotional environment for themselves.

Just as I describe typical developmental changes in emotional competence over the toddler and preschool period, and its intrapersonal supports, I explore the interpersonal roots of its individual differences (see leftmost column of Figure 1.2). In Chapters 7 and 8, I review the evidence for parents' influence on children's emotional expressiveness, knowledge, and regulation. I continue this concentration on emotion socialization in Chapter 9 by examining new evidence of how preschool teachers, broadly defined (i.e., childcare providers as well as Head Start, private preschool, or public prekindergarten teachers), contribute to the development of young children's emotional competence. Although this area of study is relatively new, it looms large because of young children's ubiquitous exposure to early educational settings.

In Chapter 10, I begin to focus on outcomes supported by the young child's growing emotional competence (see the rightmost column of Figure 1.2)—in this case social accomplishments and lack of behavior problems. I spotlight how essential these capabilities are to children's mental health, even at such an early age. In Chapter 11, I outline the ever-growing evidence for a connection between emotional competence and academic success from preschool through elementary school.

If we have a clearer understanding of the roots and nature of young children's emotional competence, we can not only examine its outcomes, but will be better able to begin the vital task of facilitating it. So, in Chapter 12, I discuss young children who develop problems in emotional competence. Some deficits in emotional competence seem to reside in the children themselves. In contrast, other deficits in emotional competence seem to arise primarily from transactions with the environment. How can such children be identified? What can be done to assist them? In Chapter 13, I outline ways of assessing and promoting emotional competence.

## A CALL TO ACTION

As concerned researchers, practitioners, and caregivers, we want to learn answers to these questions, so that we may help children develop optimal emotional skills. We are finally becoming aware of the importance of such emotional competence. We see that when children are not "smart" in this way, they are at a long-term risk for depression, aggressiveness and violent crime, problems in marriage and parenting, and even poor physical health. As adults who care about children, we need to take emotional competence seriously. As Goleman (1995) put it so eloquently over 20 years ago,

> [We must] make sure that every child is taught the essentials of handling anger or resolving conflicts positively . . . [we need to] teach empathy . . . [and] the fundamentals of emotional competence. By leaving the emotional lessons children learn to chance, we risk largely wasting the window of opportunity presented by the slow maturation of the brain to help children cultivate a healthy emotional repertoire. . . . In this sense, emotional [competence] goes hand in hand with education for character, for moral development, and for citizenship. (p. 286)

I now turn to a more detailed consideration of the nature and manifestations of preschoolers' emotional competence.

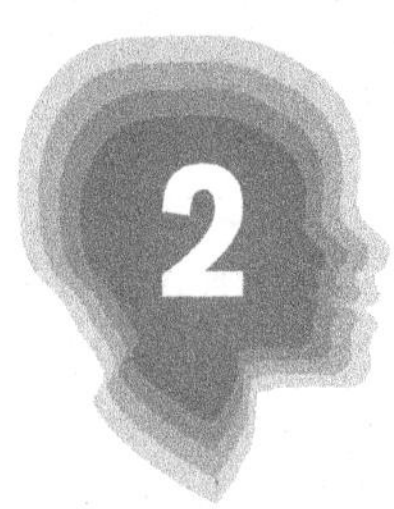

# Emotional Expressiveness

## BASIC EMOTIONS AND EMPATHY

## INTRODUCTION

Expressed emotions become ever more complex and elaborate in several ways during the toddler and preschool periods. Along with developmental change, individual children also differ in the intensity, frequency, and duration of their emotions; their own unique predominance of positive versus negative emotions; their use of pure versus mixed expressions; the speed with which they become emotional in a provocative situation; their level of understanding and attunement to others' emotions; and the time it takes them to resume their own "even keel" after being emotionally aroused (Hyson, 1994). These parameters of expression are important when one is trying to understand particular preschoolers and preschool emotional expressiveness in general. Before discussing developmental change, these factors should be delineated. From my own work, many vivid examples come to mind.

### The Balance of Positive and Negative Emotions

Some children, like Juan, show predominantly positive emotions. He grins broadly the minute he sees a friend; when his teacher reads a funny passage of a book, he is delighted. If Juan were to cry, it is certain that his teachers would take him quite seriously.

By contrast, Colin rarely shows positive emotions; he exhibits negative emotions or none at all. He often is surly and combative with peers, and scowls during circle time, reacting negatively to the slightest innocent jostle from a neighbor. Everyone just tries to stay out of his way and might not even notice a flicker of positivity from him.

By comparison, Zachary shows lots of both negative and positive emotions. He laughs uproariously on the playground when involved in rough-and-tumble play, but roars with anger when someone thwarts his building in the block corner. He keeps peers and adults alike on their toes.

## Frequency of Specific Emotion Displays

Sebi often looks sad as he enters his preschool classroom and during circle time—eyelids heavy, lips drooping. His classmates look sad much less frequently.

In contrast, Elizabeth is notable for sucking her thumb and shrinking back from the circle; on the playground she walks alone and is startled when children run by vigorously. Her behaviors mark her frequent tension, seen only irregularly in her classmates.

## Intensity of Emotion Expressions

Adults and peers need to be able to read children's expressiveness. Sometimes children's emotional intensity makes this easy; sometimes it is difficult, even when their frequency of expressiveness is relatively equal. On a bad day, Carrie's anger is explosive and is very articulately expressed. She fusses and yells at people who make her mad; her wails are audible and her lashing out is visible across the large classroom. Davis, on the other hand, is expressive in a much more subtle, muted way. When he is annoyed, his lips purse slightly, his gaze is longer in duration, and his eyebrows lower a bit. Only a fairly attentive partner could pick up on this.

## Duration of Specific Emotions

Midori's expressiveness flits from one emotion to another: One minute she is angry and struggling over a toy with a playmate, the next dissolving in laughter. Although her quick change disarms the dispute, sometimes it is hard to predict how interacting with her will turn out. But Roberto's style is different. He shows long periods of an equable but relatively neutral expression. When someone does something funny, though, he seems to retain the mood of delight and smiles for a long time. Similarly, he "holds onto" anger and grudges—even for days—when a friend does something mean. He is easier to predict than Midori is, but it is sometimes hard to modify his stable moods.

## Pure versus Mixed Emotion Expressions

Children who show very blended expressions also take more effort to "read." Chelsea's vivid emotion displays vary between exceptionally clear depictions of joy and rage: She moves from a smile that lights up her entire visage to determined, fist-clenching, foot-stomping anger. But Elena's expressiveness is much more complicated to interpret, even for a trained observer. Elements of fear, pain, and joy play habitually on her face during social interactions when happiness, if anything, is most appropriate.

## Speed of Emotion Onset and Recovery Time

When someone crosses Taylor, his wrath is immediate. There is no question about how he is feeling, no time to correct the situation before he erupts. He smolders for a long time as well.

Douglas, though, seems almost to consider the ongoing emotional situation. One can almost see annoyance building until the situation worsens just enough, and he finally sputters, "Stop that!" If his buddies respond to his outburst, he calms fairly quickly (see also Chapter 6 for coverage of emotion regulation).

Given the discussion of these features of individual emotionality, I begin this chapter with a continued examination of what experiencing and expressing emotions mean to children and the people around them. I then highlight basic emotions' emergence and change across time. Most of the basic emotions emerge before a child is 2 years old; however, their frequency and manner of expression changes with development. Personal emotional styles also become established early in the preschool period, and the development of such personal styles of expressiveness adds new complexity to young children's emotional transactions with others. Thus I discuss this complexity in young children's expressiveness and its stability as individual differences across time and situations, as well as discussing important developmental changes. As suggested by the new focus on variability and context specificity stimulated by the ideas of dynamic systems theory (Camras & Witherington, 2005), I also describe children's emotional variability across smaller timespans, pointing out the role of context and the role of change within contexts. Then I turn to another important aspect of emotional expressiveness:

## Attunement to Others' Emotions

Benji is able to discern his peers' emotions with almost uncanny ability for his age. He knows that Joelle's parents live in two houses now, and that she's very sad about it. When she slips at the snack table, knocks her elbow, and starts to cry, he runs all the way across the room to her aid.

On the other hand, Colin, along with being unemotional (except for his negativity when crossed), really doesn't attend to others' emotions at all. He plays mostly alone with toys and doesn't look up when nearby peers laugh or cry.

Thus while the expression and experience of basic emotions are being consolidated, the social emotion of empathy is also appearing. So I also consider here developmental trends and individual differences in the experience and expression of empathy. In the next chapter, I address the subsequent set of developments in preschoolers' emotional expressiveness: the unfolding of self-conscious emotions (e.g., pride, guilt, shame, embarrassment, and shyness), as well as preschoolers' growing abilities to voluntarily express (or suppress) emotions.

## Expression and Experience of Emotions

The patterns of expressiveness detailed in the examples with which this chapter begins are important in determining whether a child is a good social partner—readable, predictable, and responsive. But the internal emotional experience of each preschooler is important too. As clearly as these examples differentiate children according to parameters of expressiveness, emotion theorists still disagree about the relationship between early emotional expressiveness and emotional experience. As soon as infants exhibit the expressions associated with specific emotions, do they experience the concomitant feelings? Do infants experience emotions in the same general situations as older members of their cultures? Or instead, are early emotions experienced mostly via their valence (i.e., positive or negative) and intensity (Camras & Fatani, 2010; Lewis, 2010; Posner, Russell, & Peterson, 2005; Sroufe, 1996)? Are further cognitive development and socialization needed before toddlers and preschoolers can truly experience specifically discernible emotions? Izard (1991) favors the view that expressive patterns for basic emotions are consonant with emotional experience; they require only basic perception to be activated (Izard, 2007; Figure 1.1). Lewis and colleagues (see, e.g., Lewis, 2010; Lewis & Michalson, 1983) assert that other developments, especially that of a sense of self, are necessary for the experience and meaningful expression of certain emotions. This argument resembles the "Is cognition necessary for emotional experience?" question, addressed in Chapter 1.

In essence, the argument depends on whether expressed emotions, especially those of infants, are equivalent to a feeling state when no (or very unsophisticated) cognition occurs. In my view, this dispute often leads to a dead end in reasoning about children's emotions. It is exceedingly difficult to access the feeling states of infants (and even those of toddlers and preschoolers, for that matter); their means of self-report are extremely limited, when they exist at all (although we are making some inroads in accessing these reports[1]). Their verbal and cognitive capacities place restrictions on preschoolers' production of well-differentiated self-reports of emotion. But remember that emotion can be experienced without cognitive appraisal, although appraisal often is necessary, and becomes increasingly possible with brain development across the preschool period. My educated guess, then, is that although older persons have a more powerful combination of emotional experience, knowledge, regulatory possibilities, and increasingly varied emotion schemas at their command, even preschoolers experience and are aware of the essential elements of emotions.

In other words, there is a specific and powerful constellation of vocal/facial/bodily expressions and behaviors and associated meanings/goals/usefulness (however rudimentary) that is unique to each emotion (Campos & Barrett, 1984). An angry person, whether 3 years old or 30, lowers her voice almost to a growl, and glares, brows down,

---

[1]A few researchers have moved toward potential success in this area, however, and some parents can sensitively determine their children's "real" feelings. Fabes and Eisenberg (1992) have interviewed young children *in vivo* about the causes of their anger; Warren and Stifter (2008) and Dunn and Hughes (1998) have interviewed preschoolers about what causes their own emotions, as well as those of their mothers, siblings, and friends (see also Denham & Zoller, 1991). Of course, during these latter interviews the children are *remembering* emotions, not *experiencing* them. Nonetheless, they are at least able to consider their own emotional experience, and therein lies the possibility of somehow creating imaginative, ecologically valid ways of discussing current feelings with preschoolers. Alternatively, viewing videotapes and reliving emotion could be one way of validating a preschooler's emotional experience after the fact (see, e.g., Dunsmore, Her, Halberstadt, & Perez-Rivera, 2009). Similarly, although physiological means are not yet sophisticated enough to identify discrete emotions, there is promise in the approach of marrying convergent measurements of physiology and self-reports. Developmentalists need continued support in this difficult endeavor.

at the person or thing who made him or her mad. The person impatiently pushes at the doll's shoe that won't come off or the ATM machine buttons that are not responding. The person consciously wants to *fix this problem*, and both the expression and *experience of* anger help to mobilize his or her efforts.

As the example of anger indicates, for the basic emotions and early emotion schemas derived from them—happiness, sadness, anger, or fear—young children probably experience much the same feelings that their adult counterparts do in functionally equivalent situations, even though their rudimentary emotion schemas add some individuality. Consider a case of fear in a child and in an adult:

> Leah feels afraid when asked to stand in front of a group of adults and recite a nursery rhyme. Her heart is racing, her tummy rumbles, and she wants to run out of the room, straight into the safety of her mother's arms. As a professor, her father has a similar emotional experience each time he faces a new classroom full of students: He too wants to retreat into the safety of his wife's companionship.

Many more complex emotions, such as shame, involve self-awareness, reflection, and self-evaluation; behavioral standards established by others; and the vicissitudes of experience. For such emotions, a child may feel the core of shame, but not the full range of shameful affect felt by an adult. As Lewis (2010) and Mascolo and Fischer (2007) have noted, a sense of self and more sophisticated cognitive representational skills are necessary for experiencing and expressing more complex emotions; in experiencing and expressing these emotions, individualized emotion schemas are more paramount.

> If Leah begins to recite her rhyme, but forgets part of it, she may feel awful. The kernel of the feeling experience is there, and she wants to sink into the floor. In contrast, should her professor father forget a key element of his lecture, and stand there with a blank look on his face, he feels foolish in front of a group of students who he hopes will admire him; he also would like to sink into the floor. But more than this, he feels ashamed and embarrassed; remembering the time this happened when his department chair was observing him, he thinks "oh no, not this again!" He knows that his self-esteem has been dealt a blow and may ruminate on this gaffe for some time.

Yet the child and adult emotions have common themes: their expressive patterns, the behaviors associated with them, the attempts to understand the causes of the emotion (in this case, shame), and decisions about future courses of action. So I assert that expressed emotions have some experiential emotional continuity, regardless of the time point in the lifespan after infancy at which they occur (see also Izard, 2007), and despite the individuality imparted by accumulating emotion schemas. And again, as emphasized in Chapter 1, this emotional experience and expression impart functionally important sources of information to the child and others.

## Information Imparted by Emotional Experience and Expression

To elaborate on assertions made in Chapter 1, emotions are regulators of intra- and interpersonal behaviors: They let the person experiencing the emotions, and those nearby, know that "something must be done." This pragmatic view aids others in differentiating among expressions of early-emerging emotions based on certain features (Barrett & Campos, 1991); it can assist children themselves in appreciating the uniqueness of their own emotional experiences. Consequently, young children's expression and experience of emotions impart several important types of information, as follows:

1 ***"What emotion is this?"*** Emotions need to be identified by the child experiencing the emotion and by other people interacting with him or her. First, the basic emotions have specific vocal qualities, intonation patterns, and particular patterns of facial movement (Izard, Dougherty, & Hembree, 1980; but see Russell, 1994, for a contrasting view). These are important signals both to the child experiencing them and to others. Happiness is defined by a combination of smiles, laughter, and voices with a "pearly," relaxed pitch. In contrast, sadness is marked by crying, and with the inner corners of the eyebrows lifted, the corners of the lips down, and slow, steady-pitched speech. Anger is seen in lowered brows, tense lower lips, and staring. The speech of angry persons is clipped, abrupt, and often loud. Tightened brows raised and drawn together and a high-pitched voice indicate fear. Young children express and experience all these basic emotions and begin to recognize their expressive patterns in themselves and others (see Chapter 4).

2 ***"What should I do now?"/"What is he or she likely to do now?"*** Emotions often lead to this second question, whether implicitly or explicitly. Several theorists (e.g., Campos & Barrett, 1984; Campos, Campos, & Barrett, 1989; Izard, 2007) suggest that different emotions have particular action tendencies associated with them: fleeing with fear, aggression with anger, withdrawal or tearfulness with sadness. In general, young children develop common action tendencies for differing emotions. Fortunately, many adults are correct when they use these action tendencies to identify young children's emotions.

3 ***"Why is this emotion important to me/to the child experiencing it?"*** Emotions have adaptive functions that serve as internal teaching mechanisms. They carry personal meaning for the child experiencing them. These adaptive functions can help them to differentiate emotions. For example, the adaptive function of disgust is protection of the self from noxious substances (e.g., the tasting of a rotten apple leads to future avoidance). In contrast, the adaptive function for fear is avoidance of dangerous situations. A 4-year-old boy experiences fear when he is at the top of the monkey bars at preschool. He begins to understand that this feeling signals possible danger—"I am scared when I go a little too far"—and ideally he does something to become safer. Over time, especially as they construct emotion schemas with the aid of brain development and language (Hoemann, Devlin, & Barrett, 2020; Hoemann et al., 2019), young children also learn to better understand the experiential difference among emotions. Thus feelings of disgust are associated with getting away from "yucky" things, whereas feelings of fear are linked with avoiding potentially dangerous situations.

Discerning the adaptive functions of a child's emotions also can be helpful for adults who are involved with children. What does this emotion mean *for the child* (*i.e., what is their emotion schema*)? Is the child who rejects an unfamiliar food experiencing disgust or simply being defiant? Seeing his son's fear on the monkey bars, the 4-year-old's father should consider that the boy feels truly unsafe and respond with comfort and assistance. Reflecting about a child's previous experiences for a moment can help a caregiver understand what emotion is being experienced and respond appropriately.

4 ***"What does this display of emotion communicate to people observing it?"*** The child and observing adults also distinguish individual emotions while they are felt, based on what the feelings signify to others in the specific context. Feelings can be socially significant. When a 3-year-old girl's mother catches her playing when she's supposed to be sleeping, the child gradually understands the social meaning of the parent's frown and sigh: a return to bed and maybe even punishment are imminent. Given this understanding of her mother's annoyance, the girl's own experience of emotion centers on its social significance, which can engender her own emotion: "If I play around after bedtime, my parents will not like it. That makes me a little scared to sneak around."

Knowing the social significance of the expression or experience of emotion is important because it varies for each emotion. A 5-year-old boy shows contempt after witnessing a peer crying when he merely stumbles in the hallway of their school. He understands the social meaning of such a lapse in self-control, because he now knows the norms of his peer group and engages in social comparison: "Everyone will laugh. I say 'yuck!' "

5 ***"What am I trying to accomplish?"/"What is the person experiencing the emotion trying to accomplish?"*** Goals are very important in the experience of emotion. The seminal work of Nancy Stein and her colleagues helps illuminate children's interpretations of the significance of emotions (e.g., Stein & Jewett, 1986; Stein & Levine, 1989, 1990; Stein & Trabasso, 1989). Stein has posited that a complex process of understanding underlies emotional experience. Emotion is aroused when an event signals that something the individual wants, or does not want, is about to happen. Consider a 5-year-old girl whose drawing is destroyed by a peer. Her ongoing activity has been disrupted, and she tries to figure out what is happening. As she notices her problem, she also becomes aware of her arousal. She understands that something has happened that she doesn't want, and she feels her heart pumping in a surge of anger. An increase in heart rate is associated with arousal of this emotion.

But individual goals are crucial in determining which emotion is experienced. Again consider the child creating a drawing. She's totally absorbed in her activity. A playmate comes over and deliberately knocks her arm, hard. The emotional result of this peer's actions could conceivably be either anger or sadness. The emotion that the girl experiences depends on the lens through which she views the event—that of the peer's provocative act or the loss of the drawing. Is it her goal to conserve something she has created with her own hands? Is she sad over the injury to something personal? Or is she more concerned with the goal of her relationship with her friend and therefore angry that he did something mean?

Further examples will serve to clarify this integrated perspective. A 4-year-old girl sees a big, friendly dog. After encountering this event, she encodes it in her memory and tries to understand it. Aspects either of the external environment (e.g., the actual approach of the dog) or of internal processing (e.g., memories of an earlier encounter with a dog) can cause emotional events. These patterns of understandings can lead to two possible emotions. If the child focuses on the dog's happy "grin," she concludes, "Something new is happening, and it will be something I like"; she feels happiness. She realizes that the goal of having "a fun time" may be realized and approaches the dog. In contrast, if the child focuses on the dog's big, open mouth and prominent teeth, she thinks, "Something new is impending, and I remember that it probably will be something I don't like"; she feels fear. In this case, the child clings to her mother or runs away.

Either way, the child is aware of valuable emotional information: (a) the change in a valued state ("something I like or don't like"); (b) the conditions that caused the change; (c) the consequences of the change for goal maintenance or attainment; and (d) plans for maintaining, reinstating, or abandoning a goal. These understandings increasingly influence which specific emotion the child detects (see also Fischer et al., 1989). To illustrate, a pattern of understandings for sadness is "wanting but not having something," as when a parent departs; plans include searching for the parent or using a substitute caregiver for comfort. A pattern of understandings for anger is "not wanting but having an event," as when a peer takes away a toy; plans include getting the toy back through whatever means necessary.

Over time, the orderly pattern of these emotional experiences related to certain goals in specific eliciting situations helps the child to discern the general differences among discrete emotions (see more on Stein's work in Chapter 4). A child also comes to make plans based upon this experience of emotions and to manage emotions in increasingly organized ways (see Chapter 6).

### SUMMARY: Experience and Expression of Emotion

Preschoolers and their caring adults come to discern their emotions, the meaning of their emotions, and what actions are likely to follow. Knowing how the experience of these emotions is related to the child's goals also is crucial in distinguishing emotions as experienced and as expressed; although preschoolers may not overtly connect goals and their emotions, they eventually make connections that adults also would do well to consider. Given this foundation on the nature of preschoolers' emotions, I consider how their expression and experience change over time.

## BASIC EMOTIONS: CHANGE AND STABILITY ACROSS TIME

By the time children reach their third year, they are experiencing and expressing a variety of emotions. Their emotion repertoires include all the basic emotions—joy, sadness, anger, fear, and interest—and the ways these emotions are expressed are increasingly differentiated. Preschoolers can share positive emotions together, but they can also share negative emotions:

> Micah squeals in anger when his garage of blocks falls apart. He thinks correctly that Lan made it fall. Lan says he'll help build it up again, but then backs off, looking sad. Micah screams at Lan again; Lan backs away even further, still sad and whining. Jamell joins the fray, angrily defending Micah. In this example anger has been communicated by Micah's yelling and Jamell's scolding words. Lan's sadness is shown both vocally and behaviorally. But these means of expressing emotions have changed and will continue to change across time, since their infancy.

Malatesta and colleagues were among the first to investigate developmental changes in patterns of emotional expressiveness between early infancy and 3 years of age (Malatesta, Culver, Tesman, & Shepard, 1989; Malatesta-Magai, Leak, Tesman. Shepard, Culver, & Smaggia, 1994; see also Fogel & Reimers's 1989 commentary on Malatesta et al.'s 1989 work). These researchers expected facial displays of emotion to decrease in frequency during the period between 2 and 3 years if young children were learning to curtail expressiveness according to cultural display rules. In contrast, they expected vocal expressiveness to stay stable, because vocal expressiveness is relatively difficult to control.

But, contrary to expectations, toddlers' total vocal emotional expressiveness actually increased from the second to the third year. There was essentially no *overall* change in facial expressiveness; only interest increased, and only surprise decreased. What sense could be made of these unexpected outcomes? Apparently display rule usage to curtail facial expressiveness comes into full use in children older than those in this age range (see Chapter 3, Control of Expressiveness and Adherence to Display Rules), and the ability to use language to express emotion makes the vocal channel even more attractive as an eloquent conveyor of emotional meaning.

Changes at the level of individual emotions also were uncovered in this research. Both verbal and vocal expressions of joy, interest, surprise, and anger increased up to age 3 years. Vocal expressions of sadness decreased, while facial expressiveness of this emotion remained the same. Hence, overall children remain emotionally intense from late infancy until early in the preschool period, with both facial and verbal/vocal channels serving to communicate emotion. They do not yet limit their overall emotional expressiveness. Similarly, Mathiesen and Tambs (1999) found that children's overall emotionality actually increased from 18 to 50 months.

Several other conclusions regarding the emotional expressiveness of young children in naturalistic situations emanated from details in Malatesta et al.'s (1989, 1994) data. First, by the beginning of the preschool period, children can alternate or exchange modes of expressiveness as the situation demands. Second, they are beginning to inhibit or intensify expressiveness as needed in varying situations. They are beginning to take situational context into account and to use modes of expressiveness that suits their goals.

Other researchers have examined age changes in emotional expressiveness in older youngsters across the preschool period. As one useful example, Olino et al. (2011)

found that children's positive affect (i.e., joy, surprise, and pleasure) increased from late infancy to 9 years of age. Emotion was coded from developmentally appropriate emotion-eliciting tasks, such as puzzles, jack-in-the-box, or wiggle balls for the preschoolers. Similarly Sallquist et al. (2010) found that preschoolers' positive affect (e.g., smiling, laughter, positive vocal tone) generally increased from 18 to 42 months during free play with their mothers and during a bubble-breaking task with an experimenter (and through to 54 months with the experimenter only). Further, Barry and Kochanska (2010) observed parents and their children in everyday contexts from infancy to the late preschool age range and found that the children's joy declined early in the period, with an uptick after 38 months (presumably after emotions accompanying the "terrible twos" ebbed). In general, then, it seems that from late infancy through the preschool period, positive emotional expressiveness increases.

Negative emotionality changes over the preschool period as well. Olino et al. (2011) found that children's negative affect (i.e., anxiety, distress, disappointment, frustration, sadness, and anger) decreased from late infancy to age 9 years (see also Morris et al., 2011, for age decreases in sadness and anger between 4- and 8-year-olds). Other researchers, using varying methodologies (e.g., mother-reported temperament, Denham, Lehman, Moser, & Reeves, 1995; observed daily interactions, Barry & Kochanska, 2010) found decreases in children's overall anger from the midinfancy period through late preschool (see also Malatesta-Magai et al., 1994). Cummings, Zahn-Waxler, and Radke-Yarrow (1984) found an age-related decrease across the toddler–preschool age range in children's observed distress (including sadness) while observing interparental anger. Finally, using teacher and parent ratings, Murphy, Eisenberg, Fabes, Shepard, and Guthrie (1999) also noted a decrease in negative emotionality between children in preschool/kindergarten and children 2 years later. In sum, across many age spans and methodologies, children's negative expressiveness decreases normatively as children leave toddlerhood and continues through the preschool period and beyond (see also Gaertner, Spinrad, & Eisenberg, 2008).

Such age-related changes may be supported by self-regulation, using the ability to focus and shift attention in the service of emotion regulation. Focusing on anger, Cole, Tan, et al. (2011) found that as children matured from 18 to 48 months, their latency to anger while waiting to open a toy gift increased, and they more quickly shifted from making angry bids to their mothers to be allowed to open the gift to calmly making information-gathering bids (e.g., "when can I open the present?"), even before distracting themselves with an alternate activity. Gaertner and colleagues (2008) also found that toddlers' attentional abilities were negatively related to anger for every task and every rater in their study. We found that when children were better able to self-regulate their behavior during a delay task, they showed less negative emotion and aggression in their classrooms (Denham, Bassett, Thayer, et al., 2012). Children with more advanced self-regulation also are likely to show less prevalence of negative emotion overall (Gartstein, Putnam, & Kliewer, 2016; see also Hernández et al., 2022). So being able to shift one's attention *away from* negativity-inducing circumstances aids in the regulation of emotional expressiveness throughout the early years. Self-regulation is important to the ability to deal with and recover from negative emotions, whether this recovery was examined in real time or across longer timespans.

Further, self-regulation also supports positive expressiveness. When children who experienced alternating emotionally negative and positive tasks (e.g., being required to draw a "perfect line," or playing with bubbles) had more developed self-regulation abilities, they were quicker to show positive emotions after a negative challenge (Conway et al., 2014; see also Liebermann, Giesbrecht, & Müller, 2007). In addition, self-regulation facilitates preschoolers' expression of social and self-conscious emotions as well, such as context-appropriate sympathy and guilt (Colasante, Zuffianò, Bae, & Malti, 2014). In fact, it will become amply clear that differing aspects of self-regulation support all facets of emotional competence, and I share research supporting this notion throughout this volume. More specifically, I discuss emotion regulation further in Chapter 6.

## Context as a Moderator of Developmental Change in Emotional Expressiveness

It is hard to overestimate, however, the importance of context as a moderator of emotional expressiveness throughout the preschool period. For instance, glaring angrily at a peer during play is more appropriate, and more effective, than screaming and attracting unwanted adult attention; by contrast, a vocal signal of distress is more appropriate than a visual one when a child falls down in the yard and needs a parent to come and help (see Chapter 3, Control of Expressiveness and Adherence to Display Rules).

Recent research has begun to uncover some important ways in which context moderates the expression of preschoolers' emotion. In one excellent example, Chaplin, Klein, Cole, and Turpyn (2017) longitudinally examined age differences in 3- to 5-year-olds' anger, sadness, and happiness within three very different contexts: (1) being asked by an experimenter to draw a "perfect" circle (which was never *perfect enough*, ages 3 and 4) or solve "impossible" mazes (age 5); (2) performing a difficult task to obtain a preferred toy while alone; or (3) waiting to be able to open a toy with their mothers present. All these contexts were potentially elicitors of frustration but differed in their "pull" for different emotions based on having a social partner or the lack thereof.

Anger increased across one or both years for the impossible circle and difficult toy tasks, but not for the waiting task. In these frustrating situations, modulated anger may be summoned more frequently by older preschoolers who "use" it to persist and overcome obstacles (Cole, Tan, et al., 2011; Ramsook, Benson, Ram, & Cole, 2020). In contrast, the waiting task may be somewhat less frustrating than the other two, so that emerging emotion regulation strategies may be easier to implement; also mothers were present as useful sources of comfort during this task.

Sadness decreased over time for all three tasks. The authors interpreted the unique findings for this emotion to reflect that sadness really is not the appropriate expression for frustrating circumstances, and that there are socialization pressures to limit the expression of sadness anyway ("Don't be a crybaby"). However, despite these changes, sadness was expressed more often in the waiting task, suggesting that the expectation of maternal comfort after sadness mitigated some suppression of the emotion. Expressing sadness may signal distress to one's mother, leading at least to some sympathy for comfort.

Finally expressions of happiness decreased over time from ages 4 to 5 in the tasks with the experimenter but increased in the waiting task with the mother. Regarding the experimenter-present "impossible" tasks, preschoolers probably begin to realize that happiness is just not appropriate or useful in such frustrating settings (they probably don't feel very happy at all or even consider that a smile might make things better strategically). Nonetheless, happiness was in fact greatest when the experimenter was present, suggesting that children were adhering to social display rules to remain cheery in the face of adversity.

The waiting task with the mothers present was the same across these years, and involved at least some possibility of social interaction, which could make the wait easier—rendering happiness more justifiable as a social attractant. Expressions of happiness unexpectedly also increased from age 4 to 5 in the child-alone difficult toy task, possibly due to a change in the task that the children (erroneously) considered advantageous; however, it was still the task in which the least happiness was seen.

In sum, these preschoolers' emotions did change with age, but for all three emotions social context (especially including whether one had mother's support), and to some extent the nature of the frustrating task, also mattered. These findings remind us that developmental change in emotional expressiveness during preschool is not a unilateral issue—even this early in life, the elicitation of emotion differs depending on the parameters of the situation—whether the child is alone, with a parent, or with a relative stranger is integral to whether and how emotion is elicited, and at what intensity. Moreover, situations themselves differ in their efficacy to elicit different emotions. We should remember these tenets when evaluating preschoolers' emotional lives.

## Other Developments in Emotional Expressiveness of Basic Emotions

Along with age change in the expression of emotion, expression of some emotions also becomes more frequent than the expression of others. In peer settings, for example, happiness, and anger are expressed more often than either sadness or pain and distress (Denham, 1986, 1996a, 1996b; Denham, Bassett, Thayer, et al., 2012; Denham, Blair, DeMulder, et al., 2003; Denham & Burton, 1996; Denham & Grout, 1993; Fabes, Eisenberg, Nyman, & Michealieu, 1991; Prosen & Smrtnik Vitulić, 2018). As already noted, these "hot emotions" fill important communicative functions. Blended emotions also appear (Cole, 1985; Izard, 1991). For example, boys engaging in rough-and-tumble play can show clear signs of both happiness and anger at the same time. Blended emotions can confound adults, who ask themselves whether children in that situation, for example, need assistance or are merely having fun.

Gender differences in the expression of emotion have been noted during this period among preschoolers. These gender differences usually parallel differences in problematic emotions reported for boys and girls at later ages. For example, Fabes et al. (1991) reported that preschool boys expressed more anger than girls during peer interactions. Barry and Kochanska (2010) also found boys showing more anger with parents compared with girls, although this difference decreased across the preschool period. In contrast, girls expressed more sadness (see also Malatesta-Magai et al., 1994).

Expression of happiness also may depend on gender at times, especially in varying contexts. For example, Chaplin et al. (2017) found that girls showed more happiness in the "impossible" tasks, suggesting the socialization of girls to be polite and to make an effort to relieve social tension. Compiling dozens of works of research to summarize gender differences in emotional expressiveness, Chaplin and Aldao's (2013) meta-analysis had the following overall conclusions: (1) no gender differences in positive emotions were found during the preschool period (Chaplin et al.'s 2017 results may have been restricted to similar specific contexts); (2) girls showed more "internalizing" emotions (e.g., sadness, anxiety, and sympathy; see also Chaplin, Cole, & Zahn-Waxler, 2005); and (3) as studies already noted agreed, boys showed more "externalizing" emotions (e.g., anger). Thus, across many studies, gendered differences in the expression of basic emotions were found.

## SUMMARY: Basic Emotions' Change over Time

Overall emotion expression does not necessarily diminish over time early in the preschool period; rather, it is transformed, becoming more flexible, complex, and differentiated (Malatesta et al., 1989; Malatesta-Magai et al., 1994). The subtlety and complexity of emotional expression continue to increase markedly throughout the preschool years. The increased ability to think and solve problems supports these systematic changes in the breadth and complexity of preschoolers' emotionality (Barrett & Campos, 1991). The number and variety of interactions that the child can appreciate as significant, the variety of means by which the child can enact an action tendency, and the child's ability to modulate emotional reactions are all related to cognitive development. Preschoolers increasingly react differentially to the emotional contexts that they experience.

Regarding specific emotions, changes in positive and negative emotions during the preschool period can be tentatively interpreted as follows. The increase in positive emotions may coincide with preschoolers' experience with increasingly frequent and skillful social interaction. More specifically, positive emotion is important in the initiation and regulation of social exchanges. A child who displays more positive emotions, manifested by smiling and laughing, becomes an inviting beacon signaling "Come join me" to adults and classmates alike (see Chapter 10). Positive emotion can also render a child more open to learning (see Chapter 11).

In addition, negative emotion may decrease as brain development fuels both greater self-regulation and emotion regulation. Fortunately, then, as relieved parents and caregivers can attest, negativity decreases for most children as they advance into the preschool period. Preschoolers no doubt learn that anger doesn't always help make things better (although it can be important motivationally; Cole, Tan, et al., 2011; Ramsook et al., 2020). As I'll elaborate in Chapter 6, they increasingly have other strategies, especially communicative ones, to express their needs and meet their goals while maintaining emotional equanimity. Of note, it also is possible that emotion may be more internally experienced than externally expressed as children develop. Despite these overall generalizations about developmental change over time, the contexts in which emotions are shown, and which gender is showing them, are very important to consider.

## Individual Differences in Basic Emotions: Stability across Time

Developmental change in children's emotional expressiveness is accompanied by increasingly stable patterns of expressiveness for individual children. In other words, children tend to have distinguishable emotional styles, and these styles show stability across time. Parents and teachers talk about their children as if this were the case; they exclaim over one child's "sunny personality" and another's constant outbursts of anger over both small and large events.

Stable individual differences in enduring patterns of expressiveness are indeed apparent by 2 years of age (e.g., in irritability or negativity; see also Behrendt, Wade, Bayet, Nelson, & Enlow, 2020; Riese, 1990; Vaughn, Contreras, & Seifer, 1993, and Bornstein, Hahn, Putnick, & Pearson, 2019, for stability in overall emotionality from age 3 to 5). The work of Malatesta et al. (1989) documented the facial expressions of children's basic emotions in several contexts across the first 22 months of life. These researchers reported that "children tend to show continuity in their emotional expressive patterns across a range of discrete emotions and signals" (p. 61). In accord with Riese's (1990) data, negative emotional expressions—sadness, anger, knit brow, and pressed lips—most often showed stability from 7 to 22 months. Positive emotions were only stable from age 5 to 7 months in that study.

My colleagues and I also examined the stability of patterns of emotional expressiveness through the first 30 months of life (Denham, Lehman, et al., 1995), although our methodology differed somewhat from that of Malatesta et al. (1989) and Riese (1990). Our results indicated that emotional expressions of anger, fearfulness, interest, and joy often showed between-age stability at six measurement points between 6 weeks and 30 months; most pertinent to the age ranges covered here, anger, fear, interest, joy, and soothability showed stability from 19 to 30 months (see similar results for anger in Gaertner et al., 2008). Further, Lipscomb et al. (2012) found continuity in negative emotionality from 9 to 27 months (see also Gartstein et al., 2016, who found continuity in negative emotionality and some of its constituents from infancy to toddlerhood to early childhood).

Similar patterns of stability are seen during the preschool period. For example, Neppl et al. (2010) found stability in preschoolers' parent-rated pleasure (i.e., smiling, laughing, and positive vocalization) and anger proneness from age 2 to 3. Feng, Shaw, Skuban, and Lane (2007) observed stability in children's positivity from ages 2–3 years to 4–5 years, whereas Wu, Feng, Hooper, et al. (2019) found stability from age 3 to 4 for not only children's emotional positivity, but also for their expressions of sadness, anger, and fear. Data from LaFreniere and Sroufe (1985) extended stability findings to the later preschool years: The positive and negative expressiveness of 4- and 5-year-olds showed cross-time and cross-context stability. Negative expressiveness also was found to have moderate stability from kindergarten to second grade (Hernández et al., 2022; see also Murphy et al., 1999, for rank-order stability in negativity over a similar time span).

Covering an even broader age range from infancy to age 5, Komsi et al. (2006) found stability in anger, fear (and overall negativity), and happiness. Also infants who had been rated less happy showed more sadness at age 5. Similarly Liu et al. (2018)

found an overall stability of anger from infancy to age 6 and also isolated distinct profiles of children's emotions, which showed some rank-order change across the preschool period. Finally examining the social/self-conscious emotions rather than the basic emotions, Bornstein et al. (2019) found stability in children's shyness from age 3 to 5 (see also Armer, 2004, and Spere & Evans, 2009, for parallel findings from preschool to primary school).

Hence, clear individual differences in infants', toddlers', and preschoolers' expressive patterns can be identified, with several emotions showing significant cross-time stability over several assessments through the infant–preschool age span. What explanations can be put forward for such stability—for the emergence of such emotional styles? Expressive patterns, though flexible, can become relatively ingrained, stable components of personality (Malatesta et al., 1989; see also Tomkins, 1962, 1963, 1991; and Shiner & Caspi, 2003). Certain children are aroused particularly easily or aroused by certain stimuli through genetic pathways. Malatesta and colleagues (1989) argued that negative expressive patterns might become habitual more readily than positive patterns do, and moderate heritability of negative emotionality has been established (Goldsmith, Buss, & Lemery, 1997; Schmitz et al., 1997; Singh & Waldman, 2010).

Despite the statistically significant stability of these individual differences in emotional expressions, however, it is important to note that stability coefficients often are relatively low and are lower than those for mothers (Bornstein et al., 2019; Malatesta et al., 1989). Thus it is important not to overinterpret these emotional "styles." Young children's emotions can sometimes remain mercurial, changing across time and context. Thus, although young children's expressive styles may be partially biologically based and relatively temporally stable, they also are subject to effects of enculturation, learning, and context—in short, the development of cognition and emotion socialization.[2]

Regarding the contributions of cognition, I already have emphasized that children acquire ways of construing the events in their world, creating schemas for interpreting potentially emotional events and using these emotion schemas as foundations for ways of interacting with the world in both social and nonsocial ways. This process of emotion-schema creation promotes later stable patterns of expressiveness (Bornstein et al., 2019; Izard, 2007). For example, Carrie has come to construe a lack of response to her rather frequent entreaties to get her own way as "on purpose," whether the response is initiated by parents, teachers, or playmates. And this emotion schema has resulted in a stable pattern, known to all near her, of high-intensity anger expressiveness.

Regarding the contribution of socialization, different patterns of expressiveness "pull for" different reactions from adults and peers alike. Further, others' differing

[2] In emphasizing this view, I do not dismiss the bioevolutionary origin of emotional expressiveness, nor do I overlook the biological bases of emotional expressiveness, as will be noted in this chapter. But my background as an applied developmental psychologist drives me to look for practical ways of understanding the phenomena of development. At this point we cannot change a child's inheritance or in many cases change his or her physiology. In contrast, the functional viewpoint, with its emphasis on events in the child's life and on the child's goals and action tendencies, bolsters our understanding of toddlers' and preschoolers' lives in relation to others and suggests points of entry for change. Cognition and socialization offer entry points to maximize preschoolers' emotional competence.

perceptions of children with differing emotional profiles may trigger responses from them that maintain the child's emotional style. If Carrie's angry emotional style does result in her getting her way, her response magnifies its stability even more. Or if she is met with her parents' answering anger, she may learn from them a template for conveying anger even more convincingly, and that it is okay to do.

Also, behavior genetic studies don't only inform us about the biological foundations of behavior. They actually add to the evidence for the power that socialization responses, as well as other environmental conditions, have on children's emotional styles. For example, there are both moderate shared and nonshared environmental influences for stable negative emotionality. Positive emotionality is mostly backed by shared environmental influences (Goldsmith, Buss, & Lemery, 1997). Regarding shared environments, it is easy to imagine how the similarities in treatment by families or extrafamilial groups (e.g., siblings, other relatives, peers, and teachers) could contribute to twins' positive and negative emotional styles (see Chapters 7 and 8). Living in circumstances of frequent interparental anger would form a template for negativity for both twins.

For negative emotionality, important nonshared environmental influences might include differences in parents' treatment of siblings, birth order, illness, specific parent–child interaction patterns, and exposure to different extrafamilial interactions. For example, perhaps one root for Sebi's typical sad expression springs from the attention his baby sister gets—and which he no longer enjoys.

Thus, biology, cognitive development, and emotion socialization contribute to the stabilization of emotional styles. The culture in which a child lives also shapes his or her emotional expressiveness.

## Culture and Preschoolers' Expression of Basic Emotions

It also is important to consider how children in different cultures express emotions. The important question here is "What does expressing [a particular] emotion *mean* in this culture?" If the emotion is considered acceptable, then it may be encouraged by parents and others in the child's environment; if it is seen as unacceptable, attempts will be made to discourage its growth and development (Rubin, Coplan, & Bowker, 2009).

Thus all emotions are socialized in accord with cultural rules and expectations, even though there may be temperamental differences among children from differing cultures. In several studies of smiling, for example, East Asian infants show few differences from American infants, but show fewer negative expressions, with longer latencies to such expressions, and Chinese infants differ from both groups (Camras et al., 1998).

Over and above these very early, and likely biologically based, temperamental differences, the meaning and value of emotions, as well as how one responds to them, differ across cultures, because of the cultural rules imparted by adults. Thus, there are likely to be differences in how children in different cultures experience and express positive and negative emotions, given specific display rules, as well as temperament. Children living in collectivistic/relational cultures may learn to minimize emotional expressions that are intense or negative to preserve social harmony by being emotionally calm and balanced. In contrast, in more individualistic cultures, such expressions are more accepted because they promote autonomy and independence and the goal of maximizing happiness. Positive emotions also may be activated in different sorts of situations as well—when in harmony with others, or conversely, when asserting one's preferences, in collectivistic and individualistic cultures, respectively.

To illustrate, in terms of negative emotions, toddlers from collectivistic cultures were rated as showing fewer negative emotions (including discomfort, fear, and soothability (Desmarais et al., 2021). Further, when Chinese and American 3-year-olds experienced both resistance to temptation ("please don't touch this robot toy") and mishap (broken doll) tasks, American children were more quickly expressive of more intense happiness and sadness. In the resistance to temptation task, the Chinese children's anger, was slower to show, quicker to disappear, and milder than that of the American children, as might be expected (Wang & Barrett, 2015). However, there was an intriguing finding: Chinese children's anger decreased in latency (i.e., it was expressed more quickly) across the entire laboratory visit. This finding suggested that their attempts to suppress anger became more difficult over time, even though their last laboratory experience was one of free play. Their cultural edicts emphasizing equanimity apparently were overrun by the accumulation of frustration inherent in the situational context. Finally the Chinese children were specifically quickly angry after having felt they broke the doll, rather than being denied access to the robot. Concern (and possibly shame?) over not taking care of the doll—compared with being limited by the authority figure's explicit rules regarding the robot—may have motivated this anger; perhaps it was self-directed.

Additionally, when older preschoolers from three cultures (American, Japanese, and Chinese) were given an undesired gift (Ip et al., 2021), American children also were both more positively and negatively expressive than the Japanese children, and more negatively expressive than the Chinese children (see also Louie, Wang, Fung, & Lau, 2015, who compared Korean, Asian American, and European American 4-year-olds' emotions in response to negative and positive laboratory tasks). The Asian children were less expressive and were likely to preserve interpersonal harmony. To conclude, cultural rules strongly affect young children's emotional response to varying situations, but at times the situation "takes over," as shown in Wang and Barrett (2015), and dampens the standard cultural response.

## SUMMARY: Stability and Change in Basic Emotions

Why are these developments in expressiveness important? Adults can find it useful to recognize these developments in discerning what stays the same and what changes across this age span, both for children in general or for a particular child (e.g., Bornstein et al., 2019). It is worthwhile to pinpoint individual differences in the development of expressiveness; differing patterns of emotionality contribute to a child's relative ability to get along with others and become involved productively in the world. Knowing about specific preschoolers' personal styles and the increasing sophistication of their emotional worlds can also help adults to live with them more peacefully and fruitfully.

In sum, caregivers, parents, and early childhood educators are better informed when they know both what changes and what can stay the same in preschoolers' expressive patterns, as well as how preschoolers' increasingly sophisticated cognition affects their emotionality. They also need to consider their own contributions to preschoolers' emotionality via the emotion socialization environments that children experience, and their culture's rules regarding emotional expressiveness. Such information helps them cope well with the strengths and weaknesses of individuals and groups in this important area. Now that I have discussed basic emotion expressiveness, I turn to a social emotion, empathy.

## A SOCIAL EMOTION: EMPATHY

Empathy, or the ability to feel the emotions of another, is thought to motivate caring and concerned actions toward other persons in need. It is a social, not a predominantly a self-conscious, emotion, although it can augment, or be augmented by, the self-conscious emotion of guilt (Mascolo & Fischer, 2007; see below), and it may be influenced by older preschoolers' sense of self.

There historically has been much debate regarding the precise definition of empathy, the ways to measure it, and its likely correlates, especially in children (e.g., Lennon & Eisenberg, 1987b). A functionalist analysis of emotion could be useful in disentangling the issues raised. First, what kind of emotional arousal occurs when a child sees another person in distress? How can we distinguish children's empathy, and know it when we see it? Second, what action tendencies are associated with empathy? Third, what are the likely goals of the child experiencing empathy?

Guided by these functionalist questions, researchers have made a useful distinction between two types of empathic responses: sympathetic reactions to another person's distress and personal distress reactions (Batson, 1991; Eisenberg, Schaller, et al., 1988). Sympathy includes feelings of sorrow or concern for the other, whereas personal distress is a self-focused, emotionally aversive reaction (Eisenberg & Eggum, 2009). The facial muscle and physiological indices of these two patterns differ. Sympathetic expressions include knit brows, slightly open mouth, and heart rate deceleration (suggestive of concentration). In contrast, distress expressions are indexed by indrawn, raised brows, licking of the lips, or touching of the face, and heart rate acceleration (also often found in fear). Children who experience sympathy are likely to behave prosocially, another part of empathic concern (e.g., Edwards et al., 2015), but those who experience personal distress more often show behaviors aimed at alleviating that feeling than at helping. So, both sympathy and personal distress are components of empathy: Another's distress has aroused the child's vicarious emotion and associated action tendencies. But the child's construal of his or her own goals is central to the distinction. A focus on the other leads to a sympathetic reaction, and a focus on one's own predicament (or possible predicament) leads to a personal distress reaction. Empathy, then, has both emotional and cognitive components.

Both social-psychological and behavioral-genetic studies lend credence to the differentiation of these two types of empathic emotional responses. It is likely, then, that the observable differences between the two types of empathic response arise from differing patterns of physiological arousal, as well as from cognitive aspects of focusing on the self or on the other. Hence, children's empathic reactions are sometimes predominantly sympathetic, whereas at other times they are more indicative of personal distress. Both developmental and individual differences in these aspects of empathy are evident.

Empathy's affective and cognitive components both are very important—children experiencing empathy feel sympathetic concern or personal distress, but also often need to *know why* the other person is feeling bad and *understand* the other person's perspective, suggesting strong cognitive involvement. Often empathy is considered to include a behavioral component as well (corresponding to emotional action tendencies), which may be a prosocial response if sympathetic concern is experienced (Vaish, Carpenter, & Tomasello, 2009), or distancing if personal distress is in ascendance (Eisenberg, Schaller, et al., 1988). I will examine each of these components in what follows.

Thus preschool-age children can feel empathy; they can show it with their expressions, their words, and their actions, and empathy can encompass both feelings of sympathy and personal distress. Unfortunately, some researchers use the terminology representing this construct rather loosely. In the following sections, within this and subsequent chapters, when I can, I choose the appropriate terminology for the research presented. When researchers clearly make note of the distinction, I use the terms *sympathy* (the affective and cognitive of reacting with care toward another person's emotional difficulty) or *personal distress* (feeling aroused and upset at another person's distress, and perhaps interpreting the other's difficulty as a threat to the self). If this distinction is specifically not made (i.e., both sympathy and personal distress are included together as one entity), I use the term *empathy*. At times, as noted by Vaish (2019), researchers include prosocial behaviors that often accompany evidence of sympathy within operational definitions, and at other times they include information gathering (questioning indicating a behavioral aspect of cognitive empathy). When either of these behaviors (i.e., empathy's action tendencies) are prominent in a study's operational definitions, I use the term *empathic concern*, following the author if possible. Finally, I also use the term *empathy* when I mean the overall emotion undistinguished by any of these considerations.

Given these caveats, this social emotion deserves a more complete description. In an example of emotion, cognition, and behaviors emanating from sympathy (i.e., empathic concern), a mother and her 4-year-old child are conversing:

MOTHER: I'm kind of feeling sad.

AMY: (*facial features sobering, with furrowed brow*) What happened? Don't feel sad. I'm your friend (*patting her mother, wiping her tears away, and hugging her*). Don't cry.

Amy's facial features showed sympathy as the emotional component of empathy. Moreover, she demonstrated the cognitive aspect of empathy via her information gathering about what brought on her mother's distress. The prosocial behaviors she showed can emanate from a visceral understanding of the mother's plight and from the experience of sympathy. When does such empathy (in all its components—emotional, cognitive, and behavioral) begin, and how does it change over the course of development? How do children differ from one another in their propensity to express aspects of empathy?

## Developmental Change in Preschoolers' Empathy

### *Very Early Empathy*

In terms of the developmental progression of empathy, children as young as 2 years of age, and even younger, can (1) broadly interpret others' emotional states, (2) experience these feeling states in response to others' predicament, and (3) either attempt to alleviate discomfort in others or manage their own discomfort. Thus they may show anxious/worried and/or concerned *behaviors* in response to another's predicament, including freezing (not moving) and just looking, as well as early, sometimes clumsy, attempts at active aid (Zahn-Waxler & Radke-Yarrow, 1982, 1990).

Zahn-Waxler and colleagues' work beginning with and extending these early studies has been seminal in describing early manifestations of sympathy and prosocial responses, often examining toddlers' and even infants' emotional and behavioral reactions to the simulated distress of others. This research program has uncovered much information, and I review it here. Specifically, an early expansion of the prior work showed that empathic concern to others' simulated distress increased from 14 to 20 months, with girls often scoring higher than boys (Zahn-Waxler, Robinson, & Emde, 1992).

Next an ambitious twin study shed even more light on the very early manifestations of empathy (Zahn-Waxler, Schiro, Robinson, Emde, & Schmitz, 2001). Toddlers were observed at 14, 20, 24, and 36 months, responding to simulated distress shown by mothers and experimenters in home and laboratory visits. Sympathetic concern, self-distress, hypothesis testing, perhaps to decide how to react emotionally, and active indifference were coded in each context. Sympathy and self-distress were indexed by facial, vocal, and gestural–postural means. As the children matured, they showed more sympathy; at the same time, girls showed more sympathy and hypothesis testing/information gathering than boys (e.g., "Owie?" "You hurt?"; however, in Davidov, Zahn-Waxler, Roth-Hanania, & Knafo, 2013, this gender difference was reversed in 19- to 26-month-old toddlers). Self-distress decreased with age and was seen more in girls. Active indifference decreased but then increased between 24 and 36 months, with boys showing it more often. Thus the emotional and cognitive aspects of empathy increased through toddlerhood, with some gender differences found.

Zahn-Waxler and colleagues recently have pushed the timetable even lower to examine the roots of empathy during earlier infancy. Specifically, Roth-Hanania, Davidov and Zahn-Waxler (2011) found that modest levels of the emotional and cognitive aspects of empathy for another in distress were already evident during the first year of life; these elements increased gradually through the second year. Expanding on this study, Davidov and colleagues (2020) corroborated these findings with even younger infants, observing their responses to distress as early as 3 months through 18 months! In their study, modest levels of concern for the distressed others were evident even at 3 and 6 months, and these responses cohered across distress situations. Further, these concerned responses and inquiry behavior were more evident in the distress episodes than in neutral episodes, and the two responses (i.e., the emotional and cognitive aspects of empathy) were correlated at all ages. Both responses increased over time to 18 months, although this increase slowed with age. These early patterns also predicted a large increase in prosocial behavior during the toddlers' second year. Thus very early indicators of empathic concern emerged.

More important, self-distress reactions were rare overall in both Roth-Hanania et al. (2011) and Davidov et al. (2020). Children who are less reactive and more behaviorally inhibited may not show as much empathic concern (including concerned expressions, hypothesis testing, and prosocial behavior), however, especially in unfamiliar contexts (Young, Fox, & Zahn-Waxler, 1999). So this area of inquiry requires more scrutiny—propensity to show personal distress when faced with others' difficulties, as well as the contribution of temperament, are somewhat understudied.

Other research groups also are investigating "baby empathy." For example, an ingenious procedure allowed infants to naturalistically react to each other's distress (Liddle, Bradley, & McGrath, 2015). In trios of 8-month-old infants facing one another while seated in strollers, occurrences of one infant's distress were met routinely with discrete gazes and with socially directed behavior (waving at the distressed baby, reaching toward or touching the baby, and vocalizations directed toward the baby) on average in 54% of peer-distress episodes. Over a third of the time, these responses resulted in successful, yet brief, calming for the distressed infant.

An enhanced view of what can constitute empathic concern supports Roth-Hanania, Davidov, & Zahn-Waxler (2011) and Davidov et al.'s (2020) endeavors to study these phenomena in infants. I believe it is important to outline how empathic responses were developmentally appropriately operationalized in these inventive investigations. In both studies, infants observed their mothers and/or an experimenter separately feign pain and distress over "hurting" themselves and/or listened to an audio rendering of a crying infant. Because the infants were much younger than those in Zahn-Waxler et al.'s (2001) study, some operationalizations of sympathy, personal distress, and indifference (as well as other aspects of empathic concern, such as prosocial responding) were a bit different than in studies with older toddlers and preschoolers. Concerned affect still included sobering, sad expressions, and furrowed brows focused on the victim. Vocal cues included sad intonations, and gestural–postural cues included body alerting, leaning in, approaching, or reaching toward the victim. Self-distress could be expressed nonvocally via bodily motions or facial expressions, as well as via whimpering or crying (which terminated the session). Inquiry behavior (i.e., information-gathering, the cognitive component of empathy) included intense looking or visual scanning (e.g., looking back and forth from the victim's injury and face), vocalizing with questioning intonations (or once children were verbal, asking questions or labeling emotions). Prosocial behavior could include offering a toy or patting the hurt person, for example. These operationalizations were similar to those used in Liddle et al. (2015).

These studies showed that infants' responses to another's distress (whether expressed by their mother, an adult experimenter, or another baby) were limited to things that an infant *can do* verbally and motorically. Given these limitations, the infants made the most of their abilities to respond with empathic concern, including early links with their prosocial responses and success in helping the distressed other.

### *Preschoolers' Empathy*

Not surprisingly given the results from Zahn-Waxler and colleagues, even the youngest preschoolers show early behavioral forms of sympathy and personal distress. One of the most ubiquitous experiences of another's distress for the preschooler is a playmate's tears. Behavioral reactions to peers' crying have been tracked extensively across the preschool age period. Phinney, Feshbach, and Farver (1986) studied 28- to 48-month-olds' responses to crying peers in 290 crying episodes. The relative frequency of positive reactions to crying peers was 2.1 per hour, with older preschoolers responding more often with empathic concern to their crying peers, than did younger children. Similarly, Kiselica and Levin (1987) observed preschoolers and found that empathic concern occurred at a rate of 1.6 indicators per hour. Two-year-olds mostly showed sustained attention to a peer's crying, with 3-year-olds in transition to more behavioral intervention. The 4- and 5-year-olds most often showed empathic concern, as evidenced by comforting their friends. Thus both facial and behavioral indicators of empathic concern increase with age across the preschool period.

Considering the time span beyond toddlerhood and the early preschool years, children's self-reports of empathy also increased in the late preschool and elementary years (Lennon & Eisenberg, 1987b). It is likely that these increases are in part driven by an increased ability to not only self-reflect, but also to become more skillful in recognizing the emotions, thoughts, and needs of others.

### *Early Childhood Empathy Development: Foundations in Social Cognition*

Social-cognitive development likely fuels changes in the expressions of sympathy/empathic concern and the control of personal distress across infancy and the preschool period. Accordingly, evidence of more sophisticated indicators of empathic concern historically has been associated with self-recognition. Children who are old enough to have attained a stable notion of the self–other distinction are more likely to show empathic concern to another's condition, compared to those who have not (Bischof-Kohler, 1988; Zahn-Waxler & Radke-Yarrow, 1990; Zahn-Waxler, Radke-Yarrow, Wagner, & Chapman, 1992).

The ability to differentiate the self and other, then, may support the modest increases across the first 3 years of life in the *frequency* of facial, vocal, and gestural–postural indicators of sympathy. Building upon this self–other differentiation, the experience and expression of empathic concern might be mapped out according to a cognitive event analysis later in early childhood: "Something has happened to someone else, and this event decreases the likelihood of good feelings for them and for me. I have vicariously experienced this event and feeling, and don't want them to continue. I'd better help the person [or leave the scene to lessen my own arousal]."

However, it also should be underscored that the more recent research involving very young infants (e.g., Davidov et al., 2013, 2020; Liddle et al., 2015; Roth-Hanania et al., 2011) challenges the *necessity* of advanced self-knowledge, specifically for sympathetic responding. A simpler, prereflective form of self-knowledge based on self-perception and self-generation of action may support infants' sympathy. This caveat to earlier assertions about whether sympathy requires self-knowledge is bolstered by empirical evidence: Indicators of sympathy increase quantitatively during and after infancy (i.e., when a stable self-knowledge develops), but, nonetheless, there is qualitative continuity in its emotional nature (Davidov et al., 2013; Volbrecht, Lemery-Chalfant, Aksan, Zahn-Waxler, & Goldsmith, 2007).

## SUMMARY: Developmental Changes in Empathy

In summary, *very* young children sometimes evidence empathic concern, which includes both emotional and cognitive components, and attempts at active aid. These findings regarding toddlers seem quite remarkable, but they are well documented in both research and in more colloquial reports. For example, a 2-year-old boy attempted to soothe his older brother's distress with a multifaceted calming campaign. The younger child looked very concerned, implored his brother to stop crying, beseeched his mother to help, adopted a mothering mode himself, tried to lend a pragmatic helping hand in putting away Lego blocks, and distracted him with a toy car. Only when these efforts failed did the 2-year-old give up on caring and kindness and adopt his mother's no-nonsense style: "Stop crying. . . . Smack your bottom!" (Dunn, 1988, pp. 94–95). Most, though obviously not all, of this 2-year-old's efforts showed empathic concern.

But despite the encouraging evidence about infant and toddler sympathy, it is important to remember that some very young children have not yet developed the capacity to experience fully this complex emotion. They may show personal distress, just ignore another person's difficulty, oblivious to their emotion, or react in an emotionally anomalous manner, neither sympathetic nor distressed:

> Alberta was hurt on the playground. Mark began to cry too although he had nothing to do with the event. Michael just looked at Alberta as she cried—maybe to see what the matter was—but he showed no emotional arousal. One day, he actually laughed when Jamila fell down. He was indifferent to others' emotions in general and especially inattentive to another person's distress.

So, although personal distress decreases as children mature after 2 years of age (and as already noted, is less frequent than expected even in infancy), it still can be evoked, particularly in fearful situations. For instance, consider the stilling of motor activity and facial signs of worry when a young preschooler is trapped with quarreling parents. To illustrate how fear can block sympathy, preschoolers expressed more fear than either sadness or concern when viewing scary films of persons in difficult circumstances (Strayer, 1993; Wilson & Cantor, 1985). This lack of sympathy was not due to an inability to recognize the televised characters' emotion; rather, their own personal distress got in the way. In more naturalistic research situations, it may make more sense to ascertain whether it is reasonable that fear could be appropriately elicited and override sympathy.

In general, then, emotional, cognitive, and behavioral indicators of empathic concern begin very early, but increase in frequency during the preschool period, and personal distress reactions decrease but can still be evoked. Despite these age trends, individual children also show distinct inclinations toward one pattern of empathy or the other.

## Individual Differences in Young Children's Empathy

Children often show a predominance of either sympathetic or personal distress expressions of empathic concern. Remarkably, as early as 3 to 6 months through 36 months, individuals' emotional concern, concomitant prosocial acts, and cognitive exploration about the distress (i.e., hypothesis testing and information gathering) cohered well across situations and sources of distress and showed some rank-order stability over time (Davidov et al., 2020; Nichols, Svetlova, & Brownell, 2009; Roth-Hanania et al., 2011; Zahn-Waxler et al., 1992). The connection between empathic concern for distressed others at both early and later ages reflects a trait-like consistency (Knafo, Zahn-Waxler, Van Hulle, Robinson, & Rhee, 2008). The very earliest demonstrations of empathic concern also predicted toddlers' later attempts to help the person in distress, illustrating the early motivational role of concern for others and the continuity of the emotional aspects of empathy.

Further, although sympathetic/empathic concern and distressed styles of reacting to others' emotions often are inversely related, this is not a necessary condition (Zahn-Waxler & Radke-Yarrow, 1990); a child can show both empathic concern and distress at the intensity of another's suffering. The 3-year-old daughter of a depressed parent may treat her crying mother very tenderly, almost assuming the role of caregiver, but may also feel quite a bit of distress herself.

Finally, these styles show some developmental trends. For example, several profiles of developing empathic concern were discerned in infants from 3 to 18 months of age (Paz et al., 2021a). They included four groups with distinct developmental trajectories of empathic concern: early-onset (starting high and increasing), low-empathy (starting low with minimal increase), rising (starting low and increasing considerably), and a very small group with a negative slope (decreasing). The groups differed in terms of social competence at 36 months.

### SUMMARY: Individual Differences in Empathy

Empathic concern and its indicators are seen to occur very early and to show contemporaneous and cross-time consistency. Thus evidence is mounting for the emergence of early individual empathic styles and their connection with prosocial behavior. More research of time periods past toddlerhood would be very useful.

## Moderators of the Experience of Empathy

So any given child may be high on both empathic concern and personal distress, may be low on both, or may show a particularly distinctive type of either sympathetic/empathic concern or personal distress. But other extenuating factors may moderate such personal styles. Several parameters of an empathy-provoking experience, as well as personal attributes, have been posited as important in determining young children's empathic responsiveness.

### *Attachment and Internal Working Models*

The interplay of cooperation and turn taking, and, above all, positive affect sharing and distress relief—all hallmarks of a secure attachment—are especially vital in the development of empathic concern (Kestenbaum, Farber, & Sroufe, 1989; Thompson, 1990). Thus it seems logical that children with secure internal working models of attachment—feeling that their needs will be met when comfort is needed—would have an advantage in responding sympathetically to others (Stern & Cassidy, 2018; Zahn-Waxler & Radke-Yarrow, 1990). In fact, this advantage could be supported not only by the scripts of caring encompassed in their internal working model, but also by children's experience of parent–child discourse about emotion (see Chapter 7), the emotional and self-regulatory capacities that secure attachment fosters (e.g., emotion knowledge, emotion regulation, and effortful control; see Chapters 4 and 6), and finally neurobiological differences (Decety & Svetlova, 2012; Stern & Cassidy, 2018).

Research with preschoolers supports these theoretical propositions. For example, several researchers have found that attachment security is related to empathic concern for a stranger or a staged "baby" crying, observations with peers, or teacher ratings (Kestenbaum et al., 1989; Mark et al., 2002; Murphy & Laible, 2013; Panfile & Liable, 2012; Ştefan & Avram, 2018; Waters, Wippman, & Sroufe, 1979). In Kestenbaum et al. (1989), groups of 4-year-olds, equally distributed across secure, anxious–avoidant, and anxious–resistant attachment statuses, were observed during play. Empathy-evoking instances in which at least one child was visibly or audibly distressed, and one or more other children were near enough to be able to witness it, or someone else responded from a distance, were examined. Every child who witnessed the display was rated on affective and behavioral information largely corresponding to empathic concern and its lack. Experience in a supportive attachment relationship contributed to these youngsters' style of empathic concern: Children who had been classified as secure during infancy scored higher on empathic concern than children with anxious–avoidant histories. Moreover, 9 of the 12 incidents in which one child actually exacerbated another's distress involved children with avoidant histories.

Early relationships are prototypes for later ones, with expectations within early relationships carried forward to new ones (Sroufe & Fleeson, 1986). The secure children in this study, then, replicated the sensitive caregiving that they themselves received in times of distress. In contrast, the children with avoidant–attachment histories did not experience emotional availability in the same way; accustomed to avoiding emotions in their early relationships, and less able to regulate their personal distress (Decety &

Svetlova, 2012), they continued to do so by not responding, or responding inappropriately, to peers' emotions.

In particular, attachment figures' co-regulation with infants over time aids in, and becomes internalized as, infants' and young children's ability to deal with negative emotions, and one could assume this propensity could generalize from one's own to others' emotions (Stern & Cassidy, 2017). Thus, in accordance with this aspect of theorizing, in both Murphy and Liable (2013) and Ştefan and Avram (2018) the relationship between security of attachment and sympathy was mediated by the ability to regulate emotions. Secure attachment relationships bolster emotion regulation, which supports sympathy.

Similarly, security of attachment may ameliorate the effects of temperament upon empathic reactions. Temperamentally shy or fearful children may be overwhelmed by others' distress. However, such children may be less likely to be overwhelmed if they are in a secure attachment relationship, enabling them to respond with empathic concern despite their tendency to overidentify with others' distress (Mark et al., 2002).

In sum, the experience of responsive caregiving and emotional attunement with a caregiver, which is supportive of secure attachment relationships and internal working models, is a positive substrate for the development of both expressions of sympathy and overall empathic concern. Especially in conjunction with other positive aspects of emotion socialization and emotional competence, these relational advantages confer the child with an opportunity to learn concern for others.

### *Similarity to the Victim and Focus of Attention*

I already have stressed that children can evidence either sympathy/empathic concern or distress reactions, or no emotional arousal, to others' distress. In fact, the probability of a given reaction may depend upon the situation in which young children find themselves. Preschoolers tend to show more empathic concern when the distressed person is like them in some way (or they are at least familiar with the other's experience; Preston & de Waal, 2002) or when they focus on the other's emotional neediness.

Seeing the person experiencing distress as like oneself can be important in motivating expressions of sympathy or personal distress. M. A. Barnett (1984) told preschoolers that they had failed or succeeded at either a puzzle board or a ball-pitch game; others were allowed merely to observe the game. After either participating in or watching the tasks, children then watched a videotaped vignette of another child failing the ball-pitch game. Thus, the similarity or dissimilarity of the subjects' experience on a familiar or unfamiliar game was varied systematically (see Table 2.1). Young children's sympathy for the unhappy age-mate in the video was enhanced when children had also lost a game, a similar unpleasant experience, and could say, "I know how you feel." In particular, children who had failed at the ball-pitch game showed more facial concern and rated their own mood as less positive when seeing another child having difficulty with the same game.

Although similarity with the other's situation generally enhances sympathy and empathic concern, the story is more complicated than this. Given the similarity of shared experience, children's locus of attention also is worth noting.

**TABLE 2.1. Amount of Sympathy Shown to Videotaped Peer**

| | Outcome experienced by child | |
|---|---|---|
| **Game played by child** | Same as protagonist | Different from protagonist |
| Same as protagonist | +++ | 0 |
| Different from protagonist | ++ | – |

*Note.* Data from M. A. Barnett (1984).

Five-year-old Jason feels strong emotions while watching his friend Andrew being spanked by his mother. Depending on the situation and his focus, he feels intense sympathy for Andrew or sees Andrew's situation as a portent of his own impending distress. If Andrew has misbehaved before Jason arrives (e.g., his mother has just discovered Play-Doh in the DVD player), Jason sees the distress Andrew is feeling, focuses on his friend's pitiful tears, and feels sympathy. In contrast, if both boys have conspired to transfer much of the sandbox's contents to the flower beds, Jason witnesses Andrew's tears, thinks that his turn for spanking is next, and experiences much personal distress.

Similarly, when children see another child in a predicament, those who have been induced to focus on that child's dilemma show more sympathy than children who are induced to consider their own sadness (Barnett, Howard, & Melton, 1982; see also Barnett, King, Howard, & Dino, 1980). So, situational factors are important to consider when viewing preschoolers' sympathy or personal distress.

### *Gender and Event Context*

The gender of the victim and the context of distress also moderate empathic concern. In at least one study, preschoolers were more likely to console crying girls and criticize crying boys (Phinney et al., 1986). Thus children behaved in accordance with gender stereotypes of emotion at a young age!

In addition, the gender of the potentially empathically concerned child may moderate expressions of this emotional stance. For example, in an examination of concern for others at 14, 20, 24, and 36 months, girls were rated by mothers and observers as more concerned when the mother "hurt" her knee and the experimenter appeared to close her finger in a test materials suitcase (Rhee et al., 2013). Girls more often were coded as helping, increasing proximity to, or asking for information of the victim. Gender socialization to "be nice" may put a motivational emphasis on nascent sympathy and broader empathic concern. However, this gender-empathic concern relationship was mediated by girls' greater language ability (see also Ornaghi, Conte, & Grazzani's [2020] findings of language contributing to children's mother-reported empathic concern—emotional contagion, attention to others' feelings, and prosocial actions—but not moderated by gender). Finally, a study of much older children corroborated this relation; Eisenberg, Fabes, Murphy, Karbon, et al. (1996) found that kindergarten and second-grade teachers also reported that girls were more sympathetic.

In terms of the context of another's distress, children were more positive and prosocial as lone observers of a crying peer, than when in interaction with others (even though they were lone observers only 19% of the time; Phinney et al., 1986). Furthermore, a friend's crying elicits more empathic concern than that of a mere acquaintance's (Costin & Jones, 1992; Farver & Branstetter, 1994). Being confronted with a lone other's or a friend's distress evokes social norms and increases one's feelings of responsibility, even at an early age. Thus issues of gender and details of the situation must not be overlooked in the attempt to understand preschoolers' empathy.

### *Emotionality and Personal Emotional Profile*

Empathy is only one of many emotions experienced by young children; it makes sense to examine how the full constellation of emotions works in concert when considering preschoolers' empathy. Children need to be emotionally secure (as noted regarding attachment status) and to have experience with emotions themselves to show empathic concern for others (Denham, 1986; Strayer, 1980). Thus children's own emotional expressiveness also moderates empathic concern shown to others' emotions.

First, feeling generally positive emotions oneself makes it easier to focus on others' emotions. Along these lines, children with more positive temperaments and more positive peer interactions are more likely to exhibit empathic concern to a crying peer (e.g., comforting, mediating; Farver & Branstetter, 1994). Preschoolers who are more often happy show more empathic concern to the negative affect of their peers (Eisenberg, Fabes, Murphy, Karbon, et al., 1996). Even infants who showed positive affect while playing peekaboo or watching a puppet show at 12 months showed more of the helping and hypothesis testing aspects of empathic concern at 19 to 25 months (Volbrecht et al., 2007). Lennon and Eisenberg (1987b) went one step further: They demonstrated that preschoolers' happy displays evidenced *during* prosocial behaviors are related to the frequency of their unrequested prosocial behavior. Therefore, not only does feeling happier most of the time promote empathic concern; even more pointedly, so does feeling good when prosocial behavior is called for.

Second, several theories of empathy and sympathy also predict that negative affect, rendering the child more self-focused, hampers the ability to respond prosocially, a component of empathic concern (Eisenberg, 1986). I have found just such a pattern: Preschoolers who were observed as generally angrier or sadder show less empathic concern in response to peers' distress than do those who were more often happy (Denham, 1986; see also Strayer, 1993). Fearful toddler girls also showed less empathic concern to a stranger in another study (Mark, IJzendoorn, & Bakermans-Kranenburg, 2002). In addition, Eisenberg, Fabes, Murphy, Karbon, et al. (1996) also found that higher negative emotionality was related to less evidence of sympathy in kindergarten and second graders, especially among boys.

However, other research findings examining negative emotion and empathic concern are more complicated. In one study, adult ratings of 30- to 42-months-olds' dispositional sadness and empathic concern (including both facial concern and hypothesis testing) showed complex bidirectional relations across time (Edwards et al., 2015). These authors reasoned that perhaps proneness to their own sadness might, over time, promote children's understanding of another's sadness, activating their perspective taking and thus their experience and enactment of empathic concern. At the same time, by experiencing such empathic concern and becoming more aware of others' sadness, preschoolers also may become more aware of their own sadness and express it more themselves.

It is interesting that these results contradict the original theory that sadness and empathy should be negatively related as well as observations of preschoolers in which sadness and reactions to others' emotions were simultaneously coded (e.g., Denham, 1986). Further, in Edwards et al. (2015) sadness was rated by mothers and caregivers, rather than observed. Together, considerations of emotions *while interacting with others* and more cross-time and cross-context ratings of emotions might be telling two sides of the same story. Showing and experiencing sadness during social situations may make it hard to respond with empathic concern, but in more emotional children, *overall* sadness may contribute to observed sympathy over time, in the ways suggested by Edwards et al. (2015).

Overall emotionality similarly may allow young children to recognize others' feelings and thus to empathize with them. Children exhibiting higher overall emotionality, measured in the number of displays per minute, are more likely to show empathic concern in response to peers' emotions. They more often help, share, and/or comfort in response to peers' negative emotions (as well as matching peers' happy displays, reinforcing peers' emotions, or leaving the area of angry displays; Denham, 1986).

Thus experiencing a variety of mostly positive, moderate-intensity emotions should facilitate empathic concern reactions to others' emotions (Hoffman, 1984; Strayer, 1980). The role of sadness also could be important. Finally, an ability to regulate their emotions could assist children in focusing on the other's needs and showing empathic concern (Ornaghi, Conte, et al., 2020). In short, as noted by Decety and Svetlova (2012), " . . . children are most likely to experience empathy and concern if they are prone to at least moderate levels of affective arousal combined with adaptive emotional regulation" (p. 16).

> Midori and Benji are both in the house corner when Carrie stumbles over the doll cradle and begins to cry loudly, holding her arm and shoulder and wailing, "I hurt myself!!" Midori, who experiences emotions quickly and changeably, looks upset herself and edges away into the block area, where she smiles at Colin (who pretty much ignores her). But Benji, who also is emotionally aroused, is more skilled at focusing on someone else's distress after quickly calming his own. He crouches down and pats Carrie as she calms down. Brave boy!

### *Emotion Knowledge*

Understanding the emotions that are being displayed by others is an important substrate for responding empathically (Eisenberg, Spinrad, & Morris, 2014; see also Davidov et al., 2013; Paz et al., 2021a; Tan, Volling, Gonzalez, LaBounty, & Rosenberg, 2022). In fact, an inkling of emotional perspective taking supporting empathic responding may even exist in toddlerhood (Vaish et al., 2009); 18- and 25-month-old toddlers reacted with sympathetic concern and subsequent prosocial behavior even when a victim showed no emotion. Knowing how *most people* would feel may support empathic concern. Given the early emergence of empathy and its change across early development, a consideration of such emotional perspective taking as a possible foundation and outcome is useful.

Certainly, knowing whether another child is in pain, sad, angry, disgusted, or even contemptuous makes a big difference in how one responds. I have shown that children with higher-level emotion knowledge are less apt to merely ignore their parents' emotions. Children who are more capable of explaining emotions in conversations with parents also showed more empathic concern in response to peers' emotions; they helped more and ignored less when their peers were distressed (Denham, Renwick-DeBardi, & Hewes, 1994). Finally, understanding emotions contributed to aspects of children's empathic concern, such as acknowledging that aid was needed and offering verbal or behavioral assistance or comfort in structured situations with an adult who showed sadness or pain (Denham, 1986; Denham & Couchoud, 1991).

More recent work has somewhat qualified such findings in a potentially important way. Emotion knowledge of 44-month-olds in one study (Knafo et al., 2009) interacted with mother-rated emotional symptoms in predicting empathic concern. That is, knowledge about emotions was associated with greater sympathy toward the experimenter's feigned pain for children low in mother-rated emotional internalizing symptoms of worry, fear, sadness, and nervousness. Children high in emotional symptoms showed the opposite pattern—their emotion knowledge predicted less evidence of empathic concern. The authors considered the reported emotional symptoms to reflect emotion regulation difficulties. Thus well-regulated children may show more empathic concern when they understand another's negative emotions. In contrast, clearly understanding another person's distress could lead already dysregulated children to become even more anxious and self-focused (i.e., to feel personal distress), showing less empathic concern. The relative lack of children with such internalizing problems in earlier work may have masked this difference. Such nuances based on temperamental/behavior problem differences should be examined in more detail.

Thus emotion knowledge generally (but not always!) supports the demonstration of empathic concern. It also could be that emerging empathic concern supports growth in emotion knowledge, offering evidence of bidirectional effects. Recall that Paz et al. (2021a) found several trajectories of empathic concern's development from 3 to 18 months. These profiles of change were differentially related to the children's later emotion knowledge. The groups of children conforming to the early-onset and rising empathic concern trajectories were most proficient in later emotion knowledge, and both groups performed better than children on the low-empathy trajectory. Responding with empathic concern to another person exposes the child to emotions "close up," giving them the opportunity to learn more about emotions in general. Overall, then, the connection between understanding emotions and empathic concern appears important.

### *Culture and Empathy*

As with other emotions, cultural differences in when and how empathic concern is displayed need to be considered. In two studies, Trommsdorff (2013) and Trommsdorff,

Friedlmeier, and Mayer (2007) investigated how young children from individualistic and more collectivistic/relational cultures responded to the distress of an adult companion who evidenced clear distress over a popped balloon. Comparing and contrasting Japanese and German 5-year-old girls, sympathy (i.e., facial, vocal, and postural) was related to prosocial responding in both groups. However, the Japanese girls showed more distress, which Trommsdorff considered rather culturally appropriate given their probable lack of exposure to this adult emotion in their everyday lives. Moreover, their moderate distress was associated with prosocial responding, whereas for the German girls, prosocial behavior showed a linear decrease as the distress increased.

Trommsdorff et al.'s earlier study (2007) had used the same balloon paradigm to observe children's empathic and distressed reactions, but included 5-year-old boys and observed them from two individualistic cultures (Germany and Israel) and two South-Asian cultures (Indonesia and Malaysia). Again, sympathy and prosocial responding were positively related across cultures. But again, the children from Asian cultures displayed more self-focused distress, and in these comparisons, they also showed less-frequent prosocial behavior (in the 2013 study, this difference was in the same direction but not significant). Further, sympathy was less predictive of prosocial behavior for the East Asian children.

Sympathy did not differ in frequency across cultures in either study, and it was very infrequent at that; Trommsdorff et al. (2007) speculated that the situation of the adult victim made children feel uneasy and was not easy for them to handle. They caution that their findings may need to be replicated with a more ecologically valid condition. For example, in Denham, Mason, and Couchoud (1995), experimenters had spent over 6 hours in the classroom with each child before simulating pain, anger, and sadness during play sessions; sympathy was not measured, but children rather readily reacted prosocially to these simulations, suggesting that more ecologically valid conditions could yield profitable results.

### SUMMARY: Moderators of Empathic Concern—Attachment, Similarity to Victim, Gender, General Context, Emotionality, Emotion Knowledge, and Culture

Clearly many aspects of children's lives and ecological conditions moderate their potential expression of empathic concern. It behooves researchers and concerned adults to consider these factors when making judgments about young children's abilities.

## Biological Bases of Empathy

Given the personal and contextual moderators of preschoolers' display of empathic concern, it is important to consider empathy's even more fundamental foundations, including its biological bases. The first type of biological basis for sympathy is genetic. Regarding heritability, studies of twins have provided much support for the genetic foundations of both emotional and cognitive aspects of empathy. For example, a genetic component was found for the tendency to react either with empathic concern or with distress to others' suffering (Zahn-Waxler, Robinson, et al., 1992; Zahn-Waxler et al., 2001; see also Volbrecht et al., 2007).

More specifically, these researchers found that identical twin toddlers (14- to 25-months old across the three studies) were more similar in empathic style, whether it was sympathetic or reflected personal distress, than were fraternal twins. Heritability was suggested for both facial sympathetic concern and hypothesis testing (e.g., "Are you ok"), as well unresponsive–indifferent responses to feigned distress (Zahn-Waxler et al., 2001). This early heritability contributed to cross-time stability in these aspects of empathy, and by 20 months additional variance was explained by the twins' common environment. Mothers also reported on twins' responses to *each other's* distress, and again both genetic and common environment effects were found. Another study examining aspects of empathy in 19- to 25-month-old toddlers showed not only substantial shared environmental influences on an empathic concern composite of helping and concern, but also nonshared environmental influences. Further, nonshared environmental effects, along with heritability, influenced the hypothesis testing aspect of cognitive empathy (Volbrecht et al., 2007). Thus genetics and environment both contribute to emotional and cognitive empathy during toddlerhood.

Following upon and extending these findings with older toddlers and preschoolers, Knafo et al. (2008, 2009) found that heritability of sympathetic responding, hypothesis testing, and prosocial behavior increased with age from 24 to 36 months and continued to be present at 44 months—in fact, up to one-third to one-half of variation in these aspects of empathy and empathy-related behavior were heritable. By 44 months the nonshared environment and error accounted for the rest of variance in empathic responding. Thus the contribution of shared environment found to be important from 19 to 25 months (Volbrecht et al., 2007; Zahn-Waxler et al., 2001) had waned at 44 months. Perhaps the effect of socialization and of other shared environmental conditions and events was consolidated early, but the differential conditions of nonshared environmental conditions were still important. Finally, hypothesis testing and sympathetic reactions were moderately correlated in the older preschoolers (Knafo et al., 2009) mainly via genetic effects, confirming the theoretical connection between emotional and cognitive empathy.

Even a recent study involving twin adults confirms similar findings (Melchers, Montag, Reuter, Spinath, & Hahn, 2016); heritability accounted for over one-half of the variance in emotional and behavioral empathy, whereas heritability was less for cognitive empathy, with another important contribution made by the nonshared environment.

So early empathy has a moderate genetic foundation, which persists through adulthood. At the same time, behavioral genetics emphasizes the need to examine the environmental influences—both those shared by twins and unique to the individual child.

Another important biological basis for empathic responsiveness is brain based and neurodevelopmental. First, differences in heritability of the emotional and cognitive aspects of empathy are not surprising, because they may involve partially nonoverlapping brain regions. Brain systems relevant to the more emotional aspects of empathy, the limbic and paralimbic systems (e.g., inferior frontal gyrus, anterior insula, anterior cingulate cortex), develop earlier than those relevant to the cognitive aspect of empathy (e.g., ventromedial prefrontal and tempoparietal cortices). As Decety and Jackson (2006) note, "bottom-up" processing of the emotional empathy system by lower-level brain structures may facilitate feeling the other's emotions. Also prominent in this "bottom-up" path to empathic concern rather than personal distress are areas of the brain responsible for the self–other distinction (e.g., the right temporal-parietal junction, posterior cingulate, and precuneus, Decety & Jackson, 2006).

Although very early empathic concern exists, other aspects of emotional competence and social cognition come online with development, facilitated by development in certain areas of the brain. Two points that I have already made need to be considered. First, emotion regulation is necessary in more skilled demonstration of empathy, so that one is not flooded with personal distress. Second, there is a need for perspective taking, a central aspect of cognitive empathy, to aid in understanding the viewpoint of the distressed person. In terms of brain development, these abilities require the prefrontal cortex to come into the picture (i.e., "top-down" processing). Thus parts of the brain that contribute to self-regulation need to be activated, including areas of the frontal and parietal lobes (i.e., frontopolar cortex, ventromedial prefrontal cortex, medial prefrontal cortex, and the right inferior parietal lobe; Decety & Jackson, 2006). The ability to *understand* the other's feeling and thinking requires more "top-down" processing from higher-level brain structures.

Recent evidence confirms that there are, in fact, two such separate brain systems for emotional and cognitive empathy, although of course every empathic response may involve both emotional and cognitive aspects, depending on social context (Shamay-Tsoory, 2011). This neurodevelopmental difference could explain any divergence in developmental time lines for emotional and cognitive empathy; the cognitive aspects of empathy develop later than its affective aspects, as do the parallel brain structures. However, this assertion needs further study and clarification because Davidov et al. (2020) found a form of hypothesis testing as early as 3 to 6 months.

Another intriguing suggestion, that "mirror neurons" form a neural basis for connecting our own and others' experiences, also requires examination of both the theory and the actual results from fMRI reports. The theory suggests that viewing another's emotions activates one's own associations with that state, allowing one to react as if the emotions were one's own (McDonald & Messinger, 2011; Preston & de Waal, 2002). The road to empathic concern from mirror neurons is complex; the insular cortex connects mirror neurons in the premotor system to parts of the limbic system (e.g., the anterior insula and anterior cingulate cortex) that process the emotional aspects of the empathy-inducing occurrence (i.e., the "bottom-up" processing). The possibility of mirror neurons highlights that, although interest in the neural mechanisms involved in empathy has increased and many allied brain structures have been identified, there is still much research needed in this area.

Finally, physiological systems form another biological support for the demonstration of empathic concern. Likely physiological constituents supporting sympathy or, conversely, personal distress are as follows: (1) parasympathetic activity, exemplified by respiratory sinus arrhythmia (RSA; a measure reflecting both physiological and attentional regulation), also known as vagal tone, for the calming and focusing that could facilitate sympathy; and (2) sympathetic nervous system activity, exemplified by skin conductance, indexing heightening personal distress.

In an early look at these physiological correlates of kindergartners' and second graders' empathy (Eisenberg, Fabes, Murphy, Karbon, et al., 1996), sympathy was associated with boys' lower levels of negative emotionality, indexed by increased skin conductance following a distress stimulus. Boys' vagal tone was positively related (and their heart rates negatively related) to their self-reported sympathy. These physiological findings for boys are consistent with the view that children who are prone to negative emotionality, including personal distress, are relatively unlikely to experience sympathy, but that nervous system regulation supports sympathetic responding.

Thus parasympathetic nervous system activity played a big role in these findings. Later research supported and extended this earlier work (Taylor et al., 2015). For example, children with higher RSA under resting conditions at 42 months were later rated as higher in sympathy at 72 to 84 months (as rated by parents and teachers) via their 54 months of attention focusing, attention shifting, and inhibitory control (also rated by parents and teachers). Children's resting parasympathetic nervous system activity predicted later self-regulation, which then predicted sympathy. In this study, the coaction of both physiological and neurodevelopmental systems over time can be seen. Both work together to promote children's sympathy.

### SUMMARY: Biological Bases for Empathy

There are strong biological bases for empathy. These range from genetic, to neurodevelopmental (including potentially both brain development and more specifically mirror neurons), to psychophysiological supports, including both parasympathetic activity, involving the vagus nerve and sympathetic activity, involving skin conductance. Knowing more about these bases can further the understanding of how empathy develops.

### SUMMARY: Empathy

Empathic concern for the distress of others increases across the preschool period but appears very early in infancy. Personal distress does not disappear as children become capable of sympathy. Both facial and behavioral indices of sympathy (i.e., empathic concern) appear, and are moderated by such factors as attachment, gender, self-focus, context of the other's distress, similarity to the distressed person, and familiarity with the distressing experience. Other elements of the child's emotional expressiveness, as well as an understanding of emotions, figure importantly in empathic responsiveness, and its biological roots—genetic, neurodevelopmental, and physiological—are deep.

## CONCLUSION

Much change in emotional expressiveness occurs during the toddler-to-preschool period. Personal styles of emotional expressiveness become established, and children gain flexibility in using their expression of basic emotions strategically (e.g., using vocal and facial channels differentially). In addition to a facility with expression of basic emotions, preschoolers (and even younger children) show signs that they experience and express empathy.[3] In short, children entering kindergarten are becoming masterful in expressing emotions as goal-directed behaviors and as social signals.

> Chelsea's usual sunny demeanor draws classmates to her, and their play is full of smiles and laughter.
>
> Byron's mixture of facial disgust and goofy happiness, along with a tinge of anger in his voice, gets his message across: "I think you are weird to reject me from your play, guys. I am unfazed—but don't cross me in the future." He is showing blended emotions.

Preschoolers' increasingly multifaceted emotional expressiveness often makes interaction with them clearer and more satisfying but can also make dealing with them more complicated—compared to earlier ages, there is more going on emotionally that needs to be understood. Realizing the nature of this complexity can allow adults, and playmates for that matter, to have more satisfying interactions with children.

---

[3]They also begin to experience and express the social emotions, and purposefully modulate emotional expression, as will be covered in the next chapter.

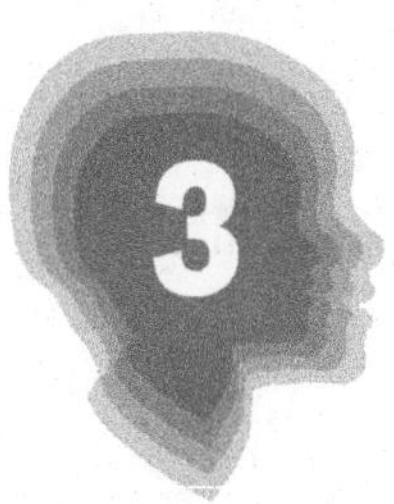

# Emotional Expressiveness

## SOCIAL EMOTIONS AND VOLUNTARY EMOTIONAL CONTROL

### INTRODUCTION

After the advent of the basic emotions and empathy, and the consolidation of emotional styles, the next major development in emotional expressiveness is the acquisition of self-conscious emotions, such as pride, guilt, embarrassment, shyness, and shame. In this chapter, I consider the developmental trends and individual differences in the expression of these emotions and differentiate among the self-conscious emotions (i.e., pride, guilt, shame, and to some extent shyness and embarrassment). Perhaps given the blossoming of the full palette of emotions—basic, social, and self-conscious—subsequent developmental change in expressiveness includes the growing ability over the preschool period to manage emotional expression voluntarily, including posing expressions, showing expressiveness according to cultural display rules and deception via hiding emotions. I address all these changes in expressive abilities in turn; they signal young children's increasing experience of a rich, complex emotional life, and herald their ability to modulate the expression of these emotions, which will be considered in detail in Chapter 6.

### THE DEVELOPING EXPERIENCE AND EXPRESSION OF SELF-CONSCIOUS EMOTIONS

Flexibility, modulation, and increased complexity in the expression of basic emotions, especially given the increasing incidence of emotion schemas, co-occur with the appearance of social and self-conscious emotions in a preschooler's expressive repertoire. I have discussed the social emotion of empathy. The self-conscious emotions include pride, guilt, shame, envy, and contempt, and, in part, shyness and embarrassment. The relatively simple patterns of understandings that usually accompany the basic emotions must be elaborated so that the child experiences these more complex emotions. Both cognitive development and specific socialization experiences allow for this elaboration.

> Joelle knows that it is not okay to break her mom's special jade horse from China and looks around furtively as she tries to force the pieces back together.
>
> Ben sees his friend Joshua wet his pants and, knowing this mishap defies an important social convention, sneers. Joshua just wants to disappear.

## Cognitive Foundations of Self-Conscious Emotions

Self-recognition and self–other differentiation that develop through the second year of life are the foundations for the experience and expression of the self-conscious emotions (Lewis, 1993a; Zahn-Waxler & Radke-Yarrow, 1990). As toddlers begin to rely on representational thought and the use of symbols, they realize that they are distinctly separate from others (Mascolo & Fischer, 2007). This distinctive self-awareness is necessary for the experience and expression of guilt, shame, pride, envy, aspects of embarrassment and shyness, and, as I've already suggested, possibly facilitates the social emotion of empathy as well (Lewis, 1993a; cf. Davidov et al., 2020).

Further, along with the ability to perceive their differences and similarities with others that is conferred by self-awareness, young children come to recognize their own success or failure at day-to-day tasks and begin to conform to the rules of their social groups. Such self-awareness, considerations of success and failure, and an understanding of standards and rules are necessary for the experience and expression of pride, shame, and guilt (Lewis, 1993a; see also Moskowitz, 1997). In fact, after attaining an objective sense of self in the latter half of the second year, toddlers and preschoolers begin to make self-evaluative comments and show shame and guilt from age 2 years onward (Stipek, Gralinski, & Kopp, 1990). For example, toddlers who understand that an object is flawed or that a standard has been breached demonstrate a nascent form of guilt by offering apologies and showing visible distress (Kochanska, Casey, & Fukumoto, 1995). The child evaluates his or her behavior against this self-standard: "*I* have done something dreadful or wonderful." Again, these self-conscious emotions would be expected early in the preschool period.

As noted in Chapter 1, emotions arise when something self-relevant happens or is about to happen, and these events mean something positive or negative for one's well-being (Tangney & Tracy, 2012). Based on the analysis above, even very young children actively interpret the arousal attendant upon success, failure, or wrongdoing. Preschoolers may experience self-conscious and social emotions according to specific patterns of understanding about their goals (cf. Stein & Levine's [1989, 1990] focus only on basic emotions).

For example, shame may be characterized by this interpretation: "I've done something [the novel event that leads to emotional arousal] that decreases the likelihood that I can continue to feel good about myself. I'm a bad person. I have experienced this event and this feeling; I don't want them to continue, but it's overwhelming. I'd better hide [or lash out, etc.]." The interpretation for pride may be the obverse of this event analysis (see also Chapter 5). The experience and expression of guilt, in contrast, might include the following interpretation: "I've done something [again, the novel event] that makes it unlikely that other people will continue to be happy with me. I've done a bad thing. I have experienced this event and feeling, but don't want it to continue. I'd better make amends in some way."

Such cognitions relevant to self-conscious emotions evolve throughout later toddlerhood and the preschool period. For shame, late toddlerhood is marked by simple, morally tinged social representations (Mascolo & Fischer, 2007). For example, during the 18- to 24-month age range, shame may be evoked by considering how the self is seen by others—"Mommy sees me [doing this bad thing]," whereas guilt may be evoked by doing something that caused another's distress. These are fairly concrete, behavior-related representations of social–moral concepts.

Later, during the third year of life, children internalize and define the self in terms of single social–moral categories. For shame, this means that the child makes stable evaluations of the self as seen through the eyes of others, anticipating adult reactions—"Mommy thinks I'm icky." Such awareness can motivate angry defiance and protest or, conversely, withdrawal and hiding. Guilt, during this age range, can be experienced without the clear contextual cues that were necessary earlier—the child can hold in mind the self's misdeed and the other's likely internal state—"when I spilled milk on Mommy's laptop, I'll bet she was mad." Finally, during the fourth year of life, the child is capable of what Mascolo and Fisher (2007) call "representational mapping," which involves understanding the connections between two or more representations, such as cause and effect, sequential order, reciprocity. Shame now can include a comparison with others, and guilt an even tighter, more detailed, connection with the harm caused to others.

## SUMMARY: Cognitive Foundations of Self-Conscious Emotions

In summary, very specific cognitive attainments, including self-understanding/awareness, attention to standards against which one's behavior can be evaluated, and rule internalization, as well as an increased ability to perform the social–cognitive event analyses above (even though it is unlikely to be conscious), are central to preschoolers' new experience and expression of self-conscious emotions (Lagattuta & Thompson, 2007).

One key way in which children begin to structure these cognitive interpretations of their emotional arousal as self-conscious or social emotions is no doubt via internalization of socialization messages from the adults in their world. Everyday contexts, even daily routines, are replete with disciplinary and achievement experiences in which toddlers and preschoolers are exposed to behavioral expectations and standards of their family and culture (see Chapters 7 and 8).

## Differentiating among Self-Conscious Emotions: Guilt, Shame, and Pride

Young children are impulsive, sometimes do not comply with rules, and are often not competent enough to succeed at certain tasks. So they experience (and express) guilt or shame. However, it may be difficult to tease these two emotions apart, both for parents and teachers, and for researchers as well. Shame and guilt reactions are often correlated and share critical defining features, including self-consciousness, self-evaluation, internal attribution, moral overtones, and interpersonal jeopardy concerns (Ferguson & Stegge, 1995). Further, both shame and guilt have some similar functions; they can regulate interpersonal behavior and social life, prompting moral, socially appropriate behavior in day-to-day social interactions as well as in close relationships.

Because of these commonalities, the measurement of shame, guilt, and even pride in young children poses numerous challenges. Unlike the basic emotions or even the concerned expression of sympathy, there are no unique facial indicators for these emotions, so that investigators must rely heavily on behaviors to infer their experience and expression. The problem is, there is likely to be some overlap between shame and guilt behaviorally. Moreover, asking young children about their own experience of shame, guilt, or pride is complicated by their lack of verbal ability and less-mature cognitive understanding of the two emotions. Thus that direct route to measurement is blocked.

To circumvent some of these difficulties (and despite the potential behavior overlap), investigators have created the operational definitions that rely on cultural consensus about body movements and postures as well as verbalizations. Unfortunately, these definitions have varied somewhat across research programs, so that care must be taken in comparing studies.

Further, because of their shared features and functions, some investigators also lump guilt, shame, and even embarrassment into one "feeling-bad-about-performance" emotion, as contrasted to pride, the "feeling-good-about-performance" emotion (e.g., Kochanska & Aksan, 2004; Kochanska, Gross, Lin, & Nichols, 2002). It is instructive to consider their findings first before examining those of researchers who have more clearly differentiated shame and guilt.

Kochanska et al. (2002) examined children's reactions to two mishap situations, each at 22, 33, and 45 months, in which the child inadvertently damaged items said to be of personal significance to the experimenter (e.g., a broken doll and stained T-shirt at 22 months). After the damage, the experimenter evidenced dismay, asking what happened and who did it, and then fixed the object. The construct that these investigators termed *guilt* had several shame indicators as well; it included avoiding the experimenter's gaze and the duration of such avoidance, bodily tension, such as squirming, hanging the head, backing away, hunching shoulders, covering the face, as well as more global ratings of distress and overall negative emotion. Interestingly, efforts to repair the damage (an accepted indicator of guilt) were not coded, probably because the procedure did not allow the child time to make such efforts.

Even though the construct as operationalized appeared to be undifferentiated self-conscious distress, its behavioral and emotional constituents showed several important relations: (1) each cohered across the two mishaps at each age, and were interrelated and negatively related to positive emotion; (2) each showed stability across all times of assessment; and (3) each corresponded modestly with maternal reports (e.g., ratings of "my child feels bad after wrongdoing; becomes quiet; feels bad when reminded of the wrongdoing"). Guilt as operationalized here also was predicted by mothers' ratings of children's early self-awareness at 18 months. So it seemed that the indicators appeared to index a stable style for self-conscious emotional responding to the mishap situation emerging from their self-awareness.

There also were developmental changes in specific indicators. Over time, children showed less gaze aversion, as well as less distress and overall negative emotion. In contrast, bodily tension and positive emotion increased with time. Possibly the children were anticipating the experimenter's negative evaluation and tried to look less distressed, trying to ingratiate themselves (maybe too they remembered that the experimenter could "fix" broken objects).

Finally, in this study children's fearfulness was observed during a "risk room" laboratory situation, in which 22-months-olds were exposed to strange objects like plastic reptiles and masks and asked to perform risky acts like climbing a ladder; their temperamental fearfulness in these admittedly weird situations was related to an index of guilt at all three times of measurement. Although fearful children react with discomfort, worry, or concern to many stressful events, it may be that this predilection supports activation of self-relevant emotions in a situation where personal responsibility is emphasized.

This aggregate of self-conscious emotion indicators then predicted children's later self-reports of a moral self (e.g., "When I'm by myself, I usually don't do what Mom says not to do"), as well as their observed violations of rules in the laboratory (e.g., cheating, not following experimenters' rules when alone with toys), at 56 months. In fact, a mediational model was supported: a fearful temperament contributed to "guilt" proneness, which in turn served to inhibit children's tendency to violate rules.

Whether these results from this research program are evidence for guilt, shame, or both is not clear, however; self-conscious emotion was indexed by signs that are prototypical of shame (avoiding gaze) and by signs that are associated with both guilt and shame (bodily tension) in a context that could elicit either or both emotions. And reparations were not measured. Nonetheless, these results are important not only as an example of how researchers struggle to study guilt and shame in young children, but also for their very thoroughness. Furthermore, they strongly suggest the importance of self-conscious emotions in the context of moral development.

However, even given the difficulty of measurement and the issue that some investigators do not differentiate guilt and shame, other research repeatedly underscores that there are important unique functional aspects of the self-conscious emotions of shame and guilt (Tangney, 1998; Tangney & Tracy, 2012). Further, recent work (da Silva, Ketelaar, Veiga, Tsou, & Rieffe, 2022) has confirmed that parents can indeed reliably differentiate indicators of guilt, shame, and pride. Thus, henceforth I look more closely at these emotions as separate entities.

### *Guilt*

In guilt, the key concern is with a particular behavior. Guilt involves a feeling that "I *did* that horrible *thing*." Young children often try to "fix" or make amends for what they did.

A mother describes an incident of her preschool son's guilt: "James [age 4] hit his 5-year-old cousin. In a firm and probably angry voice, I told him, 'We don't use our hands to hurt.' He said, 'I'm sorry, it was an accident.' He then sat on the stairs alone for a couple of minutes, then got up and apologized."

According to Hoffman (1984), the experience of interpersonal guilt results from the simultaneous feeling of sympathy toward another's distress and the awareness of being the cause of that distress—such as James realizing that his misbehavior dismayed both his parent *and* his cousin (Zahn-Waxler & Radke-Yarrow, 1990). However, whether sympathy is a precondition for guilt, whether guilt is a precondition for sympathy, or whether both arise together is a matter of some debate. In any case, the propensities to show each emotion are related by middle childhood; in fact, Roberts, Strayer, and Denham (2014) found that empathic concern led to guilt during middle childhood, supporting Hoffman's theoretical prediction.

More recent work has addressed the link between the two emotions in very young children: Vaish, Carpenter, and Tomasello (2016) observed 2- and 3-year-olds' reparative behavior in three conditions: (a) the child unintentionally caused a ball to knock down a tower the experimenter had built (guilt condition); (b) another person did the same damage to the experimenter's tower (sympathy condition); or (c) no harm. Three-year-olds showed more physical and verbal repair in the guilt condition than in the other conditions. Two-year-olds did show a broader effect of empathic concern—they helped the experimenter build back the tower more in both conditions in which harm was done than in conditions in which there was no harm, but did not show the specific motivating force of guilt. Thus, the effect of sympathy emerged developmentally before that of guilt, suggesting that at least over time sympathy may precede guilt in even very young children. In any case, *causing* harm led to motivations to repair, and the authors concluded that the experience of guilt can help to repair disrupted interactions even very early in life.

Regardless of the linkage with sympathy or empathic concern, evidence of guilt appears during the second year of life (Hoffman, 1984). During Barrett, Zahn-Waxler, and Cole's (1993) mishap paradigm (see also Cole, Barrett, & Zahn-Waxler, 1992), 2-year-olds showed more negative emotion during free play while experiencing these mishaps (e.g., a doll breaks and a cup of juice spills, ostensibly through the fault of the child). They also often attempted to make reparations. The authors took this pattern of responses as evidence of guilt. Those children who avoided via gaze aversion or moving away from the experimenter after this event were classified as "avoiders," or more likely to experience and show shame. These children also were slow to try to make any kind of reparation or to tell the experimenter what had happened. Convergent evidence from a maternal report questionnaire indicated that in nonlaboratory settings as well, amenders manifested greater guilt relative to shame than did avoiders.

More recently, these results were corroborated; clear differences were found in children's responses to the mishap paradigm—some toddlers showed quicker, more frequent gaze aversion and bodily avoidance and less frequent repairs, distinguishing shame-prone, as opposed to guilt-prone, 2½-year-olds (Drummond, Hammond, Satlof-Bedrick, Waugh, & Brownell, 2017). Results from both Barrett et al. (1993) and Drummond et al. (2017) bolstered the assertion that even early in life, guilt and shame can be differentiated.

In another study of older preschoolers (Bafunno & Camodeca, 2013), 3- to 5-year-old children were observed in situations that involved both moral and achievement contexts. These researchers also attempted to distinguish shame and guilt. For the moral context, the mishap situation was adapted. Children were introduced to a robot or wand, which was rigged to break in the presence of an experimenter, or a paper house created by a peer, also modified to be damaged when the child picked it up in the peer's presence. In the achievement situation, coded only for shame, children failed at an easy task (building a wooden train with the experimenter or working on a jigsaw puzzle with a peer) because the experimenter did not give them enough time. The facial/gaze (e.g., looking away), bodily tension, reticence, and repair, as well as verbalization (e.g., self-evaluations, confession) responses of the children were coded.

Responses were sorted into clear guilt versus shame configurations in the moral mishap situations; the results were similar to those in Barrett et al. (1993) and Drummond et al. (2017). Children categorized as guilt prone showed negative affect and scored higher than the median on the duration of their repair attempts. Those categorized as shame prone spent less time on repair and showed at least one facial/gaze response (e.g., turning away), bodily tension, and/or reticence indicator of shame, all of which were all intercorrelated. In the achievement situations, shame-relevant behaviors were seen especially when the audience was the adult experimenter, perhaps because of the authority wielded by adults and their propensity in some cultures to use shaming as a socialization tool. Further, positive associations between guilt and both pride and empathy showed coherence among the self-conscious emotions. Finally, older children and boys in this study showed more guilt than younger children and girls.

Narrative story methods also have been used to elucidate young children's experience of guilt. In these methods, children use dioramas and dolls to complete stories about fighting with one's sibling over a bicycle, an angry mother, a crying baby, and their mother's crying. They express their own experience of guilt in the themes they enact. These themes, including negative emotion, self-blame, and desire for reparation, become more frequent with age from 5 to 9 years (Zahn-Waxler, Kochanska, Krupnick, & McKnew, 1990), dovetailing with and extending Bafunno and Camodeca's (2013) naturalistic coding with preschoolers. Children acted out feeling bad and being responsible about these actions and seeking to make amends. When the mother doll cried, a girl might have the child doll give the mother doll a kiss and say, "Mommy, I am sorry, I didn't mean to hurt your feelings." In sum, in all of these studies, young children already realize their wrongdoing and have an emotional reaction to it. Varying methodologies point to an early emergence of the emotion of guilt.

### *Shame and Pride*

Feelings of shame also can arise from a specific behavior or transgression. But the ramifications of shame extend well beyond those of guilt (Lewis, 1992). The "bad behavior" is not seen as needing a simple reparation or apology; in fact, a reparation may not be sufficient to assuage this feeling. Rather, the offensive behavior is seen as a reflection of an equally offensive self. From a cognitive attributional perspective (Lewis, 1992; Lewis & Michalson, 1983; Mills, 2005), the development of a sense of self-awareness, and the ability to evaluate the self vis-á-vis learned standards and rules, together facilitate the experience of shame as a sense of global failure. Thus the key concern when feeling shame is with one's worth as a person; shame thus involves a feeling that "*I* am an unworthy, bad person."

And, seen from the functionalist perspective, shame's adaptive purpose is to maintain others' acceptance and preserve self-esteem—it signals the need to learn social standards and comply with others (Mills, 2005). Because adaptation to social standards and the need to comply is so difficult in the heat of the moment of experiencing shame and its aftermath, children paradoxically may show specific, potentially maladaptive, behavioral action tendencies, such as withdrawing, avoiding others, and hiding the self or parts of the self, such as the face. Older individuals amid a shame experience often report a sense of shrinking, of "being small." They feel worthless, powerless, and exposed, often reporting a desire to flee from the shame-inducing situation, to "sink into the floor and disappear." Shame is generally more painful than guilt.

Moreover, although shame does not necessarily involve an actual observing audience (i.e., no one needs to see the act one feels ashamed of), one's ideas about how one's defective self would appear to others can easily motivate shame. Not surprisingly, then, shame also is related to a history of socializers' disappointment, anger, disgust, or contempt in response to certain behaviors (see Chapter 7). And the shamed discomfort around such socialization messages can be lasting: The little girl explorer who journeys into the unlit fireplace with her teddy bear—inciting her mother's wrath and ridicule—may remember her shame even years later.

To expand upon the more maladaptive attributes and sequelae of shame experiences more fully, shamed individuals frequently become angry, with self-reported maladaptive anger management strategies (Tangney, 1995). For instance, as the sooty little girl and her equally sooty teddy bear are forcefully extracted from the ashes, she feels rage at the parent who is shaming her; she even kicks, bites, and squeals as she is dispatched to the tub. These behaviors do not endear her to her frustrated mother; in fact, they just make the situation worse.

Shame-prone individuals also often lack empathy and blame others for the shame-inducing event (Tangney, 1995). Hence, shame can motivate behaviors that interfere with interpersonal relationships. In fact, the tendency to feel shame about the entire self has been consistently linked to a range of psychological symptoms in older individuals (Stuewig et al., 2015). The sparkling clean little girl may ruminate about being "caught" in the fireplace and react by retreating to her room for the rest of the afternoon. If such shaming events occur rather often, she may even retain negative evaluations of both herself and others, and later symptoms of anxiety and depression.

Hence, the self-conscious emotion of shame stands in contrast to that of guilt in its behavioral manifestations. Instead of promoting these maladaptive behaviors that may separate the child from others, guilt motivates corrective action rather than avoidance:

> Three-year-old Erica, after clambering successfully to the top of the kitchen counter, dropped the top of the cookie jar and it broke. Then she turned to see her father's serious face at her current eye level. Knowing that her climbing was a "big no," and that she'd broken the special Pillsbury Doughboy cookie jar, she quickly picked up two pieces and tried to shove them together. She whispered, "I'm sorry, Daddy," and quietly but quickly climbed down, with her

father's help. He said, "You shouldn't have climbed up here, but we can glue it—I'll help you." After making the repair, they then engaged in reading a picture book together.

Thus, in sharp contrast with shame, guilt is more likely to keep people constructively engaged in interpersonal situations. The tension and regret of guilt are more likely to lead to a desire to confess, apologize, and/or amend, even in very young children. This motivation for reparation derives from guilt's focus on the offending behavior and its harmful consequences to others.

As opposed to shame, then, the self also remains relatively intact during guilt; it is unimpaired by shame-related global devaluations, thus allowing for reparative action. Older children's and adults' "shame-free" guilt is linked to a range of more positive interpersonal dimensions, including other-oriented empathy, a tendency to accept responsibility for harming others, constructive responses to anger, and self-reported adherence to conventional standards of morality (Tangney, 1992, 1995). This rather clear picture of guilt's greater adaptiveness when compared to shame becomes murky, however, when it fuses with shame or becomes so persistent that it immobilizes an individual.

Further, a somewhat clear picture also can be painted to differentiate the early manifestations of shame and pride. Much of the earliest research in differentiating pride and shame was conducted by Lewis and colleagues (e.g., Chen, Sullivan, & Lewis, 1995; Lewis, 1992; Lewis, Alessandri, & Sullivan, 1992) and by Stipek and colleagues (e.g., Stipek, Recchia, & McClintic, 1992). Both research groups presented young children with easy and difficult tasks and then observed the emotional responses of shame and pride that are implicit within success and failure experiences. For both groups, shame was coded when the child's body seemed "collapsed." In their coding of shame, the child's shoulders were hunched; the hands were down and close to the body; and their arms or hands were placed in front of the face or across the body. Also shame was coded when a child showed avoidant postures, with the head and chin down, the body leaning to the side or squirming, turning away, lowered eyes with gaze downward or askance, pouting, frowning, the lower lip tucked between the teeth, withdrawal from the task situation, or negative verbal self-evaluations, such as "I can't do it."

Erin wet on the bathroom floor because she waited too long to get to the bathroom. Her mother cried in exasperation, "Why did you wait so long? Now look what you've done!" Erin shrank down, turned partly away, and began to cry She was experiencing shame.

Pride, conversely, was coded when the child adopts an open, erect posture, with shoulders back, head up, and/or arms open and up. Other behaviors included smiling, pointing at the outcome, applauding, verbalizing positive self-statements ("Look what I did!" "I did it!"), calling attention to the product, or looking up (presumably for confirmation).

Later the day of her "accident," Erin counted all the numbers in a book. Her mother exclaimed, "Very good! You knew every one of those!" Erin smiled, danced around, and read the numbers again. This time she felt proud.

Task success and failure conditions, as well as task difficulty, moderated the occurrence of shame and pride. The constellation of indicators for pride was shown most often after success and was seen especially often after success with difficult tasks. Children showed shame only after failure, not success, and especially after failure on easy tasks. Sadness and wariness did not differ across task conditions. Hence, according to their definitions, both pride and shame were observed by these research groups as early as 27 months, and all children in their research showed these emotions by 42 months (see also Reissland & Harris, 1991).

So the expression of self-conscious emotions differs in conditions with differing implications for the self. In contrast, because their expression and experience are not intimately tied to a foundation of self-development, basic emotions, such as sadness and fear, are not expected necessarily to differ according to success or failure and task difficulty conditions. Empirical evidence as reported here strengthens the interpretation that shame and pride are unique, self-conscious emotions, not merely derivatives of the basic emotions (Chen et al., 1995).

Along these lines, a new set of experiences was used to capture 3- and 4-year-olds' shame reactions in both achievement and moral contexts (Ross, 2017). For the achievement task, children completed a "beat-the-buzzer" task, in which they were to put the correct color stickers on top of animal drawings. They were told that there were easy tasks most children their age would pass, but also ones that would be difficult. In reality, the tasks were "rigged" so that each child succeeded and failed once at both the easy and difficult task. For the moral task, the experimenter gave the child her "favorite" toy, which broke when the child attempted to replicate movements that had been demonstrated with it.

The operational definitions for shame and pride used in Ross's (2017) study were very similar to those of the Lewis and Stipek groups discussed earlier, with the coding rule for shame being negative emotion expression plus at least one sort of shame indicator (i.e., social withdrawal, closed posture, and negative verbal self-evaluations). An additional indicator of shame in the moral situation was the lack of making reparations quickly. For pride, the decision rules included the expression of positive emotion and at least one sort of pride indicator (i.e., social approach, open posture, and positive verbal self-evaluations). Guilt was coded if the child was quick to make amends following the mishap in the moral situation, along with showing negative emotion.

The findings revealed that most children showed negative self-evaluation in the moral context, but that in most cases this behavior was associated with the other indicators of guilt; this result does not surprise me, as I did not consider the operationalization of shame in the moral (mishap) context to be a strong one. A large majority of children showed both pride and shame in the achievement contexts. Failing an "easy" task was associated with shame indicators, implying that falling short of a social standard elicited an emotional response; the converse was true for pride at succeeding at a difficult task (although most children showed pride at succeeding at both easy and difficult tasks). Children also showed more pride in the achievement context than in the moral one. The children's responses were not related to age. These findings corroborate and extend the earlier assertions from Lewis's research.

Several of Bafunno and Camodeca's (2013) findings also bolster the assertion that task success and failure help to differentiate shame and pride. In their study, children showed more reticence and negative self-evaluation verbalizations in the achievement situation, suggesting that they saw the tasks as one of success or failure that could induce shame. Convergent results thus allow for distinguishing these two emotions, an important endeavor.

Finally, there has been some progress toward asking children about their own experiences of shame (and guilt). Ferguson, Stegge, Miller, and Olsen (1999) instituted a scenario-based measure, like that devised by Tangney (1990) for adults, which probes children's distinctive proneness to experience shame, guilt, and ruminative guilt. Stories such as spilling juice on an aunt's rug are presented to children as young as 5 years old. Children's predominant responses—in the case of the spilled juice, feeling bad, feeling so bad one can think of nothing else, or feeling dumb—were mapped onto guilt, ruminative guilt, and shame, respectively.

Thus progress has been made in differentiating pride, shame, and their correlates. But there may be important moderators of their experience.

## Moderators of the Experience of Pride and Shame

### *Age*

Although researchers have uncovered very few age trends in preschoolers' expression of shame, Stipek et al. (1992) found that children under 42 months of age were more likely to look away from the experimenter when they failed, suggesting their concern with social evaluation and anticipation of a negative reaction. Further, the behavioral/emotional codes for shame in Bafunno and Camodeca (2013) also were more frequent in 3-year-olds than in 4- and 5-year-olds. So 3-year-olds were more likely to be classified as shame prone; these authors added to Stipek et al.'s (1992) interpretation, speculating that these young preschoolers hadn't yet learned to control their negative reactions to such situations; they were not yet totally proficient at voluntary control of their emotions (see below).

In contrast, the older children in Stipek et al. (1992) were twice as likely merely to pout or frown after failure, consistent with "a more independent or internalized self-evaluation" (Stipek et al., 1992, p. 58). Thus the experience of shame may change from being more externally to more internally based—reflecting a more "*self*-conscious" emotion. Additionally, similar changes may occur with guilt. Older preschoolers in Bafunno and Camodeca's (2013) study showed more guilt in the mishap situations, perhaps due to a growing internalized sense of personal responsibility, a better comprehension of rules and others' feelings, and a knowledge of how to make things better. Again self-development was implicated.

### *Internal Working Models*

Malatesta et al.'s (1989) early results emphasized that early expression of a *positive* self-conscious emotion, such as pride, is associated with not only a stable concept of the self, but also a sense of one's inherent worthiness, as captured in the internal working models of secure attachment relationships. In contrast, supportive theorizing places the origins of shame in *mis*attunement between infant and caregiver; that is, infant expectations that caregivers facilitate emotion regulation and allow for sharing positive emotions are dashed (Mills, 2005; Muris & Meesters, 2014).

In accordance with this theorizing, insecurely attached toddlers expressed more shame than securely attached toddlers, while attributing negative emotions to photographs of other children and parents (Malatesta et al., 1989). Perhaps these toddlers internalized the negativity of their early parent–child interactions as follows: "I am not worthy of the care and positive regard of others; these people in the pictures probably think I am bad." Such an internal working model of self is certainly shame promoting. Hence, Malatesta and colleagues (1989) reason, when insecure toddlers observed the negative emotions of the photographed children, their own very internally based shame is activated.

However, Stipek et al. (1992) offer a slightly different argument that is still consistent with the notion that shame originates from internal conceptions about relationships with others. They reason that toddlers and preschoolers will rarely have experienced direct criticism for failing at developmental tasks, such as putting a puzzle together or embedding plastic cups (this may not be true for all children!), but that even very young children want to please grownups. These researchers say that youngsters experience shame not only when the self is threatened, but also when they are not following rules or living up to adults' expectations. Although this assertion does ground the young child's experience of shame within relationships and points to emotion socialization as important, as in Malatesta and colleagues' (1989) work, it also again obfuscates the differentiation between shame and guilt. Presumably, simply not following rules would result in guilt—not the shame-like patterns evidenced after failure by so many of the participants in Stipek et al.'s (1992) studies—unless breaking an adult's rule was seen as *failing in the relationship, being a bad relationship partner, unloved.*

Perhaps the arguments of Malatesta et al. (1989) and Stipek et al. (1992) can be integrated by asserting that shame is experienced when a child with a shame-based internal working model of the self fails another person or does not follow rules. Like the internal working models of others postulated by attachment theory, this internalization could happen during the preschool age range. The experience of shame could be more dependent on the actual response of adults in these situations earlier in the preschool period, but relatively stable and independent of adults' reactions later on.

Little further investigation has been done with young children to give firmer evidence of a connection between either attachment styles or other relationships and shame. However, results that support the attachment analysis have been found with adults (Akbag & Imamoglu, 2010; Lopez et al., 1997; Wei, Schaffer, Young, & Zakalik, 2005). As noted by Lagattuta and Thompson (2007), further study is needed to flesh out the likelihood that children's attachment relationships set the stage for proneness to *any* of the self-conscious emotions. Furthermore, extra effort should be expended to integrate the work of Stipek et al. (1992) and Malatesta et al. (1989) empirically, and to define more clearly the roles of age and internal working models of the self in the experience and expression of both shame and pride.

### Gender

Gender differences in the expression of shame, pride, and guilt also emerge early. Under some conditions, preschool girls show more shame than boys do (Lewis et al., 1992; Mills, Arbeau, Lall, & De Jaeger, 2010; Stipek et al., 1992). There are also gender differences in pride, with girls showing more positive expressions after success (Stipek et al., 1992). More recently, Bafunno and Camodeca (2013) corroborated these results, finding more girls in the shame-prone group; especially in the moral situation of the broken toy, they expressed more shame-relevant behaviors. In contrast, boys showed more reparative behaviors (see Kochanska et al., 2002), although as already noted their definition of guilt was rather overinclusive.

Moreover, the pattern of associations among self-conscious emotions differs for boys and girls. In Lewis et al.'s (1992) study, guilt- and shame-proneness were related for girls; if a girl expressed one of these negative self-conscious emotions, she also was likely to exhibit the other (see this association not moderated by gender; Ross, 2017). In Lewis et al. (1992), boys' self-conscious emotions did not show this pattern of association; their expression of guilt was unrelated to evidence of their shame. Instead, shame-prone boys were *less* likely to show pride, as if their bad feelings about themselves precluded their good feelings of pride. It's as if girls' "I feel bad about what I did and about myself" has more porous emotional boundaries than those of boys.

Another way that boys and girls may differ is in their physiological responses associated with the stress of failure and associated shame. Mills, Imm, Walling, and Weiler (2008) examined preschoolers' experience of shame across time after a series of failures and associated physiological responses (i.e., change in cortisol). The high initial shame of boys and only some girls was associated with greater cortisol reactivity and slower regulation of it.[1] This emotion- physiology pattern in boys predicted later shame even after recovery from the cortisol response. For girls, only high initial shame predicted subsequent shame. An explanation for *why* these gender differences exist remains to be given; girls may be socialized to feel more responsible for failure, and boys to be empowered to repair transgressions and move beyond failure, but boys' physiology may belie these differences. More research to replicate these differences and uncover some reasons for them would be useful.

### Culture

The frequency and implications of shame and pride (and guilt) for one's evaluation of self may vary across collectivistic/relational and individualistic cultures (Wong & Tsai, 2007). In one study (Lewis, Takai-Kawakami, Kawakami, & Sullivan, 2010), Japanese children expressed *less* shame and pride in response to both success and failure than African American and White American preschoolers. These findings correspond with other work suggesting that a low range of expressiveness, especially for negative

---

[1] Earlier work by Lewis and Ramsay (2002) found a gender difference of girls showing more shame than boys after success and failure tasks. Further, although they found shame expression to be related to elevated cortisol response, this effect was not differentiated by a child's gender.

emotions, may have cultural roots. Also, in terms of the implications of shame for children in collectivist/relational cultures, its inherent negative views of the self may inform and motivate individuals; because these reactions to shame can further social cohesion, shame may be viewed more positively. Specific research on this hypothesis remains to be performed with preschoolers, to my knowledge.

### SUMMARY: Moderators of the Experience of Pride and Shame

Although much has been learned about preschoolers' experience of pride and shame in recent years, it would be a mistake, as is usually the case, to ignore the contributions of age and gender to this emerging understanding. Older preschoolers increasingly show indications that their experience of shame is truly self-referent. Some self-conscious emotions are more easily discerned and more interrelated for girls. Additionally, there are tantalizing suggestions that a child's internal working model of attachment may be related to experiencing these self-conscious emotions. Finally, differing cultures are very important contexts for the experience of shame and pride, given the specific cultural values for each emotion. These moderators should be given even more attention in research on preschoolers' experience and on the expression of the self-conscious emotions.

## Summary: Guilt, Shame, and Pride

Overall, then, much work has been done to differentiate guilt, shame, and pride during the late toddler and preschool years. In sum, my reading of the extant research suggests that shame and guilt (and pride) can appear as separable emotions during the toddler and preschool periods in situations appropriate to the experience of such feelings. Their prerequisites are in place, but a continued effort to delineate the specific patterns of expressing these complex emotions is warranted.

If guilt has a powerful association with reparations and prosocial behavior, then it is incumbent upon adults to assist children in its experience and successful resolution. Similarly, the potentially deleterious effects of persistent or shame-fused guilt need to be specified; adults want to remedy the negative social relationships that may inspire shame in young children, to avoid any difficult outcomes associated with shame, and to foster the positive self-experiences that can engender pride.

To further these goals, even more precise investigations of the possibility of guilt- and shame-proneness would be useful. The current state of research points to the difficulties in differentiating and measuring guilt and shame. It is concerning that Kochanska et al. (2002) coded "bodily tension" in the mishap situation as guilt, and Bafunno and Camodeca (2013) coded it as shame, even though they used the same operationalizations. Operational definitions for self-conscious emotions obviously still require attention.

Nonetheless, despite many methodological challenges, many theoretical assertions about guilt, shame, and pride have been upheld (e.g., da Silva et al., 2022). Because of the potential beneficial or ill effects their experience may prompt, more research could help expand knowledge of the sequelae of these early-occurring manifestations of self-conscious emotions. Such research has begun and is reviewed in Chapter 10.

## COMBINATION SOCIAL AND SELF-CONSCIOUS EMOTIONS

Typically, emotions are classified as either social (as in empathy) or self-conscious (as in shame and guilt), but I argue that both shyness and embarrassment can (and often do) involve both social relationships and interactions, as well as evaluations of the self. I first consider shyness.

### Shyness

Shyness is defined overall as inhibited social contact, but sometimes is distinguished in dual fashion as (1) wariness, fear, and anxiety in the face of social novelty and/or (2) self-conscious behavior in situations of perceived social evaluation (Rubin et al., 2009). Although theoretically closely related and not always distinguished in empirical studies, these two types are distinguishable by form and function and possibly by biological roots. The first subtype, fearful shyness, appears during infancy as crying and other forms of distress, such as wary/fearful reactions, inhibited responding to strangers, attempts to retreat or escape, and seeking comfort. It is often measured by assessing the reaction to a stranger's approach or via ratings of behavior (e.g., "When introduced to an unfamiliar adult, how often did the baby/child cling to a parent?"). The experience of this emotion likely serves to motivate vigilance and the avoidance of threat (Schmidt & Poole, 2019).

The second subtype, self-conscious (or conflicted) shyness, appears later in toddlerhood after self-awareness is well in place; it is very similar to, if not co-occurring with, embarrassment, and is distinguished by fidgeting, lip biting/tongue protrusion, and gaze aversion. Possibly it emanates from an approach/avoidance state regarding social experiences or the tension between showing interest and fearing negative evaluation in social situations (Asendorf, 1990; Schmidt & Poole, 2019). It may serve the function of allowing more time for the child to evaluate what is going on.

The foundations of this emotion may include poor social experiences or rejection by peers and others. If these negative experiences occur frequently, they might prompt feelings of inadequacy or negative expectancies regarding others, which may contribute to the development of self-conscious shyness. Often self-conscious shyness is assessed by asking a child to stand on a podium to have photographs taken, to accept a compliment, or to sing a song, or it is assessed by parental ratings.

Stability in this second type of shyness has been found throughout toddlerhood (Eggum-Wilkens, Lemery-Chalfant, Aksan, & Goldsmith, 2015). In Eggum-Wilkens et al., self-conscious shyness showed stability from 19 to 28 months. These authors remark that this stability is similar to that found by Lewis, Stanger, Sullivan, and Barone (1991) regarding embarrassment from 22 to 35 months. A large majority of children in Eggum-Wilkens and colleagues' (2015) study showed self-conscious shyness at 19 months, and their expression of this emotion increased over time. Perhaps as children's sense of self matures, being "in the spotlight" becomes more aversive; stably negative social experiences could also contribute. Notably, no relationship between the two types of shyness was found in this study even though an association between them initially might be expected when children are relatively new at self-recognition.

However, these two types of shyness are not always differentiated. In reports in which the two types of shyness were *not* distinguished (i.e., generally defining shyness with temperament questionnaires featuring items such as "When approaching unfamiliar children playing, how often did your child watch rather than join in"), shyness also often showed stability across age periods. For example, maternal and caregiver reports of such shyness in toddlers showed moderate stability between 18 and 30 months (Eggum et al., 2009). Using similar methods, there was again moderate stability in shyness, this time from 1–2 years to 5–6 years (Sanson, Pedlow, Cann, Prior, & Oberklaid, 1996). Including an even greater time span, Karevold, Ystrom, Coplan, Sanson, and Mathiesen (2012) found moderate stability in shyness from 1½-to-12½ years. In this last study, shyness increased most steeply and was more variable during early childhood, implying that after the preschool years, shyness more resembles a trait than a situational emotional experience.

The findings regarding possible gender differences in shyness during this age range have been mixed. Studies that did not differentiate the types of shyness either found gender differences in toddlerhood favoring girls (Eggum et al. 2009) or no such differences during early childhood (Doey, Coplan, & Kingsbury, 2014). However, a tiny but significant difference favoring girls encompassing this age range was found in Else-Quest, Hyde, Goldsmith, and Van Hulle's meta-analysis (2006).

Although the fearful and self-conscious subtypes of shyness allow for theoretical and some empirical differentiation, other ways of conceiving of shyness might be useful, as they more fruitfully capture the differences between aspects of this earlier conceptualization. In one interesting analysis, shyness in 4-year-olds was conceived of as *positive* and *negative* (Colonnesi, Nikolić, de Vente, & Bögels, 2017). Children we asked to stand on a podium and sing a song while being videoed (usually considered a context for self-conscious shyness). Shyness was coding as aversion of gaze, head, or both, but positive or negative emotion displayed during these behaviors distinguished two types of shyness. Preschoolers who showed more negative than positive shyness also were rated by both parents as higher on social anxiety; in fact, children who showed *only* negative shyness were rated as more socially anxious than those who showed only positive, or no, shyness. Moreover, those who showed both types of shyness were more socially anxious than those who showed only positive shyness.

"Coy" or positive shyness was related to understanding the beliefs and false beliefs in this study. And, in contrast with experiencing only negative shyness, children's theory of mind skill and positive shyness together were associated with their *lower* levels of social anxiety. Perhaps understanding others' intentions renders a mildly aversive situation less so or gives children a route to "win over" the adult who is asking them to do a socially exposing task. Being coy (smiling, hanging the head, looking slightly away) may be useful to charm others.

Contrastingly, negative shyness seemed more related to fear and did not augur well for the children's adjustment (see Chapter 10). Colonnesi and colleagues (2017) draw a parallel between this negative shyness and the similarly positive connection between behavioral inhibition (i.e., biologically based wariness during exposure to novel people, places, and things, not just novel social experiences, as in shyness) and social anxiety.

Finally, Coplan, Prakash, O'Neil, and Armer (2004) draw another important distinction, that between shyness (e.g., "My child seems to want to play with others but is sometimes nervous about it") and mere social disinterest (e.g., "My child is just as to play quietly by him- or herself than to play with a group of children," as rated by parents). In their investigation, self-conscious or conflicted shyness (i.e., social fear and anxiety despite a desire to interact socially) predicted temperament ratings of fearful shyness and overall negative emotionality, as well as observed reticent play behavior, parallel play, lack of social initiations, and teacher ratings of anxious–fearful behavior, anxiety with peers, and lack of prosocial behavior with peers. Also, the conflicted shyness of boys was related to teacher ratings of exclusion by peers and observed solitary–passive play.

In contrast, "social disinterest" was negatively related to temperamental negative emotionality, observed social initiations, and teacher ratings of prosocial behavior with peers. But it was positively related to attention span and to teacher ratings of asocial behaviors and the probability of being excluded by peers. In short, two very different pictures emerged, which I think are important to capture (see also Rubin, 1982). Social disinterest may not necessarily be problem, except for peer exclusion, which could lead to increasing difficulties as children enter school. Further, conflict shyness *is* a risk factor, at least contemporaneously, and perhaps particularly for boys, as I expand upon in Chapter 10.

### *Biological and Cultural Foundations*

I would be remiss not to mention the potential biological roots of shyness. Buss (1986) theorized that fearful shyness involves a sympathetic autonomic nervous system response (i.e., a desire to "flee"), but that, in contrast, self-conscious shyness could activate a parasympathetic autonomic nervous system response (i.e., a means of calming). Moreover, Eggum-Wilkens et al. (2015) found a high genetic contribution to variability in self-conscious shyness. Schmidt and Poole (2019) mention evolutionarily newer brain circuits for conflicted shyness than for fearful shyness, whose roots would more likely be found in the limbic system. This makes sense to me, because conflicted shyness incorporates a conflict—"I want to interact, but I'm scared to"—that might require higher brain structures to resolve.

At the same time, shyness and social withdrawal may be strongly influenced and differentially evaluated in different cultures (see Rubin et al., 2009). Earlier research (e.g., Chen, Rubin, & Li, 1995) suggested that in collectivist/relational societies like the Republic of China, shyness was accepted, even actually encouraged, by mothers, teachers, and peers. Their interpretations seemed to equate shy, inhibited behavior with the reserve and respectfulness that promoted the cultural values of social harmony and the restraint of personal desires. Additionally, shyer children in China showed greater social competence, peer status, and academic success. Not surprisingly, then, as late as the early 2000s, Chinese children showed shyer, more inhibited behavior than children in other cultures (Rubin et al., 2006).

In contrast, in individualistic societies that encourage assertiveness and competitiveness, shyness was related to peer rejection. Furthermore, parents in such individualistic cultures were much less accepting of such shy, withdrawn behavior. The cultural differences made sense according to the meaning assigned to the behavioral expression of shyness.

However, more recent research suggests that cultural changes have fueled concomitant changes in the cultural meaning of shyness. The vast economic and political changes in China may have led to parents' desire for children to be more assertive and self-assured, with the implementation of more child-centered parenting, and thus changed how being shy impacts young children's lives (Liu, Harkness, & Super, 2020). In fact, very recently, Chinese mothers' ratings of their child's shyness was related to preschoolers' self-reported loneliness, lack of peer acceptance, mother-rated social anxiety, and teacher-rated internalizing problems (only the last two remained as significant predictors after receptive vocabulary was entered in regression equations; Zhu, Li, Wood, Coplan, & Chen, 2019). This change in the correlates of shyness, consonant with macrosocietal change, was dramatic. In Zhu and colleagues' (2019) study, importantly, receptive vocabulary acted as a buffer for the deleterious outcomes of shyness; when this language ability was low, shyness predicted all four negative outcomes. Being able to communicate may give shy children more confidence and also change how others react to them.

## Embarrassment

Embarrassment, like shame, appears early in life, and is not a pleasant experience (Miller, 2010). But it differs from shame in certain ways. Unlike shame, it is often not terribly intense and doesn't usually disrupt thought or language or elicit a wish to hide (Lewis, 2010); because it usually seems to be experienced somewhat lightheartedly, it is usually seen as a less negative emotion than guilt or shame.

As with shame and pride, researchers link the emergence of embarrassment to requisite self-knowledge. However, unlike either of these self-conscious emotions, embarrassment also is affected by the quality of an audience's behavior. It is characterized by an acute, surprised, awkward chagrin emanating from events that signal possible negative evaluations from a real or imagined audience. Embarrassed adults and children feel foolish, exposed, and conspicuous. Thus children are unlikely to be embarrassed before they have a sense of self, but to experience embarrassment, they must also perceive that they are exposed to an audience who might make fun of them (Bennett, 1989).

Lewis and his colleagues were among the first to delve into the short-term developmental course of and necessary conditions for toddlers' embarrassment. In two investigations, four embarrassment-eliciting situations were assessed: viewing oneself in a mirror, being praised overmuch, being pointed at, and being invited to dance with one's mother or an experimenter (Lewis et al., 1991; Lewis, Sullivan, Stanger, & Weiss, 1989). Clearly, each eliciting situation contained elements of self-consciousness and the possibility of an audience that might ridicule a child.

Embarrassment was indexed by silly smiles, giggling, hand gestures, and body movements—especially by smiling followed by averting one's gaze or touching one's hair, clothing, or face, and lip biting or other signs of a tense or suppressed smile. This emotion was more evident in the four situations of self-exposure just noted than in any other experimental situations and was more often seen in older toddlers and in children who recognized themselves in the mirror. However, although Barrett (2005) found embarrassment in 17-month-olds during a mishap task (i.e., the broken doll), its occurrence was in fact negatively related to self-recognition for boys. Thus such self-referential ability may be necessary, but not sufficient, for the expression of embarrassment.

The emotional and behavioral indicators of embarrassment seem to indicate an approach/avoidance stance. Recently two types of embarrassment were identified: exposure embarrassment and self-evaluative or "less-intense shame" embarrassment (Lewis, 2010; Lewis & Ramsay, 2002). Exposure embarrassment does emerge around the acquisition of a stable sense of self during the latter half of the second year of life. It involves exposure of the self when being the object of attention of others; as already noted, Lewis's research group has investigated it mostly during success experiences or other nonevaluative contexts (Lewis et al., 1991). The experience of such embarrassment is not associated with an elevated physiological stress response (in fact, it is negatively correlated with cortisol response to stress; Lewis & Ramsay, 2002), and is associated only with being the object of another's attention. Boys have shown more exposure embarrassment than girls (Lewis & Ramsay, 2002; see also Barrett, 2005).

In terms of the need for an audience cited in the definition of embarrassment, it may be that this tenet is likely to be an aspect of particularly exposure embarrassment. Bennett (1989) asked children to report how they would react in situations involving either a rule violation or a solo performance. The situations involved either no audience, a passive audience, or a derisive audience. Children ages 5 to 8 years said that they would be unlikely to be embarrassed in the presence of a passive audience, but they felt quite differently about the ridiculing audience. Hence, imagining the actual reactions of other persons is important to young children; in this emotional reasoning, as in their understanding of the physical world, they are quite concrete. Exposure embarrassment then may be more acute when preschoolers feel ridiculed, and does not necessarily involve any negative self-evaluation (Bennett & Gillingham, 1991).

Self-evaluative embarrassment emerges later than exposure embarrassment—the latter half of the third year of life, probably after greater experience with and knowledge of standards of behavior and the rules and expectations of important others. Lewis's research group has investigated this type of embarrassment most during failure experiences. Thus self-evaluative embarrassment is experienced because of failure to meet a social, rather than a moral, convention. In that sense, it is related to the experience of shame, but as Lewis (2010) and Lewis and Ramsay (2002) describe it, a "lesser shame." In contrast with exposure embarrassment, evaluative embarrassment is related to higher cortisol responses to stressful events. In a pattern opposite to that for exposure embarrassment, girls have been observed to show more shame and self-evaluative embarrassment than boys (Lewis & Ramsay, 2002).

Cultural differences again are important to consider. In contrast to their findings regarding shame, in Lewis et al. (2010) Japanese children showed greater exposure embarrassment than African American and White American children and showed more self-evaluative embarrassment after failure than White American children. Japanese children showed an equivalent embarrassment after success or failure, unlike the other groups. Thus the audience is likely even more important for Japanese children, who are not pleased even about being singled out for praise instead of being part of a cohesive group. In short, embarrassment may be a somewhat more serious event in collectivist/relational cultures than it is in individualistic cultures (Miller, 2010). Nonetheless, Miller asserts that embarrassment does seem to operate similarly in differing cultures, with similar circumstances eliciting similar feelings and interactive consequences.

More investigations of how embarrassment relates to other patterns of expressiveness and to social competence are warranted. Are easily embarrassed children more prone to the even more pernicious experience of shame? Does the experience of embarrassment put young children at risk of negotiating social interactions poorly?

### SUMMARY: Shyness and Embarrassment

Shyness has been examined by focusing on it as a fearful, self-conscious (conflicted) and even a positive (coy) or negative emotion, and has been distinguished from social disinterest. The first two distinctive patterns appear to have biological roots. However, most research does not differentiate among the types of shyness, so reconciling the different types could help caring adults to understand how and when to help shy children.

Embarrassment is generally less intense than although similar to shame; it is theoretically related to self-recognition, like self-conscious shyness, but empirical evidence for this relationship is mixed. Embarrassment too consists of two types: exposure and self-evaluative (i.e., shame-like). Exposure embarrassment is influenced by an audience's behavior (or the perception of it) and emerges earlier than self-evaluative embarrassment.

Both shyness and embarrassment also are strongly influenced and differentially evaluated according to cultural rules. More research has been done on the contributions of shyness to social and preacademic success; it might be useful to move forward to find any sequelae of a tendency toward embarrassment.

## VOLUNTARY MANAGEMENT OF EMOTIONAL EXPRESSION

Voluntary management of facial expressions also emerges during the preschool period (Field & Walden, 1982; Lewis, Sullivan, & Vasen, 1987; Malatesta et al., 1989). One of the first manifestations of voluntary expressive control is children's ability to pose specific emotional expressions, whether at an adult's request or during play.

> Manuel displays very contrived anger, brows down and mouth in a snarl, while pretending to be a police officer with Bobby and Andrea: "Move it, buster." They seem to know he is just feigning anger, and although they do flee (they are robbers, after all), his "anger" doesn't actually upset them.

So young children have sufficient voluntary control of their emotional expressiveness to display specific expressions, but this ability does change over the toddler-through-preschool age range. In research by Lewis's group, 2- through 5-year-olds, as well as adults, were asked to pose happiness, sadness, anger, fear, surprise, and disgust

(Lewis, 1993b; Lewis et al., 1987). Two-year-olds did not accurately pose any of the expressions. Three-year-olds, termed a transitional age group, posed happiness and surprise; the accuracy of posing happiness did not increase after this age (see also Bailey Bisson, 2019; Field & Walden, 1982, for early high accuracy in posing happy faces). More improvement occurred between the ages of 3 and 4. The 4- and 5-year-olds were less skilled than adults only in producing surprise and anger expressions in Lewis et al.'s (1987) results. No age group, including adults, was able to pose fear or disgust well according to discrete emotion criteria, but preschoolers tended to err by making a "scary" rather than a "scared" face.

Other researchers have asked children to pose the expressions that a protagonist would feel in a specific situation, such as "Tommy is followed home by a mean dog, and Tommy is afraid. Can you make a face to show how Tommy feels?" (Boyatzis & Satyaprasad, 1994, p. 44). Profyt and Whissell (1991) also asked preschoolers to demonstrate how they would feel in various situations calling for happiness, sadness, anger, fear, and disgust. The ability of others and the child to decode these encoded expressions was high for happiness and disgust and above chance level overall (see also Boyatzis & Satyaprasad, 1994, who found 61% accuracy of 4- and 5-year-olds' encoding of happiness, anger, sadness, disgust, surprise, and fear from situations, not separated by emotion). Recognizability of the encoded expressions increased linearly with age from 4 to 6 years old in Profyt and Whissell (1991), but Boyatzis and Satyprasad (1994) found no age differences in 4- and 5-year-olds.

More recently, Baily Bisson (2019) combined both methods. In her study, 3- and 4-year-olds also were best at posing happiness and sadness and had more difficulties with anger, fear, surprise, and disgust, whether they were asked to "make an X face" or "show how X would feel" in response to vignettes. However, the children's performance in posing the emotion for vignettes was lower for happiness, sadness, and disgust. In the methodologies using vignettes (Bailey Bisson, 2019; Boyatzis & Satyaprasad, 1994), children not only had to understand an emotional label (e.g., "happy") and know how to show that facial expression, but they had to accurately understand the vignettes' emotional import, and *then* know how to show that facial expression. Perhaps producing an emotion from a request to make a specific face is easier.

It could be instructive to examine these phenomena in a more discrete way. In the original Lewis et al. studies (Lewis, 1993b; Lewis et al., 1987), children's videotaped posed expressions were grouped into complete expressions, which included all the components of the target expression, and partial expressions, which included only some of the components of the target expressions. In part echoing trends found by Profyt and Whissell (1991), partial poses were consistently more frequent than complete poses for sadness, fear, and disgust across age groups. These results suggest how this ability develops for these more difficult-to-pose emotions.

Thus, although there are some differences in which emotions were well posed at each age across these studies, it is clear that at least some negative expressions are consistently difficult, especially for the youngest children, to demonstrate at will. Why would this be? One plausible explanation is that negative expressiveness requires more control of facial muscles, and that happy expressions can be demonstrated using only the lower half of the face, whereas negative emotions require at least both mouth and eye regions. Yet another credible interpretation is that children have deficiencies in differentiating how negative expressions look or are made (Cole, 1985; Denham & Couchoud, 1990b). A third explanation for these developmental patterns is that children are already exposed to socialization pressures to suppress negative expressiveness. Perhaps preschoolers are showing us their capabilities to both to suppress and to dissemble expressiveness when they demonstrate difficulty posing negative expressions in these investigations. Even when asked, they may be reluctant to generate or even to acknowledge expressions of sadness and anger; some flatly state, "But I'm not mad," or "I don't want to be sad" (Cole, 1985).

Although these spontaneous verbalizations hint at a socialization hypothesis, rather than the hypotheses of emotion knowledge or facial muscle control, this link is not irrefutable. The children's comments also highlight their efforts to avoid the uncomfortable felt experience that is for them still inextricable from their expressiveness. In support of this argument, even emotionally knowledgeable and motorically skilled adults have more trouble simulating negative expressiveness. Thus, it likely that all three hypotheses have some foundation. In any case, the research presented here reveals that young children's growing ability to pose expressive patterns can be taken as evidence of their increasing voluntary control of their own expressiveness.

### SUMMARY: Posed Expressions

Importantly, some of these new skills in voluntary control of facial expressions serve the function of *maintaining* rather than *derailing* social interactions. Children also learn when to display emotions that facilitate social interaction. Such voluntary management of expressiveness is important because it aids even very young children in their emotion regulation. Control of facial expression is a vital contributor to social competence, then, through the ability to manage the nuances of emotion-laden interactions (see Chapter 6). With these intentional abilities, the child feels better and more in control and also is more able to enact appropriate social interaction. Thus the consideration of display rule usage is an important next topic.

## Control of Expressiveness and Adherence to Display Rules

More specifically, this voluntary modulation and control of expression through posing form a foundation for the modification of emotional expressiveness in the service of display rules or deception (Lewis, 1993a, 1993b). Children's first attempts at intentionally and successfully posing facial expressions often occur when a rule of self-display or social display, or deceiving others about one's "true" feelings, is necessary.

> A prosocial display rule is functioning when a 5-year-old boy, given a tiny portion of meatloaf, smiles rather than yelling at Grandma that he wants more. To protect herself and avoid punishment, a 4-year-old girl may behave according to a self-protective display rule, feigning an unconcerned expression when she is discovered atop the kitchen counter (unlike Erica in an earlier example). Maybe she can get away with it!

As voluntary management of emotional expressiveness expands, display rules come to be employed. Children learn to use affective displays strategically—to substitute, mask, minimize, or maximize patterns of expressiveness according to cultural expectations for self-preservative or prosocial purposes (Ekman & Friesen, 1975). All these abilities involve knowledge of when, where, and how to control the display of emotions. Children may first minimize or maximize expressive patterns that are already within their repertoire. The mastery of substitution or masking strategies is achieved later because a greater cognitive ability to understand the difference between appearance and reality in people's thoughts, feelings, and desires (i.e., "theory of mind"; Harris & Gross, 1988), as well as facial muscle control, are required to change the expression of emotion from that which is experienced (Saarni & von Salisch, 1993).

A surge in both the understanding and utilization of display strategies takes place during the elementary school years (understanding of display rules is considered in Chapter 5). Three possible reasons exist for whatever difficulties preschoolers do have in using display rules. First, although they learn *verbal* strategies to discount emotions early, young children obtain less feedback on how to modify *facial* and *vocal* displays. They can learn facial and vocal display rules more readily through observing others and through indirect feedback. Second, even after knowing display rules and potential strategies to enact them, they need to learn *how* to inhibit both facial muscle movement and vocalization. Third, preschoolers also experience relative difficulty in making critical self-evaluations (e.g., "I need to change my angry display here for Grandma's sake"). Complete acquisition of the skills inherent in all these factors takes time.

Nonetheless, preschoolers' usage of both self-protective and prosocial display rules is more sophisticated than at first assumed. The use of naturalistic rather than laboratory contexts allows researchers to witness preschoolers' true abilities in this area. Because of this need for more ecologically valid investigations, researchers created ingenious paradigms to identify how very young children use display rules. In studies using these methods, evidence appears very early that expressiveness patterns conformance with cultural display and self-display rules. Toddlers already show expressive patterns that signal the dampening of negative emotions, such as wrinkled brows, compressed lips, and lip biting (Malatesta et al., 1989). They are minimizing emotions that could potentially cause problems for themselves and others. From this very young age onward children also maximize expressions that serve to dramatize distress to get assistance, such as the anger exhibited during a sibling conflict (Dunn, Bretherton, & Munn, 1987), or to dominate, as indicated by their rage shown on the playground (Blurton-Jones, 2017). They are modifying the expression of their emotions to serve specific goals.

## *Functions of Display Rule Usage*

Thus maximization serves the self-protective function of enlisting aid and/or gaining adults' attention and compliance with their wishes. For instance, a 3-year-old girl may begin to cry loudly several moments after she trips and falls over blocks in the block corner—that is, when her teacher reenters the room. Toddlers also use substituted or masked expressions strategically for the self-serving functions of joking and teasing (Dunn et al., 1987; Dunn & Munn, 1985; Lewis, 1993b). For example, after a 2-year-old boy holds his sister's blanket in his hand and feigns a sad look, he may begin to laugh at his own mockery.

Display rules also are used by preschoolers to smooth "bumpy" social interactions with peers and adults. Knowing when to minimize anger by showing only furrowed brows or pursed lips could help avoid a fight. Empirical data indicate that the upper facial muscles' "social" smile increases in frequency across the 2- to 4-year-old age period, but only when the child is interacting with same-gender peers (Cheyne, 1976). Presumably, this smile is voluntarily controlled to initiate contact and optimize the fun of shared activity.

Display rules are also used in the service of kindness by preschool-age siblings (Reissland & Harris, 1991). Five-year-olds mask their pride more often than their 3-year-old younger brothers and sisters do during competitive game-playing interactions. Likely, they do not want to make their younger siblings feel inept or to "rub it in" when they win.

### *Moderators of Display Rule Usage: Context, Gender, and Individual Differences*

But all this maximization and minimization and masking are complicated. How does the young child know when to enact which pattern of voluntary expression management? There must be some guides along the way! Along with the learning of display rule strategies and their enactment that I have already noted, three such guides could be (1) one's social partner, (2) the cultural rules of context, and (3) the gender of oneself and others in an interaction.

As children develop, the identities of their partners in interaction become increasingly important for the use of display rules (Zeman & Garber, 1996). First-graders endorse more emotional control around peers than around parents or when they are alone. Peers often reject, ridicule, or reprimand a friend who shows sadness, anger, or pain. Thus there is probably a complex association between children's understanding of emotions and display rule usage. As children age, they become better at reasoning about the antecedents and consequences of, for example, crying in front of a friend. They also learn to distinguish the emotional experiences of themselves and others; for instance, they feel scared while they cry, but their friends feel amused. Finally, they better implement their emotion knowledge, when appropriate, in the service of display rules (Fuchs & Thelen, 1988). Preschoolers are just beginning to discern these understandings, which I explain further in Chapter 5.

Making these contextual distinctions is a tall order. Young children may be controlling the expression of emotion, but not necessarily its experience, to conform with their culture's "feeling rules." But conforming to cultural "feeling rules" by using display rules in general (especially true for girls) is even more flexibly context sensitive. In one situation, display rules may pressure children to show socially appropriate expressions despite their emotional experience ("Don't show what you feel; show what you don't feel"). In another, display rules may allow and encourage children to show what they experience so that they can obtain support. For example, Layne slipped and fell while exuberantly skipping in a parking lot on the way to the car with her parents. She cried lustily, knowing that it was okay to show how it hurt and that then her father would pick her up and carry her. In contrast, when her grandmother's cat nibbled on her finger a little bit, she did not cry because she knew her grandmother would appreciate her not showing weakness or implying that the cat was at fault!

In neither case would display rules have been necessary if Layne were alone with no one receiving the managed emotional signal. Which sort of display rule is invoked when someone *is* around also depends on who that someone is (Zeman & Garber, 1996). And sometimes situations elicit strong emotions that preclude using display rules. These complexities also depend on gender, conforming to gender stereotype expectations for emotional expressiveness and its control.

To examine how context, cultural rules, and gender act upon display rule usage, in what is now a ubiquitous paradigm, preschoolers were given a disappointing toy as a gift (Cole, 1986). Their ensuing facial expressions were microanalytically coded. Girls were already spontaneously controlling the outward expression of emotion. Boys showed the only sad expressions, whereas girls showed more positive and neutral displays, conforming to cultural rules about girls being polite and socially appropriate. But when the experimenter queried the children about how they felt about the gift and their willingness to trade it for something better, most children—both boys and girls—reported actually feeling sad or mad. They said that they would be happy to trade the disappointing gift for a more attractive one. The experience and expression of emotions were differentiated only by girls at this early age.

In a second study, only girls participated; the examiner remained in the room with some of them after giving the unattractive gift, but for others she left the room (Cole, 1986). This procedure introduced a new and important context—whether to show emotions or not around other people. Girls smiled more when the examiner remained, suggesting that the function of such smiling is indeed to conform to expectations of "appropriate" social behavior by masking a negative emotion in the service of politeness. Again these girls may have modified their expressiveness to conform more closely to a cultural standard of socially appropriate behavior, a gender-related expectation impressed upon them early in life.

Thus, social context—wanting to enhance or minimize an expression to maintain social order—is really the whole point of using display rules, but boys and girls may interpret the social context and emotional elicitor differently. Josephs (1994) found that both 4- and 6-year-olds regulated their disappointment at receiving a broken pencil rather than their desired gift. They enacted display rules via both emotionally positive expressions and verbalizations when the experimenter who had given them the "gift" was present. Extending the Cole (1986) study, girls were more emotionally positive while the experimenter was present rather than absent, whether the gift was attractive or unattractive. Boys showed a bigger difference in expressiveness depending on the presence or absence of the experimenter when the gift was *un*attractive; in fact, in contrast to Cole, they showed as much positivity as the girls to the experimenter when the gift was unattractive. Perhaps German boys learn earlier than American boys to regulate expressiveness via display rules, taught early to be polite or not to reveal hurt feelings. Girls reacted only to the social aspects of the situation (i.e., experimenter present or absent), but boys' reactions depended both on the social and nonsocial (i.e., attractive or unattractive gift) aspects.

So it seems that young boys' use or nonuse of display rules is differentiated along different dimensions than their use or nonuse by girls. To respond supportively to young children's emotions, caring adults need to be conscious of how boys and girls differ in their perceptions of the acceptability of certain expressive patterns and in their notions of how others react to these displays.

Other issues may impact how children deal with the necessity of using display rules. For example, already showing a risk of externalizing behavior disorder at age 5 may make it difficult to demonstrate developmentally appropriate display rule usage abilities. In one study (Cole, Zahn-Waxler, & Smith, 1994), children at such risk showed some specific patterns of response in the disappointing gift task. At-risk boys showed more negative emotion than boys not at risk of behavior problems, when the experimenter was present after giving the unattractive gift; this group difference disappeared when the experimenter left the room (i.e., everyone, boys and girls alike, was unhappy with the gift!). In contrast, at-risk girls' minimizing of negative emotion was related to their diagnoses of attention deficit and conduct disorders, perhaps an *over*-regulating of their emotions.

This study also highlighted how emotions in the disappointment procedure were related to other behaviors shown by the children. The ability to show happiness when the experimenter was present was related to self-regulated behavior, like trying to fix or play with the unwanted gift, or verbalizing self-reassuring statements. However, showing negative emotions in varying ways while the experimenter was present (e.g., intensity of negative emotion, total anger) was related to mere passive toleration of the unwanted gift and even disruptive behavior (e.g., throwing the gift, making rude remarks).

These results suggest a link between self-regulation and display rule usage. Two studies have examined the support that self-regulatory abilities may provide to such control of expressiveness. Preschoolers showed more positive emotion when given a desirable gift and more negative emotion when given the undesirable gift, as expected (Liebermann et al., 2007), and older preschoolers were able to show more positivity toward the undesirable gift (i.e., they evidenced less difference in their positivity between desirable and undesirable gifts; see also Carlson & Wang, 2007). More important, in Liebermann et al. (2007), children with poorer inhibitory control (i.e., the ability to suppress dominant, automatic, or prepotent responses, via tasks like performing well in playing Simon Says, not touching a forbidden toy, and waiting to open a gift) especially showed a decrease in positive expressiveness during the disappointment procedure. In Carlson and Wang (2007), stating that one liked the gift and suppressing negative emotional expressiveness (e.g., nose wrinkled, pursed mouth, avoidance of eye contact, negative noise emitted, negative comments uttered) also were related to inhibitory control. Again the importance of self-regulation to these emotional processes is clear as early as the preschool period.

### *Display Rule Usage and Culture*

Differences and similarities across cultures also are crucial to consider when investigating display rule usage. When observing American, Chinese, and Japanese preschoolers (Ip et al., 2021), *all* children showed elements of positive expressiveness (e.g., especially a "fake smile" after receiving a disappointing gift)—but only, as seen in earlier studies, when either unfamiliar or familiar examiners were present. All were able to mask their disappointment. They all also showed a decline in negative, and an increase in positive, expressiveness when a familiar examiner, who had not given them the undesirable gift, returned and acknowledged the mistake. However, Japanese preschoolers also masked negative emotions both when asked to put toys away by their mother and when given a disappointing gift in the experimenter's presence (similar to Cole, 1986, especially girls) (Takahashi, Kusanagi, & Hoshi, 1998). Thus the usage of display rules in early childhood may be relatively equivalent across some cultures, at least when trying to remain polite while being disappointed.

But differences also exist, fitting cultural norms. In Ip et al. (2021), Chinese and Japanese preschoolers *verbally* reported more negative emotions in response to the disappointing gift, but showed more neutral facial expressions in comparison with the Americans. There were even differences between the Chinese and Japanese children's responses, with Chinese children showing even more of a "poker face" across different parts of the task. According to Ip et al. (2021), the Chinese culture emphasizes preschoolers' educational preparation, mastery, and self-improvement, views strong emotional displays as a sign of immaturity and actively discourages an overt expressiveness. Japanese parents also discourage overt expressions of emotions, more because their culture values emotional contentment and social relatedness. These differing values may help to explain the differences found in this study.

## **SUMMARY:** Display Rule Usage and Its Moderators

Display rule usage appears during the preschool age range. Much attention needs to be given to its moderators, because many instances in which it occurs depend on the context of the emotional situation. One moderator that is especially important is whether others are present, given the essentially social and cultural nature of display rules themselves. Girls and boys already differ as to how they exhibit manifestations of display rules. And there are some intriguing differences, as well as similarities, in display rule usage according to the culture in which children live. These issues point to the power of emotion socialization as an engine for display rule usage, but as explained in Chapter 7, more research is needed in this area.

Individual differences also are seen in preschoolers' abilities to enact display rules. Preexisting behavior problems impact preschoolers' display rule usage, again with gender playing an important role. Finally, the ability to exert self-regulation to modify one's natural emotional expressiveness to conform with display rules also differs across individual preschoolers. All these aspects of display rule usage would benefit from deeper study.

## Deception, or Self-Protective Expressiveness

The foregoing examples of display rule usage highlight the strategic control of emotional expressiveness to attain a personal goal, render a dyadic interaction more successful, or minimize another person's discomfort. *Deceptive* masking (or, in some cases substituting) of expressiveness also takes place within the preschool period; this possibility was presaged by earlier observational research with infants and toddlers (Dunn et al., 1987; Dunn & Munn, 1985; Lewis, 1993b; Malatesta et al., 1989). In a way, such emotional expression masking is lying—2- to 5-year-olds use their emotions to support deliberately untrue statements, to deny rule violations, or to otherwise conceal their own transgressions (Talwar & Crossman, 2011).

Thus such deception serves the function of avoiding guilt, shame, and possible punishment (Lewis, Stanger, & Sullivan, 1989). In Lewis and colleagues' studies, children watched an experimenter set up an elaborate toy. They were told that they were going to be allowed to look at it and play with it later, but that they were *not* to look at it while the experimenter left to do some work. Each child was given nothing else to do during this period. Five minutes later, the experimenter returned, stared pointedly at the child, and asked, "Did you peek?" The children's actual behavior with the toy, as well as their facial and behavioral responses to the experimenter's question, were monitored via video and coded.

In reality, only 10% of the children complied with the experimenter's instructions not to look at the attractive toy—but of those who did peek, two-thirds either lied about doing so or did not respond to the question. It is vital to note that coding of the videotaped facial expression of deniers and nondeniers did *not* differ. No one showed guilt—and deception really did occur. At the moment of questioning about peeking, the deceptive children did not show any expressive differences from those who told the truth. Facial expressive elements such as relaxed face, smiling, frowning, nervous touching, biting of the lips, and gaze aversion did not distinguish deniers from nondeniers. Moreover, judges could not reliably identify deniers versus nondeniers, regardless of the age or gender of a child or the age, gender, and experience of the judge. It is a bit disconcerting to see how adept these young children were at lying!

There were many children who were deceptive, but again there was a gender difference in those who chose to mask their guilt and fear: Girls followed the experimenter's orders much more often than boys, but boys were far more likely than girls to admit their transgression. Hence, girls formed the vast majority of deniers and nonresponders—that is, deceivers. Lewis and colleagues' (1989) and Cole's (1986) findings are convergent therefore: Young girls precociously use both display rules and dissemblance.

Lying is a more expansive topic in terms of its inception during the preschool years—it does not always involve emotions, but does, as noted regarding display rule usage, appear to require some understanding of the difference between appearances and reality (Talwar & Crossman, 2011). In a temptation-resistance paradigm like that of Lewis et al. (1989), children were left alone in a room with a music-playing toy placed behind their back. The children were told not to peek at the toy, but, as with Lewis et al. (1989), most could not resist the temptation (Talwar & Lee, 2002). When asked whether they had peeked, about half of the 3-year-olds confessed to their transgression, whereas most of the older children lied. Naive adults watched video clips of children's responses and again could not discriminate lie tellers from nonliars based on their nonverbal expressive behaviors, including emotions (although the preschool-age children tended to make self-incriminating verbal statements).

Hence, preschoolers, often mostly girls, can effectively mask expressions of apprehension about the discovery of their transgressions. Lewis (1993b) suggests that the function of this dissemblance is self-preservative, masking a fear of punishment and guilt over disobeying. The notion of "prosocial lies" also was underscored by Talwar and Crossman (2011); these actions could involve substituting emotional expressions (e.g., smiling instead of looking angry) to be kind to others. Whether this is a lie or deception or falls more clearly into the use of display rules is a matter of judgment. Nevertheless, as Talwar and Crossman (2011) note, this positive form of deception is likely to be promoted by the important socializers in children's lives, who may model the behavior or exhort children to perform it (see Chapter 7). At the same time, socializers may initially ignore negative lies during toddlerhood, but increasingly discourage them and view them as signs of maladjustment through childhood.

Other origins of deception, whether negative or positive, may be the child's self-consciousness (perhaps an amalgam of shame, shyness, and embarrassment), but also empathy, social desirability, emotion knowledge, and theory of mind (i.e., understanding one's own and others' mental states and behaviors, while learning to control theirs). Empathy and emotion knowledge would be especially important for prosocial lies. In short, deception is an emotional expressive behavior that is in part reflecting children's own predispositions and abilities, especially cognitive; at the same time, it is highly socialized. Much more research could be done on the early inception of the emotional aspects of lying.

## SUMMARY: Voluntary Display of Emotions, Display Rule Usage, and Deception

After young children become able to voluntarily produce emotional expressions, conformity to display rules clearly surfaces during the preschool period (see also Cole, Zahn-Waxler, et al., 1994). There is evidence of maximization, minimization, masking, and even deception, following the proscriptions and prescriptions of children's cultures, as well as their individual self-serving goals. However, as Cole (1985) asserts, the findings suggest that most of the evidence consists of "*nonconscious* adjustments [in expressive patterns] implying tacit personal and/or cultural display rules. The preschooler's cognitive limitations in self-reflective, inferential, and abstract social reasoning may render such tacit knowledge inaccessible" (p. 285; emphasis added).

At the same time, it is important to underscore that young children are beginning to comprehend that emotional displays may be modified; more is said on this topic in Chapter 5. They also evidence some specific strategies to do so, especially in naturalistic investigations. Because of the potential importance of maximization, minimization, masking, and substitution of emotions to social competence (or their lack), more research is needed to flesh out the intriguing results of the studies reported here. Nevertheless, adults should be aware of young children's potential for display rule usage and deception when discerning their charges' true feelings is necessary.

## CONCLUSION

In sum, self-conscious emotions appear during the preschool period—in fact, some arguably exist during toddlerhood. At the same time, the voluntary management of emotions also increases, as evidenced through the posing of expressions, the following of cultural prescriptions and proscriptions about expressive patterns, and personal dissemblance. These developments render kindergarteners' emotions ever more useful as social and internal signals.

> Andrew's preschool teacher enters the room to see a huge, squelchy mess by the water table. She doesn't have to exclaim "Who did this?," because Andrew's demeanor, both facial and physical, shows her that he is the guilty party. Self-conscious emotion is part of his repertoire.
>
> Sandra's exaggerated fear expression while her teacher reads a scary story conveys a different message; it invites other kindergartners to join her in the delicious experience of "courting" fear in a safe environment. She can make voluntary use of emotional expressiveness.

These changes hold implications for parents and teachers alike. Children of early grade school age are often much more difficult to "read" than preschoolers because some of their emotions are masked, dissembled, or blended. More effort is required to know what these older children are experiencing emotionally. Their emotional lives are also more complex, with guilt, shame, and embarrassment requiring the full attention of the adults in their lives. Supportive care from these adults when children are of preschool age can have far-reaching effects.

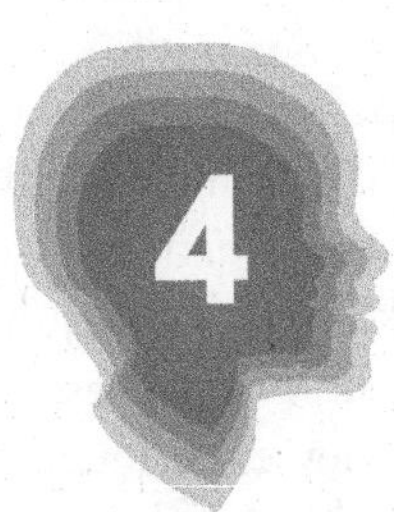

# Developing Knowledge of Emotions and Emotion Regulation

## INTRODUCTION

It is important that children be able to recognize emotions in themselves and others, label them, and associate them with appropriate expressions (Kusché & Greenberg, 1995b). Without an understanding of emotion, no distancing occurs between feeling and action, and both dealing with one's own feelings and sympathizing with others are more difficult. Among other components of emotion knowledge, preschoolers can show knowledge of common emotions' causes and consequences:

> Rosie is playing with a girl doll, who is in her bed in the dollhouse. She speaks for the doll: "I'm having a bad dream! A big scary tiger is chasing me! Mommy! Mommy!" Rosie quickly whisks the mother doll into the room. "Wake up, sweetie, wake up! There's no more, there's no tigers chasing you." There was a loving consequence in response to the doll's fear.
>
> Rosie then brings the mother and daughter dolls into the dollhouse kitchen. The girl doll says, "Thank you, Mommy. I want to make you breakfast to make you happy!" Here the doll clearly knew what would cause her mother to be happy.

As noted in Chapter 2, toddlers and preschoolers express emotions vividly and frequently. Their own and others'—age-mates' and adults'—emotions are central experiences in their lives. Children are interested in emotions as early as 2 years of age. Emotion knowledge yields information not only about emotional expressions and experiences in the self and others, but also about environmental events, especially social ones. It conveys crucial interpersonal information that guides interaction. Inability to interpret emotions can make the home, neighborhood, and classroom confusing places, hindering social and academic adjustment (see Chapters 10 and 11).

So the unfolding of emotion knowledge is quite critical for young children. First and foremost, this understanding supports preschoolers' attempts to deal with and communicate about the emotions they experience and those they witness. In spontaneous conversations, even young children talk about and reflect upon their own and others' feelings and discuss causes and consequences of these emotional experiences and expressiveness (Dunn, Brown, & Beardsall, 1991; Fabes, Eisenberg, McCormick, & Wilson, 1988). Despite his generally limited use of words, a 3-year-old boy can speak with great intensity about his sadness when he lost his favorite stuffed cat: "Wow gone. I cried."

Second, particularly because of their verbal limitations, emotions are extraordinarily important social signals for young children. Emotions are immediate and salient in their social transactions. Thus, as their cognitive and language abilities mature, preschoolers almost unwittingly construct coherent understandings about their own and others' feelings (Bretherton & Beeghly, 1982; Bretherton, Fritz, Zahn-Waxler, & Ridgeway, 1986; Harris, 1989, 1993). Young children learn the facial expressions, vocal patterns, goals, and likely behaviors associated with a variety of emotions (Campos & Barrett, 1984). According to a functionalist analysis, they work out the meaning of emotions by focusing on the connection between desire (i.e., attaining their goals) and reality: "Sadness is when I want something but can't have it, like when Mommy says I can't have pie" (Denham & Zoller, 1991).

Even 2-year-olds begin to understand that wanting and getting lead to happiness, whereas wanting and not getting lead to sadness (Harris, Johnson, Hutton, Andrews, & Cooke, 1989; Wellman & Banerjee, 1991; Wellman & Woolley, 1990; Yuill, 1984). Children of this age also come to know that the anger felt by themselves and others often involves being in an undesired state, along with a gruff vocal tone, lowered brows, and a tendency to attack physically or verbally. For example, an understanding of anger allows young children to interpret high-level anger in others as a signal to "get out of the way" (Denham, 1986).

A coherent body of knowledge begins to emerge. In sum, many preschoolers can infer basic emotions from their expressions or from the situations in which they are elicited, with an earlier emerging understanding of happiness compared to negative emotions (Bassett et al., 2012; Bosacki & Moore, 2004; Bullock & Russell, 1984; Denham & Couchoud, 1990b; Fabes, Eisenberg, et al., 1991; Pons et al., 2004; Sette, Bassett, Baumgartner, & Denham, 2015). Even 2-year-olds are beginning to understand emotions in this manner (Fernández-Sánchez, Quintanilla, & Giménez-Dasí, 2015). Through the rest of the preschool period, children gradually differentiate among the negative emotions of the self and others (e.g., Denham & Couchoud, 1990b). Using emotion language (e.g., reminiscing about family sadness when a pet died) becomes more available to them.

They also begin to identify others' emotions even when they may differ from their own (e.g., realizing that a friend feels sad rather than angry when receiving "time-out" from her preschool teacher; Denham & Couchoud, 1990a). Toward the end of this developmental period, they begin to comprehend the complex dimensions of emotional experiences, such as the possibility of hiding emotions or dissembling, simultaneous emotions, and the waning of emotions over time. They acquire an understanding of display rules and even begin to comprehend some of the underpinnings of the self-conscious and social emotions. Overall preschoolers across many cultures become able to discern their own and others' emotional states, talking about them somewhat fluently, and beginning to understand the more advanced aspects of emotion (Pons et al., 2004; Sawada, 1997; von Salisch & Janke, 2010; see Chapter 5 for elaboration on culture).

Given this broad picture, it is of further importance to conceptualize and organize these various developmental accomplishments in emotion knowledge. Several theoretical models of such change in emotion knowledge have been proposed (e.g., Denham, 1998; Hadwin, Baron-Cohen, Howlin, & Hill, 1996; Pons et al., 2003, 2004). Both Denham's (1998) and Pons and colleagues' (2004) models consist of nine age-related levels. Table 4.1 shows each theory's levels of understanding. Although specific levels and theoretical foci are somewhat different for each of these models, each one is organized to reflect the age-related progress of emotion knowledge from toddlerhood through childhood. Also both models put recognition of emotional

**TABLE 4.1. Theoretical Views of Emotion Knowledge**

| Skill area | Denham (1998) | Pons, Harris, & de Rosnay (2004) |
|---|---|---|
| Recognizing | Level 1 | Level 1 |
| Identifying emotion-eliciting situations | Stereotypical: Level 2<br>Nonstereotypical: Level 5 | Level 2 |
| Inferring the causes and consequences of emotions | Level 3 | n/a |
| Using emotion language | Level 4 | n/a |
| Understanding desire-based emotions | n/a | Level 3 |
| Understanding belief-based emotions | n/a | Level 4 |
| Reminder/time course | n/a | Level 5 |
| Becoming aware of emotion regulation strategies | Level 6 | Level 6 |
| Developing knowledge about display rules | Level 7 | Level 7 |
| Developing knowledge about mixed emotion | Level 8 | Level 8 |
| Developing social and self-conscious/ moral emotions | Level 9 | Level 9 |

expressions at the first level and understanding of situation-based emotions at the next level.[1]

Integrating these theories, I describe the following aspects of emotion knowledge in this chapter. First, there are a series of emotion knowledge skills that Pons and colleagues (2004) refer to as "externally based," plus those that we know occur in 3- to 4-year-olds:

- Labeling emotional expressions, both verbally and nonverbally.
- Identifying emotion-eliciting situations.
- Inferring the causes of emotion-eliciting situations, as well as the consequences of specific persons' emotional responses (e.g., the self, peers, and parents, Denham, 1997; Dunn & Hughes, 1998).
- Using emotion language to describe their own emotional experiences and to clarify those of others.
- Knowing that emotions change with time, but that elements of a new situation may serve as a reminder of the original emotion.
- Becoming able to describe emotion regulation strategies.

Then, in Chapter 5, I discuss the mentalistic aspects of emotion knowledge, such as recognizing that others' emotional experiences can differ from one's own, along with developing a knowledge of display rules, simultaneous emotions, and complex emotions.

Before launching into describing what we know about these emotion knowledge subskills, it is useful to point out that many studies note that overall emotion knowledge changes as children age (usually both in labeling and recognizing expressions and in understanding emotional situations, e.g., Kujawa et al., 2014; Merz et al., 2015; Morgan, Izard, & King, 2010). Facial emotion identification, expression matching, and situation knowledge all increase with age, with pronounced changes between 4- to 5-year-olds and 6- to 7-year-olds.

Development across early childhood for the more comprehensive model of Pons and colleagues (2004), or its more elementary "external" set of skills, has been shown several times (Grazzani & Ornaghi, 2011; Pons et al., 2003, 2004; Voltmer & von Salisch, 2019; von Salisch, Denham, & Koch, 2016; von Salisch, Häenel, & Freund, 2013; Weimer, Sallquist, & Bolnick, 2012). Further, there is documented stability of individual differences between these aspects of emotion knowledge assessed early in the preschool period and later (e.g., between age 3 and 4, Blankson et al., 2013; Lucas-Molina, Quintanilla, Sarmento-Henrique, Martin Barbarro, & Giménez-Dasí, 2020; Merz et al., 2015; O'Brien et al., 2011; or even between age 3 and 6, Brown & Dunn,

[1]Some of Pons et al.'s (2004) levels showed age progressions that were empirically different from their theoretical predictions shown in Table 4.1; here I adhere to their theoretical chronology, *except for* placing the knowledge of emotions' time course earlier, as they uncovered. I also elect to keep desire-based understanding, which they also found to occur earlier than expected, together with its parallel component of belief-based understanding.

1996; Dunn, 1995). Thus the important developmental questions of "what changes?" and "what stays the same?" have found support—early-emerging emotion knowledge increases across age spans during the preschool period but also exhibits clear individual differences, many of which I elaborate upon in Chapters 10 and 11.

## LABELING AND RECOGNIZING EMOTIONAL EXPRESSIONS

To show that they understand emotions and the cultural scripts associated with them, children must first distinguish among and name the common expressions associated with emotional experience. Preschoolers are already somewhat adept at recognizing and labeling emotional expressions and become increasingly skilled over the preschool period. A knowledge of basic emotional expressions is solid by the end of preschool, whether evaluated by expressions that are presented pictorially (e.g., Camras & Allison, 1985; Denham & Couchoud, 1990b), in photographs (Field & Walden, 1982; see Kujawa et al., 2014, who also included a listening task), or in real time (Felleman, Barden, Carlson, Rosenberg, & Masters, 1983). More recently, Pons et al. (2004) found that most 5-year-olds could correctly answer items regarding emotional expressions.

Specifically, preschoolers' abilities to verbally label and nonverbally recognize emotional expressions increase from 2 to 4 years of age (e.g., Denham & Couchoud, 1990b). I developed a contextually valid measure that involved puppets, both to capture children's attention and to embed a realistic situation within ongoing social interaction.[2] Children were first shown four flannel faces on which prototypical emotion expressions of happiness, sadness, anger, and fear were drawn. Our findings with this methodology revealed that 2- through 5-year-olds could point to or name emotional expressions. However, older children identified emotional expressions more accurately than younger ones, and for both groups receptive identification (pointing) exceeded expressive identification (naming).

In a more recent study examining only nonverbal recognition, Pons et al. (2004) have corroborated the ability to identify at least four out of five pictures of happiness, anger, fear, and "just all right" increased from 55% of 3-year-olds, to 75% of 4-year-olds, to 90% of 7-year-olds (see also the age change in emotion labeling and recognition in Downs, Strand, & Cerna, 2007; Salmon et al., 2013; Shin, Krzysik, & Vaughn, 2014; Strand, Downs, & Barbosa-Leiker, 2016). Further, cross-time stability in this aspect of emotion knowledge has been shown (Downs et al., 2007; Strand et al., 2016).

In addition, in my early and subsequent work, recognition of happy expressions was greater than recognition of negative emotions, and verbal labeling of happy and sad expressions exceeded labeling of either anger or fear (see also Bailey Bisson, 2019; Kujawa et al., 2014; Zsido et al., 2021). Other researchers report a similar progression in preschoolers' identification of happy, sad, and angry faces, voices, and faces with voices (Camras & Allison, 1985; Stifter & Fox, 1987). Bailey Bisson (2019) noted an intriguing finding that suggests preschoolers' process of learning emotional expressions accentuates extracting information from others' faces even before they can voluntarily

[2] This measure is known as the Affect Knowledge Test (AKT).

*produce* the same specific emotional expressions or comprehend their emotional situations. This assertion corresponds with viewpoints expressed in Chapter 3, in that voluntary management takes time to emerge, and preschoolers' repertoire of emotions (and presumably the variety of situational experiences they can take in) becomes more complex over time.

The comprehension of both emotional situations and attendant facial expressions follows a similar developmental trajectory. The first distinction learned about both facial expressions and emotional situations is one between being happy and not happy or feeling good versus feeling bad or sad (Bullock & Russell, 1984, 1985, 1986; Grosse, Streubel, Gunzenhauser, & Sallbach, 2021; Widen & Russell, 2008). An understanding of anger and fear then later emerges from the not happy/sad category. Recent research corroborates preschoolers' accuracy in verbally identifying facial expressions and situations in the following order: happy, sad, angry, afraid, disgusted, and surprised (Bailey Bisson, 2019; Weimer et al., 2012; Widen & Russell, 2004, 2010a; Zsido et al., 2021; see also Kujawa et al., 2014, for a similar order in which, however, anger accuracy was greater than sadness accuracy).

So my early research highlighted a specific difficulty that others have upheld: Preschoolers often confuse negative emotions; Bullock and Russell too find "fuzzy borders" for negative emotion concepts (see also Widen & Russell, 2010a, 2010c, and Matthews, Thierry, & Mondloch, 2022, who documented preschoolers' specific confusions in sorting photos of sad, fearful, angry, and disgusted faces). Matthews et al. (2020), in agreement with Widen and Russell, suggest that adding emotion labels to their vocabulary helps preschoolers refine their early emerging categories to exclude exemplars of other emotions; for example, once children could correctly label a fearful face, they rarely confused sad and fearful faces. In any case, young children's initial categories of emotion also are broader than those of adults. This is so even though children and adults usually share similar sets of central defining characteristics for each basic emotion. What differs is that young children's categories include more peripheral concepts.

One likely foundation for the progression in understanding happy versus not happy/angry/fearful expressions is a perceptual one that involves the salience of the mouth (Cunningham & Odom, 1986). Kindergartners were shown facial photographs of an unfamiliar adult expressing anger, disgust, fear, joy, and shame. Recall of the photos was cued by probe photographs that varied in how the mouth, eyes, or nose was presented. Children remembered expressive information from the mouth region first, the eye region second, and the nose region last.

The happy–not happy distinction was identified by mouth expressions, which were the most salient feature isolated in this study. Eye region differences, the next most salient, differentiated among sadness, anger, and fear. Thus it is reasonable that young children first differentiate an emotion whose prominent feature is the mouth—happiness. This initial learning involving one part of the face is followed by emotional expressions for the negative emotions, which differ with respect to the eye region, while also involving the mouth region (Bailey Bisson, 2019). In sum, the progression of comprehending happy expressions first and gradually teasing apart the various negative expressions is well substantiated for both emotion faces and situations and occurs between 3½ and 4 years of age for freely produced labels of emotions (Widen & Russell, 2010c).

There may be specific reasons preschoolers have difficulty differentiating particular negative emotions (Camras & Allison, 1985). When preschoolers were given verbal labels or facial expressions to identify the emotions depicted in stories, they were more likely to be accurate in identifying fear and disgust if allowed to pick among verbal labels as opposed to facial expressions. More recently, Widen and Russell (2004, 2010a) also found that preschoolers were better able to identify fear and disgust if they were told stories rather than shown expressions.

Why would these emotions' expressions be so hard to discern? Young children do have a lot of confusion regarding the expression of disgust, and often confuse its expression with that of anger; similar confusion exists between fear and surprise (Gagnon, Gosselin, Hudon-van der Buhs, Larocque, & Milliard, 2010; Gosselin & Simard, 1999). The perceptual argument already introduced seems supported for both disgust and fear, in that they each share with other emotions several similarities in anatomical and visual qualities, especially in the eye region. Further, perhaps children see very little visual evidence of fear or disgust in their environments but have been taught about them verbally. Learning the nonverbal identification of fear and disgust can be especially difficult because these emotional expressions also may be more fleeting (Bailey Bisson, 2019). Moreover, mothers of toddlers are less likely to label disgust expressions while looking at a picture book than they are to elaborate upon and ask questions about the behaviors and context associated with disgust (Ruba, Kalia, & Wilbourn, 2022).

Methodology also needs to be considered. When asked to point to an expression most like a target (i.e., not requiring oral language), 5- and 6- year-olds were able to discriminate fear and disgust from other emotions (Gagnon et al., 2010). Gagnon and colleagues note that, given this finding and these older preschoolers' overall accuracy, it is unlikely that visual perception is the only limiting factor for their ability to discriminate.

Several important factors are involved in integrating these sources of information, each of which can play a role in the developmental progression of preschoolers' emotional expression knowledge and its assessment. These factors include children's abilities to distinguish configurations of facial features across emotions, as well as to discriminate low frequency or short-duration emotions. Mothers of toddlers also give less specific tutelage about disgust than about other emotions. Additionally, receptive language can facilitate the conceptual foundation for expression knowledge, but requiring expressive language in methodology may create an artificial difficulty.

Five-year-old Erica sees her mother take a sip from a glass of milk and make a face. Her younger sister, Lauren, asks, "Mommy, what's the matter? Are you mad?," and Erica says, "She's not mad at us. The milk is yucky." She understood the expression even though she couldn't have accurately named it.

All in all, this learning of facial expressions seems to be quite a tall order. But as young children become increasingly able to discern important differences among expressions of emotions, the differentiation becomes a vital component of their overall emotion knowledge. Comprehension of emotional expressions can be seen as the perceptual bedrock for further understanding of emotions; indeed, it has been seen as providing a "toehold" that affords children a basis for interpreting and responding to emotions in their social world (Izard et al., 2011; Strand et al., 2016). This theoretical notion has been upheld by the recent cross-sectional results which indicated emotion recognition contributing to emotion situation knowledge in the United States, Italy, and Switzerland (Barisnikov, Theurel, & Lejeune, 2022; Bassett et al., 2012; Sette et al., 2015). As such, it stands preschoolers in good stead, giving them an initial ability to think and talk about emotional issues, including their eliciting situations.

In fact, these findings on the importance of emotion expression recognition are related to part of the constructivist theoretical argument that emotions depend upon conceptual foundations, which are largely verbal (Hoemann et al., 2019). Earlier research from this perspective had suggested a "facial inferiority effect" (Russell & Widen, 2002; Widen & Russell, 2004, 2008, 2010a), in which emotion knowledge, as evidenced by young children's abilities to generate accurate verbal emotion labels, emanated from increasing conceptual differentiation. These authors suggest that this concept building consisted of children creating narrative scripts based on the emotion label, rather than relying on configural differences among facial expressions. It does seem true that young children gradually differentiate both expressions and situations and that creating narrative linguistic scripts based on each emotion's causes and behavioral consequences are likely to promote this development (Widen & Russell, 2004, 2010a).[3]

However, I believe, and more recent research supports, that discrete emotions theory, which holds that facial expression of emotion is the bedrock for differentiating emotions, and constructivist theory, which focuses strongly on conceptual and linguistic differentiation of emotions across development, can each explain *part* of the development of emotion knowledge. To elucidate this theoretical synthesis, developmental change in the way emotion knowledge is structured must be considered.

Thus, Widen and Russell (2010c) have found that *older* preschool children make better use of stories about emotions' causes and consequences to generate correctly differentiated emotion labels (like the 5- and 6-year-olds whose receptive language supported expression differentiation in Gagnon et al., 2010). In comparison, *younger* preschoolers (e.g., 3-year-olds and younger) were more correct labelers when given facial expressions as prompts (see also Giménez-Dasí, Quintanilla, & Lucas-Molina, 2018).

Going even further, Strand et al. (2016) examined these possibilities longitudinally, examining relations among receptive vocabulary, emotion expression recognition, and emotional perspective-taking (i.e., situation knowledge based on desires and

---

[3]It is important to note methodologically that almost all the studies concluding that preschoolers show a "facial inferiority effect" required the participant to use language that either (1) labeled faces and situation stimuli or (2) showed a facial expression and asked why the protagonist feels this way. Using largely verbal response requirements to support the constructivist theory that promotes narrative, language-based emotional concept development seems a bit like "stacking the deck." However, many findings in this chapter describe how important language is to emotion knowledge, so there is a large kernel of truth here.

beliefs) in 36- to 67-month-olds across a 24-week period. For the younger group (36- to 48-month-olds), time 1 emotion expression recognition predicted time 2 emotional perspective taking, supporting discrete emotions theory. For the older group (49- to 67-month-olds), results instead supported the constructivist viewpoint, in that there was an interdependence between language and emotion knowledge development: time 1 receptive vocabulary predicted time 2 emotional perspective-taking, and vice versa. Furthermore, time 1 emotion recognition also predicted time 2 emotional perspective taking, even for the older group. These results suggest a transactional process that unites both discrete emotion and constructivist theories—emotion expression recognition *does* provide a "toehold" for younger preschoolers' emotion situation knowledge, and then, as language development proliferates, older preschoolers' verbal ability and both aspects of emotion knowledge are interdependent.

### SUMMARY: Labeling and Identifying Emotional Expressions

Developmental changes in preschoolers' knowledge of facial expressions of emotions start with an understanding of happiness, followed by a slow separation of negative emotions throughout the preschool period. These changes are related to the different configuration of facial features for different emotions, as well as to their frequency and duration, and the creation of linguistic concepts. Finally, expression knowledge is a central support for knowledge of emotional situations, to which I now turn.

## IDENTIFYING EMOTION-ELICITING SITUATIONS

As is no doubt already clear from my remarks, emotional expressions and their elicitors are inextricably intertwined, and both are vital components of emotional experience (Lewis & Michalson, 1983). To be able to comprehend their own or others' emotions, children must become familiar with and recognize not only the basic expressions of emotions, but also their common eliciting situations. Overall, understanding of the causal factors in emotional situations improves within the preschool period (e.g., Downs et al., 2007; Salmon et al., 2013; Strand et al., 2016 [although Strand et al.'s situation/perspective taking measure included stories about desire- and belief-based, as well as normative, emotional situations]). Additionally, individual differences in understanding emotional situations show stability over time (Downs et al., 2007; Strand et al., 2016).

In general, as already noted, a developmental progression similar to that for perceiving and labeling emotional expressions exists for comprehending the common situations for basic emotions. As with the identification of expressions, happy and sad situations are easiest for children to interpret, whereas incorrect responses, such as "sad" or "don't know" errors, occur often for other negative emotions (Denham & Couchoud, 1990b; Fabes et al., 1991).

Young children first differentiate situations they call "happy" from those they call "not happy" or "sad," then begin to distinguish "angry" situations. In my studies, children eagerly and easily fasten the happy face on the puppet who is receiving ice cream or going to the zoo. Clearly, these acts mirror their own delight in experiencing these situations. Interestingly, many of the youngest children tend to use the sad face for all the negative situations—being left by a sibling who wants to play with someone else, having to eat a disliked food, or having a block construction destroyed. Little by little, however, children clearly distinguish angry situations from sad ones.

Fear expressions present preschool children with the most difficulty not only in accurate identification, but also in situation comprehension (Brody & Harrison, 1987). As with fear expressions, difficulty in understanding fear elicitors has many causes. Again the reasons include the complex brow/eye/mouth movements in the facial expression of fear and the infrequency of children's exposure to peak fear expressions, and in this case the idiosyncratic views preschoolers have of fear's causes (Denham & Zoller, 1991; Strayer, 1986). Young children talk eloquently about such causes of fear as monsters, witches, darkness, and masks (Lieberman, 1993). In contrast, they refer far less frequently to more common, reality-based fear-producing experiences, such as falling while learning to ride a bicycle. They often include these situations with sadness-inducing ones, suggesting that they know fear-eliciting events are negative; however, they seem unable or unwilling to acknowledge the potential harm involved.

### SUMMARY: Identifying Emotional Situations

Thus young children over time understand more about the common eliciting situations for basic emotions—a vital component of their overall understanding. The trend of comprehending happy situations followed by understanding sad, then angry, and finally fearful situations is clear. Understanding these basic emotions is particularly adaptive for preschoolers because, at least for the first three, they witness and experience vivid, clear demonstrations of these very feelings (see Chapter 2). Indeed, a preschool boy may experience many emotions in a day—great joy when his best friend brings in his puppy for "show and tell"; sadness when another peer tells him, "You can't play"; and finally anger when his mother comes to take him home before he is ready. But young children go even further than recognizing the expressions and eliciting situations for basic emotions. They make more complex attributions about emotions' causes, and reason more intricately about their implications for behavior.

## COMPREHENDING CAUSES AND CONSEQUENCES OF EMOTIONS

Young children begin to use the contextual information found in their everyday experiences to figure out why happiness, sadness, and anger occur. As with other aspects of emotion knowledge, children's abilities to demonstrate an understanding of the causes of emotions increases across early childhood (Denham, Zoller, & Couchoud, 1994; Lagattuta & Wellman, 2002; Salmon et al., 2013; Shin et al., 2014; Weimer et al., 2012). They elaborate upon their early understanding of basic emotional situations to create more intricate scenarios depicting specific persons' particular feelings (Dunn & Hughes, 1998). Their explanations are particularly accurate when interpersonal and environmental event themes are involved: "Getting hit makes me angry," "Going to the playground makes me happy." Young children also realize the consequences of an emotion; for instance, a securely attached 3-year-old girl knows that a parent will comfort her when she is upset. Clearly, knowing why an emotion is expressed and what its aftermath is likely to be aids a child in learning to regulate the behavior and emotion of herself and others. I now detail these important abilities, with particular emphasis on understanding the emotions of the self, their peers, and their family.

## Comprehending Causes of Specific Emotions

Preschoolers' understanding of the causes of emotion is impressive, particularly when their knowledge is compared with that of toddlers. They form reasonably coherent, internally consistent categories of emotion–situation linkages describing the lives of themselves, their peers, and their parents. Although these linkages often correspond at least broadly to the causal understandings of older children and adults, there are distinct differences. Young preschoolers' notions about the causes of emotions may not specifically match those of adults. Sometimes 3-year-olds, but not 4- and 5-year-olds, give idiosyncratic reasons for emotions, such as "I was sad when we had snack," "I was scared about the lost baby in the forest," or "I was angry because I get angry" (Curenton & Wilson, 2003; Denham & Zoller, 1991; Fabes et al., 1991; Strayer, 1986). Some of these idiosyncratic reasons make good sense phenomenologically when the situation is analyzed in detail. For instance, the child who claimed she was sad when a snack was served had in fact disliked the day's offering, and being scared about a lost baby in the forest was a response to a fairy tale that her mother had just read.

Older preschoolers, especially, go further than just recognizing expressions and eliciting situations for discrete emotions. Using everyday experiences to create theories about the causes of happiness, sadness, and anger, they cite causes that are similar to ones given by adults (Fabes et al., 1991; Lagattuta & Wellman, 2002). Jessica notes that her brother gets mad because he doesn't want to go to school, but that Daddy is happy to go to work.

Clearly, preschoolers are acquiring a foundation of knowledge in this area; in fact, Pons et al. (2004) found that by age 7 all children in their study could discern the causes of emotions. This budding awareness of the individuality of emotional experience makes it important to examine the contributions made by different people to preschoolers' emotion knowledge (see Chapters 7 through 9). Obviously, young children glean unique information about emotions from their own experiences and those of others. Varied sources of emotional understanding add to children's accumulating information.

### *What Causes One's Own Emotions?*

Over the course of the preschool period, young children begin to realize that the causes of an emotion can vary, depending on who is experiencing it, and that potential elicitors have uniquely individual effects. One child is saddened by seeing her mother leave for work, but another becomes sad when someone wrecks his Legos. Vegetables for dinner make one child happy, whereas another registers disgust (see "Use of Personalized Information," Chapter 5).

As they develop, preschoolers can talk about what would make them happy, sad, angry, and afraid, especially when encouraged to do so within the context of play. For example, when an examiner says, "This puppet is so-oo sad . . . Let's pretend it is you. What would make you feel this way?," children often identify with the puppet (Denham & Zoller, 1991). Their conceptions of the causes of their own emotions are more complete than those they give for either peers or parents (Dunn & Hughes, 1998). They ascribe different causes to different emotions as well; their responses are not random across emotions.

Thus in my research I have found that children often cite nonsocial events for their happiness, such as playing with toys; social causes for their sadness and anger, such as wanting Mom and being punched, respectively; and fantasy causes for their fear, such as seeing a dinosaur. These results are largely consonant with those of Strayer's (1986) investigation, although we have studied even younger children within the preschool age range. Further, children talk about the causes of emotions as early as 2 years old. For example, when talking with parents about personal experiences, they provide more causes for negative than for positive emotions (Lagattuta & Wellman, 2002). Negative emotions are likely to be more compelling, requiring thought and explanation.

### *What Causes Peers' Emotions?*

Preschoolers also have been interviewed about their peers' naturally occurring emotions (Dunn & Hughes, 1998; Fabes et al., 1988, 1991). As with their own emotions, young children can perceive and report on a variety of causes for peers' emotions. They refer to social, nonsocial, and internal causes for displays of happiness, sadness, anger, and distress. For example, nonsocial reasons for happiness, sadness, and anger, respectively, include "A sunny day," "Something is broken," and "Not getting to watch TV." In contrast, social reasons given for these same emotions include "Playing with friends/by myself," "Her dad spanks her," and "Someone doesn't do what he wants," respectively. Importantly, the causes given for their peers' emotions often parallel those given by adults who also have witnessed the peers' displays (Fabes et al., 1988). Thus both children and adults rely on context—namely, events that are taking place—to accurately determine the causes of others' anger and distress.

Children, like adults, also are sensitive to internal causes of others' emotions (see also Stein & Trabasso, 1989). In fact, when intense emotions are displayed, children are more likely to focus on internal factors associated with the target child's goals. In describing the cause of a peer's intense anger, a preschooler says, "He wanted his block tower to stay up," instead of "She knocked down his block tower."

Even more important, preschoolers focus on different causes for their peers' differing emotions (Denham & Zoller, 1991; Fabes et al., 1988). Children most often supply social reasons for anger, sadness, and distress or pain; older preschoolers more likely to do so than younger ones (Curenton & Wilson, 2003). Physical and material interactions with other people, such as being punched or having a toy taken away, are often noted. This finding is not surprising given the frequency of conflict in peer play.

It is understandable that preschoolers may cite similar themes and persons as causes for anger and sadness (although some researchers report more differentiated responses; see Dunn & Hughes, 1998). Both emotions can result from the same events, with anger evolving from a focus on the other person's obstructing one's goal, and sadness from a more solitary focus on the unachieved goal state (Fabes et al., 1988). In fact, this complementarity of goal states may be one reason that sadness and anger comprehension in general takes time for preschoolers to differentiate, as already noted.

When giving social causes with respect to happiness, preschoolers often give social physical, verbal, and nonverbal causes, such as being tickled, getting a compliment, or making a funny face, respectively. But they also cite impersonal contexts to explain happiness, such as having a big playroom full of toys (Strayer, 1986). Young children do find it trickier to come up with causes of peers' happiness and sadness than to identify causes of their anger or distress/pain. In fact, even though young children are most accurate in identifying the *existence* of happiness, they are least accurate in identifying its *causes* (Curenton & Wilson, 2003). Thus most findings suggest, like the causes they give for their own emotions, that preschoolers are more successful in identifying the causes of others' negative emotions than of their positive emotions (Dunn & Hughes, 1998; Fabes et al., 1991; Lagattuta & Wellman, 2002). And among the negative emotions, sadness is more difficult for them to identify than anger or undifferentiated distress.

Why might these difficulties exist? Perhaps others' happiness and sadness can be less powerful and salient than their anger and distress. A peer's smile, or a friend's tears as he or she huddles alone, are undeniably powerful social communicators; most preschoolers would be able to identify the feelings expressed. But a response to these emotions is not almost mandatory, as it is to a friend who pushes another in anger, or to a child who falls off the jungle gym and screams in pain. Others' anger and distress may produce more threatening and adverse consequences, so that it is adaptive for children to be more attentive to and concerned with these emotions and especially their causes. Moreover, peers' happiness and sadness also may have more abstract, complex causes than their anger and distress because they are more often internally caused (Fabes et al., 1991). Thus it may not be surprising that causes given by preschoolers for their peers' anger and distress are more sophisticated than those for happiness and sadness.

To reiterate, children become more able to understand the causal complexities of emotion throughout the preschool period, and they start to focus on others' emotions later in this time frame. Through their increased social sensitivity and experience, older preschoolers are also developing more complex strategies for appraising others' emotions when available cues are less salient and consensual. Five-year-olds are more likely than 3- and 4-year-olds to focus their explanations of emotions on personal dispositions as opposed to goal states: "She had a bad day," instead of "She didn't want Billy to play with her." Obviously, also aspects of such reasoning can be very useful in actual interaction with friends. I address this important corollary of preschoolers' growing understanding of emotions more comprehensively in Chapter 10.

### *What Causes Parents' Emotions?*

Over and above the unique emotional information that different relationship partners provide, the very nature of the parent–child relationship puts a spotlight on parents' emotions. Not only are parents' emotional displays ubiquitous in children's daily lives

(Patterson, 1980), but children are also motivated to understand feelings in such an important relationship. Parents are special social partners: They are in a position of authority, so that children are likely to attend to their emotions and want to please them. At the same time, parents tend to be clear and emphatic in their displays of emotions around their children for both strategic and didactic reasons. Parents' emotions also are likely to differ in some important ways from those of peers and of children themselves. Consequently, children learn a great deal about the causes and consequences of emotions from their parents (see Chapter 8).

Children ages 4 and 5 can demonstrate a coherent understanding of the differing causes for parental happiness, sadness, and anger. Children assessed via their play actions and verbalizations during a semistructured dollhouse play interview do not see themselves as causing most parental emotions (Denham, 1996a; see also Dunn & Hughes, 1998, for a conversation-based methodology). Methodology may be particularly important in teasing out preschoolers' actual competence in this area. At play or in conversation with someone they know well they may be able to demonstrate comprehension of a variety of circumstances and events that could cause their parents' emotions, in contrast with the difficulty they have when assessed with predominantly verbal, more abstract, procedures (as in Covell & Abramovitch, 1987, 1988).

The overall pattern of our research findings is qualified, however. First, preschoolers, especially 3-year-olds, still have a good bit of difficulty specifying causes of parental sadness and anger; about 30% of all preschool participants give no causes or uncodable ones (compared to 40% "don't know" responses from 4- to 5-year-olds on Dunn & Hughes's [1998] verbal measure). Second, preschoolers, especially boys, do see themselves as causing the emotions of their mothers, but not their fathers. Given the sometimes confrontational and sometimes lighthearted nature of children's interactions with their mothers, this assumption on their part is not entirely egocentric. Preschoolers *do* cause a lot of happiness, anger, and distress for their mothers!

In general, however, young children can give some specific causes for specific parental emotions. Their causal conceptions are well articulated and even poignant, corresponding with culturally understood scenarios. They are often able to enumerate causes that can be put into categories, as they do for their own and their peers' emotions—social and nonsocial physical, social control, social verbal, social and nonsocial material, and nonsocial events. Table 4.2 depicts some of their descriptions. Most also dovetail with causes of their own emotions given by children in other studies (e.g., Covell & Abramovitch, 1987; Dunn & Hughes, 1998).

## **SUMMARY:** Causes of Emotions

Thus young children are processing even relatively fine nuances about the emotion–event linkages in their daily lives. Although the categories children use to understand their own, their peers', and their parents' emotions are similar, the actual content of the scenarios they describe for each group often differ. They say, "He's feeling mean," or "Daddy yelled at her," to describe a parent's anger. In contrast, they say, "Billy took Mike's Power Ranger," or "My brother called me names, and Mommy said I couldn't hit him," to talk about themselves or their peers. Moreover, as might be expected, their explanations of the causes of emotions are most adequate when referring to themselves rather than to their peers or parents (Dunn & Hughes, 1998). These distinctions amid similarities prompt a search for the logical foundations of young children's solid understanding of emotions.

Further, older preschoolers' descriptions of the causes of emotions are becoming more abstract. Younger preschoolers, like their older counterparts, also are learning to understand the causes of emotions with respect to goal states, but they also cite more apparently idiosyncratic cases (Fabes et al., 1991). Finally, although both girls and boys develop an understanding of the causes of emotions during the preschool years, they sometimes have differing foci. Girls sometimes cite more interpersonal causes of emotion, presumably because of their experience in relationships and their reasoning about the social world (Fabes et al., 1988; Strayer, 1986).

| **TABLE 4.2. Examples of Children's Conceptions of the Causes of Their Emotions** |
|---|
| ***Causes of happiness*** |
| *Social nonverbal:* "Neighbors moved in," "The boy's cleaning up the mess," "I love him." |
| *Social verbal:* "I told him something funny," "Mommy says 'I love you.' " |
| *Nonsocial events:* "She took a nice bath," "She likes cooking dinner." |
| *Social physical:* "Because I gave her a kiss, a hug," "I tickled his back." |
| *Social control:* "Because I didn't bother her," "Because I eat all my supper." |
| *Social material:* "How about we go to the store and buy Mom stockings! Yeah! Buy her high-heeled shoes!" |
| *Nonsocial material:* "She has a teddy bear," "He has lots of candy." |
| ***Causes of sadness*** |
| *Nonsocial physical:* "He fell down," "She fell off the roof," "She wants a baby." |
| *Social physical:* "Someone hit her," "I kicked him," "I fell down." |
| *Social nonverbal:* "When a stranger comes," "Daddy's/Mommy's angry." |
| *Nonsocial material:* "Something broke," "The sink won't work," "We have no sandwich." |
| *Nonsocial events:* "Maybe he got in jail," "Because she had to move to a new house." |
| ***Causes of anger*** |
| *Social verbal:* "They're fighting over whose turn it was to cook dinner." |
| *Social control:* "Because I ran away," "Because I go to bed with gum in my mouth." |
| *Social physical/internal:* "Brother hit sister," "I spanked him," "Daddy pushed Mom." |
| *Nonsocial physical/internal:* "He's feeling mean," "He's had a bad day," "Maybe she sat on wet paint." |
| *Nonsocial events:* "He drove to the zoo and back and got mad at everybody," "She almost got run over." |
| *Note.* From Denham (1996a). |

## Understanding the Consequences of Emotions

Another aspect of preschoolers' emotion knowledge is their understanding of the consequences of different emotions. Children use such recognition of the consequences of emotions in their behavioral decision making, just as they use their comprehension of the causes of emotions; and, as with the other "external" emotion knowledge skills (to use Pons et al.'s [2004] theoretical demarcation), this ability increases with age; Lagattuta and Wellman (2002) found that children's descriptions of the consequences of emotions increased between age 3 and 5.

Discerning the consequences of emotion can help a child know what to do in social situations, such as "How do I respond when my friend is mad?" In fact, an understanding of the outcomes of their own emotions, and the reactions of others, may form the substrate of preschoolers' responses to emotions in general (whether sympathetic or insensitive). Despite this potential importance, this topic has not received as much attention as preschoolers' knowledge of the *causes* of emotion. This lack is somewhat curious, as this thinking could be pivotal in emotion-related social information processing (Lemerise & Arsenio, 2000).

In any case, preschoolers can distinguish the causes of emotions from their consequences when completing stories about why a protagonist felt an emotion and what the protagonist did as a result (Russell, 1990). What *do* people do as a consequence of someone else's emotions? I asked 4- and 5-year-olds to enact dollhouse vignettes depicting the consequences of the children's own emotions (Denham, 1997). Children attributed plausible, nonrandom parental reactions to their own emotions. They saw their parents as matching their own happiness or reacting in an irrelevant way to it; performing pragmatic action after sadness or punishing a sibling who caused it; punishing anger; and comforting, acting to alleviate, or discussing a fear-eliciting stimulus. Parents were seen as unlikely to comfort happiness, to perform pragmatic helpful action after anger, to punish happiness or fear, or to match any negative emotion.

They can also tell the difference between the causes of parental emotions and the subsequent actions of parents when they felt happy, sad, or angry (Denham, 1996a). Table 4.3 depicts examples of their explanations of the consequences of their parents' emotions. Clearly, preschoolers hold some quite accurate ideas about

**TABLE 4.3. Examples of Children's Conceptions of the Consequences of Their Parents' Emotions**

| |
|---|
| ***Means of expressing happiness*** |
| *Shared activities:* "He dances," "She makes a pie," "She would buy things for us." |
| ***Means of expressing sadness*** |
| *Withdrawal:* "He goes to sleep," "She lays in her bed."<br>*Other:* "She went to the doctor," "Daddy wants a new kid." |
| ***Means of expressing anger*** |
| *Negative expression:* "She goes and breaks all the furniture," "He gives spankings," "Daddy goes out the door, bye-bye, and SLAM!" |
| *Note.* From Denham (1996a). |

the behavioral consequences of emotion—what people do when they experience different emotions.

### SUMMARY: Consequences of Emotions

Taken together, my investigations suggest that preschoolers have solid conceptions of how even adults behave after experiencing their own emotional arousal and of the specific responsiveness of caregivers to child emotions. So they are beginning to understand the behavioral consequences of emotions for both themselves and others. Children who understand what happens when emotions are experienced are better equipped to regulate their own emotions and react to those of others; I consider preschoolers' understanding of emotion regulatory strategies in a later section. Before presenting those ideas, however, it would be important to understand whether preschoolers could comprehend that being reminded of an emotion could trigger it again, even after the passage of time, the next step in the increasingly complex aspects of emotion knowledge put forward in Table 4.1.

## UNDERSTANDING REMINDERS OF EMOTION

In one study (Lagattuta, Wellman, & Flavell, 1997), 3- to 6-year-olds were able to demonstrate that environmental cues can prompt memories of past emotions and thus influence current emotions. For example, if a dog previously chased away the rabbit belonging to the protagonist in a story, seeing the dog later could remind the protagonist of the lost rabbit and trigger sadness (6-year-olds even understood how seeing a *similar* dog could evoke past feelings). Further, even 3-year-olds could explain why a protagonist felt happy, sad, or angry by linking past events with current emotions (Lagattuta & Wellman, 2001). Similarly, Pons et al. (2004) also found that children, including nearly half of 3-year-olds and 80% of 5-year-olds, were aware that thinking about past events can influence current emotions.

Findings about preschoolers' awareness of how memories of emotions can reawaken them may be more complicated. That is, children during the preschool period have trouble understanding that a protagonist in a negative emotional state could be reminded of a positive emotion and feel better (Lagattuta & Wellman, 2001). In fact, one preschooler said that one would need to be a "professional, adult mystery spy" (Lagattuta, 2014, p. 91) to figure this out. This lag has implications for understanding emotion regulation strategies (see later in this chapter); it is supported by evidence that adult socializers more often talk about negative emotions than positive ones with young children (Lagattuta, 2014; see Chapter 8).

Nonetheless, it also is true that, rather surprisingly, preschoolers also can imagine that emotions can be caused by imagining possible occurrences—worrying (Lagattuta, 2007). That is, almost all 4-year-olds, and some 3-year-olds, could explain that a protagonist felt worried because of thinking that something bad would or could happen. Four- to 5-year-olds expected the protagonist to feel worried when being reminded of past harm when encountering similar people or animals. In short, the idea that reminders can change emotion is evolving during early childhood.

## USING EMOTION LANGUAGE

### Development in Patterns of Emotion Language Use

Many of young children's initial understandings about emotions can be seen in their emotional vocabulary. Young children do converse about emotions, although such conversation is a small portion of their entire discourse (Lagattuta & Wellman, 2002). They show substantial ability to use emotion-descriptive adjectives and to understand these terms when used by adults (Bretherton et al., 1986; Ridgeway & Kuczaj, 1985). Even very young children refer to internal emotional states (e.g., distress, pain, joy, anger) and to their causes and consequences. During their second and third years, toddlers begin to employ emotion language to influence others to meet their own emotional needs (Dunn, Brown, & Beardsall, 1991). They use emotion words to obtain comfort, support, or attention ("I cried in bed"); to express pleasure or affection ("Give me a kiss! I love you!"); to maintain a happy state ("I like this merry-go-round!"); or to anticipate, achieve, or avoid other affective states ("No *Jurassic Park* movie; too scary").

Thus, over 75% of 3-year-old children use terms for feeling good, happy, sad, afraid, angry, loving, mean, and surprised (Ridgeway & Kuczaj, 1985). By the end of the preschool period, over 75% of 6-year-olds also use terms for feeling comfortable, excited, upset, glad, unhappy, relaxed, bored, lonely, annoyed, disappointed, shy, pleased, worried, calm, embarrassed, hating, nervous, and cheerful (Ridgeway & Kuczaj, 1985). Finally, although kindergartners produce fewer synonyms for emotion words than grade school children do, they give similar proportions of synonyms across all emotions (i.e., the largest variety of terms for happiness and sadness, and the fewest for guilt and pride; Whissell & Nicholson, 1991). Again, preschoolers show substantial understanding of emotion.

Preschoolers test and refine these understandings of emotional expressions, situations, causes, and consequences while talking with important persons in their lives. Emotion language "provides children with an especially powerful tool for understanding emotions" (Kopp, 1989, p. 349). They state their own feelings to people who need to know about them, obtain these persons' feedback about these feelings, and process causal associations between events and emotions.

> When Anson says, "I hate it when Daniel hits me all the time. It makes me really mad," his mother can sympathize and tell him it sounds as if he is justifiably offended. When he next asserts, in a puzzled voice, "But I don't know why he hits me. He's never mad," his mother is then able to point out that Daniel indeed sounds unpredictable, and to help him decide what to do. Perhaps in his next encounter with Daniel, Anson can use emotion language directly in interpersonal negotiation to get the problem solved.

It also is important, however, to note that preschoolers' emotion vocabulary is much more concrete that older children's and adults' (Nook et al., 2020). They tend to describe emotions by providing examples of situations in which the emotion, or the physiological feeling of the emotion, occurs, rather than using the more abstract synonyms that older children and adults use. Of course, this makes sense given what we know about their emerging comprehension of emotional expressions, situations, causes, and consequences. In addition, 4- and 5-year-olds' emotional vocabulary is both smaller and not as deep as that of even 6- through 9-year-olds (Streubel, Gunzenhauser, Grosse, & Saalbach, 2020; see also Grosse et al., 2021).

Nonetheless, their recognition of emotional expressions and knowledge of emotion regulation strategies were both related to the size of their emotion vocabulary (see also Raikes & Thompson, 2006, who found that the number of emotion words used by 3-year-olds in conversation with their mothers was related to overall emotion knowledge). So these more concrete uses of emotion language appear to be good building blocks for growing emotion knowledge. As noted by Grosse et al. (2021), language allows for representations that children can store, allowing then access to culture-specific features and boundaries of emotion categories, as well as the causes, consequences, and regulatory strategies for emotions. Language facilitates their ability to conceptually connect emotions' bodily sensations, facial expressions, and possible situational causes. Preschoolers make good use of this developing emotion language with their family.

## Using Emotion Language within the Family

As the previous example of Anson and his mother suggests, young children do not construct their vocabulary of emotion in a nonsocial vacuum; other people participate. Over time, preschoolers have conversations about emotions with parents, grandparents, other caregivers, siblings, and peers (Bretherton & Beeghly, 1982; Bretherton et al., 1986; Howe, 1991; Shatz, 1994). Parental verbalizations about emotions undoubtedly assist young children in learning about expressing and understanding emotions. Individual differences in mothers' usage of emotion language in its various functions give children unique understandings about emotion. (See Chapters 7 and 8 for an extended discussion of especially mothers' contribution to young children's use of emotion language within the family.)

Developmental changes can be discerned in the content and context of young children's usage of emotion language in the family (Brown & Dunn, 1991, 1992). Dunn and her associates have observed naturally occurring conversations about feelings between mothers and their 18- to 36-month-old children (Brown & Dunn, 1991, 1992; Dunn et al., 1987; Dunn & Munn, 1985). Children are not passive participants in such conversations. Between 24 and 36 months of age (Brown & Dunn, 1991), children already refer to emotions. The content and context of emotion discourse both change—as toddlers near their third birthday, they begin to use emotion language in reflective discussions. These discussions especially center on (1) the causes and consequences of emotions ("I miss Mom-Mom, I get sad"); (2) manipulating the feelings and behaviors of others ("Talk nice, Mommy, don't be so mad"); and (3) even teasing (R: "I'm going to eat you all up! And I'll tell Grandpa you died." G: "You will! And will he be happy or sad?" R: "Sad."; Shatz, 1994). Further, emotion language used with parents continues to increase with age from 3- to 5-years-old (Fabes, Eisenberg, Hanish, & Spinrad, 2001; Lagattuta & Wellman, 2002; Melzi & Fernández, 2004).

Thus young children and their mothers, who admittedly are the most often studied conversation partners, use emotion language to fulfill a variety of functions. These linguistic functions include socialization (i.e., imparting rules, like "Big kids don't cry"), explaining, guiding behavior (e.g., "Stop yelling!"), and questioning (Bretherton et al., 1986). When 3- and 4-year-olds talked with their mothers about photographs of infants expressing peak emotional expressions, they averaged almost one emotion term per photo (Denham, Cook, & Zoller, 1992); in other free discussions of emotional experiences, children from age 3 to 5 averaged from one-to-five emotion terms (Cervantes & Callanan, 1998; Melzi & Fernández, 2004).

The linguistic function of children's emotion language was not simply to comment on the pictures ("He's crying"), although this function often predominates in their conversations (Cervantes & Callanan, 1998; Denham & Auerbach, 1995). In our work, which has included talking about photos of babies showing peak emotional expressions, discussing an emotion-laden picture book, and reminiscing about personal emotional events, the preschoolers also used emotion words to explain causes ("She's happy because she likes her mom"), to infer consequences ("If you were sad, I would ask Daddy to hug you"), to ask questions about the infants' emotions ("He's making a sad face—what's the matter?"), and to guide another's behavior ("He's sad, he needs his mommy"). The variety of linguistic functions young children use in their conversations is testimony to their motivation to discuss emotional issues and to their considerable body of knowledge about emotion.

There are, however, clear patterns of usage in this early emotion language, in both parent–child and peer–peer emotion-related discussions. In general, young children refer to emotions, as early as age 2 years, in the present tense (Fabes et al., 2001; Lagattuta & Wellman, 2002). With parents, they mostly refer to negative emotions, especially their own; when they do use the past tense or refer to others' emotions, it also is mostly about negative emotions (Lagattuta & Wellman, 2002).

In contrast, when observed in interactions with peers, 4- to 5-year-olds referred, again in the first person, to unelaborated "preference" emotions, such as liking and loving (Lagattuta & Wellman, 2002); anger, sadness, and fear accounted for less than 10% each of emotion terms in Fabes et al. (2001). The older children in that study did talk more about peers' emotions in longer utterances referring to explanations, questions, and deception (see also Cervantes & Callanan. 1998; Denham & Auerbach, 1995). Thus, as suggested by the Fabes et al. (2001) work, young children talk not just to parents about emotions, but what they discuss may differ with parents and others.

In fact, between 33 and 47 months of age, Dunn and colleagues have found that mother–child conversations about feelings decreased in frequency, whereas those between siblings increased, reflecting the increased ability of the growing younger sibling to engage in emotion conversation independent of the mother (Brown & Dunn, 1992). As interaction partners, older siblings are very different from mothers; they give preschoolers a new set of experiences in the use of emotion language. They are less likely to view their younger siblings' edification as a goal, less apt to be patient, and less able to "scaffold" conversations so that younger siblings can keep up. Not surprisingly, they focus more often on seeing that their own needs are met and talk more about their own feelings than mothers do, perhaps pushing their younger sibling to take their perspective (Brown & Dunn, 1992). Hence, emotion conversations with older siblings serve different functions than those with mothers do.

Preschool-age siblings, especially those who are good perspective takers, sometimes do use language to focus on their toddler siblings' emotions, particularly during maternal absences, conflicts, or play. Such use of emotion language allows older siblings to regulate interactions with toddlers and to construct shared meanings about their world (Howe, 1991). An older sibling says, "You'd better stop that before you make me mad!" to regulate interaction, or "It made me cry, too, when I hit my head. Do you need Mom?" to construct shared meanings about caregiving. Siblings also engage in emotion talk centered on themes of play and humor, creating complex shared jokes and pretense narratives.

Thus naturalistic investigations of conversations about emotions in the family convincingly demonstrate toddlers' and preschoolers' increasing understanding of the emotional scripts of their cultures (Brown & Dunn, 1991, 1992; Dunn et al., 1987). It should also be noted that the family conversations transcribed by Dunn and colleagues contain much self-referential emotion language used even by *very* young children; this observation calls into question the notion that the self-awareness of young children is severely limited. Caregivers and parents can capitalize on this ability, sensitively discussing the child's own experience.

### SUMMARY: Emotion Language

In summary, language is an essential part of the development of young children's emotion knowledge (Strand et al., 2016; Widen & Russell, 2004). Emotion language in conversations with parents, siblings, and peers differs in form and function, but all conversation partners serve as important listeners and teachers about emotions.

## EXPLAINING CHILDREN'S EARLY EMOTION KNOWLEDGE

Before discussing more advanced aspects of preschoolers' emotion knowledge in Chapter 5, it is useful to consider how to characterize their early understanding. What is the basis of children's early comprehension of the causes of emotion? How does this understanding develop? Currently there are three models that address young children's causal reasoning about emotions: the prototype, event structure, and desire–belief approaches. The descriptions of each model and an attempt at synthesis follow.

### Prototype Approach

A "prototype" describes general types of events that correlate with specific emotions; it links emotion and the common situations that cause it. Children ages 4 to 12, when interviewed and asked to tell what would make them happy, mad, sad, and scared, gave elements of adult emotion prototypes (Harter & Whitesell, 1989; Whitesell, 1989). Table 4.4 depicts the prototypical events that preschoolers think cause emotions, along with many specific quotes from children. These prototypes make it clear that even 4-year-olds know a lot about the typical causes of emotions. Their creation of clear, conceptual prototypes is reminiscent of the linguistic constructs proposed by the constructivist perspective.

**TABLE 4.4. Prototypical Causes of Basic Emotions, with Quotes from Children**

| Emotion | Causal event (general) | Example (specific) |
|---|---|---|
| Happiness | Pleasurable stimuli | Tickling, a kiss |
| Happiness | Getting or doing something desired | Playing with dolls<br>Daddy coming home<br>A birthday present |
| Sadness | Harm to self | "Daniel hits me."<br>Falling off the bike |
| Sadness | Loss of a relationship | Someone won't play |
| Sadness | Undesirable events | Moving to a new house |
| Sadness | Powerlessness | Having a bad dream |
| Anger | Physical harm | "Bullies fight with me."<br>Being bitten by a baby sister |
| Anger | Psychological harm | Being made to eat liver<br>Having a block tower knocked down<br>"Someone hurt my feelings." |
| Anger | Something not working<br>Insurmountable obstacles | "My toys wore out."<br>"I didn't get my way." |
| Fear | Anticipated harm | "I thought tigers were in my room."<br>"Monsters were going to gobble me up." |
| Fear | Unfamiliar situations | Being left alone |

*Note.* Data from Denham and Zoller (1991).

But the specific prototype exemplars provided by children at different ages reflect age-appropriate content that is not usually found in the reports of adults; most adults, for instance, no longer consider the fearful possibility of tigers in the house. And not all features of prototypes available to older children and adults are necessarily in place among younger children. Preschoolers are likely to give one or a few very concrete causal examples of an emotion within one particular prototypical category. If asked, "What made you sad?," a preschooler can probably give an answer referring to harm to the self: "I got a boo-boo on my knee." In contrast, older children can give multiple examples within a single prototype. In talking about harm to the self, an older child reports all the following: "I got hurt on the playground," "My best friend said something mean to me," and "I was sick last week and couldn't breathe." Still older children and adults show an even more abstract understanding of the general prototype categories. They ask themselves, "What makes me sad?," and then answer, "When something happens to hurt me in any way."

In essence, the prototype approach characterizes the social cognition of emotions by referring to clusters of exemplars that share specific meanings and themes. Young children begin to grasp the thematic ideas by using the perspective of their own limited experiences. Caregivers' awareness of these themes, and of young children's capacity to comprehend them, can be useful.

When Joelle says she is sad because she had an argument with her sister, her mother can empathize and make helpful suggestions, because she has felt the same way after arguments. In contrast, a childcare provider may have no idea what Martin is talking about when he asserts, "I'm mad because I missed the snow." Nonetheless, an astute caregiver who can discern the theme of "things not working" can engage Martin in a more fruitful discussion to help him manage his feelings and become positively involved in play.

## Event Structure Approach

Whereas the prototype approach encompasses emotional themes, the event structure approach focuses on processes—on the changes in goal states that result in emotion. The emphasis is on the information-processing steps that are taken to come to an experience of emotion and especially on the goals that are operative when emotions are elicited by events. The details of the "story" behind the experience of emotion are not crucial elements, as they are in the prototype theory.

Event structure analyses are useful because they capture the processes children use to determine the causes and consequences of happiness, sadness, anger, and fear (Stein & Jewett, 1986; Stein & Levine, 1989, 1990; Stein & Trabasso, 1989; see also Chapter 2). For happiness, four causal dimensions exist. First, children must perceive some aspect of the event as novel with respect to the ability to maintain, attain, or avoid a particular goal state. Next, they must infer that a valued state has been achieved. In other words, children must realize that something new has happened, and that because of it, something good will happen or something bad will be avoided. Then children must realize that attaining or maintaining the goal has a high probability. Last, they need to recognize that the enjoyment of the goal state or goal maintenance will follow the event's outcome. A child reasons that getting candy will lead to happiness because a valued state has been achieved, and will no doubt be enjoyable.

In contrast, both anger and sadness can occur (or co-occur) because of loss and aversive states, or failing to attain a goal state that is wanted or failing to avoid the unwanted. The causal dimensions for sadness include novelty, inferences that a valued state is not achieved and cannot be reinstated, and a belief that the goal will not be enjoyed. One preschooler may reason that another child is sad because his mother has left him at the childcare center, even though he wished and expected to stay with her, and that his valued state of "staying with Mommy" is not achieved. When this child cries and cries, the other child may reason that the child who is crying wants his mother even though he cannot rejoin her now.

In anger, children focus on the conditions that cause the failure to attain a wanted state or to avoid an unwanted one; they respond to the loss or aversive state by inferring that the obstructed goal can be reinstated. Then, as a consequence of anger, they may enact a plan to reinstate the goal. Hence, a child may reason that another child is angry because he did not get to keep all the blocks and is fighting to get them back.

In fear, children are aware that maintaining a desired state is now very unlikely. Their attention is focused on the cause of this probable failure to maintain the desired state and the consequences of it. For instance, on seeing a boy crying and backing up at the top of the slide on the playground, a preschool girl may reason that the boy thinks he is probably going to fall and that he is hanging on tight to keep this from happening, so he won't get hurt.

In determining the causes and consequences of emotions, an ability already discussed in this chapter, even 3-year-olds can make accurate judgments using the two sources of information critical to event analyses. They recognize internal goals, such as wanting to keep a toy, and external outcomes, such as losing a toy. Reasoning from these premises helps them differentiate emotional possibilities. They distinguish fear from anger and sadness by the external outcome expected, associating anticipation of harm only with fear. Those who express sadness over an obstacle in their way, instead of anger, focus on the permanent, irreparable loss of the goal. In a more abstract sense, when children of this age are deciding how they would feel in a situation, they seem to use the two necessary conditions for distinguishing among emotions (Stein & Jewett, 1986; Stein & Levine, 1989): (1) the goals of wanting/having, versus not wanting/not having, states and (2) the outcomes inherent in the certainty or uncertainty of attaining these internal states. The desire of the goal condition and the belief inherent in the outcome condition lead to the next possible explanation of young children's first steps to emotion knowledge.

## Desire–Belief Approach

Thus although the language of the models differs, the desire–belief approach actually shares its emphasis on beliefs and desires with the event structure model. What the person in an emotion-eliciting situation *wants* as well as what she or her *believes* will happen are key. Children between the ages of 3 and 6 become significantly more accurate and consistent in understanding that emotional reactions depend on both desire and belief (Harris, 1989, 1993; Lagattuta et al., 1997). Very young children base their reasoning about the cause of happiness on their awareness that being pleased or happy is a function of the match between desire and reality, such as when they receive a gift (Hadwin & Perner, 1991). That is, happiness occurs when actors anticipate getting what they desire (Harris, 1989).

Understanding of desire generally precedes that for belief (Pons et al., 2004). But along with their understanding of desire-dependent emotions, children as young as 3 years also begin to comprehend belief-dependent emotions, such as surprise (Wellman & Banerjee, 1991). If a preschool girl *believes* she is staring at a large decorative block, and suddenly a boy bursts from his hiding place within his box, the discrepancy between her belief and reality causes her surprise. In this case, surprise occurs when what the girl expects or believes does *not* happen. It is important to note that even though preschoolers accurately report this false-belief basis for surprise, they also report surprise when they merely gain knowledge where they were previously ignorant (Ruffman & Keenan, 1996). Nonetheless, they do not merely understand the simple links between various situations and associated emotions but are already capable of more abstract conceptions (Wellman & Banerjee, 1991).[4]

## Integrating the Three Models

The three approaches to explaining children's causal understanding of emotions are all persuasive, but their proponents consider each to be unique and to have more explanatory power than the others. Stein and Trabasso (1989) assert that the information-processing focus inherent in the event structure perspective is incompatible with a prototype approach, and Harter and Whitesell (1989) are similarly discouraging from their opposing viewpoint.

Even so, a rapprochement among the approaches can be proposed. A synthesis of viewpoints describes children's means of understanding their emotional world better than any single perspective does. Perhaps the event structure (with the novelty experience suspending ongoing thoughts, the wanting/not wanting and having/not having goal states, and the certainty of attaining or maintaining these states) may actually overarch prototypical examples or form their logical basis. That is, event prototype exemplars may provide the thematic content of the event schema (see also Fischer et al., 1989). To paraphrase Stein and Trabasso (1989), both the underlying concept structure of the event, and the event itself, are important aspects of preschoolers' knowledge of emotions.

Distinguishing emotions both by event structure, and by thematic similarities among the events that cause them and the consequences that ensue, is important. We (Denham & Zoller, 1991) and Fabes et al. (1988, 1991) used both approaches, and the results are consistent with Harter and Whitesell's (1989), Whitesell's (1989), and Stein and Trabasso's (1989) analyses. It seems reasonable that we need to know both how a child is reasoning and what the child is reasoning about, so that we have a clear picture of development from either theoretical or practical standpoints.

This synthesis of approaches, as illustrated in Figure 4.1, adds to our understanding of the reasoning both children and adults go through when trying to make sense of their emotional world. Caregivers can benefit from knowing the "how" of their children's thinking about emotions, *along with* their sometimes-idiosyncratic reasoning about the "what" of their emotions. Such knowledge can assist caregivers in intervening to aid children in emotion regulation.

> Alex's preschool teacher, seeing his angry face, may accurately infer that he is focused on something he wants but does not have. She has isolated the important aspects of the event—goal and outcome. But what exactly is his goal, and what is the problematic outcome that's making him mad? Accordingly, her understanding of the event could prompt her to hypothesize and then pinpoint the prototypical source of Alex's anger—a friend's misdeed. Alex

---

[4]This desire—belief aspect of emotion knowledge does become elaborated more clearly later in the preschool period, as noted by Pons et al. (2004) and others, and is considered more deeply in later sections of this chapter.

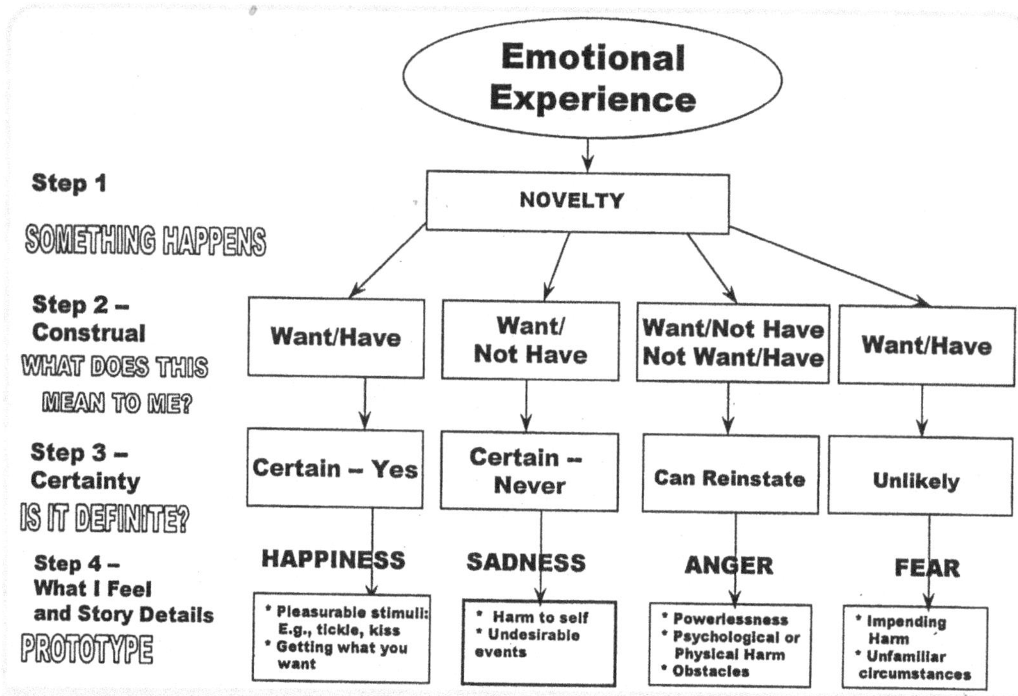


**FIGURE 4.1.** Resolving the event structure and prototype analyses of emotions' causes.

considers that his friend "stole" the blocks, even without realizing that Alex considered them "his." Focusing again on Alex's goal, his teacher can also predict that he will probably swing into unbridled action to get the blocks back. Clearly, Alex can profit from his teacher's assistance on the "how" and the "what" of his emotional event. She can help him, first, to refrain from hurting his friend and then perhaps to reconstrue the whole event.

The cognitive information processing that takes place during appraisals of emotional experience (see Chapter 1, Figure 1.1) may proceed according to an event structure or desire–belief formula but may be *about* prototypical experiences that happen often to people of all ages.

This synthesis is useful in understanding preschoolers' emerging emotion knowledge. At the same time, given their foundation in cognizing emotion generally, young children also are beginning to understand how emotion is regulated.

## BECOMING AWARE OF EMOTION REGULATION STRATEGIES

People experience emotion when valued goals have been either attained or thwarted. We feel happy when we get a present that we wanted, and sad when we fall off a new bicycle. The emotions that signal the attainment or thwarting of a goal act as intrapersonal regulators. When we feel negative emotions, we want to feel better; when we feel positive ones, we want to continue to feel good, but without letting the good feelings "run away with us." We want to maintain or achieve a valued state and avoid an aversive state; we want to regulate our emotions. Young children are learning about strategies to regulate their own and others' emotions. That is, they are learning how to change emotions, both negative and positive (Stein & Levine, 1990). In this chapter, I discuss how young children report on how to change *others'* emotions, and, in Chapter 6, describe how they conceive of changing their *own* emotions. This demarcation is admittedly somewhat artificial, but the phenomena that I report on here may be more cognitively mediated, conscious, and intentional.

Prior to understanding specific emotion regulation strategies, it would be important to know whether preschoolers comprehend that emotions typically change over time. In fact, there are limits to preschoolers' such understanding. For example, young children are just beginning to understand that the *intensity* of an emotion often changes with its duration (Brown, Covell, & Abramovitch, 1991). Brown, Covell, et al. found that 4- to 6-year-olds were able to describe change from one emotion to another over time (happiness, sadness, or anger), but asserted that emotional intensity would remain high over time, even though they could differentiate the high and low emotional intensities inherent in stories (e.g., the high-level happiness of getting a present vs. the calmer, lower-level happiness of listening to music and singing with Mommy). However, Harris (1989) reported the opposite regarding preschoolers' understanding of emotions' waning; in his work they did understand that allowing time to pass helps to alleviate emotions.

In any case, this controversy suggests that at best preschoolers are just beginning to acquire more complex notions about emotional regulation across time. The whole idea of time is rather foreign to them, and superimposing it upon another difficult set of concepts, emotion regulation, may result in "overload." Thus more than just "time heals all wounds" may be important in preschoolers accumulating knowledge about emotion regulation.

## Ways to Change Negative Emotions

Young children are motivated to change certain emotions (Carlson, Felleman, & Masters, 1983), although they are more likely to want to change the situation rather than the internal feeling (Cole, Dennis, Smith-Simon, & Cohen, 2009). The simplest approach to accessing young children's ideas about changing emotions is to name an emotion and ask them to tell or to act out how it could be changed. In line with what adults expect, they deem anger and sadness the most change worthy and happiness the least. In early studies with various methodologies, preschoolers showed that they comprehend specific nurturant and aggressive strategies to change sadness and anger, including physical, verbal, social, material, and helping/hindering strategies (Denham, 1996a; Fabes et al., 1988; Fabes & Eisenberg, 1992; McCoy & Masters, 1985).

In these studies, children cited physical and material strategies to remediate sadness, material and verbal strategies for reducing anger, and verbal and physical strategies for alleviating distress; see Table 4.5 for quotations referring to changing their parents' sadness and anger (Denham, 1996a). I found that the prevalent intervention

**TABLE 4.5. Examples of Children's Conceptions of Ways to Change Parents' Negative Emotions**

| |
|---|
| ***Changing sadness*** |
| *Nurturant physical*: "Give a kiss/hug," "Rub his back." |
| *Nurturant material*: "Give her something to eat." |
| *Nurturant helping*: "Let her sleep," "Clean up the mess." |
| *Nurturant verbal*: "Say sorry." |
| ***Changing anger*** |
| *Nurturant physical*: "Give a kiss/hug." |
| *Nurturant material*: "Give him an apple." |
| *Nurturant helping*: "Clean up the house," "Not bother him." |
| *Nurturant verbal*: "Say 'Don't be mad, Mom,' " "Say 'I love you.' " |

*Note.* From Denham (1996a).

for changing parental sadness or anger was nurturant physical ("Give a kiss/hug"). The youngsters knew that these are disarming, cheering strategies. For changing both sadness and anger, girls were more likely than boys to cite nurturant physical interventions. In short, these early studies showed that preschoolers can identify strategies for regulating emotions.

More recent work largely corroborates earlier findings. In one study, both parents and children were asked how the children would change the emotions of someone feeling bad, to help them feel better (López-Pérez, Wilson, Dellaria, & Gummerum, 2016). Both parents and their early grade schoolers more often cited emotion-related (e.g., sympathy, talking about problems) and cognitive strategies (e.g., explaining the event, reappraising a positive outcome for the event, giving advice) than especially the 3- to-4-year-olds. Parents and children of the younger group, in contrast, more often reported that the child would change another's negative emotions by showing the distressed individual affection, smiles, comfort objects, or getting help. These more concrete, behavioral strategies were within the younger children's cognitive "reach."

Another approach to examining children's strategies for changing emotions is to tell them story stems and ask how to aid the protagonist in changing emotion. In one study, children ages 4 to 9 were told increasingly complex stories about losing a parent's radio, parents' anger after a bad day at work, or parents' arguing (Covell & Miles, 1992). All the children said that the child in the story could change a parent's anger. This is a hopeful sign for families!

But the youngest group cited more indirect (again concrete, behavioral) means that did not address the cause of the parents' emotion, such as painting a parent a picture, doing well in school, or buying a parent a gift. Direct strategies were cited by the younger children only for the least-complex story, where the problem was easily solved—getting another radio. Similarly, when children in López-Pérez et al. (2016) were given specific scenarios to evaluate a child protagonist, 3- to-4-year-olds more often cited giving the distressed person attention by drawing a picture, for instance.

They too were unlikely to suggest cognitive means, like helping the other by reappraising the situation, or emotional means, like comforting via talking.

These indirect strategies may appear less useful on the surface, but in this case, preschoolers may have shown unwitting wisdom. Another group of children and parents in Covell and Miles's (1992) study rated the actual effectiveness of these indirect and direct strategies. Both parents and children endorsed certain indirect strategies (e.g., being good, smiling, showing affection) as *more* effective than direct ones. Other indirect strategies, such as doing well at school or buying a gift, were seen as less effective (cf. Denham, 1996a).

In other words, children considered strategies that would generally elicit parental happiness to be effective in reducing parental anger. They thought that directly addressing the anger-producing stimulus would be less useful, maybe even risky. So, interestingly, the youngest children in Covell and Miles's (1992) first sample would likely have been most successful in alleviating parental anger. Even though they were required to answer verbally—a difficult mode of response for them—these young children knew how mothers' anger is best diffused. The older children's more direct, cognitively more adequate responses might have gotten them in trouble!

More recent investigation has expanded knowledge in this area (Cole et al., 2009; Dennis & Kelemen, 2009; Sala, Pons, & Molina, 2014; Waters & Thompson, 2014); these studies will be considered when I discuss the *cognitive* means of changing emotions.

## Ways to Change Positive Emotions

Knowing what actions to avoid to maintain happiness and other positive states is important too. Children know that material, social, and physical aggression can change happiness to negative affect (McCoy & Masters, 1985). In the Denham (1996a) study, the prevalent intervention to change parental happiness was antisocial physical means (e.g., the boy doll punches the father doll twice and says, "I'll kick your butt"). Preschoolers also know that a person feeling "just okay" will feel worse if exposed to material aggression and better if exposed to material/social nurturance.

Sometimes, however, preschoolers become confused when asked about changing happiness: Why would this ever be a goal? I found that girls, especially older ones, were more likely than boys to cite nurturant social means to change parental happiness (Denham, 1996a). Often when giving such a response, children seemed puzzled, concretely assuming that if an emotion needed changing, then nurturance was called for. In general, preschool-age children find the idea of changing happiness somewhat outlandish. Apparently, researchers also feel this way, as most research deals with changing negative emotions for the better—no studies found discuss knowledge of how to down- *or* up-regulate positive emotion.

## Cognitive Strategies for Changing Emotions

So young children do have some ideas—rather effective ones at that—about changing their own and others' negative emotions. As noted, they are less skilled at how to change or maintain positive emotions. Over time, they come to understand that the means of regulating emotions differ in effectiveness.

Moreover, they are developing some more internal, mentalistic strategies to deal with emotions, especially negative ones. For example, Lagattuta (2014) reported that between 4 and 10 years, children begin to understand that minds can cause, augment, reduce, or change emotions, even without altering the objective situations. But these sophisticated means of changing emotion may never predominate, especially during early childhood. In fact, cognitive strategies to change emotion were given less frequently than behavioral strategies across the whole age range of 4 to 15 years (Brown, Covell, et al., 1991; see Chapter 6).

Although 4- to 6-year-olds recognized cognitive control strategies (e.g., remembering a happy time or telling themselves how to feel better) when reminded of them, they did not generate them on their own. This inability to generate strategies spontaneously was parallel to preschoolers' inability to take personalized information about emotion into account spontaneously, suggesting that less-sophisticated cognitive development is the root of these limitations. Perhaps, to help her weeping Mom feel better, Lauren is more likely to offer her a grape from the fruit bowl than she is to advise her to "think about something pretty."

As I have argued previously, however, a more engaging methodology could more clearly elucidate preschoolers' strategies, even cognitive ones, for changing emotions—finding more evidence of preschoolers' actual competence rather than their performance deficiencies. It would be specifically geared for maximizing the performance of preschoolers, with task demands tailored for the age range. In one of the first studies using such methods, 3- to 5-year-olds were presented with stories in which the characters were experiencing sadness, anger, or fear. The stories were presented as puppet plays. The puppet's feelings were common to children's experience and were explicitly stated. For example, Jacob was angry because his teacher told him there wasn't enough time for his show-and-tell. Although he was very mad, he wanted to enjoy his time at school and not feel so angry inside (see Banerjee & Eggleston, 1993; see also Banerjee, 1997a, 1997b). Children did not have the added response burdens of independently inferring the character's emotion or of puzzling over the story. They also were engaged fully in pretend play with the puppet.

One group of children was asked to generate strategies for coping with the emotional situations presented in the stories. Another group was asked to choose from the following strategies:

- External strategies, such as changing the external situations, location, or emotional expression, or seeking external help (e.g., Jacob should put a smile on his face).
- Mentalistic strategies involving thought processes, such as redirecting thoughts, reinterpreting the situation, or engaging in pretense (e.g., Jacob should think about how much fun it will be to do his show-and-tell tomorrow).
- Ineffectual strategies that would not work, such as merely repeating the story

facts, doing something that would exacerbate negative feelings, or simply accepting the emotion (e.g., Jacob should stay in class and just sit there).

In both methodologies, children reported effectual external or mentalistic strategies approximately 90% of the time. Furthermore, mentalistic strategies were reported at least once by half of the children in the open-ended group and were chosen more often than ineffectual strategies in the forced-choice group. Even without the benefit of forced-choice strategies, the oldest children in the open-ended group provided more mentalistic than ineffectual responses. More important, the oldest children in the forced-choice group even chose mentalistic strategies more often than external ones.

Building upon this earlier research, investigators interested in how preschoolers understand emotion regulation strategies that they themselves could use have implemented more child-friendly methodologies and expanded knowledge in the area. For example, Cole et al. (2009) enacted puppet vignettes, in which the protagonist's sadness or anger was clearly noted, and the easier question "How can we help X stop feeling sad/angry?" (Denham, 1997) was used.

Both 3- and 4-year-olds were able to recognize and generate spontaneously strategies to regulate sadness (i.e., on average they generated around one strategy and recognized more than two); 4-year-olds showed an advantage in generating strategies to regulate anger, which was accounted for by their greater language ability. However, between half (of 3-year-olds) and two-thirds (of 4-year-olds) recognized cognitive strategies for sadness (about a lost puppy), such as thinking about something nice or something else. Eighty to 90% of children recognized such a cognitive strategy for anger (fighting over a toy). The percentages of children who recognized *doing* something to feel better or changing the situation (i.e., looking for the puppy, sharing toys) were at or above 69% for both age levels. In short, preschoolers were able to show their understanding of emotion regulation strategies, even via verbal generation, and even regarding cognitive strategies.

Other research has upheld and expanded these findings. Again, using puppets and encouraging children to interact with them and using Cole et al.'s (2009) wording on "What can the dog/turtle do to stop feeling sad/mad/scared?," Dennis and Kelemen (2009) asked children to rate the puppets' enactment of six emotion regulation strategies. Even the youngest in the group of 3- and 4-year-olds viewed cognitive and behavior distraction, as well as repairing the situation, as relatively effective (see also Gust, Koglin, & Petermann, 2014). However, the younger children also endorsed the ineffective strategies of venting and ruminating.

The children also operated from a functionalist position, endorsing different strategies more depending on the emotion; they endorsed repairing the situation for anger, but chose behavioral distraction for sadness and fear. In a similar vein, Waters and Thompson (2014) asked 6- and 9-year-old children to rate the effectiveness of eight emotion strategies. They too chose different strategies as appropriate, depending on the emotion—for example, problem-solving for anger and support seeking or venting for sadness. Again, the younger group did rate cognitively sophisticated strategies as relatively effective, although they still also endorsed ineffective strategies more than the older group.

Finally, explicating even more specifically the use of cognitive strategies, changing one's thoughts or goals to alleviate negative emotion, Davis, Levine, Lench, and Quas (2010) found that 5- and 6-year-olds made surprisingly sophisticated cognitive suggestions for emotion regulation. In a first study, children heard stories in which the protagonist's goal was thwarted (e.g., the protagonist couldn't play baseball because of an injured leg); the procedure involved asking for justifications of strategies and probing for more than one strategy. After identifying the protagonist's emotions, goal reinstatement and goal substitution were the most frequent strategies mentioned by almost all the children. Metacognitive strategies, which involved changing one's thoughts or goals (e.g., forgetting; changing one's mental state by sleeping, fainting, or dreaming; pretending things are different; positively reappraising the situation) constituted the next most frequent strategy. Over half the children gave at least one strategy that involved changing thoughts.

When asked to generate strategies for protagonists in stories involving more varied emotions (i.e., happy, sad, angry, afraid, ashamed, and guilty—such as being sad when getting lost or feeling guilty over breaking a friend's toy), 5- to 6-year-old children generated more cognitive reappraisal strategies (i.e., modifying the meaning of the situation) than younger preschoolers, as well as more valid answers and a greater variety of strategies (Sala et al., 2014). Children's nonverbal intelligence and overall emotion knowledge were related to endorsement of cognitive reappraisal, whereas verbal ability was related to endorsement of behavioral (i.e., engaging in an action to manage the emotion), and social support (i.e., another story character helps the protagonist overcome the emotion) strategies. These findings corroborated older preschoolers greater proficiency at demonstrating an understanding of cognitive strategies and pinpointed important correlates of this ability.

Some gender differences seem important. Boys endorsed behavioral strategies more than girls, with girls favoring support-seeking strategies (Sala et al., 2014). Waters and Thompson (2014) also found that girls rated emotion-focused strategies more highly than boys. Young girls appear to focus on strategies to both feel better (rather than to do something to fix the emotion-eliciting problem) and to get help in that effort. Lagattuta (2014) goes further by summarizing findings on girls as young as 4 years old who proposed more avoidance and fewer approach strategies for reducing fear.

These gender differences in choices of emotion regulation strategies could have broader effects. In fact, Lagattuta (2014) reported on a series of studies that together suggested that girls' early understanding of emotion regulation, as well as aspects of their emotional thinking in the form of memories and predictions of the future, could affect their emotions. That is, girls as young as age 4 also (1) knew, more than boys, that future-oriented thoughts affect emotions (Lagattuta, 2005) and (2) more often than boys predicted that thinking about ambiguous past risky situations, or conversely, future harm, can lead to worry (Lagattuta, 2007). Such a pattern could be related to girls' choice of emotion-focused and support-seeking regulation strategies, leading to worrying and even later rumination and anticipation of a negative future—all factors associated with girls' more prevalent depression and anxiety. Thus gender differences in understanding emotion regulation, as well as time-based reasoning about emotions, could have deleterious effects for girls.

### SUMMARY: Awareness of Emotion Regulation Strategies

In sum, preschoolers seem to understand that something can be done to regulate emotions; they know a great deal about external strategies. Mentalistic strategies are becoming increasingly important to them. Children have notions of cognitive emotion regulation strategies at a younger age than researchers previously thought. Finally, important gender differences exist, which are worthy of further study.

## OVERALL SUMMARY AND CONCLUSION

Preschoolers' understanding of emotion is not complete, but it is surprisingly acute in several domains of emotional experience. During the preschool years, children become increasingly able to use emotion language to fulfill a variety of functions in their everyday lives. They label emotional expressions and identify emotion-eliciting situations, along with their causes and consequences. Ways of changing their own and others' emotions are becoming clear to them.

Many situations elicit similar feelings among different people, and facial expressions tend to stand for specific emotions, even cross-culturally, although there are important cultural and income-related differences in aspects of emotion knowledge. These regularities make it simpler for preschoolers to make inferences about basic emotions; they comprehend situations and facial expressions that are simple and familiar. Children during the period from toddlerhood to late preschool age generally label and recognize happy expressions first, followed by sad, angry, and fearful expressions in that order. This developmental progression appears in many studies. Receptive recognition often supersedes expressive labeling, as is often the case in language development in general. Young children also demonstrate considerable knowledge of the causes and consequences of emotional situations.

Young children are also aware that emotions may be change worthy and are becoming capable of citing effective means of doing so. Although they more often choose behavioral rather than cognitive strategies to change emotion, preschoolers can generate mentalistic strategies. During the preschool period, children also begin to generate the means to change parental emotions, especially their anger. Overall, then, notions of both self–other regulation and prosocial reactions to others' emotions are developing.

In short, emotion knowledge is extremely complex and particularly important. Preschoolers do have major limitations in this area—aspects of emotion knowledge that will improve as they grow—but their accomplishments in their short lives are worthy of our great respect, especially considering the emergence of the even more complex aspects of emotion knowledge I consider in the next chapter.

# 5

# More Advanced Emotion Knowledge during Preschool

## INTRODUCTION

Chapter 4 focused on the most basic—and increasingly advanced—early childhood knowledge of basic emotions and emotion regulation. Given this framework establishing the more foundational components of preschoolers' emotion knowledge, it is time to move on to consider what Pons et al. (2004) consider the more mentalistic aspects of emotion knowledge—for example, emotions based on desire or belief and an understanding of hiding emotions. I will broaden these concepts to include the finer nuances of young children's understanding of personalized bases of emotions.

In this chapter I explore more advanced, mentalistic aspects of emotion knowledge that are mastered—at least to a degree—later during early childhood:

- Recognizing that others' emotional experience can differ from their own (including Pons et al.'s [2004] categories of understanding desire-based emotions and belief-based emotions).
- Beginning to develop a knowledge of emotion display rules, or the ability to hide emotions.

Finally, there are emotion knowledge skills that are only emergent during early childhood. Pons et al. (2004) refer to these skills as "reflexive" abilities.

- Beginning to develop a knowledge of how more than one emotion may be felt simultaneously, even when these emotions conflict or are ambivalent.
- Beginning to understand complex social and self-conscious emotions (e.g., guilt).

After detailing these subskills of emotion knowledge, I discuss intrapersonal foundations of this overall ability, such as self-regulation, cognitive ability, verbal ability, security of attachment, and even locomotor ability. I then consider the connection between emotion knowledge and the allied set of skills, theory of mind. Finally, I begin a discussion of emotion knowledge and culture, which is continued in Chapter 8.[1]

## MORE SOPHISTICATED UNDERSTANDING OF OTHERS' EMOTIONAL EXPERIENCE

Sometimes knowing about emotion vocabulary, expressions of emotions, emotion-eliciting situations, and even the causes and consequences of emotions is not enough to permit an individual to interpret the emotional signals of others accurately. Information specific to a particular person in a particular situation or person may be needed. Through their increased social sensitivity and experience, older preschoolers develop strategies for appraising others' emotions when available cues are less salient and consensual and may differ from their own.

In an early series of thought-provoking inquiries, Gnepp and colleagues used a processing model to describe the information needed in deciding what emotion another person is experiencing or will experience in a given situation (Gnepp, 1983, 1989a, 1989b; Gnepp & Chilamkurti, 1988; Gnepp & Gould, 1985; Gnepp, Klayman, & Trabasso, 1982; Gnepp, McKee, & Domanic, 1987; see also Lagattuta, 2007). To interpret emotions even more accurately, information specific to a particular person in a particular situation may be needed. Important emotional information includes whether (1) the situation is equivocal (i.e., could elicit more than one emotion), (2) the person's expressive patterns and the situation conflict, and (3) person-specific information, such as the individual's unique desire or belief, is needed. Only toward the end of the preschool age range do preschoolers even begin to attain these skills (Harris, 1989; Harris et al., 1989; Pons et al., 2004).

### Equivocal Situations

To identify the emotion another person is showing, the first question is whether the situation has a single strong emotional determinant that is the same for everyone. Young children are clearly capable of such determinations, as shown in my own group's work and that of Gnepp, Stein, and their colleagues (e.g., Denham & Couchoud, 1990b; Gnepp et al., 1982, 1987; Stein & Jewett, 1986; Stein & Levine, 1989, 1990; see also Borke, 1971). They imagine how they themselves would feel or how people in general feel in such situations.

[1] In the decades ensuing since the publication of *Emotional Development in Young Children* in 1998, many more investigators (including myself!) have focused on how emotion knowledge contributes to social competence and school success (see Chapters 10 and 11). In this chapter I update and corroborate information on the emergence of emotion knowledge itself with newer research.

But some situations do not have a strong emotion–event association. Different people feel different emotions in response to some emotion-eliciting events. One child is happy to encounter a large, friendly-looking dog, panting and "smiling" with an open mouth. Another child is terrified in the same situation. More personal information is needed to know how the person is feeling.

Preschoolers are becoming aware that specialized information is sometimes needed to interpret emotions. They are beginning to recognize the equivocality inherent in some emotion situations—that is, the fact that some situations commonly elicit different emotional reactions in different people. In one study, we showed children a puppet expressing an emotion contrasting with the child's own likely emotion in vignettes designed to be equivocal; each child's job was to hold his or her own likely emotion in abeyance and to pick the correct emotion for the puppet (Denham & Couchoud, 1990a). For example, if a mother reported that a child was happy to go swimming, the puppet enacted fear.

The children in the study struggled to make such specialized inferences, and over the years we continued to see preschoolers score at least somewhat lower on identifying the emotions in such equivocal situations as opposed to unequivocal ones (e.g., Bassett et al., 2012; Denham, Blair, DeMulder, et al., 2003; Denham, Caverly, et al., 2002). Nonetheless, they can do so more frequently than expected by chance. They are most successful when a positive and negative emotion is contrasted, rather than two negative emotions. Thus, for example, they are often able to comprehend and indicate that the puppet was sad to go to preschool when they themselves would be happy. Even making these inferences has required some effort, however.

> Toma looked mystified while applying the happy face correctly on a puppet anticipating an oatmeal breakfast made by the mommy puppet. Personally, Toma would be angry about—in fact, would hate—an oatmeal breakfast. After he secured the puppet's happy face, he started talking rapidly to it with great zeal: "I'd be mad! Oatmeal is yucky. It gets lumps, it's cold, it has no taste!"

Assessing equivocality *and* differentiating between the more troublesome negative emotions was a task burden, which meant that choosing between two negative emotions was more difficult than choosing between happiness and one negative emotion. Preschoolers struggled with situations that pitted two equally plausible negative emotions, as when the puppet was angry at anticipating punishment, instead of fearful as they themselves would be. In agreement with earlier results, error analyses indicated that vignettes involving fear, and to some extent anger, were the most difficult for the children to interpret (Denham & Couchoud, 1990a).

In the same vein as my studies, Gnepp et al. (1987) told children stories describing different situations, some unequivocal and some equivocal. The children were asked to say they were thinking of only one feeling if they were sure how the protagonist felt, but to say they were thinking of two feelings if two were possible. Spontaneously acknowledging equivocality by saying that they were thinking of two feelings for vignettes, such as a dog's walking down the street toward the protagonist, was difficult for them.

After these free responses, however, the experimenter probed for more information. When questioned about the dog vignette, many 5- and 6-year-olds were able to say, "Some kids like dogs, and some don't," thereby acknowledging that equivocality exists. This task may have underestimated preschoolers' knowledge of equivocality. Gnepp et al. (1987) also were unwittingly asking children to acknowledge both the simultaneity and ambivalence of emotions, and thus were mingling two difficult areas of emotion knowledge.

In sum, preschoolers are beginning to deal with equivocality, especially if the necessary inferences jibe with their earliest distinctions among emotions—"good" feelings versus "bad" feelings, with sadness and anger included among the "bad" feelings. For the preschoolers in Gnepp et al.'s (1987) study, the notion of equivocality was just emerging, whereas in our work (Denham & Couchoud, 1990a), preschoolers seemed to be further along in dealing with it. Methodological differences often fuel such discrepancies; as seen in myriad other areas, preschoolers' ability to differentiate equivocal emotional situations can be concealed by performance issues in tasks that require more effort than the children can give.

## Conflicting Expressive and Situational Cues to a Person's Emotion

Even if there is a strong emotion–event association in a situation, the person experiencing the event may react atypically. For instance, a person may smile when seeing a spider dropping into the room on a strand of web. Personal information is needed, then, not only when a situation is emotionally equivocal, but also when an emotional reaction is atypical. However, interpreting a reaction as atypical requires a rather sophisticated decision—namely, *resolving* conflicting expressive and situational cues to emotions, rather than relying on one cue or the other.

The view that sources of emotional information are resolvable is a new one. This perspective stands in contrast to a long-standing debate about age changes in the relative weights children assign to facial and situational information about emotion. As early as 1979, Abramovitch and Daly asserted that 4-year-olds can decode the emotional aspects of the facial expressions of a wide range of stimulus persons, such as classmates, unfamiliar peers, and adults. Furthermore, they contended, this expression identification increasingly enables children to recognize the emotional content of situations. That is, when children are confused, they utilize emotional expressions to understand situations. This reasoning seems plausible, although the converse could be equally true: Children may take in expressions that are common in certain situations and recognize them as angry, for example. In other words, when children are confused, they use situational information to discern specific emotional expressions.[2]

This interconnection between expressions and situations is almost unavoidable. But which type of cue is most important in children's judgments as they become more emotionally competent? Situational cues may become more important than expression

[2]These assertions too are evocative of the notions of the constructivist perspective—which cue is more important, facial expressions or conceptualizations of situations?

cues in discerning how someone *really* feels, as children begin to understand the salience of display rules. But expression may also become more important as children become more sensitive to the equivocality of situations (Gnepp, 1989a). The question of whether facial or situational information is *always* primary when choosing between conflicting cues may be unresolvable.

Perhaps a more fruitful line of inquiry would involve the assumption that both sorts of information are important, with the weight given each type in specific contexts the most illuminating. Children may learn to weight each source of emotional information strategically, much as they come to utilize multiple sources of information in cognitive tasks, such as balance scale problems (Richards & Siegler, 1981; Siegler & Jenkins, 1989). This possibility is especially credible because cognitive ability has been related to emotion knowledge, as indexed both by talking about emotion and by the results of our puppet measures studies (Denham & Couchoud, 1990a, 1990b, 1991; Denham, Zoller, & Couchoud, 1994; Smith & Walden, 1998).

The relative weights preschoolers assign to expressive and situational cues of emotions were examined using a series of pictures in which facial and situational information were conflicting (Hoffner & Badzinski, 1989). Children indicated the type (happy or sad) and intensity of each character's emotion. When situational and expressive indicators are discrepant (suggesting differing emotions), young concrete thinkers infer the most recognizable, simplest emotion, rather than relying solely on either type of information. However, reliance on situational information increased with age from preschool to fifth grade and reliance on facial information decreased after the preschool period (see corollary arguments in Strand et al., 2016; Widen & Russell, 2010c). Children's ability to resolve conflicting information also increased with age. Thus, the relative influence of situational and expressive information on 4- through 8-year-olds' emotion recognition shows a developmental trend, from noticing only one type of information to considering both expressive and situational evidence (Wiggers & Van Lieshout, 1985).

The valences of expressions and situations probably make a difference, too. At all age levels in the Hoffner and Badzinski (1989) study, children were less able to resolve an anomalous positive expression paired with a negative situation (e.g., smiling while getting an injection), than a negative expression paired with a positive situation (e.g., crying at a birthday party). They could conceive of masking an emotion or substituting one emotion for another in a negative situation less readily than they could envision the extenuating reasons for feeling bad during a normally pleasant time (see also Gnepp, 1983). This pattern of findings is reminiscent of the difficulties in believing that a person in a negative emotional state could feel better when reminded of a positive emotion.

To describe *how* children weigh sources of emotional information, Gove and Keating (1979) presented 3- and 5-year-olds with stories in which the outcome was the same for each character, but the facial expressions of the characters differed. For example, in one story a child was happy to receive a dog as a gift, but in another the child was afraid. In one-third to one-half of the responses, these young subjects were able to explain the differences psychologically ("*She* likes dogs, but *he* is really scared of them").

They demonstrated an understanding that the same situation can give rise to different emotions, and thus expressions, in different people; they were weighing multiple sources of information. Children who could not give such sophisticated explanations demonstrated their inability to recognize that different people could feel different ways about the same situation. They tended to reconstruct the situation ("This dog doesn't have big teeth, so she likes him a lot").

Given vignettes involving only one person, rather than two persons in one situation (e.g., a girl smiling while getting an injection in the doctor's office), children told stories about the conflicting facial and situational information (Gnepp, 1983). The 3- and 4-year-olds were able to reconcile the conflict to form a coherent explanation of the person's circumstances about half of the time, albeit by attributing an idiosyncratic perspective to the character ("She likes shots"). Such attribution of idiosyncrasy may be a precursor of understanding the psychological causes of personalized reactions to emotion-eliciting situations (Gnepp, 1983, 1989b). Some 3- and 4-year-olds gave even elaborate explanations of idiosyncratic reactions in specific situations, often by introducing information that would change the character's emotion ("This is a special shot that won't hurt"; Gnepp, 1983). Despite the strangeness of their answers, such children are starting to see the personal complexity of situations that even appear, on the surface, emotionally unequivocal.

But even older preschoolers are often unable to ask spontaneous questions to help them resolve emotionally conflicting situations (Gould, 1984). Apparently, they can sometimes use information to solve the conflict, but do not automatically search for it, or even notice that they need to do so.

In summary, many preschoolers are still working on the ability to recognize the complex details of differing perspectives—the fact that desires and goals often differ from person to person, and why. All these considerations bear on their ability to reconcile conflicting expressive and situational cues, and it's not an easy task. Sometimes especially young preschoolers still prefer simple, script-based analyses of emotions. They may also have a vague notion, based on their experiences, that a person can encounter negative emotions within normally positive situations (or even vice versa), but this knowledge is imperfect. Moreover, these youngsters may not have been exposed to display rules for substituting positive emotional expression in negative situations. Taken together, investigations reveal two major obstacles to a preschoolers' ability to create a sophisticated union of expressive and situational indicators of emotion: cognitive limitations and experiential/socialization limitations. Clearly, the ability to understand psychological causes of emotional reactions, given conflicting information, is just emerging in some children during the preschool period.

## Use of Personalized Information

Older preschoolers do become capable of focusing on personal dispositions as opposed to goal states when identifying emotions (e.g., "She had a bad day"; instead of "She didn't want Billy to play with her"). What kinds of personal information would they use in interpreting emotions? First, unique normative information is often important:

"Sarah lives in Green Valley, where all the people are friendly with tigers and play games with them all the time" (Gnepp et al., 1982, p. 116). When asked what feelings Sarah would experience, preschoolers used unique normative information about liking tigers to modify their responses to a normally unequivocal situation. Preschoolers also are becoming aware that normative cultural categories such as age and gender moderate the emotions experienced in differing situations. For example, a boy may not be overjoyed to receive a doll as a gift.

Second, information about personality characteristics that are stable across time and situations can be especially useful. Gnepp and Chilamkurti (1988) told children stories in which the protagonist was honest, a clown, helpful, cruel, shy, or selfish. Even 6-year-old children used such information to answer questions about feelings in situations that normally could be considered unequivocal (e.g., "How would a clown feel if he wore one black shoe and one white one to school, and everybody laughed?"). No studies have examined the use of personality characteristics to determine emotion in children younger than 6, so it is impossible to say when the ability first appears.

Third, immediately present person-specific information is sometimes needed. Gnepp et al. (1982) provided stories in which the characters' behavioral dispositions modified normally strong emotion–event associations: "Mark eats grass whenever he can. It's dinnertime and his mother says they're having grass for dinner. How will Mark feel?" Children ages 4 and 5 utilized such information; their responses reflected the unique perspective of the story character ("Mark will be happy to have grass for dinner"). The children also gave more weight to such person-specific information than to normative information when the two kinds of information conflicted; these findings, where older preschoolers attain some success, are similar to our findings with our puppet measures studies (Denham & Couchoud, 1990a).

Third, another type of immediately present person-specific information must be mentioned for preschoolers. Just after Gnepp's seminal early work (1989a, 1989b), increasing attention began to be given to young children's theory of mind as it relates to their emotion knowledge (e.g., Harris et al., 1989; Wellman & Banerjee, 1991). The foundations of theory of mind—children's understanding that others' desires and beliefs affect their behavior—formed the basis of much research in the area that I call personalized information of others' emotions. Thus, around 3 years of age children begin to understand that the emotions of a protagonist in a story would differ depending on their desires, as I have already noted. For example, Wellman and Banerjee (1991) asked children questions about getting juice for a snack or a visit from Grandma (for happiness), seeing rain out the window or going to a library that had no picture books (for sadness). They also heard stories in which the protagonist was surprised (finding that Grandma's house was purple) or curious (finding a closed box in a closet). They asked the children why the protagonist felt these ways and then what the protagonist wanted and thought.

Even 3-year-olds differentiated the stories, substantiating them based on desires for happiness and sadness and on beliefs for surprise and curiosity. Two follow-up studies supported and extended these initial findings. The authors concluded that as young as 3 years, children begin to understand that discrepancies between beliefs and outcomes can engender specific emotions, such as surprise. However, this understanding is just beginning, and 3-year-olds still tend to interpret emotions based on what the protagonist *wanted*, their desire. By age 5, however, this nascent understanding of emotion and (sometimes mistaken) belief solidifies and becomes more consistent (see also Hadwin & Perner, 1991; Harris et al., 1989; Pons et al., 2004; Rieffe, Meerum Terwogt, Koops, Stegge, & Oomen, 2001). As suggested by Harris et al. (1989), during this period children come to understand that the emotions felt in a situation depend not only on its objective features, but also on the individual's desires and beliefs. Desires and beliefs vary from person to person despite what the observing child may feel.

However, adding another level of complexity may render it more difficult to transition from a focus on desire to a focus on including a belief in understanding others' emotions. As noted earlier, discerning atypical emotional reactions is difficult. Even 6-year-olds may revert to desires when trying to explain why a protagonist feels angry at getting a present from his mother (Rieffe, Meerum Terwogt, & Cowan, 2005). However, in Rieffe et al., children as young as 4 years readily used belief explanations for fear, such as being afraid to go outside and play hide-and-seek. These findings suggest that event structure for fear includes the *belief* that something bad will happen.

A fourth source of personalized information is an individual's history. Young children use such information, but less frequently than adults do, because much inference is needed to coordinate it with the current emotional reaction. Gnepp and Gould (1985) told stories in which personalized information was embedded in descriptions of the person's past experiences: "Robin's best friend said she didn't like her anymore. The next day, Robin saw her best friend on the playground. How did she feel?" Despite earlier suggestions here that young children understand that memories may evoke emotions (Pons et al., 2004), 5-year-olds made more situational inferences ("Robin was happy to see her friend because they could play together") than personalized ones ("Robin felt sad because she knew her friend didn't like her anymore"). Only older elementary-age children made more personalized inferences in a condition in which they were asked to explain such a character's atypical emotion. Although it could be important to compare methodologies between Gnepp's work (e.g., Gnepp, 1989b) and that of Pons et al. (2004), it seems that use of this type of personalized information is basically beyond preschoolers' capability.

## SUMMARY: Reconciling Unique Emotional Information

Preschoolers are beginning to understand how the causes of an emotion can differ from person to person as well as from situation to situation—trying to comprehend equivocal situations, conflicting expressions and situations, and personalized information. They are starting to unite expressions and situations in a more sophisticated way. Many of these complex judgments about emotions remain difficult, however. Understanding that young children cannot always make these inferences yet is as important as knowing how proficient they are in many other areas of emotion knowledge. A mother can't expect her 4-year-old son to comprehend completely the complex history of her personal aversion for chocolate ice cream. And a preschool girl's inability to refer in an abstract way to emotion-related aspects of her own personality may account for her answer to the question "Why are you so mad?": "Because I am."

## DEVELOPING KNOWLEDGE OF COMPLEX EMOTIONS

Another big accomplishment in the domain of emotion knowledge is understanding the more complex emotions, particularly the self-conscious and social emotions—guilt, shame, pride, embarrassment, and empathy. Because young children and their peers are beginning to express complex emotions, they have some understanding of them, but it is still emerging and develops slowly. Even the oldest preschoolers are unable to cite pride, guilt, or shame specifically in relevant success, failure, and transgression experiences—pride at a gymnastic feat or resisting temptation, or guilt for stealing a few coins out of the coin jar in their parents' bedroom (Arsenio & Kramer, 1992; Barden, Zelko, Duncan, & Masters, 1980; Berti, Garattoni, & Venturini, 2000; Harter & Whitesell, 1989; Nunner-Winkler & Sodian, 1988).

Children do not use correct emotional terms, or even descriptions, of their own and others' pride or shame until at least age 6. Preschoolers report simpler emotions, such as happiness, gladness, or excitement, rather than pride, for the gymnastic feat. Even older children report feeling bad, scared, or worried about the detection of stealing and the likelihood of punishment. They do not use terms referring specifically to guilt. Partial concepts of complex emotions predominate (see Chobhthaigh & Wilson, 2015), perhaps in part because of children's incomplete appreciation of societal rules and obligations that evoke them (Harris, 2008).

Other issues, many noted in Chapter 3, make it difficult to learn about these emotions. These include (1) facial expressions for these emotions, when they exist, are not as universal as those for "basic" emotions and are accompanied by other physical or behavioral indices, making learning more complex; (2) the experience and expression of these emotions often involves the development of the self; (3) a complete understanding of such emotions is cognitively complex in other ways, often requiring a comparison of one's own and others' perspectives; and (4) usage of the words representing these emotions emerges later in development than those for emotions like happiness and sadness (Tracy, Robins, & Lagattuta, 2005). In short, expectations for children to understand these emotions as early as "basic" emotions are unreasonable; as always, getting a fair estimate of the emergence of such understanding requires developmentally appropriate methodology.

### Understanding Guilt

Much of the research on young children's understanding of complex emotions involves guilt; some evidence about preschoolers' notion of this emotion, or at least emotions they consider to occur in conjunction with transgressions, has been uncovered. Instead of presenting children with situations and asking how the protagonist would feel, however, Russell and Paris (1994) were among the first to come at this problem from another direction: They told children how a story character felt, and then asked them to complete the story by saying why the character felt that way and whether the character felt good or bad. They found that 4- and 5-year-olds have a partial conceptualization of complex emotions such as pride, jealousy, shame, and gratitude: "They understand the [valence] associated with the emotion but have no knowledge of the kind of situation that evokes it" (p. 349) and cannot accurately explain causes. These findings fit well with the issues already mentioned about the difficulties young children *should* have regarding guilt and other complex emotions.

Further, 4-year-olds through kindergartners usually judge a wrongdoer's feelings on the outcome of his or her actions, harkening back to their incomplete understanding of social rules and obligations. They tend to use a naive desire-based causal analysis when describing the emotions felt after a transgression: A person is happy if he or she does not get caught, but is angry if he or she does. They give what has been dubbed the "happy victimizer" response, and the occurrence of this error has been replicated many times (for overviews, see Arsenio, 2006; Arsenio, Gold, & Adams, 2006; Krettenauer, Malti, & Sokol, 2008; Lagattuta, 2005).

However, young children do not expect a character, even an ill-motivated one, to feel good if he or she harmed another person by accident or observed someone being hurt. So related to guilt, one's own transgression, if it helps meet a goal, generates positive feelings, in contrast to harm unrelated to one's goals. Related to shame-inducing circumstances, children this young also indicate that they would be sad if they failed at a task.

It is important to note that the very nature of wrongdoing realistically elicits mixed emotions, even into adulthood (Murgatroyd & Robinson, 1993). For example, a 5-year-old boy does in fact feel happy that he now "owns" another boy's Power Ranger, even though he stole it from the other boy's cubbyhole. He may also feel scared that he might get caught, sorry when he sees the other boy crying, or guilty when a teacher chides him for the theft. An adult who cheats at cards may also be glad to win, but worried that the casino will summarily usher him out. For preschoolers but not adults, as already noted, the *understanding* of such mixed and ambivalent emotions is far from perfect. Adding complex moral themes to the mix just makes cognitively reasoning about such events even more difficult.

In sum, preschoolers distinguish between feeling bad and being bad. That distinction is a most basic one, a low-level generalization about the emotional consequences of moral events. They show that they know emotions are determined not exclusively by goal attainment, but also by limited moral considerations and empathic concern. *Being* bad actually can lead to *feeling* good (and often does!) as well as *feeling* bad, but witnessing or accidentally causing harm (*being* "good") also can lead to *feeling* bad. In studies using probes such as "Could he or she feel another way?" (Arsenio & Kramer, 1992), even preschoolers could acknowledge feeling both happy and sad feelings after a moral transgression.

More recent research on understanding guilt has taken a somewhat different tack. For example, if one examines the action tendencies related to guilt, considering *when* children begin to express these action tendencies might indicate early evidence of knowing what situations cause guilt (see Chapter 3). Thus, even 2- and 3-year-olds made more attempts to repair a broken toy when they had been responsible (the "guilt condition") rather than when they merely saw the breakage happen (the "sympathy condition") (Vaish et al., 2016). The authors assert that this finding implies a basic, very elementary understanding of the emotional consequences of their own wrongdoing, resulting in actions representing guilt. I find these claims interesting, but they are not exactly what I mean by *knowledge*—perhaps they are akin to procedural knowledge—whereas I focus more on declarative knowledge.

Nonetheless, children later come to understand more complex action tendencies associated with guilt. They learn that apologies are part of guilty behavior, and that an apologetic transgressor is less worthy of blame and punishment than an unapologetic one (Smith, Chen, & Harris, 2010). But even when the routinized (and thus maybe less than meaningful) wording "I'm sorry" was not included or was substituted with the words "I didn't mean to do it; it's my fault," 4- and 5-year-olds preferred the remorseful transgressor and understood that the person felt bad (Smith et al., 2010; Vaish, Carpenter, & Tomasello, 2011). So, appropriate guilt-related behavior and judgments are acquired through the preschool period, even if preschoolers cannot properly name situations of guilt.

## Understanding Pride

Preschoolers' pride at an achievement is a complex, self-conscious emotion that also has been studied recently. It does appear that preschoolers can recognize its situational antecedents (Kornilaki & Chloverakis, 2004) and facial/bodily expression (Tracy et al., 2005), although methodological differences are important, as often occurs. In their first experiment, Tracy and colleagues showed arrays of three photographs depicting facial and bodily emotion displays of happiness, surprise, and pride (i.e., expanded chest, shoulders pulled back, head tilted slightly back, small closed-mouth smile, and arms either raised above the head with fists or hands on the hips). Children were asked to "point to the photo where Joe/Jan is feeling X." By age 4 children performed at better than a chance level on identifying pride, and 45% of even 3-year-olds identified pride correctly at least half the time, with 90% of 4-year-olds meeting this criterion. In a second experiment, children were asked to point to the picture depicting pride, but also to say if they *didn't* see any picture. With this modification, pride recognition accuracy increased, and did not differ significantly among 3- to 6-year-olds.

However, in another study (Nelson & Russell, 2012) preschoolers viewed 5-second video clips including head and face only (tilted head and small smile), body posture only (moving from a neutral to an expanded posture with hands on hips, changing to arms above head), or all cues at once. The question asked regarding the videos (involving, in the entire procedure, videos not only for pride, but also for happiness, fear, surprise, disgust, and embarrassment), was "How did she feel?" For this method, it was not until children were 6 to 9 years old that they specifically identified pride at all, and then only to the multicue expression.

Like the studies already reviewed showing that preschoolers do not use language specific to complex emotions, these investigators found that preschoolers were unable to name what they saw. It is important to note that in Tracy and colleagues' (2005) study, although the pride display was static, it involved all the multiple cues in Nelson and Russell's (2012) study, and only nonverbal recognition was required. As already noted, recognition precedes expression in knowledge of emotions, as in much of preschoolers' verbal knowledge. Thus the conclusion can be reached that younger preschoolers are beginning to recognize pride, but as with earlier research, cannot verbally identify it until early in the primary school years.

Nonetheless, in two other studies, researchers in this group noted that young children were more capable of discerning pride, as well as other social emotions (e.g., embarrassment and shame) when they heard stories, rather than by examining faces (Nelson, Hudspeth, & Russell, 2013; Widen & Russell, 2010a). Although this finding was taken as support for the constructivist view that language and conceptual foundations are more important in emotion identification than are facial expressions, it seems to me not at all surprising that stories would "work" better for emotions where there are fewer, or somewhat more nebulous, unclear expressions (although Widen & Russell, 2010a, did find this effect for fear, as well).

Delving further into this question, a recent study ingeniously combined an examination of the happy victimizer effect, with the possible experience of guilt or pride (Hasegawa, 2021). Stories about pushing a peer off a swing or stealing doughnuts were created where the protagonist felt happy after such behavior (i.e., the "happy victimizer"), sad after such behavior (i.e., guilt), or happy after *not* transgressing (i.e., pride). In simplifying the task demands of the procedure, children were able to see the protagonist's emotional expression and were told explicitly how the protagonist felt (making the method more developmentally appropriate); social desirability also was avoided. Children were asked how the protagonist would feel the next day, and why.

Preschoolers (ages 5 to 6) predicted that the protagonist would perform the transgression again (especially pushing the peer off the swing) when he or she had shown a happy victimizer emotion. They were more likely to explain their prediction for the protagonist's future actions using his or her emotional state when the story mentioned the protagonist feeling sad about the transgression (for both situations, but especially theft). Thus, they thought that a happy victimizer would repeat his or her actions, but referred to emotions most in their explanations of next-day behavior when the transgressor had felt guilty. However, happy feelings were not used as a judgment in avoiding transgression, suggesting that pride was less well understood than guilt for these stories.

Based on the complexity of the results, a second study was conducted using forced-choice questions about the stories, which were changed to include two stories each in which the protagonist felt happy and sad, respectively, after transgressing, and happy and sad, respectively, after avoiding transgression. Questions included (1) "will the [transgressor] [transgressed against] push or steal?" and (2) "Why?"

Except for avoiding transgressing for pushing, preschoolers gave equivalent, prevalently correct answers compared to third graders. That is, they said that the happy transgressors could commit the offense again, and the sad ones would not. Preschoolers mentioned emotions in about half of their explanations for transgressing or avoiding transgressing for both situations. Thus at least in understanding the *valence* of guilt versus happiness when victimizing, preschoolers demonstrated a beginning understanding. The association of happiness or pride with *not* transgressing was not found.

## SUMMARY: Understanding Guilt and Pride

Regarding guilt and pride, preschoolers appear to understand the basic breakdown of moral versus nonmoral behavior and feelings, following emotional distinctions that they know best. Whether they are working from the moral situation to the moral emotion or the moral emotion to the moral situation, preschoolers' understanding is limited to elemental distinctions, such as those that supported their earliest understanding of emotional expressions and situations. They still describe the consequences of achievement and moral situations in terms of basic, rather than complex, emotions. Basic emotions are, for them, the most logical as outcomes for situations that could (or should) elicit the moral emotions of shame and guilt. And an overriding concern over wrongdoing does not always "register" with them in situations where moral issues are central. Finally to some extent the happy victimizer lives on in their judgments.

Adults who are attuned to children's abilities in this area will be less likely to mismatch their socialization messages to the child's capability to comprehend them (Arsenio & Lover, 1995); using the appropriate words for guilt and pride should not be avoided, necessarily, but simpler emotions should form the springboard for discussing morally tinged emotions.

Because the emotional consequences of a social–moral act are undoubtedly mixed, and it takes time to acquire an understanding of emotions and events, young children can benefit from adult support to show what they do understand (Arsenio et al., 2006). Their understanding of guilt and pride will take time to consolidate.

## Understanding Gratitude

What about the emotion of gratitude? This emotion has not yet been discussed, but it is surely a complex emotion. Gratitude involves positive feelings toward a benefactor, or more simply, someone who does something positive for the self. Like the early manifestations of guilt's action tendencies, 3-year-olds begin to recognize that they've been the recipients of goodwill and are motivated to prolong the prosocial interaction by showing reciprocity. As with guilt, this is not a true "understanding" of gratitude, but it is a start. Extending these early understandings, Vaish and Hepach (2020) describe a study in which preschoolers heard stories about a benefactor and two beneficiaries—one who displayed gratitude and the other just happiness. Gratitude included acknowledging the generosity of the benefactor, expressing appreciation for the gift, and affirming the relationship. Five-year-olds preferred the grateful beneficiary; 4-year-olds also showed a trend toward this choice, suggesting an emerging understanding of gratitude toward the end of the preschool period.

In a logical extension of this work, Nelson, de Lucca Freitas, et al. (2013) told 5-year-olds stories about dolls as protagonists being helped by a benefactor (i.e., to find a lost cat or being lent a sweater when cold) and were asked how the protagonist felt and why. They were prompted to give more than one answer about how they felt and also were asked specifically how they felt about the benefactor. They also were asked how the benefactor felt and the reason for helping. Presumably the investigators considered the stories engaging enough to enlist these older preschoolers' verbal abilities.

The positive feelings of the protagonists, connecting positive emotion with the benefactor, and whether the protagonists should help the benefactor were each scored for both stories. Over half said the protagonist would feel positive because of the benefactor's actions, but only for the sweater story. A large percentage of the children said that the protagonist could help the benefactor later, but fewer than 20% expressed a full understanding of reciprocity, helping in return for having been helped. Thus most of the children did not have a complete understanding of gratitude at age 5. Significantly, however, Nelson, de Lucca Freitas, et al. (2013) found that an understanding of "basic" emotions at age 3 predicted mental state understanding (theory of mind) at age 4, which then predicted an understanding of gratitude at age 5.

### SUMMARY: Understanding Gratitude

Together these studies on the understanding of gratitude suggest that at least by the end of the preschool period, children are beginning to understand gratitude, in contrast to earlier work that indicated that this development was delayed until age 7. Overall, especially regarding more recent investigations of guilt and gratitude, preschoolers are acquiring an increasing knowledge of emotions that help in monitoring and maintaining prosocial relationships (Vaish & Hepach, 2020).

## DEVELOPING A KNOWLEDGE OF EMOTION DISPLAY RULES

As stated in Chapter 3, children's expressive patterns become more complex as they grow older; they more often neutralize, intensify, mask, minimize, or substitute one emotion for another. It is important for children to not only know how to modulate emotions in this way, but also to acquire knowledge about, and follow, cultural, familial, and personal rules for expression of emotion (Josephs, 1994). Again, as Saarni (1987) noted, reasons to show emotions that are different from those one feels can be prosocial (e.g., changing an emotion to be kind to another person) or self-protective (e.g., showing a different emotion than felt to reach a goal, protect one's feelings, or avoid negative consequences). Even though there is evidence that young children *use* such rules (see Chapter 3), less empirical research examined preschoolers' *understanding* of both emotion dissemblance and display rules, which seems to evolve later (e.g., Banerjee, 1997a; Josephs, 1994; Misailidi, 2006).

As a foundation for display rule knowledge, young children must recognize situations that call for dissemblance—the act of expressing an emotion that in fact differs from what is felt. This appearance/reality understanding continues to develop through grade school; it is an important element of learning the "feeling rules" of one's culture. Knowing when and when not to show emotions is immeasurably valuable in maintaining social relations, and knowledge of when to dissemble adds to the child's growing emotional competence.

## Dissemblance: Real versus Apparent Emotions

The most elementary notion about the reality and appearance of emotion is that of dissemblance. Hiding emotions by neutralizing or masking emotional expression or substituting one emotion for another can be advantageous to young children as early as they can pose expression voluntarily (see Chapter 3). Dissemblance does not require knowledge of display rules that are normative to a family or culture, but merely the need to send an emotional signal that differs from the one that is felt—to minimize or substitute the felt emotion, for example. Along these lines, Pons et al. (2004) found that 50% of 5-year-olds realize that inner and outer emotions can differ, and that by age 7, 65% of children demonstrated such understanding.

An early, ingenious investigation of young children's understanding of dissemblance was among the first to adopt theory of mind methodologies to assess emotions' reality and appearance, as well as beliefs about them (Gross & Harris, 1988). Four- and 6-year-olds were asked to say how the protagonist in stories *really* felt and *appeared* to feel, as well as how each of two bystanders *believed* the protagonist felt. They heard stories about a protagonist who experienced emotion-eliciting situations. Sometimes this protagonist showed other characters his real feelings; at other times he hid his true feelings (i.e., dissembled). Stories in which the protagonist showed how he really felt were termed *nondiscrepant* stories, whereas stories in which he dissembled were called *discrepant* or deception stories. Not surprisingly, given the timetable for understanding emotion situations and causes, all the children understood the *real* feelings of the protagonist in both nondiscrepant and discrepant emotion displays (see also Josephs, 1994). If the protagonist felt sad about getting an injection or being teased, children demonstrated that they understood what emotion the situation would evoke—even though the protagonist showed his sad feelings about the shot in one story, but in the other story deceived his brother about his sadness about the teasing.

In more complicated discrepant stories, the bystander also gave the protagonist a situation-specific reason to dissemble to the other (e.g., "You should not hurt Grandmother's feelings by showing what you feel"). However, in these discrepant stories, even determining the protagonist's *real* feelings was more difficult than in nondiscrepant stories. This methodology highlighted the skills of the older children: The 6-year-olds were more accurate than the 4-year-olds in identifying the real and apparent emotions of the protagonist in the discrepant stories. Perhaps the younger, more concrete children thought that such an injunction could really change the protagonist's internal state. They may have interpreted the reason to dissemble as "You should not hurt Grandmother's feelings by *feeling that way*."

In terms of knowing how the protagonist *appeared* to feel ("How would he look on his face?"), again nearly all the children gave accurate responses for nondiscrepant emotions; this was expected, given preschoolers' general understanding of emotional situations. But the 6-year-olds again were more accurate than the 4-year-olds at telling how the protagonist *appeared* to feel for discrepant emotions. They understood that where there was deception, the protagonist would *appear* to show an emotion that was different from his true emotions. His face would not show the same emotion he felt (e.g., "She looked like she felt okay, not sad, so that the other children wouldn't laugh and call her a baby"; Gross, 1993).

In contrast, younger preschoolers were again more likely to think that appearance could not differ from reality—that "what you feel is what you see." Their attention more often was riveted on observable phenomena, such as the emotional events themselves. They then err by overlooking dissemblance (e.g., "She looked sad because they squirted her with the hose"; Gross, 1993). This limitation suggests that younger preschoolers' difficulty in understanding deception is more broadly based in their somewhat less developed theory of mind.

The inaccurate beliefs of witnesses underlie the perception of dissembled emotions. Thus, for beliefs, the children in Gross and Harris's (1988) study were asked what the bystander *believed* the protagonist was feeling: Children of both ages were more accurate in judging what the bystander believed for nondiscrepant than for discrepant emotion displays, in which they were asked, "Did David's friends think he was happy, sad, or just okay [when he was really sad but his face looked happy]?" But the 6-year-olds again were more accurate than the 4-year-olds in making either judgment.

To follow up on the potential underestimation of younger preschoolers' understanding of how emotions may be hidden, Gross (1993) investigated 3- and 4-year-olds' understanding of both false beliefs and false emotions, using a more developmentally appropriate methodology for these younger children compared to those in the earlier study (Gross & Harris, 1988). Children were asked to determine a puppet's beliefs about a doll with a sad or happy mask and about felt-tip markers with the wrong color caps. The children, but not the puppet, witnessed the doll putting on a mask to cover its real feelings as well as the incorrect placement of marker caps (e.g., the blue cap was placed on the red marker). Despite their own privileged information, 4-year-olds and many 3-year-olds understood that the information available to the puppet led it to believe in both a false emotion for the masked doll and false colors for the markers. They were beginning to be able to use information about how beliefs influence what is understood about someone's emotions.

At the same time, however, protagonists' real emotion's valence had an impact (Banerjee, 1997a, 1997b; Josephs, 1994). In Josephs's study, 4-year-olds had more difficulty than 6-year-olds in tempering the real emotion in positive discrepant stories—for example, they were more likely to say the protagonists were happy when they won a race even if their best friend lost, or even when they ate chocolate but then their mother "caught" them. They had more trouble invoking either prosocial or self-protective reasons to dissemble or hide positive emotions. As with knowledge about emotion regulation, changing happy emotion is especially difficult. But boys in particular have evidenced difficulty conceiving that positive emotions could be dissembled (Banerjee, 1997a, 1997b).

Overall these findings support and elaborate upon Pons et al.'s (2004) later findings, already cited; similarly, Josephs (1994) also found 5- and 6-year-olds performed above chance on comparable stories, and these children's performance improved with age. So, although improvements occurred, inferring perceptions of a person's dissembled emotions was admittedly difficult for all young children.

Although 4-year-olds exhibited difficulties in explaining dissemblance, the overall results of these studies suggested that 6-year-olds' failures to understand dissemblance were not solely due to difficulties in determining a person's real and apparent emotions. Perhaps these tasks rendered it just too difficult for preschoolers by adding one more level of inference to the task— to ask a younger preschooler to *think* about how another person *thought* about what the protagonist was *trying to project* about what he was *feeling*. Although these cited experimental procedures were intended to reflect common situations in which preschoolers might dissemble, and to make queries simply, they still may have been taxing, especially for 3- and 4-year-olds.

Several studies have attempted to reduce response burdens to get closer to better understanding what preschoolers know about dissemblance. In a more recent study, children were given more information so that less inference was required. Misailidi (2006) asked children to identify and justify the appearance–reality distinction, in stories where a protagonist's real emotion was revealed, as was a prosocial or self-protective motive to conceal with another emotion. If they were told, for example, that Mary's grandmother gave her a "horrible sweater" for her birthday, 4- to 6-year-olds could answer how Mary *actually* felt (sadness) and what her face *showed* (happiness), *and why* (to spare her grandmother's feelings). Such prosocial and self-protective motivations (e.g., not wanting to be considered a crybaby when squirted with a water gun; see also Gnepp & Hess, 1986) were justified with equivalent accuracy. The ability to identify and describe dissemblance increased from age 4 to 6, but all age groups performed at better than chance level.

This author's methodological efforts to minimize memory and verbal requirements on the task suggested that the age differences, in which 4-year-olds tended to equate "feeling" and "showing," were real and not confounded. Her methodology also may have made it easier for children to justify both prosocial and self-protective reasons to hide emotions and rendered this more truly a study of appearance–reality than one of display rules. However, it is of note that prosocial and self-protective reasons for dissemblance, which form the basis of culturally sanctioned display rules, were specified in Gross and Harris (1988), Josephs (1994), Banerjee (1997a), and Misailidi (2006). So even young preschoolers have some coherent ideas about the distinction between real and apparent emotion.

> Alex has watched his older sister near tears as she practices the piano before the big recital—he knows she's scared as she walks onstage. When he sees how calm she is while playing almost triumphantly at the event, he wonders if she still has butterflies in her tummy. What she is showing doesn't match what he knew she was feeling earlier; he is learning about dissemblance.

To find out more about such understanding in an even more ecologically valid way, Banerjee (1997a, 1997b) told 3- to 5-year-olds that the central character in each of six stories about emotions "might really feel one way inside but look a different way on her face. Or she might really feel the same way inside that she looks on her face. I want you to choose the pictures for how she really feels inside, and how she looks on her face" (1997a, p. 115) This central character was motivated to hide an emotion, whether it was positive or negative: "Diana wants to hide her brother Bill's toy because he hasn't been very nice. She does so and feels happy, but she needs to hide this happiness so that Bill will not shout at her" (1997a, p. 115).

Given the clear guidance in this study, even 3-year-olds were able to distinguish real and apparent emotions in these situations. Banerjee had implemented several methodological simplifications, compared to Gross and Harris's (1988) original study. These included (1) use of pictures to aid the children's responding; (2) fewer questions (i.e., no probes for memory of the story); and (3) explicit statements of how the protagonists really felt, so that the task *only* involved identifying the dissembled emotion.

However, although 5-year-olds performed better than 3- and 4-year-olds, all performed at a better than chance level, and greater than 50% of all age groups gave appropriate responses on four or more of six stories. Creating a more developmentally appropriate methodology allowed preschoolers to demonstrate greater competence.

### SUMMARY: Dissemblance

Again, as already considered, discrepancies between competence and performance—where children can show an ability with some methodologies, but not with others—alerts involved adults that this period is a time of emerging skill in understanding dissemblance. Even 3-year-olds can distinguish between emotional experience and expression and know that a dissembled emotion can create a false belief in another person, when they are given concrete examples of, rather than just stories about, misleading emotion displays.

Hence, knowledge of dissemblance and deception is beginning to develop in this age range. Methods that circumvent their concreteness allow younger preschoolers to show that they are discovering and beginning to acknowledge the potential differences between emotional reality and appearance. But the transition to a fuller understanding is probably still not complete until the end of the preschool period.

## Knowledge of General Display Rules

As noted in Chapter 3, dissemblance is not the only way in which children modify their expressiveness; they also modify their emotion displays to conform with their understanding of culturally, socially, or personally appropriate display rules, and their justifications for the appearance–reality distinction can help uncover such knowledge. Young children may begin to consciously understand such display rules as they begin to use them. After all, they comprehend that objects may really not be as they look, know that emotions are personal internal states, and actually use display rules (Cole, 1986; Wellman & Banerjee, 1991; Wellman & Woolley, 1990; see Chapter 3). They may learn display rules first for those emotions subject to more socialization pressure, such as anger; when admonished not to show anger, preschoolers may also learn a "Don't show anger" rule (Feito, 1997).

Following this line of reasoning, Banerjee (1997a, 1997b) thought that methodological simplifications would better unveil preschoolers' true understanding of display rules. In Banerjee's display rule assessments, a stuffed doll described an emotional experience and asked the child whether it should express the emotion. Four of the stories were restrictive; that is, social norms suggested that the emotion be hidden (e.g., "Grandma made a 'yucky' casserole and the doll wanted to scrunch up his or her face and spit it out, but Grandma was standing right there"). The remaining three stories were permissive; that is, social norms allowed emotional expressions (e.g., "The doll was happy at Dad's birthday party and wanted to shout, 'Happy birthday!' and give him a big hug").

Approximately three-quarters of the preschool-age children responded appropriately to the stories. They knew that emotions should be modified more often in restrictive, rather than in permissive, stories and for the expression of negative emotions (see also Josephs, 1994). Four- and 5-year-olds, compared to 3-year-olds, gave more appropriate justifications for their answers and cited avoiding negative consequences most often.

More recently, Pala and Lewis (2021) told preschoolers nine stories in which the protagonists, if they were to follow prosocial display rules, needed to mask their disappointment so as not to hurt another's feelings. Importantly, in the developmentally appropriate portrayal of these stories, children saw all possible combinations of both what the protagonists were thinking about (the disappointingly thwarted goal or the actual outcome) and the possible differing emotions (happy or sad). Four- and 5-year-olds were able to show how the protagonists would not show their disappointment even when thinking about their goal that had been thwarted. Even the 4-year-olds could "explain how duty and politeness dictate display rules" (p. 512). They could understand how what one feels on the inside may need to differ from the emotion one displays to social partners.

Some researchers have found gender differences in these early abilities. In Banerjee (1997a), girls responded more accurately than boys (see the discussion of girls' *use* of display rules in Chapter 3 and their understanding of dissemblance discussed earlier); in fact, boys sometimes said the doll should not show emotions even in the permissive stories. In Josephs (1994) study, girls were better able than boys to identify the emotion that "should" be shown in prosocial stories. Such evidence suggests that girls' socialization of emotion, even at this relatively early age, is implicated in their understanding.

## SUMMARY: Display Rules

Thus older preschoolers understand a great deal about display rules, although there apparently are gender differences in this ability. Despite this increasingly positive evidence of young children's developing understanding of dissemblance and display rules, especially when developmentally appropriate methodologies are used, it should be recognized that such knowledge does continue to improve during grade school (Gross & Harris, 1988; Jones, Abbey, & Cumberland, 1998; Wu, Wang, & Liu, 2017). Remember: When a friend wears an ugly sweater, you do not laugh; when your grandma accidentally breaks your toy, you do not show anger; when you lose a contest, you do not cry; and when you steal a cookie, it is best not to look guilty! Learning these rules is part of living felicitously in society.

## DEVELOPING A KNOWLEDGE OF SIMULTANEOUS EMOTIONS AND AMBIVALENCE

It is not uncommon for older children and adults to experience "mixed emotions," as when a father is amused at his 2-year-old daughter's antics, but also annoyed with the mess she makes, or when 3-year-old Maddie is amused at her baby brother's antics as he lurches to grab her Dora the Explorer backpack, but is also annoyed when he tries to bite it. Because young children's expressiveness is becoming more intricate as they leave the preschool period, they may become conscious of such simultaneous emotions and of ambivalence. They may begin to experience simultaneous emotions and ambivalence themselves, and thus to know more about them—but it isn't likely to be an easy process; as noted by Pons et al. (2004), this ability requires reflective abilities and more abstract thinking than even the mentalistic emotion knowledge abilities just described.

Several theorists emphasize how difficult it is for children to identify and comprehend situations in which simultaneous but opposite emotions occur. Harter and colleagues proposed a cognitive-developmental sequence based on the valence of two felt emotions and the number of targets toward which the two emotions are directed (Harter & Buddin, 1987; Harter & Whitesell, 1989). In this model, children progress through four levels of understanding. The first begins at age 7, when children comprehend that two emotions of the same valence can be directed toward the same target—for example, sadness and anger when a peer wrecks a just-completed puzzle. By age 11, children can acknowledge that feelings of opposite valences can be expressed toward the same target—for example, anger at one's mother for taking away a privilege while loving her all the same. In Harter and colleagues' model, preschoolers' understanding of these emotional issues is embryonic at best.

Yet there is mounting evidence that this model underestimates younger children's actual understanding of multiple or conflicting emotions. Again asking questions using more age-appropriate methodology could reveal that preschoolers have more knowledge than previously supposed (Donaldson & Westerman, 1986; Kestenbaum & Gelman, 1995; Peng, Johnson, Pollock, Glasspool, & Harris, 1992). Research from the 1980s and 1990s, as well as more recent work, confirms that younger children are beginning to understand others' mixed emotions.

First, in a downward extension of earlier work (Wintre, Polivy, & Murray, 1990), Wintre and Vallance (1994) investigated 4- to 8-year-olds' abilities to judge the existence, intensity, and valence of multiple emotions. Participants were asked, "How would you feel?" after hearing 15 stories, including "For your birthday you get a brand-new bicycle," and "You lose control of your bike and almost crash" (see, e.g., Wintre & Vallance, 1994, pp. 510–511). Children were given the opportunity to rank, on an abacus-like frame, how intensely they would feel happy, sad, angry, scared, and/or loving (depicted pictorially on one axis of the frame). The structure of the task made it easy for children to indicate simultaneity of emotions; instead of their having to spontaneously envision simultaneity, it was almost assumed. The children's most sophisticated responses to the 15 stories were used to categorize their developmental level in judging simultaneous emotions.

The results indicated that at about age 5, children could predict experiencing multiple emotions of the same intensity and same valence to affect-eliciting situations. At about age 6, they began to predict experiencing multiple emotions of the same valence but differing intensities to affect-eliciting situations. It was not until about 8 years of age that children predicted multiple emotions of both varying intensity and opposite valence. Thus, Wintre and Vallance's (1994) procedural improvements preserved but accelerated Harter's group's chronology.

Another constructive methodological refinement involves techniques that elicit, rather than spontaneously require, mentioning of conflicting emotions (Peng et al., 1992; see also Donaldson & Westerman, 1986). Children heard stories in which a pet or a possession was lost and was then found in an injured or partially damaged state. This sequence of events would typically evoke both happiness and sadness.

Children were placed in two groups, an "events" group and an "emotions" group. They were then asked two questions about the events in the story. Those in the events group were asked only about events—for example, for the lost-pet story, "Does the child find his pet?"; "Is the pet hurt?" In contrast, for the emotions group, the events were assumed. The protagonist's concomitant emotions were elicited: "When the child finds the pet, how does he feel?"; "When the child knows that the pet is hurt, how does he feel?"

For both conditions, the third question asked about the child's feelings. For the events group, however, the events were again repeated with only the added question, "How does the child feel?" In contrast, for the children in the emotions group the third question included two causal statements that linked events and emotions, such as "When the child holds the pet, he is happy that he has found the pet, but he also is sad because the pet is hurt. How does the child feel?" When experimenters highlighted the specific emotions for this group, 6- and 7-year-olds, but not 4- and 5-year-olds, agreed that emotions of different valences were directed at the same target and, what's more, could explain them. The strategy that involved being told about the simultaneous, mixed emotions for all three questions gave the older group of children the scaffolding they needed to respond correctly. The younger group could not make use of this aid.

In a similar study, kindergartners had much more trouble in *detecting* simultaneous opposite-valence emotions than in *explaining* them (which they could do in 75% of cases; Gordis, Rosen, & Grand, 1989). When these children were told stories like "Amir feels happy but also a little sad going to the airport," they were able to explain that Amir was excited to see the airplanes but felt bad that his father was going on a business trip. In contrast, they could not spontaneously assert that Amir would feel happy and sad at the same time after merely hearing a story describing the same events. Furthermore, when the explaining task was administered prior to the detection task, it highlighted the nature of the task for the children, who then performed better on detecting the simultaneous emotions on their own. In a later study, Brown and Dunn (1996) documented a gender difference in this capability that favored kindergarten girls.

These converging results suggest that young children can be sensitive to opposing positive and negative feelings aimed at the same target event. Specifically, preschoolers can recognize and explain conflicting emotions at a younger age than previously reported, although doing so can still be a challenging task, especially when their own emotions are involved (Larson, Yen, & Fireman, 2007). In particular, they perceive what it means to have conflicting feelings without being able to spontaneously talk about them. They need priming to discuss these emotional occurrences.

Along with its methodological shortcomings, earlier research also neglected to discern *why* young children have difficulties with mixed emotions. When children are beginning to comprehend so many sophisticated aspects of emotional life, why is this one topic so difficult? Young children's reliance on facial expression to interpret emotions ("Faces can't go up and down at the same time") and on their still-growing theories of mind ("You can't think two ways") gets in their way (Harris, 1983). They may need to "unlearn" some of their most cherished propositions about internal states to move forward in this area of emotion knowledge.

Even more highly scaffolded experimental conditions than those already illustrated might shed some much-needed light on these issues, by "dissect[ing] the task in order to isolate where problems may occur" (Kestenbaum & Gelman, 1995, p. 446). These investigators set up a series of increasingly scaffolded studies to do just this. In the first study, they asked 5-year-olds open-ended questions about feeling happy and sad, happy and angry, or sad and angry, at the same time. Sixty-four percent of the children acknowledged that feelings could be mixed. However, their justifications were not especially adequate. Even when their justifications addressed mixed emotions, few children cited the actual simultaneity of feelings or the juncture of two eliciting events. So verbal response demands without any type of support elicited the least understanding about mixed emotions. These results squared with other work in the area.

Accordingly, the second study required less verbal production. Children heard stories about two distinct but simultaneous events leading to either mixed basic or single basic emotions. Five-year-olds, but not 4-year-olds, were able to discern multiple emotions in the stories, especially when they had visual information. Separation of the emotion-eliciting events did make the task easier.

As in weighing expressive and situational aspects of emotion, however, the 4-year-olds' difficulties may have emanated from language and/or cognitive constraints and from lack of experience. Children of this age think more concretely than 5-year-olds; they have trouble with the notion of time and with the linguistic concept "at the same time." Perhaps, too, they have had less experience with the more subtle personal and social experiences that lead to mixed emotions. Even greater scaffolding might help to uncover their emergent competence.

In the third, most scaffolded study, these investigators continued their efforts to pinpoint where problems occurred in reasoning about mixed emotions. They capitalized upon and extended the salutary effect of visual stimuli found in the second study. Children were given three types of visual examples of mixed emotions: photographs of adults modified to include the eyes from one emotion and the mouth of another expression; cartoon "aliens" with a similar mix of eye and mouth regions; and cartoon "aliens" with two heads, each expressing a different emotion. Children answered how each stimulus felt in both open-ended and forced-choice formats. In a forced-choice format, 4- and 5-year-olds willingly identified and acknowledged mixed emotions in facial expressions, especially for the two-headed alien; in open-ended questions, they acknowledged mixed emotions *only* for the two-headed alien.

So given special assistance in visualizing how mixed emotions are experienced and expressed, young children are capable of identifying and talking about them. The methodological addition of the two-headed alien helped the children overcome the disturbing conflict between the existence of mixed emotions and the precept "You can't think/feel two ways."

Despite these encouraging findings, disagreement among developmentalists continued for a long time: Can late-preschool-age children detect only multiple emotions of the same valence and intensity, differently valenced emotions, or even only sequential emotions directed at the same target (see Peng et al., 1992; Wintre et al., 1990)? Nonetheless, early research suggested strongly that preschoolers at least are beginning to be able to explain conflicting emotions (Gordis et al., 1989). Further, children's earlier mastery of basic emotion knowledge and their growing skill at talking about the causes of emotions support this budding ability (Brown & Dunn, 1996).

After these earlier studies, investigations have continued to test young children's understanding of mixed emotions and have confirmed evidence of their understanding earlier than at first discerned. Several researchers have employed yet another methodology, asking questions about very emotionally evocative movie clips or rigged computer games. For example, Larsen, Yen, and Fireman (2007) showed children from ages 5 to 12 scenes from the film *The Little Mermaid* (e.g., the father and daughter's bittersweet farewell), and asked them not only how the characters felt, with probes to elicit the possibility of more than one emotion, but also how they themselves felt. More than half of the 5- and 6-year-olds were able to report that the father in the film clip experienced opposite-valenced mixed emotions. This percentage increased in the older children, but nonetheless even a quarter of 5- and 6-year-olds mentioned these mixed emotions without probes (see also Zajdel, Bloom, Fireman, & Larsen, 2013, who found 5- to 7-year-olds' pattern of response not differing from 8- to 9-year-olds). However, very few of these younger children reported experiencing mixed emotions themselves, and analyses suggested that children must first recognize others' mixed emotions before experiencing them (see also Zajdel et al., 2013).

In later refinements, similar findings again were upheld. In a study of 3- to 5-year-olds, the film was less gender slanted than *The Little Mermaid*; a robot was both happy to be following his dream of becoming an inventor but sad to leave his parents (Smith, Glass, & Fireman, 2015). Children were asked how the robot felt, and if they did not report both happy and sad, they were probed for the other emotion. Even 4½ -year-old children could recognize the robot's mixed emotions.

Again, fewer children this age reported experiencing mixed emotions themselves, and the same trend toward understanding others' mixed emotions first was again found, even within this truncated age range. Smith et al. (2015) suggested that preschoolers' discomfort at self-reporting negative emotions may be one confounding feature of this lag. Another plausible, and documented, reason for the difference in reporting mixed emotions for the self versus the character is that empathic concern for the film character facilitates acknowledging their mixed emotions (Zajdel et al., 2013).

A following study explored the issue of understanding one's own mixed emotions more directly. Experiencing a nonsocial situation in which mixed emotions would be likely—winning a $3 prize in a computer game in which both $1 and $9 payouts were possible (one could be happy to get more than $1, but sad not to score the $9)—children were asked about their own mixed emotions and another child's likely emotional responses to the same experience (Fergusson, Hopkins, Stark, Tousignant, & Fireman, 2020). In this procedure, children's responses were again coded as spontaneous, needing prompting, or no reference to mixed emotions. As an extension of earlier work and harkening back to Wintre and Vallance (1994), children also rated their emotions using four faces with increasingly intense happy or sad emotions. Two thirds of 5- to 7-year-olds reported mixed emotions for another child, whereas only 40% reported their own mixed emotions. Again these percentages increased with age for 8- to 9-year-olds and for 10- to 12-year-olds. Thus even very young children can report on another's mixed emotions, but although the abilities are related (Fergusson et al., 2020), they appear to understand less about experiencing their own across several paradigms.

### SUMMARY: Mixed Emotions and Ambivalence

A foundation for understanding mixed emotions is being laid during early childhood, even though comprehending such intricate nuances definitely isn't easy. As seen with other aspects of emotion knowledge, using developmentally appropriate measurement techniques allows a better view of these emerging skills, but also highlights the difficulties that exist. Preschoolers' developing understanding of this complexity in their own and others' emotions undoubtedly facilitates a leap in both children's self-awareness and potentially in their ability to get along with others. And, knowing that children may require some scaffolding to attain this new component of emotion knowledge, parents and caregivers can begin fostering it very early.

## CONTRIBUTORS TO EMOTION KNOWLEDGE DURING EARLY CHILDHOOD

There also seem to be important potential foundations (or at least strong correlates) of emotion knowledge. I discuss how socializers contribute to the development of preschoolers' emotion knowledge in Chapter 8. Here I examine how emotional expressiveness, self-regulation, language and cognitive abilities, attachment, theory of mind, attachment, and culture all play a role.

### Emotional Expressiveness

If children between 2 and 5 years old are acquiring such a solid corpus of basic emotion knowledge, do any other aspects of emotional competence contribute to it? Importantly, children's own patterns of expressiveness contribute to this basic understanding of emotions. Preschoolers first reflect on and make judgments about their own emotions, and then generalize these judgments to others' feelings (Smiley & Huttenlocher, 1989). Thus, they need to experience moderate levels of a variety of emotions to construct social scripts about emotions. Experience of emotion may even help to explain some developmental trends: Even infants clearly experience positive affect sharing and distress relief. Given this experience of their own emotions, then, it is not surprising that toddlers evidence comprehension of happy—not happy states so very early.

Accordingly, following Smiley and Huttenlocher's (1989) reasoning, overall expressiveness should contribute to the understanding of emotion. I have found this to be true: Children who showed more emotions during free play were more adept at understanding both emotional expressions and situations (e.g., Denham, 1986). Having experience with emotions became a foundation of knowledge.

Further, the specific emotions children express and their social cognition about emotions also are related. Children who feel generally happier are better able to contemplate emotional issues. Again my early work (Denham, 1986) supported this prediction: Children who were more emotionally positive showed greater comprehension of basic emotional expressions and situations. Conversely preschoolers who experienced much negative emotion (sadness, anger, or pain) appeared less able to focus on emotional experiences to acquire this basic-level knowledge.

But links among aspects of emotionality and an understanding of emotions are not quite this simple. The experience of at least *some* negative emotion is necessary for children to understand feelings. Children who more often experience anger and fear are also more fluent in verbally enumerating causes for these emotions than are children who rarely experience them (Denham & Zoller, 1990). Thus parents and caregivers need to consider their children's expressiveness patterns when trying to appreciate, or facilitate, their ability to comprehend emotions. Allowing children to experience emotions rather than suppressing them, encouraging positive emotion, and assisting them in their experience of negative emotion are important socialization themes in Western cultures, to which I return in Chapter 8.

## Self-Regulation

Various dimensions and measures of self-regulation, which has already been implicated here for its connection to emotional expressiveness, quite often (almost overwhelmingly!) is related to emotion knowledge (Blankson et al., 2013; Carlson & Wang, 2007; Denham, Bassett, Brown, Way, & Steed, 2015; Denham, Bassett, Way, et al., 2012; Denham, Bassett, Zinsser, & Wyatt, 2014; Gündüz, Yagmurlu, & Harma, 2015; Hudson & Jacques, 2014; Ip, Jester, Sameroff, & Olson, 2019; Klein et al., 2018; Lee, Chang, Ip, & Olson, 2019; Mann, Hund, Hesson-McInnis, & Roman, 2017; Martins et al., 2016; Schultz, Izard, Ackerman, & Youngstrom, 2001; Thompson et al., 2020; von Salisch, Häenel, & Denham, 2015; von Salisch et al., 2013). Some of these relationships are found longitudinally (e.g., Denham, Bassett, Way, et al., 2012; Schultz et al., 2001; Wang, Liu, & Feng, 2021). Specifically, Wang et al. (2021) found that cognitive flexibility predicted emotion knowledge at two later time points, but that the relationship was mediated by language ability; that is, early cognitive flexibility contributed to later emotion knowledge by improving children's verbal ability.

Thus both "cool" (e.g., inhibitory control, attention focusing, and shifting) and "hot" (e.g., delay of gratification) aspects of self-regulation support the acquisition of emotion knowledge, at least contemporaneously. In fact, an admittedly small intervention focusing on self-regulation showed clear advances in preschoolers' emotion knowledge; in particular, increases in inhibitory control and working memory were related to improvements in emotion knowledge (Li, Liu, Yan, & Feng, 2020). It is not hard to picture that inhibiting prepotent responses in situations where tasks are difficult or emotions are activated, remembering how expressions and situations reflected emotions during interactions, and even shifting attention to the emotional aspects of the situation, might allow one's mental space to perceive one's own or others' emotions.

However, whether emotion knowledge could predict aspects of self-regulation rather than, or in addition to, the reverse also should be considered. For example, preschoolers' emotion knowledge and a composite of working memory and inhibitory control each predicted the other during preschool (Blankson et al., 2013, 2017; Farrell & Gilpin, 2021; Ferrier, Karalus, Denham, & Bassett, 2018; Rhoades, Warren, Domitrovich, & Greenberg, 2011). The same bidirectional effects may be seen for the emotion knowledge—emotion regulation relation (e.g., Lucas-Molina et al., 2020).

After the preschool period, however, emotion knowledge focuses on distinguishing more complex emotions and reading the social cues of the situation. These new developments may depend less on inhibitory control; inhibiting one's own feelings to label others' emotions may be useful during preschool, but later emotion knowledge and self-regulation become more domain specific (Farrell & Gilpin, 2021).

### SUMMARY: Self-Regulation

The take-away message here is that for preschoolers, self-regulation appears to promote emotion knowledge, and the converse may also be true. Thus, aspects of self-regulation, both "hot" and "cool," but particularly inhibitory control and cognitive flexibility, are related to preschoolers' emotion knowledge. These connections may diminish after early childhood. Finally, language ability is often implicated in this connection.

## Language, Cognitive, and Motor Ability

Hence verbal ability, especially receptive language, also has been implicated as related to young children's emotion knowledge. Much recent research continues to corroborate the emotion knowledge/language association (Bosacki & Moore, 2004; Conte, Grazzani, & Pepe, 2018; Conte, Ornaghi, Grazzani, Pepe, & Cavioni, 2019; de Rosnay et al., 2014; Kujawa et al., 2014; Martin et al. 2015; Martins et al., 2016; Morgan et al., 2010; Pons et al., 2003; Salmon et al., 2013; Schultz et al., 2001; Seidenfeld et al., 2014; Streubel et al., 2020; Tang et al., 2018; von Salisch et al., 2013). In fact, verbal ability specifically enhances growth over time in emotion knowledge (Kårstad, Wichstrøm, Reinfjell, Belsky, & Berg Nielsen, 2015). Further, some research holds that verbal ability especially contributes to the earlier, external forms of emotion knowledge (De Stasio, Fiorilli, & Di Chiacchio, 2014).

Beck, Kumschick, Eid, and Klann-Delius (2012) extended this relationship to examine various age-appropriate aspects of grade schoolers' emotion knowledge (e.g., knowledge of mixed emotions, expressive emotion vocabulary, situation knowledge, including questions about bodily sensations and thoughts during emotions) and language/literacy (e.g., narrative structure and reading comprehension). Although the ages of these children were older than the ages of children discussed in this book, an interpretation of the findings is useful. The two constructs—emotion knowledge and language ability—created well-fitting latent variables that nonetheless were so highly correlated as to be better explained by a common factor. This finding highlights the centrality of language to emotion knowledge, a tenet of the constructivist perspective.

Further, as noted by Martin et al. (2015), children with language difficulties may be particularly vulnerable to emotion knowledge deficits, as well as to missed opportunities for social interactions and conversations that might support its growth (see also Ogren & Johnson, 2020). The message here is to consider how the lack of linguistic ability limits not only the acquisition of emotion concepts, but also language-rich social experiences that contribute to their acquisition.

At the same time, nonverbal intelligence or cognitive ability is associated with emotion knowledge, as well. For example, both Bennett, Bendersky, and Lewis (2005) and von Salisch and colleagues (von Salisch et al., 2013, 2015) found cognitive ability positively associated with emotion knowledge. It may be that the more mentalistic aspects of emotion knowledge are related to nonverbal, fluid intelligence (De Stasio et al., 2014).

Even more specifically in the area of cognition, Lewis and Minar (2022) have shown that self-recognition at 18 months is related to 4- and 5-year-olds' emotion knowledge, independent of IQ's significant contribution. The metacognitive understanding that the self and other are unique entities, with knowledge of others' minds, may support the emergence of early emotion knowledge. Such understanding of the self and others could make it easier to focus on separate persons' emotions, especially one's own. Such a possibility points toward the need to examine emotion knowledge—theory of mind linkages (see the"Theory of Mind" section).

Finally it has been postulated that being motorically active can aid in the development of brain regions that are key to cognitive processes, and furthermore that being motorically able boosts the social interaction that can fuel preschoolers' emotion knowledge (Cavadini, Richard, Dalla-Libera, & Gentaz, 2021). These authors noted that locomotor play allows children to interact while chasing, running, jumping, climbing, or engaging in rough-and-tumble or pretend play, and that such experiences would be rife with opportunities to experience and witness emotions. Again, as with language ability, motor ability can give access to social interaction that facilitates the development of preschoolers' emotion knowledge.

## SUMMARY: Language, Cognitive, and Motor Abilities

Preschoolers' language ability rather understandably relates to emotion knowledge, which partly supports the constructivist viewpoint (albeit with the boundary conditions elucidated here earlier). Language affords not only the ability to create emotion schema and constructs, but it also, along with motor ability, facilitates social experience that is full of emotions during early childhood. Moreover, aspects of nonverbal intelligence and self-knowledge may also support acquisition of the more sophisticated aspects of emotion knowledge. These foundational abilities underlie, and no doubt also are reinforced by, emotion knowledge.

## Theory of Mind

As suggested by the idea that self-understanding promotes emotion knowledge, there also is evidence that the cognitive ability to understand other people's minds, their desires, and beliefs—"theory of mind"—is associated with emotion knowledge (De Rosnay et al., 2014; Lee et al., 2019; Leerkes et al., 2008; Tang et al., 2018). This connection may be especially true for external causes of emotion such as understanding expressions, situations, and causes of emotions (Weimer et al., 2012), and obviously it will further the development of emotion knowledge revolving around one's own and others' desires and beliefs. This connection is found even among children as young as 2 years (Conte et al., 2018).

However, it would seem likely that each type of understanding could predict the other. But which would be ascendant as a causal factor? Although many of these investigations assess both theory of mind and emotion knowledge contemporaneously, some longitudinal research has found that emotion knowledge precedes and is related to theory of mind (Brock, Kim, Gutshall, & Grissmer, 2018; Eggum et al., 2011; Hughes & Dunn, 1998; O'Brien et al., 2011; Sarmento-Henrique, Quintanilla, Lucas-Molina, Recio, & Giménez-Dasí, 2020).

Why might these results be true? One can speculate that emotions may be more readily understood than others' minds, given their internal physiological and facial expressions, especially compared to the more subtle, less uniform indicators of others' thinking (O'Brien et al., 2011). Further, children with more sophisticated, earlier emerging emotion knowledge, especially with an emerging understanding of emotions in equivocal and personalized situations, may have a better platform of attentiveness to subtle social cues, so that they may notice discrepancies between their own and others' experiences, beliefs, and desires.

This direction of effect may reverse at later ages, as older children well versed in parsing others' beliefs and desires might be more adept at learning the nuances of complex social and self-conscious emotions (Eggum et al., 2011). Also, this opposite direction of prediction, with theory of mind predicting later emotion knowledge, has at times been uncovered during the preschool period (e.g., Seidenfeld et al., 2014). So although support is converging around emotion knowledge supporting theory of mind rather than the other way around, this conclusion is not yet universally accepted. What is widely accepted is that the two constructs are definitely related. It is not surprising that each may contribute to variation in the other at different times.

Other aspects of mentalization may be important to consider in concert with the association of theory of mind with emotion knowledge; for example, understanding deception may be part of a broader configuration of social cognitive development during early childhood. For example, Nancarrow, Gilpin, Thibodeau, and Farrell (2018) found that theory of mind was greatest for children who understood both emotions and deception. As well, the intimate linkage of language with both theory of mind and emotion knowledge was highlighted by its status as a mediator between emotion knowledge and theory of mind abilities (Sarmento-Henrique et al., 2020).

## SUMMARY: Theory of Mind

In short, these two aspects of social cognition are intimately interrelated. Indeed the desire and belief aspect of Pons and colleagues' (e.g., 2004) theoretical model of emotion knowledge and methodological innovations include emotional attributions based on children's ability to understand desire- and belief-based emotions. Continued work on formulating an even clearer interpretation of the interrelationship of these abilities is likely to further the study of young children's social cognition more broadly.

## Attachment

Another candidate for a foundation of emotion knowledge is having a secure attachment with at least one attachment figure; emotional security and a close, warm relationship with one's parent can contribute to emotion knowledge (Cummings, 1995a; Dereli, 2016). It seems logical that feeling secure—that one's attachment figure will keep one safe and also share positive interactions—would render the world of emotions less intimidating and facilitate important conversations about emotions with the attachment figure. These considerations have found empirical support; in fact, a recent review asserts the contribution of a secure attachment to emotion knowledge, often mediated by mothers' conversations (see Chapter 8; Pavarini, de Hollanda Souza, & Hawk, 2013). Some of the results in this area are contemporaneous, but longitudinal trajectories also have been found; secure attachment status at 1 year was related to understanding mixed emotions at 6 years (Steele, Steele, & Croft, 2008; Steele, Steele, Croft, & Fonagy, 1999).

In my work (Denham, Blair, Schmidt, & DeMulder, 2002), both children's secure attachment to their mothers and lack of negative themes expressed in a series of attachment story completions were related to their understanding of equivocal emotions, both in simple correlations and in a structural model. Similarly other, more recent research on secure base scripts demonstrated in attachment story completions (e.g., elaborated and coherently ordered stories, especially showing the attachment figure as a haven of safety and base for exploration) were related to equivocal emotion knowledge and overall knowledge of emotional expressions and situations (Fernandes et al., 2019; Ştefan & Avram, 2018, 2021).

Another aspect of my and others' reasoning—that conversations about emotions in the context of a secure relationship would advance emotion knowledge—was supported by Raikes and Thompson (2006, 2008). In their 2008 study, security of attachment at age 2 was related to children's use of emotion terms 1 year later in conversations about the times when the child had been happy, sad, and angry. Then, the ability to label emotion terms in conversations with their mothers predicted their emotion knowledge (expressions and situations). These authors took these notions one step further by noting that securely attached preschoolers' abilities to remain engaged during discussions about negative emotions with their mothers (i.e., *not* changing the subject, evading mothers' questions, refusing to talk, or even running away) was related to their knowledge of negative emotions, especially when their mothers also were validating their conversations (Waters et al., 2010). Scaffolded demonstrations of emotion knowledge in conversations predicted more structured assessments.

In fact, secure attachment has been related to even more sophisticated components of emotion knowledge. Being able to identify belief-based emotions, for example, was related to security of attachment (de Rosnay & Harris, 2002). Further, the ability to generate comforting emotion regulation strategies (Ştefan, Avram, & Miclea, 2017) or an aggregate of comforting, problem-solving, distraction, and reappraisal strategies (Ştefan & Avram, 2018) was related to children's secure responses to attachment story stems.

### SUMMARY: Attachment

The benefits of having a secure attachment relationship reverberate throughout emotional competence. In the case of emotion knowledge, being secure can render one more open to emotional experience and can be emblematic of greater, more useful, emotional communication with socializers.

## Contributions of Culture to Emotion Knowledge

Very recently, Harris and Cheng (2022) reviewed evidence concerning the developmental trajectories of young children's situational and more personalized emotion knowledge and found robust support for similarities in this progression across diverse cultures. Despite such relative similarity in developmental change, ignoring the contribution of children's particular culture on specific aspects of their developing emotion knowledge would be a mistake. There have been several within- and between-culture studies of emerging emotion knowledge during the preschool period, and they often focus on specific cultures' underlying beliefs that bear upon the type of emotion-related learning children acquire by age 5 years.

For example, some reports have focused on the differences between more and less collectivistic/relational cultures. Specifically, Chinese preschoolers showed less understanding of emotions from age 3 to 5 than their American peers, especially for negative emotions (Wang, 2003). Such knowledge also improved less rapidly for Chinese children, especially for anger and fear. Further, Chinese preschoolers (and adults) rated emotions as less intense than their American counterparts. Finally although most story situations were identified with the same emotions across the two cultures, consonant with the existence of emotion prototypes, differences occurred for several situations, such as the approach of a stranger or being falsely accused by one's parents. Considering culture, emotional meaning is not necessarily tied to specific situations. The findings that East Asian preschoolers were more sensitive to implicit contextual cues to emotion, with children from Western cultures relying more on explicit semantic information, suggest a possible foundation for these differences (Möller, Bull, & Aschersleben, 2022).

In general, it can be posited that in collectivist/relational societies like China, emotion knowledge is less critical than in individualistic cultures like the United States.

Such a difference is likely because in China there is an emphasis on social harmony and group interests, rather than on individual internal subjective experiences like emotions (Doan & Wang, 2018). In the United States, emotions are considered important aspects of one's self and well-being. Consonant with these beliefs, Chinese parents talk less about emotions and more about behavioral standards. Thus, differences across cultures concerning the value of and teaching about emotion go far in explaining the differences in preschoolers' emotion knowledge.[3]

It also is important to point out that, even within cultures considered as similar as Italy and Germany, there may be cultural differences in preschoolers' emotion knowledge. Thus, Italy can be seen as more collectivistic/relational than Germany, with an emphasis on interdependence, the importance of kin, and less fostering of autonomy. In contrast, there is more emphasis in Germany on independence and individual achievement. Despite these dissimilarities, the two cultures share many Western, individualistic cultural values, so that understanding, comparing, and contrasting children's emotion knowledge in these two cultures could promote even greater understanding.

In one study (Molina, Bulgarelli, Henning, & Aschersleben, 2014), Italian preschoolers actually scored higher on emotion knowledge than German children, seemingly contradicting Wang (2003). However, the specific subskill that drove this difference was the *knowledge of hiding emotions* or understanding of real versus apparent emotions. This specific skill may be more important in a culture, such as Italy, where adults' roles require children's deference and respect (see also Joshi & MacLean, 1994). Similarly, Naito and Seki (2009) found Japanese 6-year-olds proficient in display rule knowledge; these authors suggest that this skill was likely to be promoted via the children's immersion in a culture where a very strong distinction was drawn between one's private thoughts and feelings and the face shown to the world. Children acquiring emotion knowledge in such cultures may be less free to express emotions and become better versed in understanding hiding of emotions.

In fact, recent research has confirmed that both Chinese and Italian preschoolers performed better on their knowledge of hiding emotions rather than on knowing that reminders can bring back emotional experience, whereas German and British children showed the opposite pattern (Tang et al., 2018). These results support the relative focus on real and apparent emotions in specific cultures, consonant with results already mentioned, but add the notion that individualistic cultures might promote children's understanding of emotion reminders. Again these results point to differing approaches regarding emotions in the family—parents in collectivist/relational societies are less likely to talk about past emotional events, and when they do, discussion occurs in a more judgmental tone (e.g., Wang, 2001).

So cultural meanings regarding emotions, and, more broadly, cultural beliefs about children's place in the world and core values for the self in society (Halberstadt & Lozada, 2011) contribute to the development of preschoolers' emotion knowledge. However, the contributions of other aspects of children's demographic status may be masked

[3]See Chapter 8 for more detail on how specific socialization experiences (i.e., modeling, reacting to, and teaching about emotions) contribute to how components of emotional competence vary across cultures, and for suggestions on why this is so.

by national/cultural differences. Thus, one large-scale cross-national study (Kårstad et al., 2015) compared the emotion knowledge of preschoolers in Brazil, Norway, Italy, and Peru; these authors found similarities between more economically advantaged children in Brazil and those in European countries with stable, relatively high living standards (i.e., Norway and Italy). These children demonstrated greater emotion knowledge than economically disadvantaged children in Brazil and others living in poverty, such as those from Peru, particularly from the Quecha tribe (Tenenbaum, Visscher, Pons, & Harris, 2004). Although there were other between- and within-culture nuances in this study, the main message was that differences in emotion knowledge varied according to living circumstances.

What might fuel these differences in young children's emotion knowledge attributable to socioeconomic status? Kårstad et al. (2015) and Tenenbaum et al. (2004) mention the issue of parental socialization—especially that poorer parents may use more punitive discipline and do not discuss emotions with their children. For the Quecha children in Peru, other factors included their lack of access to formal schooling, where they may have gained experience with pictures and photographs (such as those used in the research methodology) and may have become more familiar with being tested by adults. Thus, these children did not have socialization experience in school, and may have been hampered in even understanding the emotion knowledge assessment. Further, in the Quecha children's life in a remote agrarian society, the cultural emphasis on control of certain emotions and being cared for by older siblings may not expose them to extended discussion of emotion. Similarly Roma preschoolers in Spain, who live in a highly collectivist/relational culture, and are poor, not well educated, and largely socialized in their peer groups, performed less well on emotion knowledge than non-Roma children (Giménez-Dasí et al., 2018).

### **SUMMARY:** Culture

Different cultures value emotion and its expression differently, as noted in Chapters 2 and 3. These differences can translate into varying ways that emotion knowledge, too is valued and socialized, with concomitant differences in the development of young children's emotion knowledge. Thus, it behooves both researchers and caring adults in children's lives, such as early childhood educators, to be aware of the varying ways that emotion knowledge may be valued, socialized, and developed in the lives of children in their care.

## OVERALL SUMMARY AND CONCLUSIONS

Preschoolers are beginning the long progression toward understanding personalized aspects of emotions, mixed emotions and ambivalence, and complex emotions such as guilt and shame. Initially when confronted with complex emotional situations, they center on the salient qualities of the eliciting situations and of the individuals displaying emotions. When these sources of information conflict, children of preschool age are strongly influenced by facial expression in judging emotion but are beginning to transition toward reconciling the two sets of cues. In the absence of an emotional expression, these children tend to infer the emotion that they associate with a situation. The qualities they focus on in inferring causes of emotions fit well within the prototype and event-structure explanatory approaches put forward in Chapter 4.

Preschoolers are also starting to use personalized information to infer how someone is feeling and sometimes to explain conflicting cues to emotion. That is, when person-specific information readily suggests how that person feels, preschoolers can use this information rather than conflicting normative or situational information. But young children prefer immediately present emotion cues to information about a person's past experience. This preference makes sense, given their limited comprehension of the time course of emotion.

Considering even more sophisticated aspects of emotion knowledge, methodological intricacies have made it difficult to access young children's comprehension of dissemblance, display rules, and mixed emotions. But when measures are more ecologically valid, preschoolers' nascent abilities in this area are discerned.

Finally, because expressive patterns of guilt, shame, and pride occur later than those of the basic emotions, the lag in understanding complex emotions or emotions expressed in moral situations is not surprising. More research should be initiated to explore these foundations of children's moral sense, because these social and self-conscious emotions have important ramifications for children's developing abilities to feel good about themselves and to interact with others.

# Emotion Regulation

## INTRODUCTION

Preschoolers are learning to regulate their own emotions. Various strategies to regulate emotions surface during the preschool period. One is self-talk.

> Emily repeats emotion language her parents have used with her to help herself calm down at nap time, which she despises: "Big kids like Emmy and Carl and Linda don't cry. THEY big kids . . . the baby cry at Tanta's . . . babies can cry but . . . big kids like Emmy don't cry . . . they go sleep. . . ." (Engel, 1995, p. 39).
>
> Similarly, Ella has twisted her ankle while dancing on the patio. The discomfort wakes her in the night, and her mother comforts her and talks to her about what is bothering her. She asks whether she should kiss the hurt foot. "No, I do it," Ella replies. She lies back down in bed, holds her foot, and whispers over and over to herself, "Nice and better. Nice and better." Soon she is asleep.

Both girls successfully regulated their emotions using their developing language, a topic I turn to again. However, the topic of emotion regulation during early childhood is much more multifaceted than these evocative examples suggest. As I elaborate in much detail, when an emotion is elicited, the experience of emotion often changes in intensity, duration, or type—this *change* in the experience and expression of emotion is *emotion regulation* (Bailey, Denham, Curby, & Bassett, 2016). There are many developments that govern when and how young children enact emotion regulation.

Thus, more broadly, emotion regulation (hereafter abbreviated as ER) is a crucial aspect of emotional competence. One view of ER is that it is recruited when emotions exceed children's resources. When emotions occur, children's neurobiological processes, thought processes, and/or behavior can become disorganized, instigating a need for ER (Barrett & Campos, 1991; Eisenberg & Fabes, 1992; Thompson, 2011). Emotions need to be managed to recapture an "even keel." But not all toddlers and preschoolers are as capable of managing emotions as Emily and Ella are.

Two-year-old Chuckie, tired and hungry already at 5 o'clock, demands that his mother turn on the television as she tries to stow groceries in the kitchen cupboard. Upon receiving a curt "Not yet," he begins to cry, thrashing and kicking on the kitchen floor. What can he do? He wants his show right now, but Mom looks mad too.

Three-year-old Melissa is approached by a Rottweiler and cringes in fear. What are her options?

Four-year-old Roberta and her friends are pretending in the house corner. She starts crawling around on all fours and barking—she's the family dog. Somehow this strikes everyone funny—it's so unexpected. Together, they laugh hard and loud, over and over, until they fall to the ground in a heap. As their preschool teacher calls to them to calm down because it's time to transition to small-group work time, they are still chuckling and playfully slapping at each other; they don't even hear her.

ER plays a role in each of these situations.

Emotional arousal is unavoidable. Children and adults alike register emotion at all times. Negative emotions need to be managed especially often, but as in the example of Roberta's glee, positive emotions can require regulation as well. There are many ways to modulate emotion, as called for in these three examples. People learn ways to tolerate and endure experiences of emotions that are just a bit "too much"; this modulation, toleration, and endurance of emotions are essential aspects of ER (see Kopp, 1989).

Sometimes too the experience and/or expression of emotion need to be "up-regulated"—"whistling a happy tune" when afraid, showing more anger than is felt to "win." Susie cries louder to get help when she hurts herself on the swing; Joey smiles more broadly to make Huynh feel welcome when he approaches the block corner.

Usually when ER is discussed, however, much more emphasis is put on the "down-regulating" of emotions. This distinction is probably a fair one, because I think that down-regulation is more often necessary than up-regulation, especially during the preschool years. In this chapter, I most often follow this line of thinking. Nonetheless, it is important to consider situations where augmentation of emotional experience and expression is important and to acknowledge clearly that positive emotion can also require regulation. Both positive *and* negative emotions may require down- *or* up-regulation (Gross, 2015).

Clearly, preschoolers already are working at all of this. Even very young children begin to deal with emotions and emotional situations, and to consider managing emotions through both down- and up-regulation. In fact, even infants and toddlers are already beginning to try to deal with their emotions (August et al., 2017). For example, 3-month-old infants exposed to their mothers' flat or depressed affect demonstrate negative affect of their own, but they also show various behaviors that may be precursors of more sophisticated attempts at ER, such as sucking on a pacifier, averting their gaze, or seeking attention (August et al., 2017; Tronick, 1989). Eighteen-month-olds self-soothe when upset if their mothers are absent (Garner, 1995), and 2-year-olds are beginning to use well-differentiated, independent ER strategies. As discussed in Chapter 3, preschoolers are learning to dissemble emotions and use display rules to regulate emotions in social situations, and these experiences also may require the down- or up-regulation of either positive *or* negative emotions. Regardless of age, then, ER occurs constantly in some form or other: Whether consciously or unconsciously, all people are aware of and are fine-tuning their emotional experience and expression (Bridges & Grolnick, 1995; see also the "self-monitoring" path in Chapter 1, Figure 1.1).

In this chapter, I first put forward a working definition for ER. I then describe its affective, cognitive, and behavioral components. While discussing these strategies, I examine developmental change and individual differences. Next it is important to address ER's biological roots. Given these biological roots, it is logical to next consider how emotional experience and expression and general self-regulation work together to contribute to ER. Finally, the roles of children's language ability, emotion knowledge, and culture are also topics of interest.

## DEFINING EMOTION REGULATION

The concept of ER is a slippery one to define and operationalize, however. Many highly regarded investigators in developmental psychology have struggled with this task. It is notoriously difficult to separate emotions, as expressed, from their regulation. After all, the model of emotional experience put forward in Chapter 1 describes a process that takes place very rapidly, and all components of emotion, occurring after the initial arousal and lower brain centers' activation, also could be considered regulatory. Indeed, persuasive arguments can be made that ER is part of emotion itself (Campos, Mumme, Kermoian, & Campos, 1994; Thompson, 2011), that the experience of emotion itself cannot be disentangled from the neurobiological, cognitive, and behavioral ER processes that accompany it. But at the same time, as asserted by Cole, Martin, et al. (2004), and as depicted in Figure 1.1, emotions' activation can be inferred first, with the regulatory processes, such as cognitive appraisal and behavioral action tendencies, being at least somewhat independent aspects of the emotional experience.

Thus perhaps a unification of these opposing views is possible and can form the foundation for discussion here: Emotions are always regulated, as suggested by the feedback path in Figure 1.1—regulatory processes inherent *within* the emotion experience can take place, so that emotional arousal and the very experience of emotion itself, as well as emotional expressiveness, can change, or be *regulated*. But the activation of emotion also can be pinpointed, whether it is as simple as the limbic-driven arousal, feelings, and behavior in the leftmost column of Figure 1.1 or as complex as that seen in the rightmost column—either way, children's expression and/or experience of emotion can be measured, and many of its inherent regulatory processes can be examined separately.

I again return to a functionalist definition of emotions themselves in the effort to delineate ER more clearly: "Emotions, from a functionalist perspective, equal the attempts by the person to establish, maintain, change, or terminate the relationship between the person and environment in matters of significance" (Campos et al., 1994, p. 256; see also Barrett & Campos, 1987). That is, emotions represent processes that allow individuals to relate to the environment based on the significance of an event for their well-being (Cole, Lougheed, et al., 2018). Consonant with this overarching definition of emotion, ER is necessary when either the presence or absence of emotional expression and experience interferes with a person's goals, whether conscious or nonconscious. Emotions are constantly monitored, and they must be *regulated.*

Further, in the integrated view of ER I propose here, and in agreement with Cole, Martin, and colleagues (2004), emotions are not only regulated but are also *regulating*—they can affect other systems—physiological, neuroendocrine, behavioral, and social. Such regulation *by* emotion is either intrapersonal—as when feedback from emotional behavior changes a related process like cardiovascular activity—or interpersonal, as when a child's emotions alter the behavior of others, affecting *their* goals (Cole, Martin, et al., 2004). It is especially crucial to note this interpersonal regulation *by* emotions in the discussion of preschoolers' ER—the adults and age-mates in their milieu often signal that intrapersonal aspects of ER are necessary because children's expressiveness has (dys)regulated *their* emotions and behaviors. In fact, the goals of the child and social partners can intersect, signaling the need for ER. Children's emotions can motivate them to seek assistance in the service of calming down, and at the same time can trigger supportive behavior from adults whose goal is to help them achieve equanimity.

In the three beginning examples, ER was necessary when circumstances interfered with goal-relevant matters.

> Chuckie is trying to change a personally important aspect of the environment—he wants his cartoons! But throwing a fit was unlikely to persuade his mother to act, especially because she had her own goal to get groceries put away. To avoid a vicious cycle of fussing at one another, it would be advisable for Chuckie to regulate his anger. Mother may need to regulate her grumpy response to Chuckie's anger too.
>
> Melissa wants to get rid of the dog; this goal is paramount to her, but she is more likely to conquer her fear by choosing an ER strategy that will enlist aid or allow her to escape the scene. The adult walking the dog is motivated by Melissa's fear to take safety precautions.
>
> And Roberta is having difficulty maintaining the state of fun with friends without being overwhelmed by it. At the same time, her teacher needs all the children to calm down to transition to a new activity; the goals of both Roberta and the teacher intersect to make ER necessary. While Roberta gulps deep breaths instinctively to calm down, the teacher may be singing a quiet "calm down" song.

In each example, the children need to down-regulate emotions to get what they (and their social partners) want. The experience and expression of emotion became too strong or too long lasting for the child and/or her social partners to achieve their goals, and emotions were both regulated and regulating for both parties.

Beyond the needed focus on both intra- and interpersonal goals, another issue needing attention when one is trying to define ER is that, as Thompson (1993) has asserted, ER has been regarded both as an outcome and as a process. Developmentalists often still consider ER as product—was Chuckie able to regulate his anger so his mother might give him TV time later? Is he usually able to deal with his feelings?—and research using this perspective is reported here. However, Thompson importantly focuses on ER as a process (see also Cole, Lougheed, et al., 2018). He suggested the following oft-cited definition: "Emotion regulation consists of the extrinsic and intrinsic processes responsible for *monitoring, evaluating, and modifying* emotional reactions, especially their intensive and temporal features, to accomplish one's goals" (Thompson, 1994, pp. 27–28; emphasis added).

Also, in the three beginning examples in this chapter, temporal and intensive features of the emotions experienced overburdened each child's immediate ability to organize thinking and behavior.

> Two-year-old Chuckie's quick latency and rise time for anger, along with its intensity, make his wanting his way (and his mother's afternoon!) quite difficult. Three-year-old Melissa's persistent fear leaves her shaky even after the dog moves on. And 4-year-old Roberta, though happy and ostensibly enjoying a positive experience with her friends, takes a long time to recover from the high-intensity experience; she acts and feels out of control.

This focus on process has been expanded via use of dynamical systems modeling, which affords a view of ER processes progressing from the activation of an emotion. Following this innovative approach, I also enumerate important new results looking at preschoolers' ER as it unfolds across small-scale time periods. These molecular trajectories of ER strategy usage change throughout children's development and give a unique view of *what develops* in ER.

Another useful process-focused view of ER to overlay on an ongoing definition of ER emanates from Gross's process model of ER (Gross, 2015; López-Pérez et al., 2016; McRae & Gross, 2020) and from my own vision of emotion as described in Chapter 1. In this formulation, it is thought that individuals may utilize several processes over time in any emotion-generative cycle (Gross, 2013, 2015): (1) situation selection (i.e., taking action that changes the probability of being in a situation, such as asking to visit the ice cream store to boost positive emotion, avoiding a scary place, or going somewhere to calm down when upset); (2) situation modification (i.e., taking action to alter a situation one is already in to change its emotional impact, such as fixing the problem that leads to negative emotion or asking for physical comfort or social support); (3) attentional deployment (i.e., changing the focus of one's attention, such as looking away from a distressing stimulus to feel better or more actively attending to an alternative activity, like playing with toys or watching a movie); (4) cognitive change (i.e., changing one's appraisal of the situation to alter its emotional impact, such as thinking about positive things, talking through the situation, or managing to think that the situation is not so bad); and (5) response modulation (i.e., directly changing one's emotional experience, be it physiological, cognitive, or behavioral, such as taking a deep breath or venting by crying).

Although Gross (2013, 2015) calls situation selection and modification, attention deployment, and cognitive changes *antecedent* to the activation of emotion, and response modulation as *respondent*, occurring after emotion activation and requiring some degree of effort, in my view young children may only utilize situation selection as antecedent. I think it is likely that preschoolers may anticipate emotional situations and adjust them accordingly (e.g., making sure to avoid the place where loud, scary noises occur). However, I think that their situation modification, attention deployment, and appraisal likely occur either during the emotion or after experiencing it. They are likely very quick ER responses, and this "tweaking" of theory does not change the further discussion here. Finally, Gross and others (e.g., Moreira & Silvers, 2018) view ER as either *implicit* (i.e., unconscious, effortless, automatic, involving bottom-up processing from lower to higher brain centers) or *explicit* (i.e., conscious, effortful, and controlled, involving top-down neurobehavioral and autonomic processing, from higher to lower brain centers). I follow this designation in what follows.

Although preschoolers do not have the linguistic and cognitive resources of older individuals, Gross's general model could be dovetailed with the processes mentioned by Thompson (1994), in that situation selection and modification and attention deployment could be seen as monitoring processes, in which the individual is viewing (or anticipating) the inception of an emotion and attempting to modify it. Cognitive change processes could be seen as Thompson's evaluating process, and response modulation could correspond to Thompson's modifying processes.

Thus just as the functional viewpoint suggests that there are specific patterns of expressiveness for all emotions, along with particular cognitive processes and behavioral action tendencies associated with them (Barrett & Campos, 1991; Cole, Lougheed, et al., 2018; see also my depiction of emotion in Figure 1.1), there are also emotional, cognitive, and behavioral aspects of ER. These aspects can be seen as the "monitoring, evaluating, and modifying" to which Thompson refers or the corresponding parts of the process model of ER. For young children, these time- and context-specific aspects of ER could include strategies such as self-soothing as monitoring or emotional ER; distraction, self-instruction, and cognitive reappraisal as evaluating processes or cognitive ER; and behaviors, such as support- or information-seeking, venting, or escaping as modifying processes or behavioral ER. To tell the full story about ER development, all these aspects must be pursued. In describing the development of ER during the preschool period, I attempt to integrate Thompson's, Gross's, and functionalist viewpoints.

## The Components of ER

The key components of ER incorporate these three dimensions—emotional, cognitive, and behavioral. Figure 6.1 depicts my view of the multifaceted nature of ER. As already noted, my view of ER is directly related to the definition of emotion I have put forward in Chapter 1. Each of the steps of emotional experience—emotional arousal, perception and cognitive construal, and behavioral action—can require regulation, and thus become parts of both implicit (more or less involuntary) and explicit (strategic) ER.[1] As stated in Chapter 1, and as shown in Figures 1.1 and 6.1, both emotional experience and ER involve the following steps, which differ somewhat across implicit and explicit ER:

### *Implicit ER*

Implicit ER then is relatively automatic and unconscious, although likely not entirely. As noted in Figure 6.1, it consists of several steps.

1 An emotional event of significance for the child's goals is identified. Then, almost immediately, emotional arousal is experienced and monitored: What are the sensations like? To regulate, the child may automatically choose to select a new situation or change the situation, as when behaviorally inhibited children avoid peer interactions when anticipating fear, or other preschoolers slip their thumbs into their mouths to self-soothe. These reactions are relatively effortless and quickly instituted.

Even very young children are aware of their arousal (see the leftmost columns of Figures 1.1 and 6.1), though not necessarily consciously. Because they are beginning to appreciate sensory information and to articulate the nature of their own sensory functioning (O' Neill, Astington, & Flavell, 1992; O'Neill & Chong, 2001; Schmidt & Pyers, 2011; Weinberger & Bushnell, 1994), young children probably start to appreciate aspects of their own emotions, albeit imperfectly. They sense how strongly they feel an emotion, how quickly it comes upon them, and when and how it peaks. Such awareness supports this ER step, as well as the next perceptual-cognitive step.

2 The means of perceptually controlling attention and cognitively "figuring out" the situation are central to children's experience of emotion itself and often occur nearly simultaneously (Barrett & Campos, 1991; Campos et al., 1989; Stein & Trabasso, 1989; Thompson, 1994; Thompson & Calkins, 1996).

Young children's perceptual and cognitive approach to ER include the external or internal means of redeploying attention when emotion either becomes "too much" or seems "too little," as well as revising their initial interpretations of the emotionally arousing events (Thompson, 1994). In this more automatic, implicit ER, preschoolers may passively turn their attention away from the emotional situation, distracting themselves rather randomly. Or they may—without conscious thought—give up on their goal or substitute another.

The choice of whether or not to pay attention to an emotional situation and its attendant arousal—that is, setting up an "emotions gatekeeper"—thus is primarily perceptual. Both a child and his or her caregiver can control whether an emotional situation is perceived at all. A child can internally change the attention given to emotion-eliciting stimuli: When confronted with the Rottweiler, Melissa may go

---

[1]This model is speculative in that its full instantiation has not been empirically tested, but it squares with theoretical definitions of ER already given, and my description of it is supported by empirical understanding where available.

into an almost dissociative state if the fear is severe enough—sucking her finger, closing her eyes, looking as if she is asleep. In contrast, the external means of refocusing a child's attention are often attempted by adults: Roberta's teacher may separate her from the crowd and help her focus her attention on a more low-key activity. At this perceptual level, the child calibrates how much of the emotional experience leaks into awareness—from totally ignoring the emotion to being focused upon it to the exclusion of all else.

When attention must be directed toward the emotional situation, it cannot be totally ignored or neutralized. At this cognitive level, children not only "take in" emotions, but figure them out, starting at a very elemental level: "I have something at stake; something bad [or good] is happening that matters to me." "What do these sensations mean to me?" (See the middle columns of Figures 1.1, and 6.1., as well as Figure 4.1's explanation of event analysis.) They then evaluate the situation's features and its potential for fitting with their goals (Eisenberg & Fabes, 1992).

Instead of internally or externally avoiding the elicitor of the emotion, or becoming fixated upon it, children can interpret the situation, even at this implicit level of ER (Bridges et al., 1994; Grolnick, Bridges, & Connell, 1996; Grolnick, Kurowski, McMenamy, Rivkin, & Bridges, 1998). Their subsequent, rather automatic, cognitive appreciations of how intensity, rise time, and latency of their emotional experience relate to their goals' success or failure aid preschoolers in seeking to diminish or augment a particular emotional experience.

In the previous examples, Chuckie sees that he is not going to get something he desires; Melissa is aware that she is going to get something she does *not* desire; and Roberta sees that she is getting something she desires, but that it is going slightly awry. These fundamental, low-level goal-related cognitions can take place within implicit ER but may not even be conscious.

These first two steps of ER—emotional monitoring and perceptual/cognitive evaluating—are often quite inextricable and can take place very quickly. What happens next, if an individual has any time for reflection, is often much more influenced by the cortical areas of the brain, and can proceed more thoughtfully, especially in explicit ER: What can *I* do about this arousal that I have interpreted? Such behavioral responding may be initially implicit (again, very automatic and immature), but with development become more explicit.

3 So finally preschoolers may choose specific responses that serve the goal of modulating emotional experience. They may choose to deal directly with the experienced and interpreted emotion and with its causes and consequences: "What can I do, if anything, about these emotional experiences I have discerned? Do I need to act, and if so, how?" Often in implicit ER, given its quick and relatively involuntary nature, the choice of behavior during and after negative emotion is to vent or escape (Blair, Denham, Kochanoff, & Whipple, 2004). If she quickly decides the Rottweiler is indeed a threat, Melissa may flee.

4 It is important to note that these steps could logically follow one another but need not occur sequentially, as suggested in Figure 6.1. Further, as already amply described, young children may require the assistance of an adult to manage

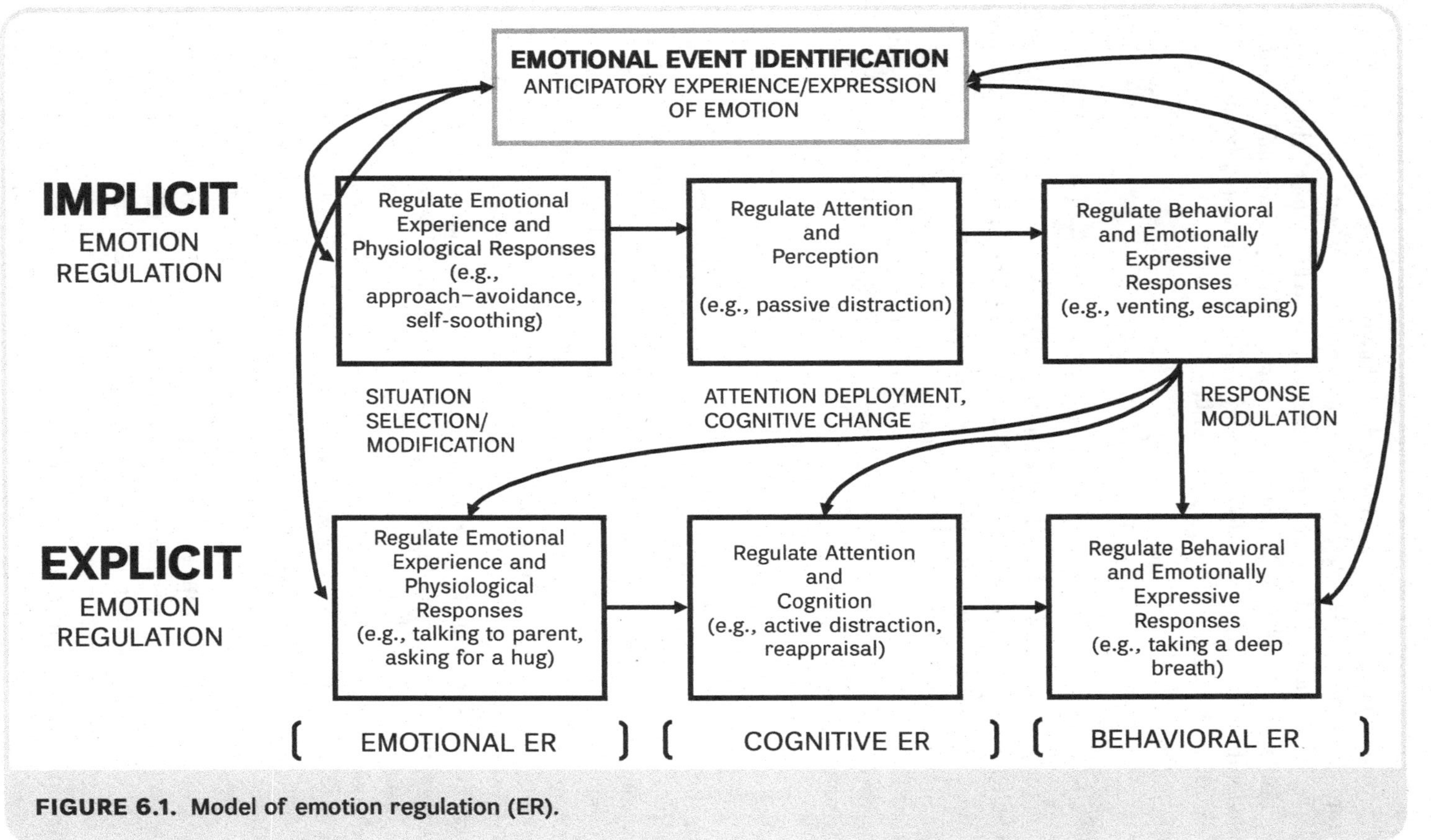


**FIGURE 6.1.** Model of emotion regulation (ER).

implicit ER successfully (Lunkenheimer, Olson, Hollenstein, Sameroff, & Winter, 2011; Moreira & Silvers, 2018). Finally, the behavioral or response modulation aspect of implicit ER may lead back to emotion identification—What am I feeling now? Did the ER efforts succeed? Is my goal anywhere nearer to being met? Then, especially as preschoolers age, explicit ER—with a full complement of emotional, cognitive, and behavioral components—may follow from less-successful initial behavioral efforts; alternatively, for these older children explicit ER may begin directly after the emotional event is identified.

### *Explicit ER*

This more effortful, controlled ER strategy also has emotional, cognitive-perceptual, and behavioral components. It works on a fast time scale, but not as automatically as implicit ER (although it may become routinized, as the top-down response system becomes more efficient as preschoolers age; Cole, Lougheed, et al., 2018). As with implicit ER, emotional, cognitive-perceptual, and behavioral efforts may be sequential, but need not be. They will feed back into the identification of whether the emotion still exists.

1 Again, an emotional event of significance for the child's goals is identified. Emotional arousal is experienced. To regulate, the child may more effortfully choose to select a new situation or change the situation. These choices are more complex than in implicit ER. For example, she or he may talk the situation over with a parent, as Ella did when her foot hurt during the night. The child may ask for a hug or other emotional support. Or the child may go to her or his room when experiencing angry feelings. These strategies help the child to select a new situation or modify the emotional situation as experienced.

Controlling emotional responses helps the child avoid overarousal: Using these newly more sophisticated strategies of explicit ER, the child can try to modulate the intensity, rise time, threshold, or latency of the emotion as expressed, or even to alter the discrete emotion being expressed. If Melissa's mother were with her, Melissa could come closer and slip her hand into her mother's. She could feel the intensity of her feeling, and its peaking, subside. As with implicit ER, these efforts within explicit ER feed back to the original state of arousal and subtly or not so subtly change it. Melissa's fear could diminish.

However, it should be reemphasized that, especially as children are capable of being more strategic with their ER efforts, minimizing emotional expression and its temporal parameters is not the only viable means of emotional responding in the service of ER. The capacity for generating and sustaining emotions can also be important as part of this emotional processing step; accentuated emotional responses can function as social regulators, especially to gain help or get one's way. For example, a sad preschooler cries out loud when his or her mother appears because this choice of behavior is directly related to receiving comfort.

Further, the choice of expressive ER responses, which allow the child to continue showing emotion in accordance with his or her goals, also depends strongly on the context of the emotion experienced, so it often is situation specific (Thompson, 1994). The child's individual expressive repertoire, his or her goals, the demands of the setting, and the values of social partners all interact. If she is accompanied by someone who will laugh at her, Melissa wants to diminish the intensity of her expression of fear of the Rottweiler, or at least to increase its latency by waiting until she can reach her mother's side. She seeks to diminish her expression and experience of fear if she is alone as well, because it feels so intense, but she will want to enhance her expression of fear if an adult is nearby and can rush to her aid. If his mother looks really annoyed at his outburst, Chuckie does not stop feeling angry altogether, but he tries to rein in the intensity of his expressed anger. Instead of screaming, he forcefully glares at his mother to change her mind by dint of his mighty will! Thus the means of situation modification can be strongly context specific.

2 Cognitive-perceptual strategies are also used in explicit ER and may follow from initial efforts to select a new situation or change the situation if these attempts are not completely successful in allowing the child to meet his or her goal (and the emotion persists). Possibly these strategies could be the first attempted ER processes. Thus preschoolers may actively distract themselves with toys or another new activity. Or they may use problem-solving reasoning about the situation: (a) figuring out a new goal ("I want to use these Legos instead of these wooden blocks," "I'll play inside instead of going out"); (b) finding a way to meet the original goal; (c) deciding to give up and relinquish their goal; or (d) deciding that they can change their thoughts by forgetting (e.g., "I'll just forget about that monster under the bed") or even by cognitive reappraisal (e.g., "I didn't want that cookie anyway").

They also may revise what they consider the causes of their own emotions—for example, "No, Mom, I'm sad because my tummy hurts [not because my friend took my toy]." In addition, the cognitive activity of pretend play can allow a preschooler to defuse anxiety through practice at solving problems, comforting self-talk, or other means (L. A. Barnett, 1984).

Toward the end of the preschool period and onward, ER strategies become increasingly cognitive and less dependent on observable behaviors in situations such as a friend's moving away, another kid's saying a mean thing, waiting for an injection, or experiencing an adult's anger (Band & Weisz, 1988). Older children can "think about" rather than "do" something else, and recent research confirms that these abilities are developing during the preschool period (Davis et al., 2010).

Thus the interpretations of children in my early examples could be different, with different implications for the regulation of these children's emotional experience and expressiveness, if the child is able to enact explicit ER. As he watches his mother, Chuckie could decide that stacking the boxes and cans of food on a low shelf is fun and begins to feel more interest than anger—he changes his goal. He may even get a cookie out of this! Melissa may notice the 6-year-old walking along with the Rottweiler and reinterpret her arousal as joy at being united with an old friend and her new dog—she put a positive spin on the event. Roberta, almost feeling pain from all the laughing, may consider her extreme hilarity a signal of interference with her goal of bodily safety. Deciding then that she is tired of crawling like a dog, she may retreat to a quieter area of the classroom—she redefined her goal. Similarly, Leah, the little girl about to recite a nursery rhyme (see Chapter 2) could see her "butterflies" as excitement rather than fear. What is important here is that arousal needs a name, and the cognitive "spin" put on physiological signs of emotions may render them more or less palatable.

For this type of ER too there are context effects. Importantly, the specific emotion elicited by the situation helps govern the likely strategies that are selected. Self-conscious and social emotions (e.g., guilt and shame) may require mostly cognitive coping, such as rationalizing, "I'll be a good boy, so I won't feel bad anymore." These difficult, complex emotions can also be dealt with by downplaying the importance of other people's opinions, the wrongdoing, or the enviable person or possession. Similarly, discerning that high-level happiness calls for ER can require a preschooler to be cognitively and perceptually aware of subtle contextual nuances—for instance, knowing what level of glee is appropriate in the preschool classroom.

3 For a more behavioral response, in explicit ER, rather than (or in addition to!) venting, the child may choose more sophisticated responses that serve the goal of modulating emotional experience, such as taking a deep breath to calm down, seeking assistance, gathering information, or turning the page when there is a scary picture in a book.

Again the emotion being experienced helps to determine which behavioral ER effort is chosen. As an example, young children do different things to deal with anger as opposed to fear. For anger, some possibilities are to strike out or resist, argue, enact revenge, retreat, or get an adult's help (Fabes & Eisenberg, 1992). For fear, the prominent alternatives are to self-soothe or seek comfort from others (as reasoned choices rather than simple situation modification).

Further, regulating such emotions as sadness, anger, and fear may require the most active behavioral strategies, which help the child to suppress, modulate, or even augment the emotions' action tendencies. A 5-year-old boy crying over losing a game tries to stop his whimpering because he doesn't want to feel bad or be ridiculed. Minutes later he may purposely roar very loudly at the "ex"-friend he supposedly caught cheating; he accentuates his anger to get his way.

## SUMMARY: Defining ER

Thus, both implicit and explicit means of ER already are developing during the toddler-to-preschool period. Although any individual could use either type of ER, younger children in this age range are more likely to use implicit ER.

The different components within implicit and explicit ER—emotional, perceptual/cognitive, and behavioral—are associated with various strategies used during late toddlerhood and the preschool period. Strategies change and become more varied as preschoolers become capable of explicit ER. So young children are increasingly able to utilize variably effective ER strategies.

These strategies allow children to become organized for coordinated action in the service of their goal. Whether implicit or explicit ER is enacted, adults, peers, and the children themselves must ascertain as much as possible about the particular emotion that is experienced to predict whether ER is necessary, and if so, its likely means and whether support is called for.

It also is important to remember that some ER strategy choices are more satisfying and adaptive than others. What satisfies the child experiencing the emotion furthermore may not please the other people in his or her social group at the time. As always, the personal experience of emotion *and* the social expression of emotion must be considered. For instance, the 5-year-old who lost the game may feel smug when he deals with his anger by hitting the "cheater"; undoubtedly though the "cheater" and his or her teacher do not consider this choice so successful! Melissa may retreat from the dog and suck her thumb on the edge of the playground; although doing this helps her to regain her equilibrium, her mother worries that she is *too* scared of new things, too uninvolved.

In addition to depending on who is involved, the success of ER is related to temporal factors. Short-term success is not necessarily accompanied by long-term success. A preschooler may have no "best" routes to regulating the expression and experience of an emotion. For example, the daughter of a depressed mother may choose to soothe both her own and her mother's sadness and fear by comforting the mother and enacting behaviors that are very empathic, at least on the surface. But there can be a long-term price to pay for this mode of ER (Thompson & Calkins, 1996; see also Chapter 12). So sometimes there is no "optimal" emotional, perceptual/cognitive, or behavioral ER mode. Keeping in mind that ER strategies can have adaptive or maladaptive results, how do these strategies that young children choose for ER change across time and how do they stay the same for individuals?

## DEVELOPMENTAL TRAJECTORY AND INDIVIDUAL DIFFERENCES IN EMOTION REGULATION

As for all developmental phenomena, the important questions to ask about ER are "What changes?" and "What stays the same?" Accordingly, in the sections that follow I review changes in supported and independent ER during the preschool age range. At first, adults need to support young children's ER efforts; little by little, though, preschoolers usually gain some independent means to regulate emotions.

Age change and stability are not the whole picture, however. Individual differences are important as well. Children differ in the types of ER they manifest in the "same" situation, and particular ER processes may or may not succeed in increasing the adaptiveness of a particular child's functioning (Barrett & Campos, 1991). So individual differences in ER also must be explored. Thus I not only explore the changes in ER from toddlerhood through the preschool age but also describe the nature and source of some individual differences.

### Developmental Change in ER Strategies

Because of its complexity as an emotional, cognitive, and behavioral process, ER consists of loosely connected abilities with differing timetables (Thompson, 1994). In general, as already noted, adult support in ER is often needed in the toddler and early preschool years. Then children become increasingly able to use independent ER strategies.

### *Supported ER Strategies*

Thus toddlers and young preschoolers often need external support to become skilled at regulating their emotions (Kopp, 1989; Thompson, 1994); their parents' and caregivers' support allows their ER strategies to be maximally effective.

Early in the toddler-to-preschool period, parents often assist their children in a cognitive ER strategy they will begin to use themselves—that is, purposely redeploying attention. This strategy can be a very useful means of regulating emotion. Other ER strategies are demonstrated by parents and caregivers as well and may be learned by children. In one study, children whose mothers used comforting, cognitive, distraction, and behavioral ER strategies were more likely to use these same strategy types (Stansbury & Sigman, 1995). Caregivers and parents can also structure a child's environment for a better fit with the child's ER abilities, enacting situation selection and modification for the child. Melissa's mother chooses not to walk down a certain path while enjoying a spring stroll because she sees, in the distance, a large dog that may frighten her daughter. Another father avoids arranging a playdate with a certain child who he knows will leave his son cranky and overstimulated.

Emotion language is an especially powerful tool for supported ER because it allows children to state their feelings, to understand the feedback to them, and to process causal associations between events and emotions, thus enabling the choice of an ER response (Kopp, 1989). Preschoolers with access to more sophisticated maternal emotion language during emotion discussion and simulation showed more efficient ER in their preschool classroom (Denham, Cook, et al., 1992; see similar results in Chapter 12 for children of depressed mothers in Zahn-Waxler, Ridgeway, Denham, Usher, & Cole, 1993). Talking about emotions with parents can enable preschoolers to stay on a more emotionally positive even keel in other situations (see also Chapter 8). Conversations about emotions play a prominent role in parents' frequent reconstruing or recasting of emotionally arousing events: How many preschoolers have heard the words "This will only hurt a little"?

Another important foundation for the success of supported ER is a secure attachment relationship between the child and the adult. For example, feeling safe, cared for, and able to enjoy good times together were associated with ER shown in the preschool classroom, especially for the father–child relationship. Fathers' role as a playmate may allow for practice in ER during active play. And, in fact, being secure with at least one parent, even when insecure with another, supported preschoolers' ER in the classroom (Fernandes et al., 2021). As well, children having a secure internal working model of attachment later regulated their emotions, especially anger, more optimally. They also were more able later to use their preschool teacher for ER support, particularly when they were sad or angry (Ştefan & Negrean, 2022).

Taken together, these studies suggest that relationship qualities, such as security and the ability to discuss emotions together, are an important underpinning for supported ER. As already seen for emotional expressiveness and emotion knowledge, adult–child relationships matter.

### *Children as Partners in ER*

Thus during toddlerhood parents take the lead in assisting ER, but individual children are likely to make some independent efforts toward ER. As the preschool period progresses, adult support is still important, but ER is more and more a partnership, as children become simultaneously more autonomous and more capable of cooperation.

Toddlers can sometimes use the independent ER scheme of simple self-distraction through varied means, such as physical self-comforting or self-stimulation, approaching or retreating from a situation, passively orienting attention toward or away from a stimulus, or even symbolic manipulations of a situation through play (Kopp, 1989). In fact, toddlers can learn to use the strategy of distraction by observing an adult (Schoppmann, Schneider, & Seehagen, 2021). Shatz (1994) evocatively reported on the ability of her 2-year-old grandson, Ricky, to distance or disengage to gain control over his emotions:

> I offered [Ricky] a banana and opened the peel just a little. Ricky's habit was to pull the peel down a bit at a time as he ate the banana, but this night he pulled the peel down too far at once. Annoyed, he tried to throw the banana on the floor, but I intervened . . . there was no compromising. Ricky was angry. He climbed down from his chair and went to stand in a corner facing the wall. . . . After about ten minutes Richard . . . found him lying on the couch in the TV room. R: [Grouchily]: Don't bodder me. I sleeping. (p. 129)

What's more, children become sensitive at quite an early age to context-dependent features of adaptive ER processes, using ER strategies differently depending on the nature of the situation (Feldman, Dollberg, & Nadam, 2011). They know when the support of their parents is available or unavailable; toddlers most often actively engaged their mothers' aid when mothers were present and not preoccupied (Grolnick et al., 1996; see also Feldman et al., 2011). They did not seek comfort when the experimenter had asked their mothers to be preoccupied with a magazine; similarly, the 2-year-olds in Feldman et al. (2011) used more self-soothing and calming self-talk (but also more proximity-seeking) when mothers were unavailable. They also used more advanced ER strategies involving attention deployment and play when on their own as well.

After toddlerhood, young children slowly build up associations between ER efforts—be they emotional, cognitive, or behavioral—and concomitant changes in their feeling states. Their exclusive reliance on caregivers' help with ER lessens and their awareness of the need for ER strategies increases. They start to appreciate the success or failure of their attempts at ER and become more flexible in choosing the most successful ways of regulating emotions in specific contexts. Behavioral disorganization resulting from strong negative affect decreases (see Chapter 2), probably because of this concomitantly increasing repertoire of emotional, cognitive, and behavioral strategies relevant to an expanding sphere of situations (Cole, Michel, & Teti, 1994).

Independent ER strategies available to youngsters during the preschool period increase primarily as a function of cognitive development and socialization. Although I discuss the influence of socialization on ER in Chapters 7 through 9, in the following section I consider the use of cognitive ER strategies and their possible foundations.

## Preschoolers' Developing ER Strategy Use

Consistent with my outline of implicit and explicit ER during early childhood, investigators have documented developmental trends in the use of various ER strategies. For example, in a longitudinal study in which toddlers' and preschoolers' ER was observed during delay-of-gratification tasks (i.e., not having any toys to play with at age 2 years, waiting for a cookie at 3 years, and waiting for a gift at 4 years) boys used different strategies at different ages (Supplee, Skuban, Trentacosta, Shaw, & Stoltz, 2011).

Even at 24 months, the boys could utilize planful, organized, goal-oriented strategies aimed at changing the source of the negative emotion—refocusing their attention while waiting (e.g., singing and dancing around the room while waiting) or asking questions to learn more about the wait (e.g., "When will they bring toys?"). However, they used such strategies less often at ages 2 and 3 years than at age 4 years.

In contrast, at younger ages they more often focused on the object of their wait (not a very productive strategy!). They also used active emotion-focused strategies (i.e., asking for or accepting comfort from a caregiver or self-soothing) more often at age 2 than they did later (Supplee et al., 2011). Similarly, when 3- and 4-year-olds were asked to refrain from playing with a group of special toys and were not allowed to eat a snack that was already available, the younger group used more behavioral strategies to help them ease their frustration—stating or restating their reasonable requests, or just playing with the toys or eating the snack (Stansbury & Sigman, 1995). Cole, Lougheed, et al. (2018) generally concur with these findings: 3-year-olds could use distraction, but 4-year-olds used it even more. Thus, although young preschoolers, just emerging from toddlerhood, could use planful ER strategies, they more often fell back on more immature strategies than the older children did.

In a study that evaluated ER at even younger ages, Deichmann and Ahnert (2021) observed toddlers (ages 15 to 39 months, average age 21 months) in a frustration task in which an attractive toy was inaccessible in a translucent plastic box. When the toddlers' frustration level was high, they made use of emotional, attentional, and behavioral strategies. Like the toddlers in Supplee et al. (2011), they tended to use self-comforting (e.g., sucking hands, fingers, or clothing, hair-twirling, holding objects close); self-distracting (e.g., looking at or reaching for other objects); help-seeking (e.g., gazing at or moving toward/reaching for parent, asking for help); or escape (e.g., standing up to leave) strategies. Moreover, there were age differences even within the age range Deichmann and Ahnert observed; younger children more often used low-level self-distraction (e.g., looking away from the desired object and looking at or reaching for other objects), but enacted pretend play less often.

In many respects the strategies used in this study were like those the toddlers used in Supplee and colleagues' (2011) work, as well as in Cole, Lougheed, et al.'s (2018), research. But an added result in Deichmann and Ahnert's (2021) work was that the duration of observed frustration was examined. Toddlers' frustration was shorter in duration when they used self-comforting, self-distraction, or pretend play (e.g., interacting with the toy even though it was inaccessible, talking to and stroking the toy through a hole in the Plexiglas, ascribing different meanings to the situation). So their relatively less-sophisticated ER strategies could be effective.

Sometimes there is evidence of gender differences in preschoolers' ER strategy usage. For example, in Deichmann and Ahnert (2021), girls engaged in more self-comforting and less pretend play. In another study of older preschoolers (mean age = 55 months), younger boys were more likely than other groups to show overt anger and seek escape after experiencing anger in the preschool classroom; older girls were more likely to actively resist the thing or person that caused their anger, as well as less likely to seek adults' help (Fabes & Eisenberg, 1992). The age groups and emotion-inducing situations differed quite a bit in these two studies, but one might conclude that girls' preferred ER strategies improved with greater maturity, and that boys still could have used adult support!

Thus the ER strategies used in Deichmann and Ahnert (2021) and Supplee et al. (2011) fit largely within the emotional, perceptual, and behavioral aspects of the implicit and explicit models devised here. Behavioral strategy usage, such as doing something to fix or tolerate the eliciting situation or alleviate obstacles, still outpaces cognitive strategy use during the preschool period (Band & Weisz, 1988; Strayer & Schroeder, 1989). However, even given this focus on emotional, perceptual, and behavioral strategies, it seems important to examine the emergence of cognitive strategy usage. Thus other studies have looked more closely at the comparison of preschoolers and early grade-schoolers, and/or expanded their research focus to zero in on whether (and if so how) preschoolers use more cognitive ER strategies.

For example, Losoya, Eisenberg, and Fabes (1998) reported on teachers' views of preschoolers' (age 4 to 6 years) and early grade-schoolers' (age 6 to 8 years) ER strategies. As Supplee and colleagues (2011) found with younger children, these investigators found that 4- to 6-year-olds sought emotional support more frequently than the older group and used venting as a behavioral strategy more often. In contrast, the older group used cognitive restructuring (e.g., cognitive reappraisal, or thinking about the situation in a positive way) more often.

A recent study also addressed the issue of cognitive strategies within a broad context, asking children, when they were 3 to 6 years old and then 5 to 8 years old, what they and a child in a photograph would do to stop feeling angry, fearful, and sad (Thomsen & Lessing, 2020). Children's responses were coded as the following strategies, *used at one or both time periods*: (1) behavioral problem solving (i.e., changing a situation though an action, such as talking to another child with whom one has a conflict); (2) distraction (doing other things, such as playing with something else); (3) mood raising (thinking about happy or nice things); (4) accepting the situation; (5) forgetting the situation; (6) cognitive problem solving (thinking about ways to solve the problem); (7) reappraisal (minimizing the problem through changing the perspective, such as "I didn't want to play with that anyway"); (8) giving up; (9) venting (arguing, saying nasty things, pushing); (10) withdrawal from the situation; (11) expressing emotion to regulate it (e.g., shivering and crying, swearing); (12) seeking social support (e.g., "I ask my grandma for help"; and (13) emotional control (e.g., "I hold in my tears"). Furthermore, the size and diversity of children's ER strategy repertoires were also calculated.

Strategies cited by at least 15% of children at one or both time periods included behavioral problem solving, distraction, social support (these first three were cited by more than 50% of children at both time periods), mood raising, accepting, forgetting, withdrawal, and emotion control. Only the strategy of accepting the situation increased significantly over time, although 11 strategies showed increases, including cognitive problem solving and reappraisal (which together increased from 7% to 16% of children citing them). Behavioral strategies were also cited more often across the two time periods (from 58% to 74%), as were distraction (61% to 72%), forgetting (from 16% to 25%), withdrawal (13% to 22%), and expressing emotion (9% to 14%). Mood raising, another cognitive strategy, was used by over a third of children at both time points. Children's repertoire of ER strategies also became more diverse over time, with the earlier size of their repertoire predicting this later diversity.

Further, López-Pérez, Gummerum, Wilson, and Dellaria (2017) asked both parents and their children, ages 3 to 4, 5 to 6, and 7 to 8 years, what strategies the children would use to regulate emotions. Regarding children's responses, the two youngest groups tended to cite attention deployment—focusing on something else, diverting attention (e.g., "When I feel bad, I play with my toys"). The 3- to 4-year-olds cited neither cognitive change (e.g., revising the way one thinks about a situation, giving it a more positive meaning), nor situation selection and modification to any extent (e.g., situation selection—making sure one will end up in a specific state, such as going to one's bedroom to calm down; situation modification—changing how one feels in the situation, such as talking to a parent, discussing the problem, asking for a hug; cf. Sala et al., 2014). All the children cited response-modulation strategies (e.g., taking a deep breath to calm down). The situation selection and modification strategies here were defined in the same way as the explicit ER strategies in Figure 6.1, and, as López-Pérez et al. (2017) note, probably require emotion knowledge and forecasting as well as the problem-solving skills of separating the goals, outcomes, and emotions that are not yet solidified at the earlier age in their study.

Overall, the studies by Deichmann and Ahnert (2021), Losoya and colleagues (1998), Supplee and colleagues (2011), and Thomsen and Lessing (2020) all confirm the predominance of behavioral, emotional (i.e., seeking social support), and perceptual ER strategies during the preschool period. However, both Losoya et al. (1998) and Thomsen and Lessing (2020) also highlight that even preschoolers sometimes may use cognitive ER strategies (see also Stansbury & Sigman, 1995). In Thomsen and Lessing (2020) such strategies included accepting, forgetting, mood raising, cognitive problem solving, and reappraisal, quite a range of cognitive possibilities.

At the same time, however, it was the oldest children at the second time of testing in Thomsen and Lessing (2020) who cited cognitive problem solving and reappraisal most often, and such strategies were generally not cited by the 3- to 4-year-olds in López-Pérez et al. (2017). So there still is some debate about preschoolers' ability to use such strategies. Reappraisal, in particular, is a complex process, involving the subprocesses of (1) selective attention to the reframeable features of the emotional stimulus, (2) mentalizing to monitor one's own emotional states as they change, (3) maintaining multiple reappraisals in memory, and (4) selecting appropriate reappraisals and inhibiting inappropriate ones (Moreira & Silvers, 2018). One can see why younger preschoolers might not be able to mobilize all these processes in real time.

However, as noted in Chapter 4 regarding understanding *others'* regulation of emotion, several studies have suggested that at least by age 5, or even earlier, preschoolers cite cognitive ER strategies as possible choices (Cole, Dennis, et al., 2009; Cole, Tan, et al. 2011; Dennis & Kelemen, 2009; Sala et al., 2014; Waters & Thompson, 2014). Moreover, Davis et al. (2010) asked children to talk about the times when they themselves had been sad, angry, and scared. For this procedure, the children tailored their responses to specific emotions (see also Dennis & Kelemen, 2009; Waters & Thompson, 2014). They mentioned cognitive strategies (e.g., changing their thinking by forgetting, changing their mental state, pretending things are different, positive reappraisal; changing their goals by reinstating, substituting, or forfeiting) more for sadness and fear than for anger (for which they preferred more active agent-focused strategies and changing their thoughts more than changing their goals). Davis and colleagues (2010) note that these young children were surprisingly articulate in reporting the use of metacognitive ER strategies—over two-thirds of the children reported that they would change their thinking.

Theoretically speaking, the increasing use of cognitive ER strategies could be expected as children make gains in language and cognition (topics to which I return). Given increasing emotion knowledge, cause–effect reasoning, and self-awareness, preschoolers begin to understand what situations upset them and become able to better organize and monitor their behavior. Moreover, they become cognitively able to absorb culturally relevant socialization of ER from adults (see Chapters 8 and 9), such as feeling rules (e.g., "Big kids don't get upset when their parents leave"); display rules (e.g., "Don't show that emotion, or show it this way"); and ER rules (e.g., "When you are afraid, whistle a happy tune to distract"). Overall, then, it seems that preschoolers' and kindergartners' use of cognitive ER strategies skills are more sophisticated than previously thought, although they are emerging mostly at the end of the preschool period and are still developing given ongoing changes in language and cognition.

## Drilling Down to Small Time Periods: Dynamical Systems Analyses of ER and Its Development

In the preceding section, I enumerated the types of ER strategies preschoolers begin to use independently—and the explosion of preschoolers' possible strategies to achieve ER seems apparent, and rather humbling. Examining ER strategy usage in this way is tantamount to viewing ER as an outcome. It would be useful also to examine young children's ER as process: when is it activated, what does it look like?

ER takes time when it is being enacted. The strategies used change, as already noted, across years, but also across very small time periods (Cole, Lougheed, et al., 2018). The success or failure of the strategies used during these small slices of time also changes with development. Cole and her colleagues have been at the forefront of looking at ER as process rather than as product, tackling the examination of how ER operates during such short time intervals.

The investigations by this research group have focused on how, when frustration is activated, regulatory processes affect ER's trajectory. In these studies, children ages 24 to 60 months were presented with a frustrating situation—having to wait to open a gift, when they had only boring toys to play with and their mothers were preoccupied with other tasks (e.g., 24-month-olds were given a pair of cloth cymbals, 36-month-olds, a car missing some wheels, and 48-month-olds, a toy horse with a missing leg). Such a situation has ecological validity given that parents are often busy, and waiting is not easy, especially if there isn't a good outlet for one's attention. Overall, from 2 to 5 years, desire and frustration (i.e., attention focused on the gift, nonverbal anger, angry bids to mothers, and disruptive behavior) declined, but never disappeared (Cole, Lougheed, et al., 2018; see also Tan, Armstrong, & Cole, 2013). What changed was not the level of frustration, but its dynamics—bouts of frustration became shorter from 3 to 5 years; frustration waned more quickly by age 5 (Cole, Lougheed, Chow, & Ram, 2020).

Microanalytic coding and analyses focused on how effective ER strategies were in this trajectory in allaying the children's desire for the gift and frustration at the wait. Three-year-olds, for example, did initiate ER strategies without adult assistance (i.e., self-soothing, distraction, and calm attention or information seeking), but their usage didn't dampen their frustration and desire very efficiently (Cole, Bendezú, Ram, & Chow, 2017). They used distraction in particular more quickly and longer than toddlers, but distraction and other ER strategies were only temporarily effective. These findings add much to the simpler tallying of overall ER strategy usage.

Although conventional static analyses in Cole and colleagues' work (2017) showed that ER strategy usage was related to lower levels of negative responses (examining ER as product), dynamic modeling (examining ER as process) expanded this finding and showed its complexity. These 3-year-olds deployed ER strategies more quickly and frequently when they were more frustrated, but only when frustration was *lower* did ER strategy usage decelerate desire and frustration and delay their reoccurrence. That is, their ER "worked" for less-intense instances of emotion; for more intense emotion, their ER strategies could not assuage their feelings.

In noting that the strength of the 3-year-olds' desire and frustration mattered, these findings elaborated on the work of Cole, Tan, et al. (2011), who had found that from 24 to 36 months of age, the latency of ER strategy usage (i.e., distraction and calm bids) decreased while its duration increased and the latency to anger increased. Over time, toddlers more quickly recruited ER strategies and used them longer, so that anger was averted for longer periods. Some success in independent ER was developing.

In sum, even though 3-year-olds used distraction more quickly than 2-year-olds, it still wasn't very useful. Greater desire and frustration, particularly in the presence of externalizing behavior problems, still dampened and overwhelmed the success of ER strategies. In short, the *successful* use of ER strategies across a short time period is just beginning in the early preschool years; these young preschoolers are learning ER strategies, even though they don't work in a lasting way and may only work when the need for them is less dire (see also Cole, Lougheed, et al.'s (2018) findings with a frustrating lockbox task).

During the preschool period, children may become more accustomed to being challenged emotionally, and less perturbed at such times, as well as able to use ER strategies more quickly (Cole, Lougheed, et al., 2018). Findings from Cole, Lougheed, Chow, et al. (2020) uphold this assertion—as already noted, from 24 to 36 to 48 months of age, children were increasingly adept at recruiting ER strategies. But when faced with the goal of removing a toy stuck in a locked box, 24- to 36-month-olds were quite variable in how they tried to deal with their emotions—trying one strategy and then another. In contrast, for 48- to 60-month olds, this variability of strategy usage occurred less often and occurred later in the task when children were tiring of their efforts (Cole, Lougheed, et al., 2018).

Recently these data have been reexamined across a longer age range—24 months to 5 years (Ratliff, Vazquez, Lunkenheimer, & Cole, 2021). Combining these two studies' findings allows a detailed look at changes in ER strategy usage and its effectiveness across the entire preschool age range. More specifically, although at 24 months the emotional ER strategies of self-soothing and support seeking led to most emotion waning, the use of these strategies declined across time. By age 5, the most useful ER strategy was attentional, in the form of longer bouts of distraction. Further, across the time period children first more often used language to ask for help and information, but this strategy's usage waned as distraction became more efficient. Overall, from the relatively inefficient ER strategy usage early in the period, by age 4 bouts of ER strategies became shorter, yet more efficient. And, in fact, the growth in the duration and dominance of distraction was related to adults' view of their ER during these experiences. In contrast, the growth in the usage of bidding for attention and information negatively predicted ratings of ER (Ratliff et al., 2021). There also is evidence that by the end of the preschool years the regulation of negative emotion is possible in other, more independent, settings; for example, older preschoolers were more capable than younger preschoolers of remaining positive during a disappointing gift procedure (Liebermann et al., 2007).

When considering developmental change in ER, it still is important to remember the intimate intertwining of emotional expressiveness and its regulation. For example, Tan et al. (2013) found differences in the ER efficacy of children whose mother-rated negative affectivity decreased or increased from 18 to 36 months: For those whose negative emotionality *de*creased across this period, the latency of calm bids to their mothers (i.e., more quickly talking to their mothers about the challenge of waiting and asking for maternal support) decreased by 36 months. At the same time, however, for those mothers whose negative emotionality reportedly *in*creased, the corresponding decrease in latency of calm bids was very steep, with especially short latencies by 48 months, suggesting a different tone and meaning to these bids. Overall, the authors considered that quickly using the calm-bids strategy at 36 months was developmentally appropriate, but that by 48 months it was a less-advanced means of ER than the more commonly used and efficient technique of distraction. Fussing at mothers by age 4 was neither useful nor appropriate.

Further, Deichmann and Ahnert (2021) also examined the efficacy, not only the prevalence, of various ER strategies when very young children were confronted with a toy in a locked box. Frustration was less at all intervals 1 to 5 seconds after self-comforting, self-distraction, and pretend play. Seeking help and attempting to escape were negatively related to frustration after 3 to 5 seconds, perhaps because these strategies required a bit more time to determine their efficacy. So in this study even toddlers used ER strategies with success.

These findings appear to contradict, to an extent, those of Cole and colleagues, in terms of the specific ER strategies that were found useful to younger children. However, the operational definitions for the strategies used by Deichmann and Ahnert (2021) with toddlers were somewhat less mature than those used by Cole—for example, distraction was similar to the briefer, less-focused attentional strategy I suggested here for implicit ER, and help seeking was merely gazing at, moving toward, or reaching for the parent, or actually asking for help. Again, drawing conclusions about toddlers' and preschoolers' ER strategy usage requires attending to investigators' operational definitions. Nonetheless, the examination of ER strategy efficacy in the moments that emotion is elicited has been very fruitful.

### SUMMARY: Developmental Change in ER

Strategy selection and its efficacy in alleviating negative emotions both as aggregated and *at the time of emotion elicitation* undergo qualitative and quantitative change from toddlerhood through the preschool period. Given the collected findings on how ER changes macroanalytically and microanalytically across this age span, it would be useful to consider what aspects of ER "stay the same" and what are the notable individual differences?

## Individual Differences in ER during the Preschool Period

Thus aside from the developmental differences in ER, it is vital to examine these individual differences. Patterns of such variations in ER may be seen from very early in life. For example, August et al. (2017) examined young infants' means of ER during a still-face paradigm, looking for ER continuity when the same children were ignored by their mothers during the preschool period. These preschoolers' ER difficulties (e.g., fretting, negative attention seeking, and overactivity) were predicted by infants' similar means of managing emotions when essentially being ignored by their mothers in the still-face paradigm (e.g., fretting, attention seeking, self-soothing). The strategies used were consistent with the process view of ER and showed evidence of stability.

Working with slightly older toddlers, Halligan et al. (2013) examined 12- and 18-month-olds' ER behaviors by rating their containment of negative emotion during a developmental assessment as well as their anger during a toy removal experience; the means for standard scores on these two indices represented *ER capacity*. At 5 years, these children took part in a "rigged" buzz-wire task, in which they tried to move a hoop along a wire without touching the wire and triggering a buzzer across three trials. The rated responses included negative affect, bids to the experimenter, self-soothing, self-directed verbalizations, behaviors focused on fixing the situation (e.g., testing a new strategy), and focused attention on the task. As the three trials progressed, children became negative more quickly, but also used more ER strategies. The ER capacity at age 5 was operationalized by mean standard scores for mean latency to negative emotion and the total strategies utilized.

The ER capacity generally indexed ER as product at both ages. Importantly regarding individual differences, there was stability in ER capacity from 12 to 18 months and from 18 months to 5 years. Thus, observations of ER at early ages can predict similar behavior throughout the preschool period.

Other research focused on individual differences has assessed ER through maternal and teacher ratings using the Emotion Regulation Checklist (ERC; Shields & Cicchetti, 1997), which includes 24 items that tap children's ER (e.g., "Can recover quickly from episodes of upset or distress," "Can modulate excitement") and general negative emotionality/lability (e.g., "Seems sad or listless," "Exhibits wide mood swings," "Is prone to bursts of anger, tantrums"). Many researchers have used this questionnaire, which instead of pinpointing specific strategies purports to give a summation of a child's ability to maintain an even keel emotionally, as well as a child's relative negativity and inability to recover from it; as such, it examines ER as product rather than as process. The questionnaire has good psychometric properties and has been translated into several languages (e.g., Ersan, 2020; Molina et al., 2014). But in some ways the construct of ER, to my mind, is not perfectly represented (e.g., the ER subscale includes items such as "Puts himself in the place of others and understands their feelings," "When others are sad or sluggish, shows interest in them") (see also Mirabile, 2014; Weems & Pina, 2010). Moreover, as Cole, Martin, et al. (2004) have cogently noted, being emotionally negative does not *necessarily* indicate dysregulation. However, the measure is so widely used that I examine it in this and the following chapters as an index of ER or lability.

Thus, using the ERC, several investigators found continuity across time with teachers or mothers as raters from 3 to 5 years (Lucas-Molina et al., 2020) and from 5 to 7 years (Blandon, Calkins, Grimm, Keane, & O'Brien, 2010). Blair and colleagues (2015) also found significant correlations of ERC ER from ages 5 to 7, but mothers were the only reporters, so that the possibility of a monorater bias should be considered. In summary, both observations of ER strategy usage and its outcome, as well as teacher and parent reports, have shown at least modest stability across time in early ER.

> When Carrie, who often has "no good, horrible, very bad days" tries to calm down, she stands apart from the other children for a while, licks her lips, and wrings her hands, perhaps to self-comfort. It is easy to envision Carrie as a very emotional, "difficult" first grader.

In addition, along with individual *stability*, there may also be individual *patterns of change* in ER strategy usage during this age range. For example, Supplee and colleagues (2011) also performed person-centered analyses of ER strategies in the 2- to 4-year-old boys they observed. For emotion-focused active strategy usage (e.g., seeking or accepting comfort, self-soothing) they found two groups—a group who used the strategy very little at all time points and a group that had high usage at age 2 with a steep decline thereafter. Perhaps using this strategy early was useful for them, but they no longer needed to resort to it later. Similarly, their analyses isolated two groups for "planful" strategies' (e.g., distraction and information seeking) usage over time —a group that generally used the strategy type only moderately over time and a group that increased their usage over time. Finally, two groups showed differential patterns of focusing on the delay (not a very productive strategy)—one group that continued to use this strategy over time, and another that used it only a little at ages 2 and 3, but even less at age 4. In essence, each strategy had individuals whose use of specific strategies remained stable or changed to be more efficacious.

### SUMMARY: Individual Differences in ER

Thus there is variable and person-centered evidence of moderate stability in the use of various ER strategies, and in ER as product, from infancy through the preschool period. Not only does usage of certain strategies and ER as product overall correlate across ages, but developmental profiles that fit groups of children also can be identified, yielding another way to conceptualize individual differences—that there are groups of children who develop in certain varying ways.

Nonetheless, Thompson, Lewis, and Calkins (2008) point out that much variability in ER is not accounted for in these conclusions, asserting that "early emerging individual differences in emotion regulation are not very stable over time because they are based on a changing constellation of behavioral and neurobiological capacities with different maturational timetables and origins" (p. 125). Hence, we must not overlook the complexity of ER and its roots in self-regulatory, expressive, cognitive/linguistic, and biological systems.

## CONTRIBUTORS TO INDIVIDUAL DIFFERENCES IN EMOTION REGULATION: EMOTIONAL EXPRESSIVENESS AND SELF-REGULATION

When discussing the experience and expression of emotion and its relation to the model of ER put forward here, it is profitable to consider emotionality in conjunction with a child's self-regulation (i.e., attention, inhibitory control, and working memory). In fact, Eisenberg and Fabes (1992) developed a model of early childhood ER that may aid in understanding how it differs from child to child. These authors posit that two important factors must be assessed to predict the ER strategies young children will use. These elements underlie, and may either facilitate or disrupt, ER attempts: (1) stable individual differences in parameters of emotionality, such as intensity, threshold, and rise time; and (2) stable individual differences in self-regulatory processes, such as attentional shifting or focusing and voluntary initiation or inhibition of action. These two factors acting together likely figure prominently in the differences seen in young children's ER.

According to this model, an individual child's relative standing on these two factors determines how successful their ER will be in social situations and how it is likely received by important persons in the social environment. The centrality of these factors makes sense because they map onto the emotional, cognitive, and behavioral aspects of ER.

One possible combination of these two characteristics will result in a very intense but also highly self-regulated individual. Intense but also very self-regulated children may appear shy, withdrawn, inhibited, and less able to enjoy social situations. Moreover, a child who is low in emotional intensity but nonetheless very self-regulated may appear affectively "flat" and unsociable, for example (Eisenberg, Bernzweig, & Fabes, 1991).

High intensity of emotion coupled with low self-regulation is even more problematic (Cole & Jacobs, 2018). Unbridled, underregulated intensity of emotional reactivity is clearly often associated with difficulties in ER. Preschoolers exhibiting more intense negative emotions (outside conflict situations) were more likely to cope with conflict through aggressive venting or acting out (Arsenio & Lover, 1997; Eisenberg, Fabes, Bernzweig, et al., 1993). Emotional intensity and more intense negative emotion are also related to acting-out modes of ER during peer interactions; for boys, such expressiveness also is negatively associated with constructive ER, such as verbal objections or leaving the situation (Eisenberg, Fabes, Bernzweig, et al., 1993; Eisenberg, Fabes, Nyman, Bernzweig, & Pinuelas, 1994). Moreover, children of high emotional intensity, especially high-intensity anger, react to adult anger with increased distress, negative appraisals, and aggression (Cummings, Iannotti, & Zahn-Waxler, 1985; Davies & Cummings, 1995). Overall these associations make intuitive sense; "hotheads" are not commonly expected to be able to deal with emotion-provoking situations in a constructive manner.

The moderately self-regulated, moderately emotionally intense child is probably in the best position to succeed at ER. Such a child is emotionally expressive, but also capable of planning, problem-focused coping, and flexibly using various ER strategies. All told, this model for individual differences in ER captures dimensions that are important to consider. First, I expand upon ER's connection with emotional expressiveness.

## Emotional Expressiveness

Not only is the level of arousal (i.e., emotional intensity) important to individual differences in young children's ER. The valence of the prevalent emotion, or even specific prevalent emotions, also is relevant. For example, expressing more prevalent negative emotionality in many situations, not just in the challenging one being observed, has been related to less-efficient ER strategy usage and focus on the restricted object during an emotionally challenging situation (Cole, Bendezú, et al., 2017).

Experiencing negative emotions can be overwhelming, challenging one's abilities to regulate them. Further, such prevailing, easily aroused negative emotion is likely to impair the development of ER strategies—while feeling negative emotions, young children can't sustain effective strategies and often resort to less effective ones that actually amplify their distress (Fox & Calkins, 2003). As a final insult, the continuity of such experiences leaves little room to develop effective ER strategies. The frequency, duration, intensity, and speed of onset of negative emotions, singly and in combination, increase the probability that preschoolers' emergent independent ER will be swamped and rendered less operative. In support of these considerations, both younger and older preschoolers' negativity/lability was negatively associated with their ER (Shewark & Blandon, 2015). With respect to younger preschoolers' ER, this trajectory may begin even earlier; that is, temperamental negativity reported by mothers of 14-month-olds predicted both the level and change of observed ER from 14 to 36 months (Brophy-Herb, Zajicek-Farber, Bocknek, McKelvey, & Stansbury, 2013).

The prevalence of specific emotions is another likely candidate for a contributor to preschoolers' development of ER. Some work has examined children's emotional profiles in association with their ER, assessed either as product or as process. Several investigators have found the prevalence of sadness, anger, and fear to be associated with lower levels of adaptive ER as assessed by the ERC (Ersan, 2020; Ersan & Tok, 2020; see also Miller, Gouley, Seifer, Dickstein, & Shields, 2004). Looking more at ER as process, mothers' ratings of their children's negative emotionality (sadness and fear) are associated with escape behaviors observed during children's bouts of anger in preschool (Eisenberg, Fabes, Nyman, et al., 1994). Perhaps their typical frequency of negative emotions renders preschoolers more susceptible to choosing less adaptive strategies and to "outrun" the bad feelings. In contrast, these investigators found that mothers' reports of children's overall low emotional intensity were related to the children's use of nonabusive language to deal with anger (Eisenberg, Fabes, Nyman, et al., 1994). Like the children examined in a more dynamic situation (Cole, Lougheed, et al., 2020), children who had a calmer "set point" were more able to use ER adaptively.

Finally, in a more complex design, Goodvin, Carlo, and Torquati (2006) found, via maternal ratings of all aspects of their study, that 3- to 8-year-olds' avoidant ER strategy usage was related to their personal distress when others experienced misfortune, such as living in an environment high in maternal anger and contempt. In this case, and somewhat like Eisenberg et al. (1994), empathetic distress for children living in frequent negativity, perhaps not surprisingly, led to children trying to escape when emotionally difficult events took place. Their emotionally negative environment made them more likely, when disturbed by others' difficulties, to want to escape the situation emotionally and physically.

Other negative emotions can be similarly problematic but with some unique qualities. The prevalence of shyness in one's emotional profile may make it that much more difficult to enact ER strategies at all. For example, kindergartners to second graders rated as shyer by their mothers and teachers were more likely to be rated by teachers as likely to do nothing in response to a conflict situation and less likely to regulate emotions by obtaining emotional support or taking constructive actions (Eisenberg, Shepard, Fabes, Murphy, & Guthrie, 1998). In short, shy preschoolers did not enact productive ER strategies; perhaps they felt "frozen."

Shyer preschoolers also were less likely to use active distraction while waiting for a cookie (Feng, Shaw, & Moilanen, 2011). Similarly, shy preschoolers in Hipson, Coplan, and Séguin's (2019) study were less likely to use active regulation (i.e., self-directed speech, information gathering, constructive action; the measures of both shyness and ER were rated by parents). Looking at a more complex emotional picture related to shyness, toddlers ages 2 and 3 who showed more behavioral inhibition (i.e., withdrawn reactions to an adult stranger, a robot, and an inflatable tunnel) demonstrated less engaged, more passive ER during a disappointing gift situation at age 5 (Penela, Walker, Degnan, Fox, & Henderson, 2015). Passive ER strategies included just tolerating the mistaken gift. Overall, experiencing shyness and behavior inhibition renders one less able to enact useful, active ER strategies during the preschool period.

In contrast, experiencing positive emotions more generally may afford the preschooler with a reservoir of strength from which to respond to emotional challenge. Thus, preschoolers' observed happiness was positively associated with ER (Ersan & Tok, 2020). Further, 3- to 8-year-olds whose mothers rated them as more likely to experience empathic concern (not distress) were reported by teachers as more likely to use support-seeking ER strategies and less likely to use aggressive, venting strategies, when faced with emotional challenges (Goodvin et al., 2006). Davies and Cummings (1995) also found that children induced to experience positive emotions were less distressed and held more positive cognitions while experiencing background anger.

### SUMMARY: Emotional Expressiveness and ER

Taken as a whole then, day-to-day prevalent emotion experiences, whether considered as overall emotionality or as specific emotions, contribute to the types of ER strategies used by preschoolers and their efficacy. The other component of Eisenberg and Fabes's (1992) model, self-regulation, also has been examined for its effects.

## Self-Regulation and ER

As noted by Eisenberg and Fabes (1992), self-regulation is clearly related to ER. In the ensuing years, more knowledge has been acquired about the aspects of self-regulation that contribute to ER. For example, preschoolers' greater working memory is related to ER, both as observed and as parent rated (Leerkes et al., 2008; Wang & Saudino, 2013). The biological roots of both self-regulation and ER are emphasized in Wang and Saudino's findings; their genetic roots in fact account for their association (see the section "Biological Bases of Emotion Regulation").

Inhibitory control also relates to ER. In one study inhibitory control was related to composite ER in a disappointment paradigm, as well as in the effort required to enact ER strategies (Hudson & Jacques, 2014). Children who could respond appropriately by pressing a button when they saw a sun, but refraining when they saw a moon, were able to show more positive facial, vocal, verbal, and behavioral responses when getting a nonpreferred gift and exerted more effort to do so (see also Kieras, Tobin, Graziano, & Rothbart, 2005; Liebermann et al., 2007; Orta, Çorapçı, Yagmurlu, & Aksan, 2013). The ability to focus and shift attention also would seem important to ER, considering that the distraction strategy is really an example of shifting attention, and problem solving requires focusing attention to enact new behaviors.

Inhibitory control assessed by an even larger battery of tasks (Simon Says, Forbidden Toy, Gift Delay) was related to an ER composite (including suppressing emotions when reacting to a disappointing gift or keeping a secret, and understanding children's true feelings; Carlson & Wang, 2007), even with age and verbal ability accounted for.

Parents' reports in this study also demonstrated associations between self-control and ER, and ratings of both children's self-control and ER were related to the inhibitory control battery, suggesting the validity of the assessments' results. The findings were similar if "understanding children's true feelings," which may have been closer to an assessment of emotion knowledge, was removed.

In an example of Eisenberg and Fabes's (1992) joint predictions highlighting both emotionality and self-regulation, ER was most effective at medium-level inhibitory control; being too controlled, these investigators hypothesized, might have blunted affect or increased anxiety (Carlson & Wang, 2007). However, when emotion is more intense, greater inhibitory control may be necessary for successful ER. The balancing act between emotional intensity and self-regulation is finely tuned even during early childhood.

Considering self-regulation more holistically, the coaction of working memory plus inhibitory control may allow for suppression of unwanted emotional experience and expression, and perhaps even physiological markers of arousal (Carlson & Wang, 2007). Since both inhibitory control and ER involve preventing impulsive behavior and carrying out an opposing action, brain development, which I discuss later in the chapter, is likely implicated.

Finally, the relationship between ER and self-regulation is likely to be bidirectional; they are distinct, albeit related, abilities (Leerkes et al., 2008). For example, successful ER frees up resources for self-regulatory processes that assure meeting a goal. In fact, this relationship may be more than bidirectional—it can be very difficult to extricate ER from self-regulation, and vice versa. Based on the maturation of neural systems, both ER and self-regulation emerge during infancy and toddlerhood, and although one set of abilities may be ascendant, they go hand in hand during difficult circumstances: The cognitive processing involved in self-regulation is at times required for ER, and ER is sometimes necessary during experiences that are commonly considered as self-regulatory (e.g., not peeking at a gift; Calkins & Dedmon, 2000; Calkins & Marcovitch, 2010). Both are embedded in overall self-regulation.

Another important self-regulatory issue in the development of independent, explicit ER, which has not been given much attention recently but could be very critical, is whether the child feels that they can control the situation. No matter which ER strategy a young child uses in a particular situation, it is important for the child to feel a sense of control over his or her own ER. No one likes feeling "out of control." Children ages 5 and 6 who watched a scary fairy tale on videotape and did not believe they had control over frightening events remembered less of a subsequent videotape on children's medical examinations (Cortez & Bugental, 1994). They felt the need to assert some measure of control, and subsequently used attentional disengagement during the second video to lessen their short-term distress. Using this mode of ER exacted a price, however: Through its use, they were insufficiently attentive and acquired only limited useful knowledge of a potentially threatening but ubiquitous event—a medical examination.

Children who feel that they have little control over ER also may vent their emotions (with varying results, depending on the target of the venting), or even sublimate through illness, compensating activity, or dissociation (Cole, Michel, et al., 1994).

Feeling a lack of control over emotional situations can impact cognitive and social outcomes.

### SUMMARY: Self-Regulation and ER

Inhibitory control, working memory, and cognitive flexibility are all aspects of self-regulation that contribute to children's individual differences in ER. However, this association also often is found to be bidirectional both contemporaneously and over time, no doubt reflecting neural contributions to both. As well, an aspect of self-regulation that has not been much studied, but may be important, is whether children *feel* that they can regulate their emotions—a sort of meta-self-regulation. More research in this entire area, especially uniting information on brain activity (see the section "Brain Structures and ER"), could be very useful.

## OTHER SUPPORTS FOR INDIVIDUAL DIFFERENCES IN EMOTION REGULATION

### Language Ability

I have already noted how adults' use of emotion language can assist in supported ER; how emotion language and conversations constitute important tools of emotion socialization of all components of emotional competence, including ER, is discussed further in Chapters 8 and 9. But it also is important to consider how young children's own facility in using language bolsters their ER. Being able to talk about one's feelings and their contexts can help enact various ER strategies, including but not limited to (1) self-soothing (as Ella did when her foot hurt in the night); (2) defusing the situation by selecting a new one (e.g., "Can we go to the park, Mom?" to feel better); (3) modifying the situation (e.g., asking for comfort); (4) cognitively reframing situations (especially, e.g., "I didn't want to go to the pool anyhow," "I'm just going to forget about that mean guy," "Broccoli is not so bad")[2]; or (5) gathering information useful to ER (e.g., "When will I get to open my present?"). These examples show how language comprises an articulate accompaniment to emotional experience and expression, in communicating one's goals, needs, and plans. Being able to reflect on one's own and others' emotions, perhaps via self-talk, can be an important part of ER, a tool for guiding feeling and action. Moreover, resolving past emotional events via language allows one to anticipate what to do should the events arise again (Cole, Armstrong, & Pemberton, 2010).

Thus it might be expected that more advanced language ability could assist preschoolers dealing with their anger in real time over having to wait for a gift (Roben et al., 2013). Toddlers and preschoolers were asked to tolerate such a wait (8 minutes) four times during the 18- to 48-month period. Their anger, ER strategies, and expressive language were captured at each assessment. Children with greater expressive language,

[2]It would be interesting to consider whether these exemplars of cognitive reappraisal are supported by the conceptual foundation suggested by Hoemann et al. (2019) and the symbolic representation upon which Holodynski and Seeger (2019) rest their assertions.

as well as greater growth in language, showed less anger by 48 months. Moreover, their anger at having to wait decreased more over time.

What process did language ability appear to aid in this situation? First, an increase in language over time was related to quicker and longer support seeking at 36 months, and support seeking at this age (although not earlier when it was more nonverbal) was related to both a lower level of anger at 48 months and a greater decrease in anger over time. Second, children's ability to distract themselves from the wait for longer durations by 48 months was similarly related to language ability, and thence to less anger during the wait. In short, as language level and growth increased, anger decreased, mediated by ER strategy use. Language was an important support in using these ER strategies, including support seeking and calm information seeking and distraction at a time of transition to independent rather than exclusively supported ER.

Why might these contributions of language obtain? Several possibilities come to mind (Cole, Armstrong, et al., 2010; Roben et al., 2013). Understanding and producing verbal information allows for more efficient ER. For example, a verbally rich inner life could help children have more distracting ideas. Regarding the link with support seeking, a child having a vocabulary that allowed them to put words together to communicate with adults could learn more easily to regulate anger, by reflecting on and coming to a shared understanding of an emotional experience. Such a child could, for example, verbalize her or his needs without expressing frustration nonverbally, calmly seeking support and information.

It is easy to see that language and ER are likely also related via their connections with more general self-regulation, such as the control of attention (Cole, Armstrong, et al., 2010). Such control allows the child to slow emotional responses and inhibit or delay actions.

### SUMMARY: Language and ER

Language ability supports the use of independent ER strategies. Verbal facility can aid their use of self-talk for distraction and can allow them to communicate with adults to solicit aid and also learn new strategies. Further, the common linkage between ER and verbal ability with broader self-regulation also is important to consider.

## Emotion Knowledge

Including another factor along with language—emotion knowledge—could make Eisenberg and Fabes's (1992) model even more complete. It makes sense that understanding more about the nature of emotions (i.e., how they feel and their causes and consequences) could play a role in enacting more optimal emotional, perceptual–cognitive, and behavioral ER strategies. At the same time, experience in enacting ER strategies could give the preschooler more emotional experience and add to his or her knowledge.

Regarding links between ER and emotion knowledge, Di Maggio et al. (2016) found a connection between a direct assessment of preschoolers' emotion knowledge and teacher ratings of ER (see also Blankson et al., 2013, 2017; Morgan et al., 2010).

In my own work, our puppet measure of emotion knowledge was predictive in a path model of children's observed ability to regulate emotions via language during classroom free play (Denham, Bassett, Zinsser, et al., 2014).

Even more specifically, preschoolers' emotion knowledge has been related to their observed effort to control their emotions during a disappointing gift situation (as indexed by self-soothing and fidgeting; Hudson & Jacques, 2014). In that study, overall ER during the disappointing gift procedure (i.e., an aggregate of facial, vocal, verbal, and behavioral responses) was related to preschoolers' knowledge of display rules. This specialized emotion knowledge may have stood the children in good stead during the disappointment paradigm—although they knew they felt negative emotion, they knew what should be done regarding display rules. They smiled in the experimenter's presence, while expressing anger and sadness and trading in the gift for a "better" one when alone.

Some work in this area has been longitudinal. For example, Thomsen and Lessing (2020) found that emotion knowledge and the size of the self-reported ER repertoire were related at age 3 to 6 years (T1). At the same time, the T1 ER repertoire size predicted emotion knowledge at age 5 to 8 years (T2), which then was related to both the size and diversity of the T2 ER repertoire. Other studies also have uncovered the ER-to-emotion knowledge cross-time prediction (e.g., Lucas-Molina et al., 2020).

### SUMMARY: Emotion Knowledge and ER

Emotion knowledge may set up a foundation for ER (Denham, Bassett, Zinsser, et al., 2014), or vice versa. Thus, it does appear that both attributes of emotional competence (i.e., ER and emotion knowledge) have important bidirectional associations with one another, even longitudinally. Each can bolster the other during early childhood, attesting to the intimate connection between understanding emotions and being able to regulate them.

These intrapersonal abilities and attributes—emotional expressiveness, self-regulation, language, and emotion knowledge—all make important contributions to ER. However, another foundation for ER remains to be considered here: its biological bases.

## BIOLOGICAL BASES OF EMOTION REGULATION

This model of individual differences in ER that I've been discussing here, with its emphasis on temperament as suggested also by Eisenberg and Fabes (1992), points to the likelihood of biological contributions to ER and emotional competence as a whole. I do subscribe to an inclusive view of the etiology of emotional competence, in which biological (species-typical, genetic, and physiological), cognitive, and social factors interweave in a complex medley. As noted by Thompson et al. (2008), ER is a diffuse network of multilevel processes that feed back and interact. So far, I have discussed preschoolers' development of ER strategy usage and individual differences that are apparent during the preschool period, with attention given to how emotional expressivity, self-regulation, language, and emotion knowledge promote or hinder this development. Given the ample consideration of other factors contributing to ER, and before covering more social factors both here in a discussion of culture, and in Chapter 8, I now turn to a discussion of the biological bases of ER. Importantly, neural structures and processes interact with and underlie both emotion generation and ER, and physiological control becomes integrated with ER in early childhood, suggesting that both aspects of the biological bases of ER should be discussed (Thompson et al., 2008). In what follows, I take a somewhat selective tour of these crucial biological bases of ER.

## Brain Structures and ER

Consider the brain structures that bear upon the model of ER I have created in this chapter. One area of the brain that is a good candidate for involvement in ER is the anterior attention system (Calkins & Marcovitch, 2010), because, along with its relation to the prefrontal cortex (PFC), it regulates many facets of functioning, including not only ER, but also cognition and behavior. In fact, the connections between self-regulation and ER that have been considered here are likely centered in just this area of the brain. As networks in the attention system mature, increased inhibitory control allows children to purposefully redirect attention via various distraction strategies.

Thus the anterior cingulate cortex (ACC), in its two divisions, regulate two aspects of the young children's functioning: (1) cognition and attention, via links with the PFC; and (2) emotion, via links with the limbic system of the brain, the peripheral autonomic central nervous system and the visceromotor and endocrine systems. These two subdivisions act reciprocally with lower brain systems. Through the "top-down" function of the first ACC division and "bottom-up" of the second division, they form feedback loops to and from the limbic system. That is, the first division may help to moderate emotional signals from the limbic system, whereas the second division uses crucial information from the limbic system. Both cortical areas function to support ongoing behavior that is both cognitive and affective (Thompson et al., 2008).

In general, then, both the PFC, especially its medial and frontal lobes, and the ACC mediate higher order processes like planning, monitoring, and goal setting, all of which are aspects of the volitional control of attention that are central to ER. These brain regions, as synaptic connections become more efficient and the pathways between them and other brain regions become more integrated, assist in children's growing ability to attend to aspects of their environment and respond quickly to specific contexts and situations (Calkins, Dollar, & Widaman, 2019). They support cognitive flexibility, inhibition of the prepotent responses that the children in Cole and colleagues' studies had such difficulty moderating, as well as reappraisal, judgment, and self-monitoring—in short, the use of flexible and effective ER strategies (Perry & Calkins, 2018; Thompson et al., 2008). These anterior attention regions of the ACC and PFC mature late, undergoing growth and consolidation from infancy to adolescence, but with the most dramatic changes in the period studied here, from toddlerhood through preschool.

Along with the ACC especially, the ventral cingulate cortex (VCC) also takes in information from the limbic system, another brain region crucial to the experience and regulation of emotions. In the limbic system, both lower brain structures of the amygdala and hypothalamus respond almost automatically to emotion cues. The amygdala is online from a very early age; this "lower" brain region moderates thought, perception, and planning in the cortex—giving the cortex "something to chew on" by detecting, decoding, and appraising emotional stimuli (Moreira & Silvers, 2018).

Thus, it is the limbic system where lower-level automatic and implicit, rather than deliberate and explicit, ER can take place. In particular, the amygdala in its "bottom-up" connections with ACC divisions and the VCC "tunes" and constrains the cortex to look at emotion meaning, tuning perception and cognition (Thompson, 2011). Fulfilling its feedback function, the ACC dampens the amygdala's message via its "top-down" action. In fact, activation of the amygdala is more consistently attenuated by ACC-related ER than any other brain system; as such, its effects may decrease with development after childhood (Moreira & Silver, 2018).

Other regions of the brain also are strongly implicated in ER, including the ventromedial prefrontal cortex (vmPFC), the ventrolateral prefrontal cortex (vlPFC), and the dorsomedial prefrontal cortex (dmPFC), and dorsolateral prefrontal cortex (dlPFC; Moreira & Silvers, 2018). The vmPFC is unique in that it is involved in both emotion *activation* and implicit ER. It moderates amygdala activation, but of course the inverse also is true. Importantly, the vmPFC assists in the integration of emotional information, making it critical for using contextual information and information held in memory during ER. It appears to be more often involved in implicit, rather than explicit, ER.

However, the developmental course of vmPFC's role in ER is somewhat controversial. Findings with children sometimes show a *positive* coupling of the vmPFC and the amygdala, implying that increased emotional stimulation via the amygdala was actually enhanced by the vmPFC (suggesting that bottom-up develop before top-down connections). However, there also is some evidence with children older than preschoolers that this structure does play a regulatory role in down-regulating amygdala activation (Pitskel, Bolling, Kaiser, Crowley, & Pelphrey, 2011), with increasing activation during implicit ER after early childhood. Further, similar results were found with young people from ages 6 to 23 years during a reappraisal ER strategy, in which both a reduction in negative affect and the inverse coupling of vmPFC and amygdala increased with age (Silvers et al., 2017). Thus increasing age predicted greater top-down regulation of the amygdala via the vlPFC. Although these results are tantalizing in that this progression (and flipping of positive to negative coupling) seems to begin just after early childhood, the region's importance should be noted. Moreover, the brain architecture responsible for changes in this circuit changes in an experience-dependent manner, further highlighting its potential importance.

The vlPFC and dlPFC are key subdivisions of the lateral PFC, and are implicated in numerous top-down processes, including working memory, inhibitory control, and planning, as well as in the distraction and reappraisal ER strategies. As such the vlPFC has a role in explicit ER. As a support for the response selection aspect of explicit ER, its function increases with age, although some of the age-related findings differ depending on strategy and emotion. In general, the vlPFC plays an important role during reappraisal, moderated by vmPFC-amygdala connectivity (Silvers et al., 2018).

These findings suggest that it too is important for explicit ER beginning at the end of early childhood (but extending into early adulthood), perhaps coming online after the earlier vmPFC structural development and involvement in implicit ER. As for the dlPFC, it is implicated in one's attention to emotional stimuli, and as such maintains reappraisal content and goals in working memory, with a shift to the vlPFC to select an appropriate strategy. Thus, it also is important in explicit ER.

Finally, the dmPFC also is implicated in explicit ER, particularly in reappraisal strategy usage, monitoring its effectiveness; however, it also has been noted in implicit ER. Moreira and Silvers (2018) report that its function increases over age, with children as young as 4 years possibly recruiting it within their consideration of their own and others thoughts and feelings. However, much evidence suggests that its responses peak in adolescence, pointing to older youths' and adults' abilities to represent emotions cognitively.

In short, ER is obviously supported by brain processes that develop over time, especially in the attention and limbic systems. Many of the networks mentioned experience substantial growth after early childhood, with new interconnections developing among cells and prunings of other connections. Nonetheless, the surge in many aspects of these regions' development that takes place during early childhood support the changes in ER already reported, seen as both process and outcome. The integration of emotion, perception, cognition, and behavior depends upon coaction with activity within specific brain regions.

## The Autonomic Nervous System's Role in ER

Another key biological support for ER involves the autonomic nervous system (ANS). This system provides afferent and efferent feedback, transmitting information from peripheral organs *to* the central nervous system (CNS) and *from* the CNS to peripheral organs. The system's pathways especially integrate with other neurophysiological and neuroanatomic processes, linking cardiac activity with CNS processes in a reciprocal fashion (Calkins & Marcovitch, 2010). Both parasympathetic and the sympathetic branches of the ANS play a role in this heart–brain connection (Perry & Calkins, 2018).

Actions of the parasympathetic nervous system (PNS) have garnered much attention in the last few decades because its pathways are especially involved in regulating the biobehavioral state, motor activity, attention, and emotion. First, much attention has been given to how this connection promotes the regulation of the biobehavioral state, motor functions, attention, emotion, and cognition (Porges, 2003). In particular, consideration of ER has focused on the vagus nerve, which originates in the brainstem's nucleus ambiguus and provides input to the sinoatrial node of the heart. The vagus nerve thus promotes changes in cardiac activity, allowing for transitions between the maintenance of metabolic homeostasis and active responses to environmental events.

Thus, both the vagal regulation of the heart (vagal tone, as measured by variability in heart rate that occurs at the frequency of breathing, i.e., respiratory sinus arrhythmia, or RSA) during relatively calm situations (i.e., baseline vagal tone) and especially in response to challenges have been studied in relation to ER. Vagal tone is generally greater during baseline homeostatic conditions and is *withdrawn* or *suppressed* during challenging conditions. When experiencing calm conditions, the vagus nerve inhibits sympathetic nervous system (SNS) via activation of the PNS and thus promotes relaxation. So baseline vagal tone characterizes one's general level of arousal and capacity to respond. Low baseline vagal tone might represent hypervigilance, whereas overly high baseline vagal tone might reflect a 'too relaxed' state. For example, moderate (i.e., "just right") baseline vagal tone in early childhood predicted aspects of prosociality and empathic concern concurrently and longitudinally (Miller, Kahle, & Hastings, 2017).

In contrast, when conditions are challenging, the suppression of vagal tone allows for sympathetic nervous system predominance and increased heartbeat (Calkins et al., 2019); this increase facilitates the focused attention needed to regulate emotion. Such vagal suppression during challenging situations functions early in development and has been related to self-soothing and attention control during infancy and ER during preschool. For example, Calkins and Dedmon (2000) showed that toddlers at risk for behavior problems evidenced less vagal withdrawal after emotional challenge, and this smaller decrease was accompanied by clearly dysregulated emotional behavior. But, as with baseline vagal tone, however, there could be "too much of a good thing"—too-great suppression might denote overarousal. In fact, an intriguing idea that it is vagal flexibility—the initial RSA suppression and subsequent return to baseline—that denotes behavioral regulation (Ugarte, Miller, Weissman, & Hastings, 2021). It should be noted too that lesser suppression or even augmentation can be related to more easeful social interaction (Brooker & Buss, 2010). The picture is complicated.

Nonetheless, it has become clear that an ANS reciprocal connection with both higher brain structures and a peripheral organ such as the heart, via vagal tone, has an important connection to ER. Vagal withdrawal during an emotional challenge is now used as a marker of physiological regulation or arousal, as another way to index ER. In fact, meta-analytic findings demonstrated that children's vagal withdrawal is associated with fewer externalizing, internalizing, and cognitive/academic problems, as well as fewer social competence problems in nonclinical groups (Graziano & Derefinko, 2013). Further, relations were strongest when baseline vagal tone was already accounted for, highlighting the importance of the *change* in withdrawal.

Finally vagal recovery to baseline *after* an emotional challenge also is important. Being able to return to the calmer resting state is part of ER. For example, young children whose vagal tone remained suppressed well after an emotionally challenging situation remained focused on the desired object rather than on engaging in more positive behaviors (Santucci et al., 2008).

As already implied, the SNS also has important functions of its own that are related to ER. More specifically, for example, 4- and 5-year-olds' increased SNS reactivity along with decreased vagal tone during an interaction with a stranger demonstrated more effective ER during a subsequent disappointment task (Stifter, Dollar, & Cipriano, 2011). This reciprocal ANS activation represented an adaptive form of autonomic control that bore upon young children's ER.

### **SUMMARY:** Biological Bases of ER

Both brain structures' functions, along with the autonomic nervous system's processes, form important foundations of ER in early childhood and thereafter.[3] These biological processes, when measured, help to identify ER mechanisms that cannot be observed. As noted by Perry and Calkins (2018), however, we must remember that there are two directions of influence here as in so many areas of study: Children's behaviors influence the development of biological systems just as the biological systems' functioning affect their behaviors. We must examine this interplay at both long and short time scales (e.g., see Brooker & Buss's [2010] dynamic findings on change in vagal tone and toddlers' observed positive affect).

## Cultural Influences on ER

There are crucial issues of culture in understanding young children's ER, because the very meaning of emotions and their regulation are governed by culture. It is unfortunate that most research in early childhood ER has been done from a Western, individualistic viewpoint, because much can be learned from comparing and contrasting individualistic and collectivistic/relational cultures' approaches. However, it is instructive to consider the differences between cultures in how the adults in them—and eventually the children themselves—would ascribe meaning to children's emotions and their regulation.

For example, as already noted, the focus of collectivistic/relational, interdependent cultures is on relatedness and on preventing the very elicitation of emotions that would threaten it. Thus, where the interdependent self is more valued, ER serves the goal of preventing hurting others or threatening the group, and of enhancing relational harmony, based on shared instead of individual efficacy (Trommsdorff & Cole, 2011; Trommsdorff & Rothbaum, 2008). ER is considered important both to the self and the social group, focusing on promoting empathic, other-focused emotions that fostering relatedness, and on devaluing those that disrupt it.

In contrast, in individualistic, independent cultures, the focus is on autonomy, but also on self-goals, promotion of emotion, and self-only regulation (Trommsdorff & Cole, 2011; Trommsdorff & Heikamp, 2013; Trommsdorff & Rothbaum, 2008). More specifically, in individualistic cultures, ER serves the goal of enhancing the positivity and efficacy of the independent self. The emotions of an authentic self are valued and even promoted.

How do these important differences in worldview impact notions of ER in early childhood? First, the movement from supported to independent, *intra*personal ER has already been mentioned here. This is a very individualist viewpoint, with the child taking much responsibility for his or her own ER. In contrast, in collectivistic cultures children's ability to enact ER with the support of an attachment figure within

---

[3]Other biological functions, such as hormonal (especially with respect to cortisol) functions, are important.

parent–child interaction may not evolve into a more autonomous self-enacted use of strategies. Indeed, in such cultures the *inter*personal context of supported ER may transform into an "extended interpersonal" context of relatedness, following the internalized social expectations of an interdependent self (Trommsdorff & Heikamp, 2013). In this case, ER would be a conjoint process in which the adult socializers and the child are still very much in partnership.

Of note, these extended interpersonal or intrapersonal ER processes can be seen very early in the process depicted in Figure 6.1—at the point of elicitation of emotion or the *potential* elicitation of emotion. Different emotion-relevant situations are promoted or downplayed, and appraisals are preadapted within culturally valued relationships. For example, in a collectivist/relational culture, such as Java and Japan, because saving face and the maintenance of the group's harmony are valued social expectations, children may be protected from even experiencing some negative emotions (Trommsdorff & Cole, 2011). Situation selection and modification are undertaken for the child by socializers, a topic I return to in Chapter 7. Although adults in individualistic cultures do take part in situation selection and modification, the proactive stance of socializers in these cultures is much looser.

Thus given these cultural differences in developing ER, the situations that elicit emotions, and the very emotions that are valued, may differ substantially (Trommsdorff & Cole, 2011). Prevalent emotions of differing cultures thus reflect their differing values. For example, in more individualistic cultures, anger and pride are seen as reasonable emotions, whereas collectivistic/relational cultures value shame, sadness, and empathy instead. Children's prevalent emotions would be evaluated more positively when they "fit" within the culture; when there was a poorer "fit," the ER pressure would be greater.

As examples, the emotional reactions of Japanese and German preschoolers were measured within specific situations (Trommsdorff & Friedlmeier, 2010). Given what I've already noted here, one would expect that emotions would be differentially elicited and regulated in different situations. One situation involved an achievement of the self—children were asked to draw a picture, and their failure in terms of not finishing on time was "rigged." German preschool girls showed more intense distress expressions when they could not finish the task, and although both German and Japanese girls showed more intense distress when the experimenter took the drawing away to "evaluate" it, by the end of the task Japanese girls were again less intensely distressed than the German ones. This situation triggered self-concerns more in the German girls than in the Japanese because of their already strong socialization regarding goals of the self and its uniqueness. Thus the situation posed more of an ER challenge for the children living in an individualistic culture.

A different situation, however, sparked a different emotion in the Japanese girls. When they witnessed another's misfortune, the Japanese preschool girls, like the German girls, became relatively intensely distressed. However, when they were removed from the situation, the Japanese girls were even more intensely distressed, but the German girls' distress was waning. As opposed to the drawing situation, seeing the distress of another posed more of an ER challenge for the children living in a collectivistic/relational culture.

In making an initial foray into explaining culture's impact on developing ER, I have concentrated on the distinction between individualistic and collectivist/relational cultures, as well as, to a degree, the differing value that cultures place on the emotional experience and expression. However, there are other lenses through which to view this development in any given culture, most of which are plumbed inadequately as of now: (1) the power distance between children and socializers; (2) children's place; (3) the ways children are considered to learn (Halberstadt & Lozada, 2011). One can envision a power-distant collectivistic/relational culture, for example, in which children are expected to obey and defer to adults, and in which anger is discouraged and its regulation is promoted, whereas more egalitarian collectivistic socializers may actually value it. Further, for example, one can envision an individualistic culture that differs in the love, devotion, and indulgence directed at its children; a culture that emphasizes this value might be much more accepting of emotions and put less pressure on young children to regulate them. Finally, beliefs about how children learn undoubtedly would influence how ER "rules" are conveyed, for example, whether they are considered to be acquired via maturation or need to be taught. These values, however, require much more study, which promises to be fascinating.

### **SUMMARY:** Cultural Influences on ER

Recent research has uncovered important distinctions in how ER is envisioned by socializers in differing cultures. The need to regulate emotions in general and specific emotions in particular differ substantially given the values of differing cultures. Much emphasis has been placed on the important differences between individualistic and collectivistic/relational cultures, and it certainly is important to know what is expected of children to understand the ways in which they regulate emotions. Other dimensions that differ culturally have been raised, such as power distance, the place of children in each culture, and the ways children are considered to learn (Halberstadt & Lozada, 2011); cultural expectations of children's ER deserve more thought and attention in research.

## CONCLUSION

Enormous advances in our understanding of young children's ER have taken place since the publication of my earlier book, *Emotional Competence in Young Children*. In this chapter I've detailed our current understanding of how preschoolers' ER changes over time and of how children evidence their own style of ER; in Chapters 10 and 11, I examine the large corpus of literature on how ER contributes to social and preacademic success.

Much work still can be done, however, to examine both developmental change and individual differences in preschoolers' ER. First, definitional problems have eased substantially, but the operationalization of a richer, fuller conception of ER can still become clearer. Second, research could include all the aspects of ER. For example, work on individual differences in ER should flesh out its emotional, perceptual/cognitive, and behavioral elements more equally. At the very least, researchers who focus on only, or even mostly, one aspect of ER should acknowledge that they are doing exactly that—investigating a piece of a larger, more complex picture.

Young children can reduce, generate, or sustain emotional experience by these emotion-related, perceptual/cognitive, and behavioral means I have already described. In my view, ER represents the pragmatically useful culmination of emotional expressiveness, understanding, and socialization from all the important people in children's lives. As such, it is extremely important to children's success in their social and preacademic worlds: It helps them to reach the goals they desire, it helps them to feel better and to feel both social and preacademic mastery (see Chapters 10 and 11), and it helps them become part of their culture (Hyson, 1994).

# 7

# Socialization of Emotional Competence and Impact on Preschoolers' Expressiveness

## INTRODUCTION

How is emotional competence fostered? The components of emotion socialization theory include socializers' expressed emotions, contingent reactions to specific emotions, teaching about emotions, beliefs about emotions, and socializers' own emotional abilities. All these components of socialization directly and/or indirectly help young children acquire the components of culturally and age-appropriate emotional competence (Denham, 2019; Denham, Bassett, & Wyatt, 2014; Eisenberg, 2020; Eisenberg, Cumberland, et al., 1998). Thus preschoolers do not develop emotional competencies in a vacuum.

> Jamie is screaming at his mother, "I want my snack right now!" "It's too close to dinnertime, Jamie. I know you're mad because you're very hungry, but you need to wait," his mother answers as she scrubs carrots at the sink. His eyebrows lower. He glowers ferociously, butts his head against her, and yells again, "Give me now!" His mother remains calm, but sighs deeply. "Jamie, I don't like it when you yell at me like that. In fact, it makes me really sad." She has excellent ER skills herself (maybe she counted to 10 before her answer), and she also believes that her son's vivid emotions, although sometimes difficult to endure, represent important teachable moments.

Jamie's mother unwittingly demonstrates three important ways in which she teaches her son about emotions. First, she models not only calmness in the face of a stressor (Jamie!), but then also the appropriate facial expression of sadness when verbally attacked by a loved one. Second, she reacts to his emotions in a supportive way, while she also suggests the need for regulation. Third, she uses developmentally appropriate emotion language. Her speech can assist Jamie in figuring out that some events are often linked with specific emotions: "People get mad about not getting what they want, but people also feel sad when they are yelled at." Talking to him as she does also shows him that he can use words as tools, rather than resorting to full-blown tantrums.

Many people play important roles in toddlers' and preschoolers' lives—their parents, of course, as well as childcare providers and preschool teachers, siblings, and playmates. Information about the nature of emotions and their expression is embedded within even the most minute interactions with these significant others (Denham, 1989, 1993; Denham, Bassett, et al., 2014; Denham & Grout, 1992, 1993; Eisenberg & Fabes, 1994; Eisenberg, Fabes, Carlo, & Karbon, 1992; Halberstadt, 1991; Jones & Bouffard, 2012). In this and the next chapter, I describe the key contributions that other people make to young children's growing emotional competence. These other people are called "socializers" because, whether intentionally or not, they show young children what is acceptable in a culture.

All the people in young children's lives are potential socializers of emotions. They can make interesting events happen, have access to things that are attractive, are similar to the child in some way, or are loved by the young child. Parents are the primary socializers of young children's emotional competence; close contact with parents is important in fostering—or, unfortunately, impeding—the development of emotional competence.

Teachers also have varied qualities that make them attractive socializers. They show young children wonderful new skills, direct their play, and form close emotional bonds with them. The emotions that teachers are comfortable sharing give their pupils experience with patterns of expressiveness that are different from their parents' (Hyson & Lee, 1996). Their reactions to the emotional displays of children in their classrooms can affect how the children cope with their emotions while adapting to the new classroom experience (Denham & Burton, 1996). Whether feelings are discussed openly in the classroom or not also gives important explicit and implicit messages about the world of emotions. Teachers' important roles are discussed in Chapter 9.

Peers are similar to one another; they can control one another; and they can share enjoyable activities. They also are very attractive to other young children. And of course, anyone who has spent any amount of time in an early childhood classroom knows that preschoolers' emotions abound when they come together for play: Friends are often delighted or furious with each other, sometimes hurt each other's feelings, and occasionally get into scary situations. Aptly, peer research is focusing increasingly on the role of emotion, and from these reports some evidence can be gleaned. Patterns of expressiveness, for example, are associated with the amount of conflict a child experiences with peers (Arsenio & Lover, 1997).

In particular, if a child is often engaged in conflicts and arguments with playmates, the prevalence of the child's negative emotions increases (Denham, Mason, Caverly, et al., 2001). Frequent exposure to peers' negative emotions contributes to a child's own sadness, anger, and fear through direct imitation, disinhibition, or contagion. In the case of Jamie in the beginning example, his angry face and "head butt" are very similar to his friend's emotional behavior. Jamie may think this way of expressing anger is okay, or even may become angry more easily, after dealing with his friend's ire on the playground all morning.

Older brothers and sisters exert power over their younger siblings but also are similar to them. Because of these qualities, young children naturally look to them as experts in the feelings business, as in other areas. Preschoolers who have closer relationships with older siblings learn much about emotions from them (Dunn, Brown, & Beardsall, 1991; Dunn, Brown, Slomkowski, Tesla, & Youngblade, 1991; Strandberg-Sawyer et al., 2002). The behavior of older siblings guides young children's ideas about what emotions are appropriate for various situations and about how those emotions can be displayed.

Although intriguing research has examined the influence of nonparental socializers, nonetheless, more is known about the parental role. Much of current knowledge about preschoolers' emotion socialization rightly (to my mind) focuses on the contribution of parents. So, although many people undoubtedly make powerful contributions to preschoolers' emotional competence, the main focus of this and the next chapter is on parental socialization. As already noted, in Chapter 9, I discuss how early childhood educators contribute to young children's emotional competence. I now take up the general mechanisms of emotion socialization.

## MECHANISMS OF EMOTION SOCIALIZATION: MODELING, TEACHING, AND CONTINGENCY

Socializers contribute to young children's growing emotional competence—in patterns of expressiveness, emotion knowledge, and ER. Just how do they make these contributions? Three social learning mechanisms have been proposed as major processes involved in emotion socialization (Denham, Bassett, et al., 2014; Denham, Mitchell-Copeland, Strandberg, Auerbach, & Blair, 1997; Eisenberg, 2020; Eisenberg, Cumberland, et al., 1998; Halberstadt, 1991): "modeling," "contingency," and "teaching." These three aspects of socialization—how the socializers show or don't show their own emotions, how they react or don't react to the emotions of others, how they teach or don't teach about emotions, respectively—are the key means by which young children absorb the emotional messages of socializers. These modes of socialization are evident when parents maintain a cheerful demeanor at the pediatrician's office, react sympathetically to a tired child's irritable crying, or have a serious chat about a friend who made their child sad. Such socialization influences their offspring's emotional competence—including their child's expressiveness, emotion knowledge, and ER. In brief, parents' generally positive emotional expression (including "safe" expression of negative emotions), encouraging reactions to children's emotions, and openness to and expertise in talking about emotions, all help their preschool-age children to become emotionally competent.

Further, parents' beliefs about emotions are increasingly recognized as important to emotion socialization (particularly beliefs referring to acceptance of and/or attention to emotions and the value of emotions and their regulation; Meyer, Raikes, Virmani, Waters, & Thompson, 2014). Beliefs are related to the actual enactment of emotion socialization (e.g., parent- or teacher-reported reactions to children's emotions, Halberstadt et al., 2013; Halberstadt, Thompson, Parker, & Dunsmore, 2008; Wong, McElwain, & Halberstadt, 2009; and observed family negativity, Wong, Diener, & Isabella, 2008). Because of this belief–behavior connection, I also discuss newer research on how parents' beliefs impact the emotion socialization and even emotional competence outcomes for their preschoolers.[1]

Another important consideration is the potential reciprocal nature of emotional transactions between parent and child; children's emotionality undoubtedly affects parental emotion socialization behaviors. For example, mothers' positive emotion during a waiting task, administered four times between 18 and 48 months, increased more over time *if* their children were less angry, more content, or engaged more in positive ER strategies (Cole, LeDonne, & Tan, 2013; see also Fields-Olivieri, Cole, & Maggi, 2017). These mothers' negative emotion decreased less when their children were angrier than other age-mates. Another example of children influencing emotion socialization is 2-year-old boys' support-seeking ER strategies predicting mothers' more supportive reactions to their emotions at age 3; mothers' socialization behaviors could be seen as responses to their children's earlier emotional competence (Premo & Kiel, 2014). So it is important to remember that children's own emotional lives and emotional competencies influence their parents' actual emotion socialization behaviors.

But back to the contributions of parents: How does emotion socialization operate? Young children are active social cognizers, always trying to understand what they see, and they pick up on emotional expressions of others as very salient parts of their social world. Modeling of emotional expressiveness happens whenever a parent shows an emotion, and a child observes it; it does not have to be intentional on the part of the socializer. In the following descriptions of mothers' emotion diary entries (see Denham & Grout, 1992), 4-year-olds witnessed the emotional expressiveness of their mothers. It is easy to extrapolate to the impact of these experiences on the children's emotional competence.

> Rachel and her baby sister shared a joyous playtime—coloring, playing with Legos, and singing songs. She saw her mother's happiness and smiled even more.
>
> Tyrone learned how anger might be expressed when his mother tried, unsuccessfully, to make a telephone call. She asked him to be quiet and walked into another room, but he followed her and began chasing his sister noisily. She quit her phone call, told him she was very angry, and sent him to his room. He yelled and fussed all the way upstairs. In the same way that Rachel absorbed her mother's happiness, Tyrone took the cues of his mother's lowered brows, her distinctly lowered voice, and her verbal message. He was angry too but also more clearly recognized anger in others after this exchange.

---

[1]Unfortunately, more research has been performed regarding parents' beliefs about emotions without connection to the emotion socialization techniques I focus on, and with parents of older children.

Claire learned about anger and sadness, too. She witnessed an argument between her mother and father. Her mother began to cry out of frustration and sadness over the long-standing, apparently unresolvable conflict. Claire watched with eyes wide; she approached and held onto her mother's legs, begging, "Please stop crying, Mommy." Then, getting tearful herself, she said she didn't feel good when her mother cried. Claire became saddened through the contagion of her mother's emotions, but also added this experience to her knowledge of how sadness is expressed. She also tried to figure out ER for herself and her mom.

Similarly, parents' contingent responding to children's emotions fuels emotional competence or its lack. In the following examples (again based on mothers' emotion diary entries; see Denham & Grout, 1992), parents reacted to their 4-year-olds' emotions.

Jeremy experienced his parents' accepting, helpful reaction to his emotions. He watched the movie *Jaws*, against his mother's better judgment. He fearfully, animatedly asked many questions about the movie afterward, and anxiously discussed it in great detail (e.g., "What was that red stuff?"). His mother and father answered all the questions and supported him as he resolved these things in his mind. Jeremy's emotions were accepted, and he was able to regulate them, as well as to learn about what makes things "scary."

Stacey's mother had bought a new wading pool and had high hopes for the fun the family could have. But this was a difficult day. Whether she was told to wait, get in, or get out of the pool, Stacey cried and couldn't be consoled. Nothing could please her. Finally, she had a minitantrum—lying down on the floor, knocking over a chair, and kicking at things. Her mother told her she couldn't act like that and helped her to pick up what she had knocked over. Then after she let Stacey cry a while, she consoled her, hugging her and discussing what had happened. Then everyone went back outside to the pool and had a good time! In this case, Stacey learned that some intensities and means of expressiveness are less acceptable (or at least they don't get the desired results!), and that talking about rather than venting feelings can have a positive outcome.

Finally, parents, some more than others actively address the world of emotions with their preschoolers, teaching them about it. Here are more examples from the Denham and Grout (1992) study:

Anikka learned about emotions while looking at a picture book with her mother. A new puppy tried to run away into the path of a school bus:

MOTHER: They were frightened. . . . [They] grabbed the dog and brought it to safety. See the worried looks?

ANIKKA: They look so scared.

Annika learned some new vocabulary for the emotion of fear, new cues for fear, and a new reason to be fearful—the safety of a loved one.

Sometimes young children actually initiate clarifying conversations about emotions.

Brian's mother felt ill. She told Brian that she could not play because she felt bad. He asked her whether she felt sad or happy. She then told him neither: "I feel sick, not any other way, but I'll be better soon." He hugged her, told her he loved her, and brought her Sesame Street magazines to read in bed. Brian learned that sometimes his conjectures about others' feelings could be incorrect, and that the best thing to do is ask!

In discussing emotion socialization I adapt and somewhat simplify Eisenberg's (2020) newest version of Eisenberg, Cumberland, et al.'s (1998) model (see Figure 7.1). As already noted, both in this chapter and Chapter 2 and depicted in the figure, a child's emotional arousal in a specific situation is central to both enacted emotion socialization practices and acquisition of emotional competence outcomes over time, and is affected by child characteristics. Especially germane to this chapter, the child's emotional arousal affects and is affected by emotion socialization practices. For example, a child who is exhibiting intense fear will probably elicit different emotion socialization techniques than one showing less extreme arousal. In turn, the specific emotion socialization practices chosen can affect the child's arousal, and his or her success at modulating such arousal can mediate the contributions of emotion socialization to their emotional competence outcomes. That is, the parent who can successfully help their child moderate their emotional arousal may be more successful at delivering emotion socialization messages that bolster the development of optimal emotional expressiveness, emotion knowledge, and ER.

Moving on from this child arousal focus of emotion socialization, several other factors can affect how the three major aspects of emotion socialization—modeling, contingent responding, and teaching—transpire. First, as already noted, child demographic characteristics are important. Whether the child is just emerging from toddlerhood or ready to go to school (i.e., their age) may matter in terms of how parents enact emotion socialization. Parents likely do not expect as much of younger preschoolers, in terms of emotional competence. Likewise, emotion socialization may look different for boys and girls. Children of differing temperaments—their relatively stable day-to-day level of arousal and regulation—may elicit different emotion socialization behaviors. Furthermore, how parents' emotion socialization behaviors "fit" with the child's age, developmental level, gender, and temperament can affect the effectiveness of their emotion socialization behaviors. I discuss some of these moderators of emotion socialization in this chapter.

Second, parent characteristics certainly impact their emotion socialization practices—for example, fathers sometimes enact these practices differently than mothers do, with different effects. Moreover, as already noted, emotion-related beliefs are important precursors to parental emotion socialization practices. For example, if a mother believes emotions to be dangerous forces from which children should be protected, she will likely react quite differently to her child's emotions than Jamie's mother, who believes that emotions are important to express and talk about. And it is not surprising that parents' own emotional competence factors importantly in their emotion socialization. Finally, general parenting style and its consistency also can affect the type of emotion socialization practices a parent uses. A distant, authoritarian parent would likely exhibit different emotions, show different reactions to children's emotions, and

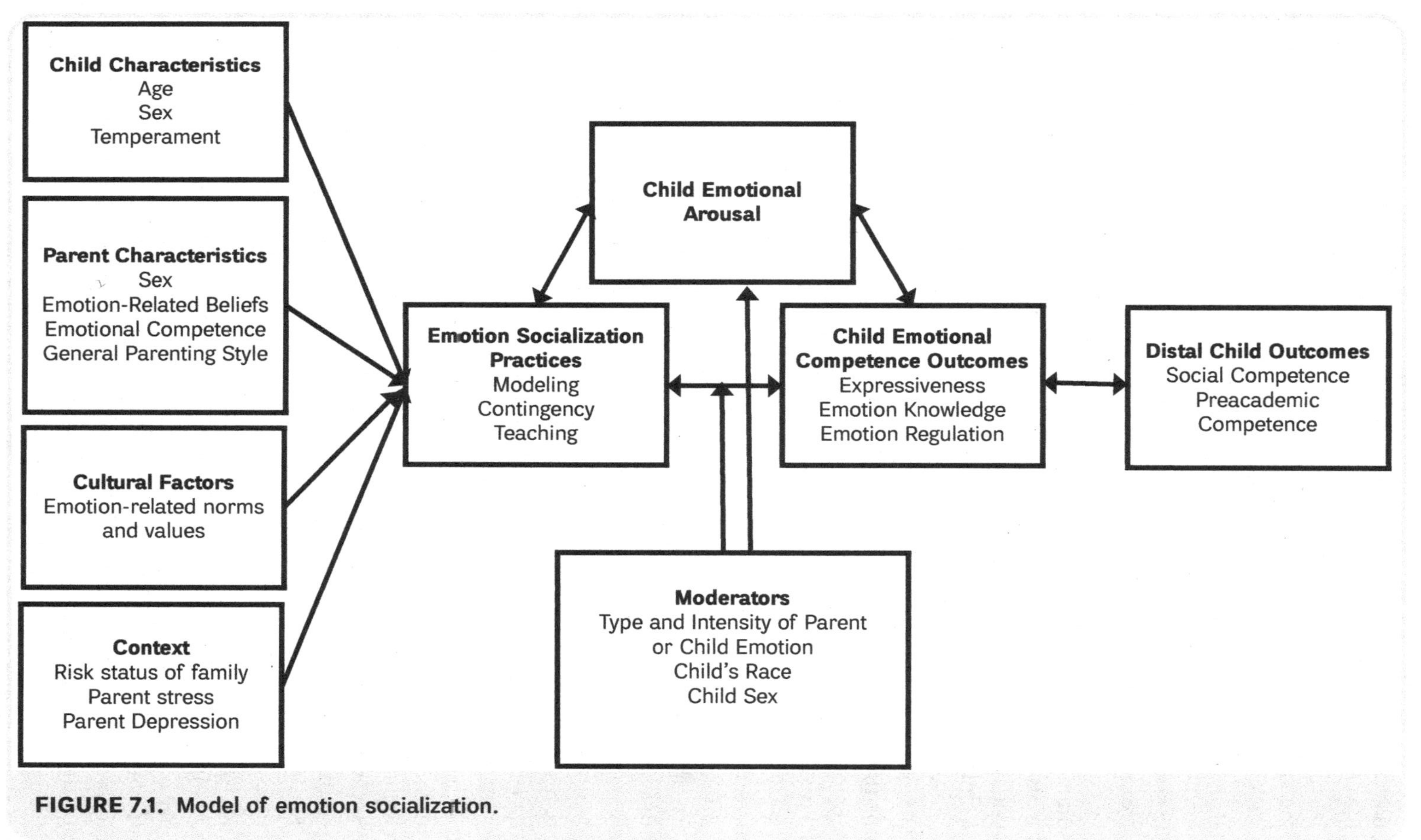


FIGURE 7.1. Model of emotion socialization.

teach differently about emotions, compared to a parent high in overall supportiveness and emotional availability, who adopts authoritative parenting approaches.

Third, culture is as always of paramount importance. The norms and values of one's culture delimit the types of emotion socialization practices deemed acceptable. For example, a Chinese parent would likely show fewer emotional displays and react to those of her child in a very different manner than those of her counterparts in the United States based on the feeling rules of her collectivistic/relational culture.

Finally, the context in which emotion socialization can occur is significant and is considered more deeply in Chapter 12. Living in poverty or other dangerous conditions, high parental stress, and maternal depression are but three conditions that affect socializers' lives and their likely emotion socialization behaviors.

Even after emotion socialization practices and parent, child, cultural, and contextual factors are accounted for, some other issues may moderate their contribution to the child's development of emotional competence. Here and in Chapter 8, where evidence is available, I consider situational moderators of how parents express emotion socialization behaviors. For example, the intensity of the parent's and child's specific emotions within any encounter can affect the parent's socialization behaviors and their effects. Jamie's mother would likely react differently to his anger if it were not so intense (e.g., she might just pat him on the shoulder and keep on scraping carrots). If *her* responding anger were intense, she would certainly react differently. Jamie's and his mother's emotions not only affect chosen emotion socialization practices, but practices *work* differently given the type and intensity of parent and/or child emotion. For example, Jamie's mother's intense anger could have deleterious effects on his acquisition of emotional competence that more mild annoyance might not.

Further, are a parent's emotion socialization behaviors clear, appropriately directed at the child, and appropriate for the current context? Are they primarily proactive or reactive? And do the child's age or gender matter in the nature and outcome of emotion socialization? As an example, using typically beneficial emotion socialization practices in contextually *in*appropriate settings (e.g., discussing feelings when the environment is not safe) could have very different consequences than its use in a more appropriate setting. Emotion socialization practices might also be more beneficial for younger preschoolers than older ones, or boys rather than girls.

With these modes of parental emotion socialization and their precursors and moderators in mind, many aspects of young children's emotional competence (or incompetence) come into clearer focus. The contributions of their social world are potent and ongoing.

Thus along with outlining these basic mechanisms of emotion socialization and the potential issues impacting them, in this chapter, I paint a fuller picture of how these socialization mechanisms contribute to preschoolers' emotional competence, focusing on emotional expressiveness. In Chapter 8, I concentrate on the socialization of emotion knowledge and ER, as well as consider the issues of how both mothers and fathers socialize emotions and how their emotion socialization contributes directly to preschoolers' social competence. I then consider peer and sibling emotion socialization, as well as the issues of culture more deeply. For now, then, I turn to the contributions of emotion socialization to preschoolers' emotional expressiveness.

## SOCIALIZATION OF EMOTIONAL EXPRESSIVENESS

In what follows, I first review modeling, teaching, and contingency as a means of socializing a central component of emotional competence—namely, emotional expressiveness. I then review the socialization of more sophisticated expressiveness (i.e., of the self-conscious and social emotions) and of display rule usage.

### Modeling Influences on Expressiveness

First, children observe emotions exhibited by people with whom they interact. The modeling mechanism of emotion socialization includes specific positive and negative emotions observed by children, along with socializers' overall emotional expressiveness. In general, parents' and children's positive emotional expression are significantly related (Davis, Suveg, & Shaffer, 2015a; Feng et al., 2007; Fields-Olivieri et al., 2017; Isley, O'Neil, Clatfelter, & Parke, 1999; Sallquist et al., 2010).

Conversely, when mothers are often angry and tense with young children, preschoolers respond in an angrier and less emotionally positive way (Feng et al., 2007; Lee & Sung, 2021; Newland & Crnic, 2011). Moreover, mothers' negativity shows continuity over time, suggestive of an emotional environment that children must tolerate (Feng et al., 2007). Well-modulated negative emotion, however, may be good templates for children's equally well regulated expressiveness, and thus have positive effects (Denham & Grout, 1992). I now consider in more detail the pathways and mechanisms by which parents' expressiveness contributes to their children's expressiveness.

#### *Prevalent Emotions*

The prevalent emotions shown by parents are rich sources of information for young children's own expressiveness. Strong experiences and expressions of emotions are common while parenting preschoolers (Garner, 2010). When events take place that really matter to parents, emotions follow (Dix, 1991; Patterson, 1980). And things that matter happen all the time; sometimes parents' concerns coincide with their children's needs, and sometimes they decidedly clash, leading to negative emotion for parents.

> A little boy must see a certain video right now, but Dad is taking a shower and simply doesn't want to trail dripping soapsuds through the house.
>
> Siblings squabble, seemingly meaninglessly, over something as incomprehensible as who can carry a certain item of clothing around the house. WHY?? Mom sighs and hangs her head, tired and frustrated.
>
> A parent presses a preschooler to begin complying with demands for simple, familiar tasks, such as putting on shoes to get ready to go to childcare. The child simply refuses, saying "No. Not 'day. I'm a dinosaur, and dey don't wear shoes!"
>
> If their child has just thrown rather than put away a toy during the twelfth negative interchange of the hour, the parent understandably feels frustrated, impatient, furious, or afraid of his or her inability to teach the child an important lesson.

Parental tension and anger are sometimes unavoidable. And often they are related; for example, Chung and Kim (2020) found that mothers experiencing more anxiety about parenting showed more anger around their young children.

Hence, feelings are ever-present accompaniments to parent–child interactions. But thankfully they aren't always negative. Perhaps negative emotions are most memorable, but at the same time, parents' and children's concerns and behaviors can often be compatible, with resultant positive emotions:

A mother feels joy as her preschooler squeals in delight at climbing a tree by herself.

A father and his preschoolers laugh together uproariously over making a rude noise.

In either case, whether parental emotions are positive or negative, they are activated and witnessed by the child. In fact, real-time momentary assessments of mothers' emotions show that they do express higher-intensity positive emotions, and more diversity of emotions, when caregiving than when not (Kerr, Rasmussen, Buttitta, Smiley, & Borelli, 2021).

Different aspects of young children's expressiveness are influenced by these parental emotions in at least four ways (Barrett & Campos, 1991):

1 Parents model the display of specific emotions and children pick up on these patterns. For instance, particular ways of expressing fear and wariness are conveyed by different parents watching the dog's approach. One parent gasps and exhibits very widened eyes, but another shows much more subtle indicators of wariness, such as pursing his lips. Young children may pick up on and mimic these differing modes of expression.

2 Parents also show children the common behaviors (i.e., action tendencies) associated with expressions of emotions. They demonstrate their own differing ways of coping with emotional situations, and children of different parents learn different behaviors for expressing and dealing with emotions. For example, one mother who feels unease at a dog's approach gets up precipitously and whisks the child and herself away from the playground, whereas another, equally wary parent quietly speaks to the dog, assesses the risk, and elects to stay at a safe distance. She is showing her child both ways of expressing emotion behaviorally and regulating it.

3 Parents unconsciously highlight and discern the emotional significance of events—their meaning—for children. Their expressive patterns implicitly teach the child which emotions are acceptable in the family and which specific emotions are appropriate for specific types of situations. For example, a 2-year-old girl observes a parent expressing hesitance, licking her lips and slowing her pace, at the approach of a large but friendly dog. Thereafter she demonstrates fear herself during similar experiences. She has learned the emotional significance of this situation. This learning impacts both her expressiveness and emotion knowledge.

4 Finally, parents provide an overall emotional environment to which the child is exposed. The emotional world view of a child (or of an adult, for

that matter) is shaped by the general emotional tone experienced day after day. For example, constant immersion in others' simmering conflicts or, conversely, typically enjoying others' positive outlooks, has an effect. Eventually the family's emotional milieu puts a unique emotional stamp on a young child's personality. Four patterns of emotional environments can be discerned (Tomkins, 1962, 1963, 1991; see also Malatesta, 1990, for an interpretation of Tomkins's work):

a. In the "monopolistic" pattern, a single emotion dominates experience. Parents, for example, may be angry individuals, rarely expressing positive emotions to each other or to their children. Children reared in such a family may be easily annoyed, often cranky, and quick to anger. They respond with anger to a variety of stimulus conditions that would not bother other children. And they may also experience and express fear if the anger seems targeted.

b. In the "intrusion" pattern, a minor element intrudes and displaces a dominant emotion. A mother may be quite upbeat most of the time but may become anxious under specific conditions. For instance, a gossipy sister visits; upon her departure the mother feels jumpy, nervous, and threatened. Her normally cheerful toddler son also adopts this response pattern and eventually reverts to wariness when socially challenged. A particular child in his playgroup evokes such negative emotion.

c. In the third "competitive affect" pattern, an emotion-based aspect of a parent's personality is often in competition with another aspect. Each interprets reality in different ways. One parent "blows up" fiercely, and then is apologetic and sorrowfully placating. The young child then interprets family conflict in terms of anger or misery. Understandably, the child vacillates between sadness and anger in conflict situations.

d. In the fourth pattern, personality styles are "affectively balanced." Parents show a rich, varied emotional expressiveness that gives flavor and zest, as well as information, to their smallest transactions. Here, parents are especially emotionally competent; they understand and can regulate the diverse emotions that arise in social interchange. In these instances, the preschooler experiences and comes to express a well-modulated, but not incapacitating, variety of emotions as his or her life experiences warrant.

According to the modeling hypothesis, then, children's expressiveness reflects their parents' own total emotional expressiveness, as well as the particular profile of emotions that the parents express—the prevalence of their happiness, sadness, or anger (Cummings & Cummings, 1988; Denham, 1989, 1993; Denham, Bassett, et al., 2014; Halberstadt & Fox, 1990). Children are exposed both passively and interactively to these negative or positive emotions. Either way, they interpret the emotional import of their parents' emotional expression and tend to express similar profiles of emotions themselves. Indeed, research reveals that certain expressive patterns of toddlers and their mothers become more and more alike across time (Malatesta et al., 1989).

So when parents and children interact together, children's emotions are associated with those of their parents (Feng et al., 2007). As already suggested, positive emotions are contagious: In one study including a series of laboratory visits to an apartment-like setting (Denham, 1989), happier mothers had children who were happier as well as less sad and angry (see also Davies & Cummings, 1995). They enjoyed sharing lunch together, and the children were less agitated when an experimenter assuming the role of a "doctor" asked them to get ready for a checkup. Importantly, more recent evidence corroborates that both mothers' and children's positive emotions were associated contemporaneously, as in my research.

And these contributions are not limited to mothers; fathers' positive expressiveness at home, assessed via audio recordings, were associated with children's emotional positivity (Gerhardt et al., 2020). In this study, fathers', and *not mothers'*, emotional positivity was associated with that of preschoolers. Perhaps in a normal day in the home, mothers are focused on stability and safety in their routine, whereas fathers, often considered "playmates," provide children in this setting with more emotional experiences. Fathers could be seen as loving buddies, and mothers as "emotional gatekeepers."

In contrast, parents' negative emotions are punishing and dysregulating, and this effect is well established by toddlerhood (Davies & Cummings, 1995; Denham, 1989, 1993; Malatesta, 1981). The relations between parent's and children's emotions can be seen easily while they interact. In my study (Denham, 1989), maternal anger and tension were negatively correlated with children's happiness, and anger was positively related to children's sadness and tension. More irritable or jumpy mothers pushed their children to sit, to eat, and to follow instructions; the experience was not pleasant for them, for their children, or even for the observers. So the scaffolding provided by maternal emotions, for better or worse, supported the children's expression of emotions within these situations.

The influence of parents' emotions can extend across time. In fact, when mothers were able to maintain positive emotions while playing with their 2- to 3-year-olds, even though one of the toys they were given was scary or provocative, the children were more apt to express positive emotions during similar situations 1 year later (Feng et al., 2007). Thus these effects of modeled positive emotions live on.

The influence of parents' emotions prevails not only across time, but also across contexts. Thus, in my early research, mothers' emotions were related to their children's emotions and their abilities to regulate them during stressful situations when the mothers were absent (Denham, 1989; Denham & Grout, 1992, 1993). Again, maternal positivity predicted more positive emotion in children; for example, mothers who showed relatively more happiness during mealtime and the "doctor's" visit had toddlers who themselves showed more happiness in several situations in which their mothers were not present.

Corroborating evidence exists. When both mothers and fathers reported on their patterns of expressiveness, in general and in their children's presence, the maternal and paternal positive emotions, *expressed around their children*, made unique contributions to their preschoolers' positivity in challenging peer contexts (Garner, Robertson, & Smith, 1997). In addition, family positive emotion, as well as sadness, discouragement, and anxiety, predicted how positively children dealt with a disappointment paradigm (Garner & Power, 1996). These investigations added incrementally to the knowledge base about how parental expressiveness socializes child expressiveness.

Conversely, parents who show negative emotions, especially anger, have children who likewise show less positive and more negative emotions in independent situations. It is more difficult for these children to deal with emotional situations on their own. In my study already mentioned, mothers who exhibited more sadness had children who expressed more anger when the mothers were not present. Maternal anger, even though it was very infrequent in this laboratory setting, was associated with children's diminished happiness in the independent situations (Denham, 1989).

It is worth noting that in Denham (1989) the contexts experienced without the mothers occurred across several days, suggesting that the contemporaneous effects of the mothers' emotions during lunch and the "doctor's" visit were not unique. There were both time and context effects. Further, these findings held up even after children's emotions with their mothers present were accounted for; aside from the bidirectional effects of children and mothers affecting each other's emotions, maternal emotions contributed to both children's specific expressive profiles and to their ability to marshal emotional resources in independent situations.

Thus maternal emotions observed microanalytically in this study were markers of the general emotional environment experienced by the children. Toddlers' emotions when on their own—alone, with another adult, or with a sibling—were reflective of the emotional expressiveness patterns they had gleaned from their emotional environment. Moreover, anger measured in a more molar way also shows relations with toddlers' own anger: Mothers' representations of anger within the mother–child relationship also are related to toddlers' expression of anger when a goal is blocked (Feldman et al., 2011).

This contribution of parental expressiveness does not cease as children grow older: the mothers' emotions expressed during interactions with their preschoolers also exert an influence on children's emotions shown during free play in their class. In another of our studies, we used interviews and diaries to allow mothers to give their own perceptions both of what emotions they displayed in their preschoolers' presence and of how they expressed them (Denham & Grout, 1992).

These mothers rated the frequency of various emotions in their daily lives. Those who reported showing not only more frequent happiness, but also less frequent tension, in their children's presence had children who showed more happiness and less anger during free play in the preschool setting. As expected, preschoolers whose emotion socialization was calmer and more positive showed more emotional competence with their playmates.

However, mothers who endorsed feeling more anger, scorn, and contempt during their everyday lives had children who showed less happiness and more anger in preschool (Denham & Grout, 1993). Those who expressed negative emotion at home had children who showed more dysregulated emotion during their peer interactions. More recent research corroborates these findings, with parent negativity related to child negativity measured very thoroughly, in terms of frequency, duration, intensity, and latency for sadness, anger, and fear (Mirabile, 2014).

### *Moderators of Parents' Prevalent Emotions*

Other ways that parents teach children about expressiveness, in addition to the mere prevalence of their emotions, also emerged as important when we queried mothers in interviews and in diary studies. Mothers described important moderators of their expressions, such as the causes and resolutions of emotional incidents. The reasons for mothers' emotions—the concerns that activated them, to use Dix's (1991) terminology—were crucial to their children's emotional competence in preschool. That is, the effect of maternal emotions differed, depending on their cause: Children were more emotionally positive when mothers reported that their anger was not predominantly caused by their children's disobedience and when they indicated that their happiness was caused by their children (see Denham & Zoller, 1990). Being the focus of mothers' happiness and not their anger made a difference in the ways children showed emotion in the peer environment.

As already discussed, and confirmed in our interviews and diaries, parents show lots of emotions, and emotional environments include unavoidable tension and anger, especially when preschoolers are key players! When these negative emotions are strongly felt, resolving them is important (see also Cummings, Simpson, & Wilson, 1993; El-Sheikh, Cummings, & Reiter, 1996). In our interviews and diary study, when mothers apologized to children for their moments of tension, the children were happier in preschool (Denham & Grout, 1992). Apologies include comforting emotion language that allows children to maintain a sunny outlook. Parents need to tell even young children, "I am very grumpy, but not because of you. And I'm sorry if I am making you miserable, too." Cummings and colleagues' (1993) work also supports the importance of resolved anger; even relatively subtle resolutions are associated with children's lessened distress.

In contrast, when mothers considered their anger *helpful* in child rearing and did *not* apologize for it, children were more emotionally positive in preschool. These mothers were citing their sometimes-justified sternness in child rearing: "I am displeased with your behavior." It is likely that these mothers showed their anger in specific ways, using firm vocal tones and serious, downturned brows—the dreaded "Mom Look"—and did not get "out of control" in anger. In short, the context of a parent's emotion, not only the emotion per se, is important in the socialization of preschool emotional competence.

The intensity of mothers' negative emotions also contributed to their children's sadness. These preschoolers were sadder during free play when their mothers reported higher-intensity tension and when they reported crying to express sadness in the children's presence. Such children were immersed in negative emotion and its contagion and also were probably learning quite specific modes of negative expression.

The contribution of parental emotion may depend on children's overall expressiveness as well. In one set of studies (Denham & Auerbach, 1995; Denham, Cook, et al., 1992; Denham, Renwick-DeBardi, et al., 1994), mothers and their children looked at and discussed photographs of infants showing peak discrete emotion expressions (from Izard et al., 1980). When the mothers considered their conversations complete, they looked back at the photos of the sad and angry babies and enacted these emotions themselves. Unexpectedly, mothers who simulated higher-intensity anger had children who showed *less* sadness and anger during free play in their preschool classrooms. Perhaps these children of high-anger mothers responded with inhibition and lessened emotional expressiveness when with peers; or, perhaps more likely, mothers of more negatively reactive children may have down-regulated their own expressiveness to protect them from anger (see also Fabes, Eisenberg, Karbon, et al., 1994; Liu, Calkins, & Bell, 2018). Mothers' and children's overall levels of emotionality undoubtedly interact in their influence on emotional competence shown in the preschool environment.

It also may be important to determine the connection between the frequency and intensity of each parental emotion; these two parameters of emotion could interact in contributing to young children's emotional competence. If a negative relation between the intensity of anger and its frequency were specified, for example, these findings could be better explained. Perhaps near-constant exposure to lower-level anger is more detrimental than exposure to occasional outbursts of intense anger. These emotional parameters in combination require more study.

Other combinations of moderating factors need to be uncovered to understand the contribution of parental expressiveness to young children's expressed emotions. For example, in the Denham and Grout (1992) study, mothers who said that their anger was frequent and caused by their children's disobedience, and who reported not apologizing for this anger, had children who were sadder when in preschool; the frequency, cause, and resolution of maternal emotion acted in concert. And the unexpected finding in the Denham, Renwick-DeBardi, et al. (1994) study might be better explained in terms of the mothers' *reason* for showing higher- or lower-intensity anger during the simulation—did they show anger as if they were teaching about it, or did they enact a scenario in which the child caused their anger?

Gender differences in parental modeling and its power as a socialization technique also have been discovered (Denham, Mitchell-Copeland, et al., 1997). Specifically, mothers' and fathers' relative balance of happiness and anger predicted their daughters', but not their sons', positivity in their preschool classroom. Parents' more internalizing emotions—their sadness and tension and/or fear—also were negatively associated with their daughters', but not their sons', positivity.

Other findings regarding emotion socialization, which I report on subsequently, also add to this picture of daughters' sensitivity to parental socialization of emotional expressiveness as both a blessing and a curse (Denham, Bassett, & Wyatt, 2010). Daughters seem to be quintessential observers of parents' emotions and also more attentive listeners to parents' teaching about emotions. The greater salience of the socialization context for girls' behavior needs to be studied more explicitly in the realm of emotional competence.

Fathers and mothers may also differ in *how* they show emotions around their children. We have found that we observed fathers as more positively expressive with their children compared with mothers, but mothers self-reported experiencing more positive emotion in the family (Denham, Bassett, et al., 2010). This finding seemed puzzling at first. Mothers reported on more positive emotions, such as gratitude, so that may be one explanation for this finding. However, fathers, as prototypical playmates, also *showed* more happiness (the only positive emotion we observed).

Ethnicity can also appear as a moderator of the relations between parental emotion and children's emotional expressiveness. In one study, mothers' and children's positive emotions were related across a year's time (Hooper, Wu, Ku, Gerhardt, & Feng, 2018). However, ethnicity moderated this association; it held true only for African American mothers and their children. African American preschoolers may be socialized to be more sensitive to others' emotions, especially in a task like the cleanup task, where emotions might be expected to be negative (see Nelson, Leerkes, O'Brien, Calkins, & Marcovitch, 2012); this sensitivity could make it easy for these children to learn means of expressiveness from their mothers. Or maybe for European American dyads this association is more child driven, with mothers' emotional sensitivity to the child more ascendant than the child's sensitivity to the mothers' emotions.

### SUMMARY: Socialization of Preschoolers' Expressiveness via Parents' Own Emotions

Converging evidence exists that parents' expressed emotions exert an influence that extends beyond the immediate interactional setting. Children learn about the emotional significance of events—whether for enjoyable "together times," or stressful, conflictual situations. They also learn how to show emotion, both expressively and behaviorally. Above all, they are exposed to an ethos, or an emotional environment, that has far-reaching effects on the emotional organization of their personalities. Along with disclosing the associations between parental and child expressiveness, research also has uncovered important moderators of these relations, including (1) the reason for the parent's emotion, (2) the resolution of the emotional event, (3) how helpful the parent *believes* the emotion to be in terms the event's outcome, (4) the intensity of the parent's emotion, (5) whether the parent is a mother or father, and (6) the ethnicity of the parent–child dyad.

Because emotion researchers most often study the frequency or duration of parents' emotions, most research has so far focused mainly on the contribution of the monopolistic pattern of emotion (and, thankfully at times, also the affectively balanced pattern). Results show the child behaviors associated with the predominance of a particular parental emotion. But it is methodologically feasible to identify clusters of parents who show either intrusive or competitive emotional organization—for example, parents who are mostly happy, but sometimes fearful or often angry *or* sad. These analyses should be undertaken. Nonetheless, the conclusions reached from the current state of research should give caregivers and parents pause. As they become aware of the effects of their own expressiveness, important adults in young children's lives can adjust their own expressiveness for their preschoolers' benefit.

## Contingency Influences on Expressiveness

Children's emotions often elicit, even require, contingent reactions from social partners. Thus, according to the contingency hypothesis (Denham, Bassett, et al., 2014; Eisenberg, Cumberland, et al., 1998; Halberstadt, 1991), parents' own expressed emotions and behaviors are likely to be contingent on their young children's emotion displays (Malatesta & Haviland, 1982). Adults respond to young children's emotions in ways that have been construed as either supportive or nonsupportive. Such reactions to children's emotions can be important vehicles for letting children know what action tendencies are appropriate when they feel different ways and what events merit emotion expression at all. Given this mechanism, specific reactions to children's emotions can either encourage or discourage certain enduring patterns of expressiveness in the children themselves, as well as their mobilization of emotional resources in social situations where they are "on their own."

> If Kelsey is terrified of entering the swimming pool—crying, eyes wide, feet pushing back from the side of the pool—her somewhat embarrassed, goal-oriented, but loving parents could act in at least two different ways. They could ignore and minimize her fear, saying something like "Oh, Kelsey, stop it, there's nothing to be afraid of! This will be fun, let's just try it! Splash!" Alternatively, they could respect the intensity of her feelings and sit down with her near the pool, saying, "I would never let anything hurt you. Let's sit here and put our feet in the water until you feel better." And if she were unable to calm down, these parents would give up on this new experience for that day, or maybe for the foreseeable future. If she could calm down, they could ask her respectfully whether she'd like to try getting in, and honor her answer.

The second reaction would help Kelsey become less fearful in other situations, first with her parents present and later on her own (Malatesta, 1990; Tomkins, 1991). Her fears need not monopolize, or even unnecessarily intrude upon, her emotional experiences. They will undoubtedly be experienced and expressed but can be modulated and dealt with. Hence, supportive or nonsupportive reactions to young children's emotions shape their emotional responses to specific eliciting situations, and in fact ultimately contribute to the emotional organization of their personalities (Tomkins, 1991).

More specifically regarding parents' reactions to children's emotions, mothers' supportive reactions (e.g., helping solve the problem, validating and encouraging free expression of emotion, and comforting or attending to the child's emotional needs) to children's emotions positively relate to preschoolers' positive expressiveness (Fabes, Poulin, Eisenberg, & Madden-Derdich, 2002). In contrast, parents using nonsupportive reactions to emotions (e.g., dismissing or belittling, minimizing, showing distress, or even punishing) are more likely to have sadder, more fearful children (Berlin & Cassidy, 2003), who show more negative, dysregulated emotion even up to a year later (McGee et al., 2022).

## SUMMARY: Supportive Contingency: Contributions to Children's Expressiveness

To elaborate on supportive reactions to children's emotions, the child's emotionally balanced, "integrated" emotional organization is fostered when caregivers exhibit primarily supportive reactions—when they assist the child in maintaining positive emotion and tolerate the child's negative emotion as valid and worthy of regard and concern rather than of disgrace.

Five-year-old Monroe feels very sad because his first "bestest" friend must move away. His emotionally supportive parents help him say goodbye, allowing him to experience the sadness, but also to know the value of relationships. They suggest ways to manage the sadness, such as helping him to write letters. They freely reminisce about this good friend and about the good times they shared, telling Monroe that this good feeling can happen again. They assist him in moving through his sadness, rather than criticizing it.

Overall, Monroe's sensitive parents assist him in enacting strategies that reduce his negative emotion, subsequent to its usefulness as a social signal. They focus on helping him to regulate his emotions. Above all, they remain emotionally engaged with him while he experiences negative emotion. They communicate this attunement facially and verbally, also nurturing his own empathic concern by their example. Supportive parents take their children's emotions seriously. "Listening attentively, asking questions to clarify what the child believes, and offering a reassuring explanation as well as the promise of protection . . . ," as well as " . . . remain[ing] emotionally available even while firm . . . " (Lieberman, 1993, pp. 35 & 39), constitute the core of successful emotion socialization.

Supportive reactions to preschoolers' positive emotions also can be important. In fact, mothers' acceptance and validation of children's positive emotions increases from age 3 to 9 (Talley, Zhu, & Dunsmore, 2021). More research in this area should be undertaken.

## *Nonsupportive Contingency: Contributions to Children's Expressiveness*

Nonsupportive emotion socialization leads to far less positive developmental outcomes than does supportive emotion socialization (Gottman, Katz, & Hooven, 1996a, 1996b). Some nonsupportive parents want to be helpful but ignore or deny their children's emotional experience—treating emotions as things that blow over, or even a trivial bother. They " . . . fail to use emotional moments as a chance to get closer to the child or to help the child learn lessons in emotional competence" (Goleman, 1995, p. 191).

Rebecca is afraid of the dark. Her parents just ignore her, focusing on their own need for sleep, so that she never really deals with the experience. In any case, she is still left with the fear.

Others may be just too *laissez-faire*; they may go along with any alternative a child selects to handle emotions or resort to distraction even when other, more effective and useful ER strategies are possible. All upsets are soothed, and even bargaining and bribery are used to stanch the flow of negative emotions.

Brandon's parents allow him to show his continuing anger about being picked on at school, but they are exhausted by the whole topic. When the anger floods him, he screams at his mother, "I'm mad at YOU! I hate you!" They distract him with ice cream for dessert, offering no means of regulation or gentle pressure to express emotions in a more useful way.

In a final, most pernicious way, nonsupportive socializers may be full of contempt, showing no respect for how the child feels. "They might, for instance, forbid any display of the child's anger at all, and become punitive at the least sign of irritability" (Goleman, 1995, p. 191).

> Scott's parents, who are punitive socializers, show disregard and even contempt when he moves away from Monroe's neighborhood. These parents tease Scott for his tender feelings, so that in the end he is let down not only by missing his friend, but by their reaction as well. Unlike Monroe, he is very lonely and still feels very bad, even ashamed. He doesn't return Monroe's letter.

Again, children's positive emotions are important; it is not just contingent reactions to children's negative emotions that require attention. Unsupportive reactions to positive emotions can also be deleterious to children's optimal expressiveness. Such parents may report feeling uncomfortable or embarrassed by their children's positivity or even reprimand them (e.g., frown at them and tell them to be quiet). Expanding on these ideas, both mothers and fathers who reported lack of supportiveness to their 5-year-olds' positive emotion had children who demonstrated more emotional negativity, perhaps suppressing their positive emotions (Shewark & Blandon, 2015).

### *Parents' Reports of Their Contingent Reactions to Preschoolers' Emotions*

Now it is time to report on even more specific research in this area. First, it can be important to glean information from parents directly about how they socialize emotional competence. Many investigators gather parents' self-reports about their reactions to children's emotional expressiveness (e.g., Berlin & Cassidy, 2003; Casey & Fuller, 1994; Eisenberg & Fabes, 1994; Eisenberg, Fabes, Schaller, Carlo, & Miller, 1991; Fabes et al., 2002). Whether via interview or simpler questionnaire,[2] parents give eloquent testimony about their own reactions to their children's emotions. They describe how they deal with their children's emotional responses in common emotion-provoking situations and mention their own specific emotions directed at their children (e.g., Casey & Fuller, 1994).

Even though the picture of supportive versus nonsupportive reactions is often very clear, the picture is not simply a matter of "be an emotionally supportive socializer, and raise super kids." Specifically, aspects of emotion socialization often are related. Thus the ability to make supportive contingent reactions to children's emotions is related to parents' predominant form of expressiveness, as well as to how parents feel about their children. Parents who themselves are more emotionally positive in general are more

[2] The Coping with Children's Negative Emotions Scale (Fabes, Eisenberg, & Bernzweig, 1990) has been used productively in many studies since its creation. It consists of 12 stories about children showing negative emotions (e.g., being scared by a TV show, or angry at not being able to go to a birthday party), with parents rating their distress, as well as reactions classified as punitive, minimizing, emotionally encouraging, emotion-focused, and problem-focused. Many of the findings reported here reflect the use of this questionnaire or slight adaptations.

capable of being supportive socializers of emotion for their young children. Specifically, those who depict their families as positively expressive are more accepting of their children's emotional responses and more likely to cite verbal reassurance as a strategy they would use to help their children regulate emotion (Casey & Fuller, 1994; Casey, Fuller, & Johll, 1993). Conversely, parents who describe their families as less positively expressive focus more on altering their children's emotional responses, are less accepting, and propose more active intervention strategies aimed at suppressing or changing their children's emotions. Feeling "bad" themselves leaves little emotional room for parents to be emotionally supportive socializers. And parents in more negative families probably do need to exert pressure on their youngsters to down-regulate their emotionality.

Further, parents who describe their children as enjoyable and easy to deal with are more accepting of their children's negative emotions. In contrast, parents who tend to feel anger toward their children are less accepting and expect conformity to parental expectations. These parents also are less satisfied with their children's emotional responses. Parents' ability to accept and foster their children's emotional experience, and whether they feel the need to control it, are rooted in the very nature of their emotional relationship with their children (Casey & Fuller, 1994).

Consonant with this emphasis on relationship, it must be underscored that parents' contingent responding also is related to their children's own enduring emotional expressiveness—in other words, to their children's temperament. Children's effects upon their own emotion socialization must not be overlooked; emotional development is very transactional in nature. Hence, it is not surprising that mothers report they are distressed by and try to minimize children's expressiveness when the children are viewed as high in negative emotion or emotionally intense (Eisenberg & Fabes, 1994). Some children pose a challenge to parental equilibrium, and parents press them to exhibit less negativity. For example, parents of toddlers they deemed temperamentally shy also reported being less supportive of their emotions than parents of nonshy toddlers (Grady, 2018). They were especially minimizing of their sons' shyness (see Chapter 3 reference to shyness in boys).

Similarly, it is easier to encourage expression of emotion and emotional problem solving when children themselves are able to focus and switch their attention easily (Eisenberg & Fabes, 1994). Thus, although in this discussion much of the onus is placed on parents' supportiveness or nonsupportiveness in response to their children's emotions, children play an active role in the very nature of their socialization experiences. The interaction of their own emotions and self-regulation with parents' emotions and feelings about family emotions can create a vicious cycle of negativity. Thus, it is important to consider child effects on parents' reactions to emotions.

### *Observation of Contingent Reactions to Preschoolers' Emotions*

So parents' reports of their own contingent reactions to children's emotions have yielded important insights. Another way of obtaining information on the contingency hypothesis is to observe parents' specific emotional and behavioral reactions to children's emotions (e.g., Denham, 1993; Denham & Grout, 1993; Denham, Mitchell-Copeland, et al., 1997; Denham, Renwick-DeBardi, et al., 1994; Malatesta et al., 1989).

These varying reactions exert their influence very early. Maternal punishing reactions to toddlers' emotions predicted the children's own emotions (Malatesta et al., 1989). Further, Malatesta and colleagues' (1989) and my own reports of mothers' reactions to children's emotions included their *emotional*, as well as or rather than their behavioral reactions. In Malatesta and colleagues' study, toddlers' sadness during reunions within the Strange Situation was predicted not only by their own sadness in similar situations when younger, but also by their mothers' earlier lack of interest (these effects were moderated by a child's gender and birth status). Likewise, children's anger during reunions was predicted not only by their own earlier anger, but also by their mothers' surprise at their earlier sadness. So, there was not only cross-time stability in toddlers' expressiveness, but also predicted stability of later expressiveness from their mothers' earlier contingent reactions. When their mothers' emotion socialization was not particularly supportive, toddlers showed cross-time continuity in their negative emotions.

I have observed mothers who responded in a way I considered optimal to their toddlers' happiness, sadness, anger, and fear; they also had children who coped better with their own emotions when the mothers were absent (Denham, 1993). Specifically, maternal positive responsiveness to children's sadness, anger, and fear during mealtime and a "doctor's" visit predicted children's happiness, fear, anger, and affiliation with others when the mothers were not present (in hypothesized directions), even after the effects of child age and gender and of children's own patterns of emotional expressiveness with their mothers were accounted for (Denham, 1993).

What did I consider the more helpful emotional reactions to young children's emotions? I operationalized a specific cluster of emotional reactions that I deemed as "optimal" to obtain these results. Optimal reactions to sadness included behaving with tenderness and *not* showing negative or happy responses. Appropriate reactions to angry displays included displaying calm neutrality or cheerfulness and not matching a child's anger. Angry responses only lead to continued angry, noncompliant behavior on the child's part (Crockenberg, 1985). Optimal responsiveness to a child's fear included calmness, cheerful caretaking, or modeling of appropriate, nonfearful problem-solving behavior. Nonoptimal reactions included responding to children's emotions with anger, sadness, tension, or too immediate and intense overplacating tenderness, which only served to prolong the child's distress in my sequential analyses. Even maternal smiling that occurs too soon after a child displays happiness can be nervous or "fake" and can overstimulate a young child (Malatesta et al., 1989). In sum, I found that positive emotionally responsive mothers assisted their toddlers in independently tolerating, confronting, and managing negative emotions, rather than minimizing them at all costs.

These patterns are not restricted to toddlers and their parents. Parents' emotional reactions to their preschoolers' emotions also are related to preschoolers' expression of emotions (Denham & Grout, 1993; Denham, Mitchell-Copeland, et al., 1997). Emotionally supportive parents fostered their preschool children's emotional competence on a variety of indices (Denham, Renwick-DeBardi, et al., 1994). For example, when mothers responded positively to their children's emotions (via their emotions, physical gestures, or comments), they helped to maintain or escalate children's positive emotion during play. A year later their 3-year-olds showed more positive and less negative emotion during similar play situations (Feng et al., 2007).

### *Moderators of Contingency*

The story on contingent reactions to children's emotion may be more complex, however. Whether emotion socialization techniques, especially supportiveness to children's emotional expressiveness, remain developmentally static has not been elaborated upon until recently. Given a developmental perspective, however, it is reasonable to expect age in socialization via contingent responsiveness. Indeed, age differences were found in mothers' reactions to their young preschoolers' anger (Kochanska, 1987). Mothers of infants and toddlers in the sample, from 15 to about 30 months of age, were more likely than mothers of children from 30 to 42 months old to provide affection, gratification, or distraction and to inquire about the cause of the anger. In acknowledgment of the growing expectations of their children's increasing autonomy and self-regulation, mothers of older children were more likely to suggest cognitive strategies to their children or to ask them to stop displaying anger.

Further, emotion socialization practices considered adaptive for younger children may become less developmentally appropriate, and even bear some relation to maladaptive outcomes when utilized with older preschoolers. Supportiveness does not fill the same function or convey the same message as children age. Whereas younger children (e.g., 3- and 4-year-olds) may be well served by parents' emotion-focused and problem-focused supportiveness, older children also at times may elicit "stricter" contingent reactions as maturity demands increase (Mirabile, Oertwig, & Halberstadt, 2018). And the meaning of these reactions, which we would call "nonsupportive" during early preschool, may impart a different message to older preschoolers. As Grusec and Goodnow (1994) have pointed out, the effect of parental socialization is dependent upon the children's own perception, understanding, and acceptance of the message—and a subtle message of "get your act together" may be just what the older preschooler needs.

There also are age-related differences in the consequences of these socialization techniques. Parental matching of their children's positive emotions predicted children's prevalence of happiness over anger, but more so for 4- and 5-year-olds than for 3-year-olds (Denham, Mitchell-Copeland, et al., 1997). Older children were more able to use this positive matching as an actual template for their own expressiveness. Perhaps their developing attentional abilities played a role here, in that they were better able to focus on their parents' expressions.

Regarding gender, there are important differences, as well as similarities, in the emotion socialization of mothers and fathers (Casey et al., 1993). Mothers were more realistic than fathers in admitting that children's emotions would not necessarily match their own wishes (e.g., that they might react to stop the emotions). Mothers also were more likely than fathers to say that they could modulate their children's emotions via their reactions. Thus, mothers' greater day-to-day experience with preschoolers made them more realistic about the volatile nature of their charges and the need to regulate their capricious expressiveness. At the same time, mothers report using more supportive reactions to their children's emotions than do fathers; this result is widely found (Denham, Bassett, et al., 2010; see also Ince & Ersay, 2022, for concordant cross-cultural results). Together, these findings align with my notion of mothers as "emotional gatekeepers," suggesting that mothers feel more responsible for emotion socialization and more often use supportive reactions to enact it.

But fathers do not come up short on all aspects of supportive reactions to their children's emotions. In the earlier study, fathers did not differ from mothers in their empathy for and acceptance of children's feelings. Fathers also exhibited a range of ways to assist children during emotional experiences that were as diverse as mothers' (Casey et al., 1993). Although these results are a bit difficult to square with our own, they do bear further study. Fathers may feel empathy and acceptance but also believe they need to be strict arbiters of emotional behavior; they also may have a range of ways to react to preschoolers' emotions but use them at different rates than do mothers.

The differences between parents were not the only evidence of gender moderation of contingent responding to children's emotions. Parents socialized the emotions of boys differently from those of girls. They wanted boys to inhibit sad and fearful responses, whereas girls were expected to inhibit angry responses (Casey & Fuller, 1994; Casey et al., 1993). These expectations dovetail well with cultural norms: "Big boys don't cry"; "Girls make nice."

At the same time, we observed both mothers and fathers reacting more positively overall to their sons' emotions (Denham, Bassett, et al., 2010). Similarly, Kochanska (1987) found that psychiatrically well mothers were more attentive to and concerned about their sons' anger than their daughters' (see the parallel finding on the teaching of emotion knowledge in Chapter 8). They more often offered angry boys affection, gratification of their perceived needs, and cognitive strategies. Depressed mothers showed a similar pattern of responses to their young daughters' anger, perhaps because of the dependent, role-reversed nature of their relationships; depressed mothers wanted to maintain their helpers' equilibrium. Again, daughters seem to be very attuned to their parents' emotions, but here it also becomes clear that sons' emotions may be more salient to parents. Child gender is an important moderator of emotion socialization, and it needs to be more fully explored.

Finally, ethnicity has recently been considered for its effects on the ways in which mothers react to their young children's emotions. Several studies point out how what I have posited as supportive contingent reactions may not always be so for all groups or for all emotions within groups. For example, African American mothers evaluated their children's negative emotions as less acceptable than their European American counterparts did; they also expected negative social consequences for their children's, especially their sons', negative emotions (Nelson, Leerkes, et al., 2012). Further, they endorsed "supportive" reactions to their children's emotions less strongly than European American mothers, and instead endorsed "nonsupportive" (i.e., punitive and minimizing) reactions to their children's anger, as well as to their sons' fear and sadness. These authors suggested that African American mothers are emotionally stricter to keep their children safe, reflective of their caring and concern that their children thrive in a discriminatory society. Thus their children's negative emotions are seen as dangerous and encouraging them could backfire. In fact, African American mothers endorsed two specific "supportive" reactions—encouragement of children's emotions and problem-focused reactions—less strongly than European American mothers (Nelson, Leerkes, et al., 2013). But they did not differ from European American mothers on endorsement of emotion-focused reactions, such as comforting.

Living in an emotional milieu in which "nonsupportive" reactions to their emotions are embedded in warm, empathic relationships, African American preschoolers may not consider this stringent approach to be punitive. Interpreting their mothers' no-nonsense approach to emotion socialization more positively, these children's social–emotional outcomes might differ from those for European American preschoolers whose mothers were similar in their contingent responding. In fact, encouragement of emotions is negatively related to African American preschoolers' social–emotional competence. In contrast, European American children, more often encouraged to show emotion, may respond to different kinds of support than their African American counterparts. That is, they benefit more from discussions about emotion and from problem solving about emotional problems (Nelson, Leerkes, et al., 2013).

Moreover, given these considerations, it might be productive to look at supportive reactions in even finer detail, moving beyond encouragement of emotions. Specifically, emotion-focused supportive reactions to children's sadness (i.e., comforting, showing understanding), reflective of the warmth of their African American mother–child relationships, were related to African American children's later avoidance of internalizing emotions (Hooper et al., 2018). Conversely, reinforcing the idea that African American children do not interpret their mothers' supposed "nonsupportive" reactions as angry and punitive, African American mothers' more overtly angry responses to their children's anger predicted their children's later emotional dysregulation, as well as their internalizing and externalizing emotions (Hooper et al., 2018). Reactions to children's emotions and their sequelae absolutely must be viewed in broader contexts and deserve further consideration.

## SUMMARY: Contingent Reactions to Preschoolers' Emotions

Parents' contingent reactions to children's emotions often figure prominently in the development of preschoolers' emotional expressiveness. Supportive responsiveness, except where ethnic and cultural norms give it a different meaning, is generally related to positive aspects of preschoolers' emotional expressiveness. Conversely, nonsupportive reactions are generally related to negative aspects of expressiveness, again except where norms change its meaning. Age and child or parent gender are also important moderators of these relations. Older preschoolers may be required to control their expressiveness more than younger children. Further, mothers show more supportive reactions than fathers, and fathers show more nonsupportive reactions compared with mothers. Boys and girls often are treated differently regarding parents' contingent reactions.

Caregivers want to help their children experience a well-modulated, rich emotional life that enhances rather than incapacitates. It is vital that they carefully consider the impact of their contingent responses to their children's emotions.

## Teaching Influences on Expressiveness

In its simplest form, teaching about emotion consists of verbally explaining an emotion and its relation to an observed event or expression. It is not surprising that adults' tendencies to discuss emotions, and the quality of their communications about emotions, if nested within a warm relationship, assist the child in expressing emotions.

"The preverbal child is at the mercy of rages and anxieties. . . . This is why the mother and father are at the center of the young child's sense of well-being or despair: they are the ones in charge of understanding the child's experience and attending to it, and they also are the ones who find a substitute to act for them when they are not there" (Lieberman, 1993, p. 47). One such "substitute" is emotion language. Talking about emotions gives the child a tool to use in modulating the expression of emotions (Bretherton et al., 1986; Dunn et al., 1987; Dunn & Munn, 1985; Greif, Alvarez, & Tone, 1984; Kopp, 1989). Parents who talk about emotions and foster this ability in their children enable their children to express certain optimal patterns of emotions, and to separate impulse and behavior. Even when the parents are not present, their conversations are recalled.

### *Functions of Emotion Language*

Emotion language has three special functions in the socialization of emotional expressiveness (Miller & Sperry, 1988):

1. It allows specificity in communicating how to feel, what to say, and what to do in certain situations.
2. It has the "capability of representing the non-here-and-now" (Miller & Sperry, 1988, p. 220), so that socializers can assist the child by reminiscing about emotional experience, anticipating it, and visualizing emotional possibilities.
3. Linguistic features, such as the unmitigated imperative to signal anger (e.g., "Get out of here right now!") and intonation (e.g., gruff, clipped speech), allow for a richness of emotional communication.

Miller and Sperry's (1987) observations illustrated many of these functions of emotion language within a very specific context. Working-class mothers of toddler girls were observed and interviewed about how they dealt with their daughters' anger. Mothers in this community anticipated the experience of their own and their daughters' anger. According to them, anger can be explained and needs to be justified by reference to its instigator's actions. Thus they taught this principle to their daughters via their emotion language: "She sassed me, so I just smacked her," "Jen ran her bike into her, and I screamed, 'Let Jen have it.' " The clear message in this particular setting was that anger is not only okay; it is necessary when one feels victimized.

The way mothers in this study used the language of emotion also provided their toddlers with subculturally important distinctions between legitimate and nonlegitimate anger. What is appropriate to feel, and how should one act to express that emotion, in this specific community? Nonlegitimate anger included acting "spoiled," showing anger merely as a function of frustration. Daughters were pressed by their mothers to act appropriately in emotionally charged situations and not to "waste" their anger over "wimpy," nonlegitimate concerns.

Even finer distinctions were made. Angry, aggressive retaliation was more easily legitimized toward peers than toward adults: "It's okay that she kicked her friend, but she'd better not try that with me. I'm her *mother.*" Differential encouragement of emotions also occurred. Sadness was much less often seen than anger in situations of intentional injury and transgression. People who had been wrong did not get sad; they got even.

The little girls absorbed these discussions and messages, and their patterns of expression were affected by the teaching of their socializers. For example, young as they were, these girls were even able to give their emotions legitimacy by generating false accusations to justify their expressions of anger if necessary: "She broke my toy" (when she had not). Although this study makes it clear that not all communities promote the same emotional messages—many middle-class families are less positively disposed toward anger—the principles used by these mothers are very common. Teaching about emotions supports a child's initiation into a social group.

Other research also reveals how emotion language helps young children learn how to express emotions. Recall that in one set of studies (Denham & Auerbach, 1995; Denham, Cook, et al., 1992) mothers looked at photos of infants showing peak emotions and then simulated sadness and anger. The frequency, function, and accuracy of the emotion language used by each dyad member were coded during these situations. The functions of emotion language included (1) commenting ("She has a surprised look on her face"); (2) questioning ("She's happy, isn't she?"); (3) explaining ("He's mad because he doesn't like nobody to touch him"); (4) moralizing ("It makes me sad to see [the baby] sad"); and (5) guiding behavior ("I'm gonna be angry if you do that . . .").

Maternal and child language, especially during the simulations, was strongly correlated with children's emotions expressed in preschool. Some functions of mothers' emotion language were associated with happier, less angry, and less sad experiences in the preschool classroom; specifically, mothers who explained their emotions in the simulations had children who were less sad in the preschool, for example.

In contrast, mothers who talked on and on about their own distress during the simulations, but without explaining it, had children who looked *more* emotionally negative in the classroom. These mothers "wallowed" in negative emotion via their language, conveying a negative emotional style. Their unrelenting, overly arousing but equally unilluminating, harping on negative emotions was debilitating to the children, in contrast to their explanations that seemed to satisfy children and give them information that helped them stay on an even keel. So not all teaching about emotions is created equal.

But perhaps neither talking about emotions in a general way while looking at baby photographs, nor while supposedly experiencing them during the simulations, is the best way of learning about emotional expressiveness via teaching. Perhaps the first context could benefit from being more personal, and the second by being a bit less personal. Instead, maybe children gain an optimal understanding of their own and their parents' expressive patterns while reminiscing about actual emotional events. Reminiscing about emotions experienced together is a special way of reflecting about strong feelings and ways that they can be expressed and regulated in a realistic, but calm atmosphere.

In a second set of studies then, my colleagues and I focused on such parent–child reminiscences about emotions. Naturalistic conversations were recorded, in which parents and children reminisced about the children's emotions (happy, sad, angry, and afraid; Denham, Mitchell-Copeland, et al., 1997). Mothers who talked more about emotions during these conversations had children who were happier and less angry during free play in their preschool classrooms. Reflecting on real occurrences of emotion at a safe remove from actual experience could be especially illuminating—learning about their own feelings gave these preschoolers information to use when expressing emotions in the classroom.

Other more recent research also has highlighted the contribution of parents' teaching to their preschoolers' expressiveness. These investigations corroborate that some mothers may have more difficulty than others in fulfilling the teaching function of emotion socialization, and that such difficulty may bear upon children's expressiveness. To flesh out the complex picture of maternal teaching about emotions predicting their children's later positive *and* negative emotional expressiveness, varying levels of maternal stress could be important (Wu, Feng, Hooper, et al., 2019). In this study mothers and 3-year-olds discussed recent events that had made the children happy, sad, angry, and scared. Teaching was captured through the following methods: (1) providing or asking for the emotion's name, (2) asking about and discussing the emotions' causes and/or experiences, (3) accepting and acknowledging the child's emotions, (4) mentioning problem-solving ER strategies, (5) discussing the nature of emotion.

Notable findings included the fact that stressed mothers who did not engage in teaching about sadness rated their children as higher in sadness 1 year later. Without helpful information and given a mother who was stressed but wouldn't describe the experience of sadness with them, children were more at the mercy of sadness themselves. As noted by the authors, "stress strengthens the reciprocal associations between maladaptive emotion socialization and adverse child outcomes" (Wu, Feng, Hooper, et al., 2019, p. 9).

In contrast, children were rated as more emotionally positive at age 4 when their highly stressed mothers had engaged in *less* teaching about positive emotions a year earlier; the association was the exact opposite for children of low-stressed mothers. Perhaps highly stressed mothers' teaching about positivity is experienced similarly to that of the mothers in our study who "overdid it" when talking about their simulated emotions. More is not necessarily better. Additional details to flesh out this relation would be very useful.

What's more, in this study, children seemed to affect their mothers' teaching too—if mothers saw their children as highly angry at age 3 *and* they experienced high parenting stress, they provided less teaching about anger when children were 4 years old. In contrast, children's fear seemed to prompt adaptive emotion socialization. So it is important to consider other factors, such as maternal stress, in evaluating teaching about emotions.

Some recent research finally has examined the role of fathers. For example, fathers' use of specific functions in teaching about emotions during a typical day at home (in this case, labeling, accepting, direct teaching, and reasoning about emotions; Gerhardt et al., 2020) affected their children's positive expressiveness in home observations and even their ability to remain emotionally positive in a laboratory-based cleanup task a year later. Fathers' emotion talk contributed to their preschoolers' later abilities to remain on an even keel, whereas mothers' emotion talk did not.

As already noted, fathers often have been considered playmates, with a style that is often emotionally positive, but also challenging for young children in terms of risk taking and exploration (Paquette, 2004). Similarly, fathers' emotion teaching may be more stimulating than mothers, giving the child practice in responding to challenges and stressors. These emotional interactions and conversations can provide the child with a wider range of both positive and negative emotional experiences, and may give the child more practice in emotional expressiveness. To test these possibilities for explaining Gerhardt et al.'s (2020) results, it would be necessary to examine such at-home conversations even more closely for their context. The activities in which the conversations take place, and even the connection between their emotion language's specific functions and the children's later expressiveness, could be important in unpacking these findings. Does fathers' emotion language during discipline encounters or during play relate to children's later expressiveness? Is their direct teaching and reasoning language more important to later outcomes than the mere verbal labeling of emotions?

### SUMMARY: Teaching and Preschoolers' Expressiveness

Emotion language that is shared by parents and their preschoolers is important because it is a means of direct teaching and learning about emotion. The information given young children about emotions can be associated with their own patterns of expressiveness. Maternal talk about emotions, especially explanations for emotions, imparts important messages about how to show feelings and how to regulate them. Less is known so far about the contribution of fathers' emotion language, although this problem has eased somewhat in the years since I wrote my earlier book. In any case, parents and caregivers need to carefully consider enacting open, though not overwhelming, discussions about feelings with their children.

## Socialization of More Sophisticated Expressiveness: Social Emotions—Empathic Concern

Empathic concern facilitates social interactions; for example, children who spontaneously help playmates are viewed positively by them (Eisenberg, Pasternack, Cameron, & Tryon, 1984; see Chapter 10). How are such emotional responses to the predicament of other people promoted?

Many aspects of parental expressiveness are central to the development of empathic concern. When children have experience with clear but not overpowering parental emotions, they have the opportunity for empathic concern for important others' emotions. They are more likely to evidence concern, and to help, comply, commiserate with, or cheer up their partner—instead of becoming upset, just watching, or doing nothing at all.

Specifically, mothers' emotionally balanced emotional expressiveness (i.e., more positive than negative emotions) is a positive predictor of empathic concern. Negative emotions shown in such an overall positive context also allow for the development of empathic concern. For example, a parent may stub their toe and act both annoyed and hurt. Such experiences may give the developing child practice in learning to care for a loved one in distress. However, more consistent exposure to parents' negative emotions is painful for young children and generally impedes the development of empathic concern (Denham & Grout, 1993; Denham, Mitchell-Copeland, et al., 1997; Denham, Renwick-DeBardi, et al., 1994).

Focusing on positive and negative emotions more specifically, mothers' prevalence of negative emotions, especially anger, during either laboratory play sessions or home visits, negatively predicts children's empathic concern and prosocial responsiveness to peer emotions during free play in their preschool classrooms (Denham & Grout, 1993; Denham, Mitchell-Copeland, et al., 1997; Denham, Renwick-DeBardi, et al., 1994). In contrast, mothers' positive emotions are related to empathic concern even during toddlerhood (Brophy-Herb et al., 2011).

But maternal emotional contributions to children's sympathy may differ for girls and for boys (Spinrad et al., 1999). Mothers' positive emotions during two emotionally challenging situations (i.e., waiting for electrodes to be put on their child, and doing a difficult puzzle together) were positively related to their 4- to 6-year-old daughters' self-reported sympathy, whereas their negative emotions were negatively related to their sons' sympathy.

Thus different maternal emotions supported boys' and girls' development of empathic concern. For girls, sharing positive emotional experiences with their mothers may prime their propensity for care; feeling good provides a substrate from which to attend to others' emotions. By comparison, boys experiencing their mothers' negativity may become more self-focused, feeling the personal distress that can block sympathy.

Other qualitative aspects of parents' emotional expressiveness around their children are central to the development of both general expressiveness and empathic concern (see Chapter 2). The intensity of maternal negative emotions and the presence of concurrent unresolved conflict also are associated, in my interviews and diary studies, with less-mature patterns of responses to peer emotions: less help and concern, but more frequent sustained attention. Hence, not only the specific emotions shown by parents, but their intensity and the resolution of negativity (as emphasized by Eisenberg, 2020), are necessary in inducing children to behave sympathetically.

Parents' contingent responsiveness to emotions also is important in the socialization of empathic concern. What do parents do when their children are distressed or anxious or show socially inappropriate emotions? Do they exhibit anxiety or sympathy themselves? How do their reactions map onto their children's reactions to their peers' distress (Eisenberg, Fabes, Bernzweig, et al., 1993; Eisenberg, Fabes, Carlo, et al., 1992)? Their reactions can give young children a guide for reacting to other people's emotion.

It makes sense that children who live in a sympathetic environment learn to follow suit. Even during toddlerhood, when mothers reacted to children's emotions with concerned attention and teaching, they reported that their children show more attention and prosocial reactions to others' emotions (Ornaghi, Conte, et al., 2020). When these mothers showed positive attention to their toddlers' emotions, they modeled empathy, providing a template for their children to follow in reacting to others' distress. The early emergence of this association is of note.

Thus children who observe optimal emotional and behavioral reactions to their own and others' emotions have guides to follow in their own empathic involvement with peers (Zahn-Waxler, Radke-Yarrow, & King, 1979). When mothers show certain benevolent patterns of reactions to their children's and others' negative emotions, preschoolers also show less egoistic distress and more sympathetic concern to the distress of others (Eisenberg et al., 1992; Fabes, Eisenberg, & Miller, 1990), as well as more prosocial behavioral reactions to the emotion displays of peers (Denham, 1993; Denham & Grout, 1993).

Along with the other positive things Monroe's parents did when his friend moved away, his mother showed him empathic concern. She found Monroe holding a toy they used to both play with a lot, and he was crying a little. She sat down beside him and rubbed his back for a while, and then gave him a hug. He not only felt much better, but also learned a lot about showing empathic concern from her.

As usual, there may be gender differences in how the socialization of empathic concern, this time via contingent reactions, registers with young children. In a series of studies about these questions by Eisenberg et al. (1992, 1993), parental self-reports about emotion socialization were often related to their reports about their young daughters' responses to others' distress. Sometimes not only their children's distress, but also their socially inappropriate emotions, were the focus.

Thus when mothers and fathers reported that they would try to downplay their daughters' expressions of emotions that would hurt others, such as contempt, they saw their daughters as exhibiting less helping and comforting behavior toward distressed peers. This parental pressure to restrict certain emotions was, however, related to their daughters' emotional sympathy unaccompanied by assistance toward another. Because of their parents' socialization, these young daughters experienced a strong empathic reaction internally, but were reluctant to enact the associated behavioral action tendency on behalf of a distressed peer. They considered *all* emotions as needing to be hidden, because their parents' messages about suppression found their mark.

Teaching also is necessary to the development of empathic concern. Particular aspects of maternal communication should be considered in relation to preschoolers' demonstration of empathic concern (Eisenberg, 2020). Parents who delineate the clearly important features of their emotions when communicating with their children proactively give their preschoolers a deeper, important understanding of others' distress. Thus the children in the Denham and Grout (1992) study were most prosocially responsive to their classmates' emotions when mothers said they (1) explained their sadness, (2) expressed their tension more positively when it affected their children, or (3) expressed their relatively infrequent anger rationally to their children. Positive and rational ways of knowing why and how their parents feel emotion are most productive in inspiring children's empathic concern. Such parental socialization can provoke other-oriented empathic concern, as opposed to self-focused personal distress.

Madeline's mother is sick and tired of her daughter's dawdling. As she feels her temper rising and hears her voice becoming sharper, she stops and takes a deep breath, so her anger does not intensify. The "fit" she feels coming on would do no one any good. She sits down beside her still-playing daughter—it is time for school—and sternly says, "Maddie, I am getting really frustrated. You must put on your shoes." Later in the car, she reflects, "You know, I'm glad we got that settled. You were really a good helper when I told you what we needed." The mother has expressed her anger rationally, and Madeline may be more empathic with others' frustrations in the future, as when Carrie has a meltdown. She knows that others' negative emotions have reasons and can be resolved. Maybe next time Carrie gets upset, Maddie will offer her a toy.

Finally, the vicarious experience of the others' emotions can also be fueled by parents' specific discourse with them. Young preschoolers just learning to move around skillfully in their play environment—and only beginning to interact purposively with peers—may be told, "It really, really hurts Johnny when you hit him like that." It is easy to see that these messages—emotional, verbal, and behavioral—could give rise to empathic concern (see, e.g., Garner, Dunsmore, & Southam-Gerrow, 2008). For example, such maternal explanations about emotions were related to toddlers' information seeking, a component of empathic concern (Garner, 2003).

### SUMMARY: Socialization of Empathic Concern

These results, taken together, suggest that exposure to parents' regulated and nonoverwhelming displeasure or distress, as well as their supportive reactions and discourse about others' distress, give young children a guide to follow in reacting to others' emotions. These techniques provide practice with empathic concern (emotional, cognitive, and behavioral) within the parent–child relationship, which can then be generalized to the peer setting. More long-lasting, intense negative parental emotions and reactions that are unexplained, undiscussed, and unresolved can so distress young children that the process is likely short-circuited through the pain of guilt, information overload, or incapacitating fearfulness. The general tenets of emotion socialization, as with positive and negative emotions and guilt and shame, are supports for the development of empathic concern.

## Socialization of More Sophisticated Expressiveness: Self-Conscious Emotions

Socialization also contributes to individual differences in the experience and expression of such emotions as pride, guilt, shame, embarrassment, envy, and contempt (Lewis, 1993a). With respect to these emotions, socializers' messages don't always fit the supportive or nonsupportive framework, partly because socializers are not necessarily reacting to emotions, but usually to behavior. Nonetheless, parental reactions do clarify for a child the emotional nature of success, failure, wrongdoing, others' suffering, and social mores. Parents react very clearly with emotional, behavioral, and linguistic messages about the child's adherence to the family's standards, rules, and goals (Lewis,

1993a). They also comment explicitly about the child's competence and behavior across a range of domains.

Parents' specific reactions to children's success, failure, and wrongdoing figure largely in which events each child considers noteworthy and emotionally arousing. This explicit content of standards and rules is communicated by parents.

> Some parents may expect children not to touch fragile bric-a-brac. The preschooler who does so despite this implicit rule experiences a parent's scowling face, a loud "No!" or even a slap, and perhaps a statement such as "Why can't you ever listen?"
>
> Or consider a young girl exploring in a pile of dirt with her teddy bear. She is met with a cold, abrupt removal to the bathtub, and with the parent's contemptuous words, "Only you can find so many ways to get into trouble!" Similarly, a boy who plays Power Ranger on his mother's new sideboard, deeply scratching it, is promptly reminded of the house rule that "it is not okay to climb on furniture," and sent for a prolonged time-out. Of course, the reactions in the first two examples would be considered nonsupportive and the last could be supportive, depending on its delivery.

Again note that the children weren't displaying emotions, but behaving in ways counter to their family's standards. Nevertheless, these parental reactions could *engender* negative emotions like sadness and anger in the child, and complicated emotions too like shame or guilt. In addition, much information about achievement is given by parents.

> Some families value early preacademic performance. When a preschooler in such a family learns to write his or her name, the child is rewarded with a parent's broad smile, a delighted hug, and a statement such as "That's super! I knew you could do it!"

Such socializing discourse not only imparts emotional meaning to everyday events, but also fuels the ways children "figure out" how to feel. Feelings of shame are natural outcomes when parents focus on a child's inadequacy and perhaps are unclear about the exact nature of the transgression. In contrast, the child playing Power Ranger on the sideboard feels only guilt rather than shame, because his mother has focused only on the importance of not breaking rules, without the accompanying contempt.

In short, socialization practices specific to early transgressions, failures, and successes affect the development of a child's tendency to feel and express complex self-conscious and social emotions. Such experiences are implicit in the following descriptions of shame and guilt.

### *Socialization of Shame*

Often the "moral" emotions—shame and guilt—are engendered by socialization that includes an amalgam of modeling, coaching, and/or contingent responding, along with attributions about the child's worth, culpability, responsibility, or caring for others. In the case of shame, the mechanisms of emotion socialization posited here are coupled with other sorts of messages that pervasively degrade the child.

> A habitually overtaxed and exhausted mother, after spending several hours with her perpetually whiny, fidgeting preschooler, Denise, finally snaps: She states venomously, "You are such an idiot!" She has acted angrily, but she also has given Denise clear and damaging information about her worth. The next day, when Denise plays quietly with a new game for an extended period, the mother says nothing.

Once children have learned the standards and rules for behavior, parental reactions like those in this example can engender shame (Lewis, 1992). Denise gets the message that she has done a bad thing by her very existence, and she feels shame. There is no emotion socialization technique at play on the next day, but neither is there any approbation for achievement and good behavior.

Self-reported shame in 5- to 12-year-olds has been clearly related to parents' expression of emotion—specifically, to the "absence of [positive] discipline, the strong presence of *hostile emotion*, little recognition of good behavior . . . [and] little in the way of concrete feedback regarding what the child had done that was right or wrong . . ." (Ferguson & Stegge, 1995, p. 190; emphasis added). The strong presence of parental anger figures notably in the development of shame, especially in the absence of positive parenting (see also Moskowitz, 1997). In parental shame induction, the anger is often accompanied by disgust, as well as by the disciplinary techniques of love withdrawal and humiliation.

Whether conveyed by modeling, coaching, or contingency mechanisms (or all three during one interchange!), such messages are extremely dysregulating to young children. They lead to another important aspect of the socialization of the experience and expression of shame—children's internalization of negative attributions about their own ability and worth, as implicit in the previous example (see also Zahn-Waxler & Kochanska, 1990, although they do not distinguish guilt and shame as sharply as Tangney et al., 1995, or Ferguson & Stegge, 1995). In such a context of emotion socialization, a child's experience of shame seems almost overdetermined.

More details on these attributional contributions to the experience and expression of shame were uncovered by Alessandri and Lewis (1993). Parent–child interactions were videotaped during easy and difficult puzzles, copying, and basketball-toss activities. Parents' verbalizations were coded as global or specific regarding their content ("You are a good ballplayer" vs. "You placed that piece just right!"), and as positive versus negative with respect to their emotional tone. Thus each verbalization fell into one of four cross-classified categories. Children whose parents made specific negative evaluations about them expressed more shame across all three activities of both difficulties, with both parents. When parents made positive specific or global statements, children evidenced less shame. Girls received fewer of these positive specific evaluations, and more of the specific negative ones, suggesting a reason for them to become more shame prone than boys.

## *Socialization of Guilt*

Both shame and guilt emerge after the child internalizes standards for behavior. Guilt, as specified in Chapter 3, is more closely allied with misbehavior than shame, which is related to deficiencies in the self. Ferguson and Stegge (1995) searched for the roots of guilt, along with shame, in young children. In contrast to shame, guilt was associated with parents' blame and anger after misdeeds and failures, and with their pride in positive encounters. Importantly, children who demonstrated guilt had parents who said that they had done a bad *thing* that caused displeasure, rather than that the children *themselves* were bad.

When parents reported a higher discrepancy between their children's actual behavior and what it ought to be, but a lower discrepancy between their children's actual self-regulation ability and what it ought to be, there also was more guilt. This constellation of parental correlates paints a picture of a child who is seen as able to self-regulate and behave well, but who does not do so in a particular morally important encounter:

> "You could have left the vase on the table. You didn't have to pick it up and then drop it. But you did. I'm so disappointed in your behavior."

The parents' communication of this view contributes, according to Ferguson and Stegge (1995), to the child's feeling naughty or sorry after a transgression.

### SUMMARY: Socialization of Self-Conscious Emotions

Caregivers' actions are related to their children's emotions of guilt and shame; in particular, their negative emotions that are strongly expressed together with personally evaluative statements or behaviors are linked to shame. More parents and teachers need to know about this connection, because they probably would not want to induce shame if they understood its pervasive negative effects. And even though a modicum of guilt probably motivates amending behavior, parents and teachers should carefully consider socialization practices contributing to either guilt or shame. Parent education programs should be fine-tuned to include a focus on emotion socialization (see Chapter 13), particularly spotlighting the problems inherent in shame induction. Along with safeguarding against the promotion of guilt and shame, however, parents and teachers also want to foster empathic concern for others that motivates prosocial behavior.

## Socialization of Display Rule Usage

Given the unfolding story of socializers' contribution to children's expressiveness, it follows that parents also are likely to convey information about when and when not to display emotional expressions. Wrinkled brow, compressed lips, and lip biting are expressive patterns that suggest dampened negative emotion. Parents' use of these patterns is associated both concurrently and predictively with toddlers' early use of the same display rules, suppressing negativity to meet cultural expectations (Malatesta et al., 1989).

The parental emotions experienced by preschoolers during interactions and in the more general emotional environment also contribute to their ability to perform according to emotional display rules. Mothers' self-reports of internalizing negative emotion (e.g., sadness) in their families were related to children's inability to show positive expressions after a disappointment, even when the effects of children's own emotional intensity and emotion knowledge were taken into account (Cole, Zahn-Waxler, et al., 1994). Children who lived in a sadder, more muted emotional environment were less able to "put on a good face" when disappointed.

In contrast, when mothers themselves maintained a positive demeanor when their child received a disappointing gift, their children were less likely to show negative expressions during the disappointment. Children whose mothers tempered the disappointment by "cheering them up" were less likely to behave in a negatively expressive, impolite manner toward the experimenter.

### SUMMARY: Socialization of Display Rules

The sparse research available, then, suggests that at least the modeling aspect of emotion socialization is important to young children's developing use of display rules. Little or nothing is known yet about the contribution of contingent responsiveness and parental teaching to young children's display rule usage. This area is ripe for investigation.

## CONCLUSION

Overall, there is much accumulating evidence pointing to various elements of parents' and other caregivers' modeling, coaching, and contingency contributions to the expressiveness patterns seen in young children. The emotions adults demonstrate, the ways they react to children's emotional experiences, and the ways they talk about emotions are important contributors to children's enduring patterns of emotional expressiveness. More research is needed to flesh out the patterns of parental socialization more fully—in Tomkins's terminology, via not only parents' monopolistic emotional organization, but also their intrusive or competitive expressive profiles. Furthermore, fuller views clarifying the moderating influences of child age and gender, culture and ethnicity, and fathers' special contributions would be very useful. Even more work also needs to be done on the socialization of more complex emotions and display rule usage.

In addition, I would like to see more on what lies behind all the correlational evidence that has accumulated. If maternal positivity predicts child positivity, for example, what actual cognitive, emotional, and social *processes* are at work to account for the association? Experimental paradigms such as those discussed by Cummings (1995b) could be used advantageously.

# 8

# Socialization of Preschoolers' Emotion Knowledge and Emotion Regulation

## INTRODUCTION

In Chapter 7, I introduced the concept of emotion socialization, with a focus on the socialization of preschoolers' emotional expressiveness. Aspects of socialization also contribute to individual differences in young children's emotion knowledge and ER. A body of evidence on the contribution of overall positive parenting techniques to children's emotion knowledge and emotion regulation (ER) also exists.

Along with this concentration on the socialization of emotion knowledge and ER, it is also important to introduce ongoing information on how both mothers and fathers socialize all aspects of their young children's emotional competence and how such emotion socialization in fact contributes directly to their social competence. I describe the small corpus of literature on how peers and siblings enact socialization of emotional competence for young children as well. Finally, the crucial ways in which culture impacts emotion socialization round out this discussion. First, I describe the contribution of emotion socialization to preschoolers' emotion knowledge.

## MODELING INFLUENCES ON EMOTION KNOWLEDGE

### Contributions of Modeling to Understanding Expressions, Situations, and Causes of Emotions

Parents' expression of emotions can teach children specifically about emotions (Nixon & Watson, 2001) or make it more difficult to address the issue of emotion altogether. By modeling various emotions, moderately expressive parents give children information about the nature of happiness, sadness, anger, and fear—their expression, their probable eliciting situations, and their more personalized causes. Family positive expressiveness (e.g., happiness and gratitude) particularly promotes emotion knowledge, perhaps rendering young children more open to learning about emotions. For example, when his mother claps delightedly upon opening the mail, a preschool boy sees that receiving a long-awaited letter calls for an expression of joy.

Conversely, exposure to negative emotions (e.g., sadness and anger) may hamper emotion knowledge by upsetting children, making reflection about emotion difficult (Burley, Hobson, Adegboye, Shelton, & Van Goozen, 2021; Denham, Zoller, et al., 1994; Nixon & Watson, 2001; Raver & Spagnola, 2003). This assertion is true especially when parents' negative emotion is intense and/or long lasting. However, exposure to well-modulated negative emotion is related to emotion knowledge. In families in which there is some conflict and negative emotion, children will "have opportunities to observe models and gain instruction about the appropriate ways to express negative affect" (Garner, Jones, & Miner, 1994, p. 624).

> Mother tears up when Aunt Joan calls to tell her of their father's (Rashida's grandfather's) grave illness. These emotions show Rashida one cause for sadness and one way to express it. As Daddy pats Mother's hand and strokes her back, the linkage between sadness and care also is reinforced in Rashida's mind.
>
> Later, her mother and father are sharing the drive to their grandfather's house. As they approach a bridge that goes up, up, up, Rashida's mother licks her lips and her eyes dart from side to side. She does not cry out, but Rashida knows that she is afraid. Rashida and her older brother—though he rolls his eyes and sighs audibly in mock disgust—see not only that even big people can be scared, but also that they have learned ways to minimize their expressiveness and perhaps their experience, of the emotion.

Research upholds these notions. When mothers reported somewhat negative feelings about their children, their children were able to verbally enumerate more causes for sadness; they were well versed at feeling sad themselves (Denham & Zoller, 1990). Mothers' internalizing negative expressiveness, such as sadness, also more broadly predicted kindergartners' knowledge of emotional expressions, even when children's age and receptive language ability were accounted for (Bowling & Jones, 1993). In fact, when mothers said they were *willing* to show emotion freely, to let their children observe and/or hear their own emotions (e.g., fear, annoyance, and frustration), their younger preschoolers demonstrated greater emotion knowledge (Abraham, Kuehl, & Christopherson, 1983; Denham, 1996b). Seeing maternal emotions exposes children to circumstances in which emotional expressions and situations can become clarified. So a moderate degree of experience with mothers' more internalizing negative emotions can contribute to emotion knowledge.

But, as already noted, when parental emotions are more frequent, intense, and negative, children are disturbed and dysregulated (Crockenberg, 1985; Denham & Grout, 1992; Parke, Cassidy, Burks, Carson, & Boyum, 1992). When dysregulation occurs, children experience heightened personal distress during emotionally charged events; this self-focus diverts attention away from facial and situational information about emotion, so that little is learned. If, instead of being charmingly expressive, Rashida's mother were constantly "blowing her top" in extreme, intense, and hurtful ways, Rashida's knowledge of emotions would probably be restricted. And for children already at risk for behavior problems, caregivers' emotional negativity and negative comments about them may be especially detrimental to their knowledge of negative emotions (Burley et al., 2021). At the same time, little information about emotional expressions and situations is imparted by parents whose expressiveness is quite limited. Balanced parental expressiveness is the most useful.

My colleagues and I conducted several studies to evaluate the contributions of socialization predictors to children's emotion knowledge (Denham, Cook, et al., 1992; Denham, Renwick-DeBardi, et al., 1994; Denham, Zoller, et al., 1994). Regarding maternal expressiveness, mothers' facial expressions of emotion were coded second by second during an approximately 90-minute laboratory playroom visit. Furthermore, as already discussed, mothers simulated sadness and anger during a structured task, and these characterizations of emotion were categorized as either highly emotional with predominantly empathic and guilt induction, or less emotional, with a more intellectualized approach to conveying the emotion to the child.

Specifically, these studies again highlighted the power of maternal anger as a *dis* organizer of social–emotional development (see also Cummings et al., 1985; Cummings, Zahn-Waxler, & Radke-Yarrow, 1981; Denham, 1989; Dunn & Brown, 1994): Maternal anger expressed during interaction with the child was negatively correlated with emotion knowledge. The mothers of children who were low and high in emotion knowledge differed in the amount of anger displayed: the "stars" of emotion knowledge had mothers who were lower in anger; the mothers of less adept children showed more anger. Children of mothers who experience higher levels of anger directed at them are specifically less able to demonstrate comprehension of angry situations (Garner, Jones, & Miner, 1994a). Maternal tension and sadness also are often modestly negatively associated with various separate indices of emotion understanding. It is easy to imagine the confusion and pain of young children who are relentlessly exposed to their parents' negative emotions. It is no wonder their emotion knowledge is compromised.

## Contributions of Modeling to Display Rule Knowledge

Little work has been done on parental emotions' specific contributions to more advanced levels of preschoolers' emotion understanding, such as understanding of display rule usage. Preschoolers' and kindergartners' knowledge of display rules—in situations such as losing a game, seeing someone in silly pajamas, not liking a present, or watching a parent leave on a trip—was associated with mothers' self-reported emotional expressiveness, even after children's age and receptive language ability were accounted for (Bowling & Jones, 1993; Jones et al., 1998). First, knowledge of self-protective display rules was related to maternal dominant negative emotions, such as anger and contempt. When children knew that their mothers could react intensely, even explosively, they also knew ways to "cover up" emotions to avoid getting into trouble (e.g., covering up their guilt after stealing a cookie). Less happy mothers might also require their children to be more in control of their expressiveness (e.g., not laughing in church). Their children's uncontrolled emotionality was the "last straw" for these dysphoric mothers. In contrast, knowledge of prosocial display rules was negatively predicted by maternal internalizing of negative expressiveness, such as sadness. Sad, morose, emotionally self-focused mothers were less able to convey to children how expressiveness can be managed for the sake of kindness (e.g., not showing disgust at Grandma's casserole).

Corroborating these notions, Wu et al. (2017) found that mothers' positive expressiveness was related to children's knowledge of display rules (i.e., via a total score that most heavily weighted justifying display rules prosocially). Adding to the earlier authors' reasoning, Wu et al. (2017) suggested that a positive, "easy and harmonious" emotional environment might give preschoolers comfort with emotions that allowed them to explore the requirements of their parents and society regarding appropriate expressiveness.

However, it would be a mistake to overlook the contributions of both mothers *and* fathers and of other socialization methods. In two of my studies, we found, collectively, that 5-year-olds' display rule knowledge was predicted over time by mothers' (1) observed and self-reported negative emotions; (2) observed negative reactions to their emotions (as in Jones et al., 1998); and (3) their discussion of negative, rather than positive, emotions while reminiscing about emotional events. These results suggest that witnessing, experiencing, and learning about negative emotions with mothers help children know when to show and when not to show emotions. In contrast, fathers' observed and self-reported positive emotions and observed supportive reactions contributed to their children's later display rule knowledge in kindergarten (Denham, Bassett, & Wyatt, 2010; Denham & Kochanoff, 2002). Some of the contributions of both mothers' and fathers' emotions were more pronounced for their daughters (Denham, Bassett, et al., 2010).

Again, it seems that nuances of mothers' emotional lives, even if negative, support the development of an aspect of emotional competence in their preschoolers. Alternatively, fathers' sometimes challenging positivity may allow children to experience instances of display rule usage safely during play (e.g., when Dad smiles even though he lost a game, or when Dad catches an older brother in a breathless game of tag, laughing uproariously, and the older brother doesn't say "Owwww," but laughs instead).

Affording children a window into the full range of emotionality appears salutary for developing the complex understanding of display rules. Fathers' positivity may contribute to children's security about considering the world of emotions, whereas mothers' input rounds out the picture of how complicated this world can be. Such a viewpoint corresponds to my view of fathers as loving playmates and mothers as emotional gatekeepers (Pavarini et al., 2013).

## **SUMMARY:** Modeling Influences on Emotion Knowledge

In general then, parental positivity promotes preschoolers' emotion knowledge. In contrast, overexposure to negative maternal emotions, especially anger, often impedes the process by which children come to understand emotion. The role of more internalizing maternal emotions, such as sadness, is less clear. Some exposure to these more internalizing emotions can be beneficial to the development of emotion knowledge. Knowing that adults' expression of emotions is pivotal to the accumulation of one more core emotional skills may motivate parents and caregivers to be more conscious of their socialization influences.

## CONTINGENCY INFLUENCES ON EMOTION KNOWLEDGE

According to the contingency hypothesis, parents' emotional and behavioral reactions to their children's emotions also help them in differentiating among emotions. Again supportive emotion socialization is associated with the most positive child outcomes. Children of parents who encourage emotional expression[1] have more access to their own emotions than do the children of parents who value maintaining a more stoic, unemotional mien, and thus begin to understand emotions better.

> Jonathan can speak about subtle differentiations in his own anger at the bully in his class. Sometimes he is just plain mad and wants to punch Donald; sometimes he is mad only a little, because he doesn't know why Donald hates him. His parents listen, and when he is angry, they validate his feelings, letting him know that it is okay to feel this way. Talking with them helps him solidify some of these ideas about emotions.

But these parents very easily could have dismissed the irritable torrent of "Donald this" and "Donald that" that emanates from Jonathan at the dinner table. Thus, parents' varying reactions to the child's expressions of specific emotions also suggest to the child those situations when they are and are not appropriate. Jonathan is learning not only when to express emotions; he is also learning about the very nature of emotions themselves.

### Contributions of Supportive Contingency to Children's Emotion Knowledge

Parents' reactions convey important messages about emotions, promoting preschoolers' emotion knowledge (Bjørk et al., 2022; Perlman, Camras, & Pelphrey, 2008; Pintar Breen, Tamis-LeMonda, & Kahana-Kalman, 2018). Supportive reactions to children's emotions may help them differentiate emotions, perhaps by making the children feel more comfortable about exploring emotions and affording them practice in successfully dealing with them (Denham & Kochanoff, 2002; Denham, Zoller, et al., 1994; Fabes et al., 2002; Fabes, Leonard, Kupanoff, & Martin, 2001).

---

[1]Given earlier discussion of ethnic differences in the working of contingent reactions to children's emotions, these findings may be more applicable to White children, but research findings do not, as far as I know, exist.

We found that mothers' emotionally positive responsiveness to children's observed emotions predicted preschoolers' emotion knowledge (Denham, Zoller, et al., 1994). As noted earlier, in this case positive responsiveness included reacting with happiness to children's happiness, with tenderness to their sadness, and with calmness to their anger. So mothers who were more tolerant and positive (i.e., who were more supportive) had children who were able to identify emotional expressions and situations, even those requiring some personalized inference.

> Claire's mother was tolerant of Claire's distress during the argument between the parents; later she talked to Claire calmly and tenderly as she tucked her into bed. Her approach to Claire's emotional experience was consistently responsive in this manner. When questioned about her knowledge of emotions in our study, Claire was able to see the viewpoint of the puppet who felt differently than she did: "Well, I really like to go swimming. But he is really, really scared, so I will put the scared face on him."

The impact of supportive reactions to emotion may interact or work in concert with parental emotional expressiveness. For example, knowledge of facial expressions and the causes of emotions and their consequences were predicted by supportive responsiveness to preschoolers' emotions in concert with higher parental negative expressiveness (Mazzone & Nader-Grosbois, 2016). As noted earlier, some negative expressiveness can be useful for preschoolers' development of emotion knowledge. An environment of general support of children's own emotions could make them feel safe enough to tolerate and learn from parental negativity. At the same time, it may be even more salutary to live within an environment of mothers' support and *positive* parental expressivity (Denham & Kochanoff, 2002).

## Contributions of Nonsupportive Contingency to Children's Emotion Knowledge

Mothers' lack of emotionally negative responsiveness predicted preschoolers' emotion knowledge (Denham, Zoller, et al., 1994). In our study, negative responsiveness included reacting with anger to children's sadness or anger or with happiness to their sadness. One pattern of responsiveness initiated escalating cycles of negativity; the other constituted "making fun" of a child or putting on a "good face" that ignored the child's needs.

Parental behaviors contingent on children's emotional displays also influence their understanding of situations that elicit emotions; we focused on these behaviors in our next series of studies. Either negative responsiveness or ignoring of a child's emotions by mother or father was a negative predictor of emotion knowledge (Denham et al., 1997). Negative responsiveness was generally indexed by directly telling or indirectly inducing the child to stop showing an emotion—for example, by distracting the child. The contributions of such negative responsiveness were significant even after we accounted for intrapersonal contributors, such as age, gender, children's own reactions to parental emotions, and cognitive and/or language ability.

Mothers' self-reports about their own negative responsiveness in emotion socialization also were revealing. Mothers who reported that they discouraged their children's emotional expressiveness ("I think children must learn early not to cry," "I do not allow my child to get angry with me") had children who were less adept at comprehending angry situations or demonstrating emotion knowledge more broadly (Denham & Zoller, 1990; Garner et al., 1994a).

Hence, parents showing behaviors that fit the nonsupportive socialization paradigm had children who were less adept at age-appropriate emotion knowledge tasks. Preschoolers of parents who demonstrate punitive reactions are likely to be motivated to avoid emotional information—emotions are risky (Denham & Kochanoff, 2002)!

Chelsea's mother reacts angrily to her emotions. When we asked Chelsea to put an emotion face on a puppet acting angry to be served oatmeal for breakfast, she crossed her arms on her chest and stated firmly, "No. I not talking about angry. I can't play 'til it's happy."

Dismissing responses (e.g., "When my child is angry, my goal is to make him or her stop") also become part of a milieu in which children learn less about emotions (Ornaghi, Pepe, Agliati, & Grazzani, 2019), probably because the very importance of emotions is downplayed.

## Children's Age and Gender Moderate Contingency's Contribution to Emotion Knowledge

*The* age of the child was also found in our work to be an important moderator of contingency's effects on preschoolers' emotion knowledge. In particular, younger children who experienced mothers' negative responsiveness following their emotional displays showed less-advanced emotion knowledge (Denham, Mitchell-Copeland, et al., 1997). Younger preschoolers especially need to be open to their own experience of emotion, and to begin comprehending complex emotions. Their willingness to consider emotional events and issues was especially stymied by this punitive, dismissing approach. Maybe if Chelsea had been closer to age 5, rather than only 38 months old, she may have been more amenable to consider negative emotional situations.

Older children's emotion knowledge, on the other hand, especially benefited from parents' matching of their positive emotions, suggesting that a positive emotional environment was more important for their acquisition of emotion knowledge. Younger children are most affected by the contagion of such reactions' negativity, whereas older preschoolers seem more able to discern such behaviors as distinctive reactions to their own particular emotions.

Child gender also moderated the contribution of the parental responsiveness to child emotion: In the study just described, maternal negative emotional responsiveness was a negative predictor of boys' but not girls' emotion knowledge (Denham, Zoller, et al., 1994). Because girls obtain more teaching about emotion than boys, boys may rely more on more indirect mechanisms of contingent responsiveness to acquire emotion knowledge. In this way, boys are especially vulnerable to such punitive socialization.

### SUMMARY: Contingent Reactions and Emotion Knowledge

Despite the complexity of the overall story, there is support for key ideas about how children learn from parents' reactions to their emotions. Supportive contingent responding allows preschoolers to experience many expressive patterns and to reflect on even negative emotions, thus promoting their emotion knowledge. Across several studies and other ways of depicting responsiveness, the effects of contingent responses to children's emotions on developing emotion knowledge were found to be consonant with theoretical notions about supportive and nonsupportive emotion socialization. As is so often found, children's age and gender are important to consider in these patterns.

Caregivers and parents probably don't realize how far-reaching are their responses to their children's emotions that they consider simple or inevitable. As with other aspects of emotion socialization and emotional competence, it would be useful to let them know more about these valuable findings.

## TEACHING INFLUENCES ON EMOTION KNOWLEDGE

According to emotion socialization theory, parents encourage children's exploration and emotion knowledge directly; they teach them explicitly about emotions. They verbally communicate to children the experiential meaning of emotions (Saarni, 1987). Such communication heightens children's awareness of emotion within parent–child interactions and motivates them to attend to and process such emotional information.

> While looking at a photograph of an intensely sad, crying infant, one mother in our studies (Denham, Cook, et al., 1992; Denham, Renwick-DeBardi, et al., 1994) had this exchange with her 3-year-old daughter:
>
> MOTHER: Have you ever felt like that? You know what I'd feel like if I were like that? I'd feel like nobody likes me at all. . . . What would you do if I was feeling like that?
>
> ASHLEY: I would ask Daddy if he could hug you.
>
> MOTHER: Give me the kind of hug you would give me. . . . Poor little [baby]. Oh, he must feel so bad. That's a real big sad. He looks like his little heart is broken.
>
> Ashley's attention was riveted on the conversation, on the photograph of the infant, and on her mother's face.

Such parent-led conversations about the names, causes, and consequences of different emotions could specifically aid the child in his or her active attempts to link expressions, situations, and words into coherent, predictable schemas about emotional experience (Bullock & Russell, 1986). Verbal give-and-take about emotional experience within the scaffolded context of chatting with a parent helps the young child gradually formulate a coherent body of knowledge about emotions' expressions, situations, and causes. Thus teaching about emotion, at which Ashley's mother so clearly excelled, in its simplest form consists of verbally commenting on or explaining an emotion and its relation to an observed event or expression.

Such conversations help to direct children's attention to salient emotional cues, and at the same time allowing them the reflective distance from their own feeling states so that they can better interpret and evaluate feelings' causes and consequences. Maternal emotion talk contributes to their preschoolers' emotion knowledge (Brown & Dunn, 1992; Denham & Grout, 1992; Denham, Mitchell-Copeland, et al., 1997; Denham, Renwick-DeBardi, et al., 1994; Doan & Wang, 2010; Dunn, Brown, Slomkowski, et al., 1991; Dunn, Slomkowski, Donelan, & Herrera, 1995; Garner, Dunsmore, et al., 2008; LaBounty, Wellman, Olson, Lagattuta, & Liu, 2008). In fact, two meta-analyses found that emotion conversations or other instruction (e.g., discussing emotion-laden picture books) were related to emotion knowledge (Tompkins, Benigno, Kiger Lee, & Wright, 2018; Zinsser, Gordon, & Jiang, 2021). Further, the general trend of these findings also holds true for low-income minority families (Garner, 2006; Garner, Jones, Gaddy, & Rennie, 1997). I return to the prediction of children's assessed emotion knowledge after discussing the important role of emotion conversations as they occur in real time.

## Family Conversations about Emotions

Conversations about emotions further the child's developing emotion knowledge (Brown & Dunn, 1991). As such, they bear greater scrutiny. First, it is useful to examine how such conversations change as children grow older. A recent examination of home conversations about emotions between mothers and their 15- to 47-month-old children showed that mothers' observed use of emotion words in the home increased with their children's age, as did their children's (Ogren & Sandhofer, 2021). However, the focus of mother–child conversations about emotions also may change with age. For example, naturally occurring conversations about feelings between mothers and their children as young as 18 to 36 months old show how maternal emotion language teaches children about feelings (Brown & Dunn, 1991, 1992; Dunn et al., 1987; Dunn & Munn, 1985). Specifically, by the time toddlers reach 18 months, mothers and children discuss the causes of emotions, particularly those of the toddlers. From 24 to 36 months, however, mothers change their feeling-state language to parallel their children's usage and increasing understanding. They refer more often to others' thoughts, feelings, and desires, and their use of emotion language to control behavior ("Stop crying," "Now calm down") decreases.

Age change in parents' and children's emotion talk also may depend on the emotion discussed. While mothers and fathers looked at emotion-laden picture books with their first-born and second-born children, both mothers and fathers used labeling, questions, and explanations of emotions and emotion-related behavior involving the child or someone else (Van der Pol et al., 2015). When children were 2 years old, both parents talked most about sadness, but by the time the children were 3 years old, they mentioned both anger and sadness. Parents' talk about anger, fear, and happiness increased between ages 2 and 3. Adding a discussion of anger when children were 3, after discussing sadness most when children were 2, follows the developmental trend of children's emotion knowledge. Parents' talk about anger, sadness, and happiness then decreased when children were between ages 4 and 5. Although emotion talk does increase in natural conversations at home through age 4 (Ogren & Sandhofer, 2021), it may be that in the picture-book-reading context parents "step back" and let the older child do more talking.

Along with age changes, individual differences in emotion talk also should be noted. Individual differences in mothers' usage of emotion language and its various functions teach children to use emotion language in specific ways. Emotion language of both mothers and their preschool-age children is embedded in discourse that fulfills a variety of functions, such as commenting, questioning, explaining, attempting to change another's behavior, and moralizing (i.e., a "little sermon"; Denham, Cook, et al., 1992; see also Bretherton et al., 1986). When viewing photographs of infants showing emotions in our 1992 study, mothers especially used more questioning and explaining than their children, commensurate with their role as teachers; however, there was no mother–child difference in the use of emotion language to guide behavior ("You're making me sad"). Apparently even young children know how to use emotion language to influence others! Further, the child's participation in such conversations, using mostly commenting, can be taken as online evidence of emotion knowledge.

Continuing examination of the function of each conversation partner's emotion language can help to elucidate findings even more (Denham, Cook, et al., 1992). When mothers asked more questions about emotions, children answered by using more emotion words in explanations. When mothers explained emotions, their children asked fewer questions and used less-frequent guiding language, suggesting that they were more satisfied with complete information. More broadly, Cervantes and Callanan (1998) found that explanations also were related to children's total emotion talk. This association suggests that not only did such explanations satisfy the children's need to understand, but also that this resultant understanding perhaps motivated them to add to the narrative. Finally, in Denham, Cook, et al. (1992) more-accurate mothers also had children who used more-accurate emotion language—that is, who described emotions more appropriately.

But an important question is: Does mothers' emotion language at one time predict children's emotion language even later? Is more going on than children's being able to carry on a conversation contemporaneously, as admirable as that may be? Will they be able to use emotion language more ably later if their mothers use it with them now? When mothers and older siblings discuss emotions with toddlers at 18 months, their children also talk more about emotions at 24 months (Dunn et al., 1987). As well, preschoolers whose mothers used more emotion language in parent–child conversations about past emotions used more emotion language themselves later; the contrasting child-to-mother effect did not exist (Adams, Kuebli, Boyle, & Fivush, 1995; Fivush, 1989; Kuebli, Butler, & Fivush, 1995; Kuebli & Fivush, 1992, 1996).

Obviously, there is a lot going on here—the conversations between mothers and their preschoolers are often content-full, but this eloquence varies a lot between dyads. Some mothers and children make ample use of the varied functions of emotion language, and talk a lot about the photos and simulations, past experiences, or picture books. Others just have less to say about emotions in general. Both contemporaneous and longitudinal relationships among aspects of mothers' and children's emotion conversations reflect these individual differences.

Of course, in conversations with young children, the parent is the experienced partner.

Nonetheless, family talk about emotions is transactional; the issues brought up by one conversation partner are tackled by the other. Children who talked to their mothers about feelings had mothers who also talked to them about feelings at both 33 and 47 months (Brown & Dunn, 1992; see also Cervantes & Callanan, 1998; Leyva, Catalán Molina, Suárez, Tamis-Lemonda, & Yoshikawa, 2021; Ogren & Sandhofer, 2021; Raikes & Thompson, 2008).

Thus, even though parents are the experts in talking about emotions, the benefits for the child of participating in such conversations can begin quite early, and the co-action of parent and child may be crucial. Mothers' elaborative conversational style about emotions, which includes not only open-ended questions but also open-ended factual and even purely informative statements, along with explanations, figures prominently in this co-action, by promoting children's best participation and growing emotion language. For example, children were more likely to generate emotion labels when mothers' emotion talk was more elaborative and validating *and* allowed the child to be an active conversation partner (Raikes & Thompson, 2008).

Further, such an elaborative style within mother–child emotion conversations is important not only for the development of emotion knowledge shown during conversations, but also for translating its use into action. When parents elicited toddlers' labels for and causes of emotions while discussing the emotion-laden pictures in a storybook, children helped and shared more quickly and more often in experimental tasks (Brownell, Svetlova, Anderson, Nichols, & Drummond, 2013; see also Drummond, Paul, Waugh, Hammond, & Brownell, 2014). It should be noted that in this study parents' own labeling and explaining were not associated with toddlers' prosocial behaviors—getting the child to talk about emotions too seemed the best approach for their social behavior, presumably due to their engagement, as well as their enriched knowledge of emotion.

Co-regulation of emotion conversations thus has far-reaching results. Emotion knowledge can grow while parents and children co-narrate emotional experiences—the content and meaning of their own, other family members', or story characters'—over time. The knowledge that preschoolers display during conversations unfolds when parents and children talk about the beginning, middle, and end of emotional experiences and link them via thematic content (Fivush, 2021). Individual differences reside not only in the amount of emotion talk the dyads generate, but also in the stories they tell and how they are structured and in the way the conversations become true dialogues. And the outcomes of such conversations also translate into a richer corpus of knowledge about emotions for the preschoolers.

## Emotion Conversations Predicting Preschoolers' Emotion Knowledge Assessed in Other Contexts

Preschoolers who are involved in these dialogues are able to demonstrate their emotion knowledge in assessment contexts. Mother–child emotion language at one time point predicts preschoolers' later indices of emotion knowledge. For example, Dunn, Brown,

Slomkowski, and colleagues (1991) examined the connection between mother–child emotion language at 33 months and emotion knowledge at 40 months. Both child-to-mother and mother-to-child emotion talk, especially a child's talk about causes of emotions, were related to the child's overall emotion knowledge. Similarly, emotion talk at 36 months—again, both child-to-mother and mother-to-child—was related to the child's later emotion knowledge at 6 years (Dunn, Brown, & Beardsall, 1991). It should be noted that none of these associations were moderated by the children's verbal fluency or general linguistic experience; the specific importance of emotion language in the family is underscored.

Again, it is important to go beyond total emotion talk and the specific linguistic functions of emotion talk, to examine especially mothers' elaborative emotion conversational style and its relation to emotion knowledge; such a style can be particularly useful in the development of preschool emotion knowledge (Laible, 2004; Laible, Panfile Murphy, & Augustine, 2013; Van Bergen & Salmon, 2010). Others also have found dyadic coconstruction of emotion narratives and children's engagement in emotion conversations to be predictive, either concurrently or over time, of preschoolers' emotion knowledge (Laible, 2011; Laible et al., 2013). In one study, these associations were apparent mainly with elaboration during the reminiscence of a negative event, and an in-depth dyadic discussion (i.e., more than three conversational turns) also was related to emotion knowledge (Laible, 2011). Mothers' emotional statements, elaborations, and questions during storybook reading also were related to their preschoolers' understanding of the causes of emotions (Schapira & Aram, 2020). Finally, underlining the child's active part in learning about emotions during reminiscence conversations, Raikes and Thompson's (2008) findings suggested that mothers' emotion talk predicted children's emotion talk, which then predicted later emotion knowledge.

As part of the elaborative conversational style, questions can also be especially important elements in emotion teaching and in promoting preschoolers' emotion knowledge (especially girls'; Bailey, Denham, & Curby, 2013). They focus the child's attention, pushing him or her to think and to formulate thoughts about the conversation's emotional content, to practice using challenging language, and to put emotional memories and experiences into words (Salmon & Reese, 2016).

> Four-year-old Craig and his mother are looking at a picture book about two children who get a new puppy. When Craig's mother asks him about the little boy's emotions when he sees the puppy run into the road while the school bus approaches, Craig pauses to think. He remembers when their dog slipped out of its collar near the road, and responds, " 'Member when Tippy got loose? I think this boy is very, very scared his dog might get hurt bad. He better get his mom to catch his dog!"

Further, the focus of such questions may differ depending on the emotion discussed (Lagattuta & Wellman, 2002). For example, in viewing images of varying self-conscious emotions, mothers asked more causal questions about shame, guilt, and embarrassment than about the positive emotions of awe and pride (Cooper, Pradera, Sorensen, & Reschke, 2021); these results dovetail with earlier work (Knothe & Walle, 2018; Lagattuta & Wellman, 2002).

Another way of demonstrating co-regulation of emotion conversations—in which both partners' input is crucial—is via mothers' repetition of their children's language. Mothers who repeated children's emotion language during the photograph discussion had children who displayed greater knowledge of emotion situations, again suggesting the importance of co-regulation (Denham, Cook, et al., 1992).[2] Accuracy in discussing emotions is necessary; the accuracy of children's emotion language with mothers was important in this context, as well; it was related to children's knowledge of emotional expressions and situations (Denham, Cook, et al., 1992). Mothers who used language that somehow did not describe the emotion depicted gave murky information that did not promote their children's emotion knowledge.

Parents' emotion talk while actually showing emotions also is likely a very helpful context for learning about emotions. Such an experience may be especially riveting for children. For example, the mothers who spontaneously explained their emotions while simulating them in our laboratory had children who were more adept at understanding emotions (Denham, Cook, et al., 1992; see also Dunn, Brown, & Beardsall, 1991; Dunn, Brown, Slomkowski, et al., 1991; Garner et al., 1997). Their highlighting of personally relevant emotion information by explaining their own feelings or repeating the children's utterances (e.g., "You make me sad when you don't sit still") aroused their children and captured their attention. Guilt-tinged, quickly processed, and salient "hot" cognitions may have ensued in the children (see Hoffman, 1984). Such cognitions, resulting from this inductive style of discipline, are fertile ground for the development of emotion knowledge (Hoffman, 1975; Hoffman & Saltzstein, 1967; Maccoby & Martin, 1983). Thus this particular emotional context is a special window of opportunity for young children to learn about the causes and consequences of emotions.

Such personally relevant discourse about emotions could center on both young children's and their parents' own experiences of negative emotion (Dunn & Brown, 1994). Unfortunately, however, less talk about feelings occurs when young children are experiencing emotion and family negativity is high. Perhaps the negative relationship between maternal anger and children's emotion knowledge, then, is due not only to the children's oversensitization to negative emotion, but also to the disinclination, outside the laboratory, for mothers who experience negative emotions to talk about them. Children likewise process personally relevant emotion information best when they are calm. So reminiscing about their own and their mothers' emotional experiences—after they have occurred—is a beneficial tactic that numerous researchers have utilized.

Finally, although my discussion has focused on emotion language specifically, it may be profitable to consider a broader context for teaching about emotions. For example, Doan, Lee, and Wang (2019) have shown the importance of a more comprehensive examination of maternal mental state language (including desire, beliefs, and thoughts, as well as emotions) because, as they reason, explaining an emotional situation requires such language as well. They found that, for European American children between 3 and 4½ years old, mothers' mental state language while reading a picture book was

---

[2] Young children also tend to repeat emotion words their mothers use during conversation (Ogren & Sandhofer, 2021).

related to contemporaneous emotion knowledge, and for Chinese immigrant children it was related to growth in emotion knowledge over time.

## Gender as a Moderator of Teaching about Emotion Knowledge

Are there gender differences in parents' teaching about emotions? In North American culture, females are assumed to be more emotional and more interested in emotion; research results, although not replicated in all studies, confirms such assumptions. Accordingly, early research suggested that, in general, parents and older siblings talk more about emotions to preschool-age girls than to boys (Dunn et al., 1987; Fivush, 1989; Greif et al., 1984; Kuebli & Fivush, 1992, 1996).

Even the type of emotion and the contexts of emotion deemed appropriate to discuss are exposed to gender-related pressures. To pursue this line of argument, Fivush et al. (1989) also explored ways in which mothers and their 30- to 70-month-old children discussed emotional aspects of their past experiences; mothers directed more total feeling language and more unique emotion words to girls and placed emotions in an interactional framework to a much greater extent with daughters. Regarding specific emotions, they discussed anger much more often with sons and sadness more often with daughters (Fivush, 1989; Kuebli et al., 1995; Kuebli & Fivush, 1992, 1996).

Similarly, in my own work, fathers also talked more to their daughters than they did to their sons about emotions during a reminiscence task, and mothers talked more to their sons about negative emotions, especially compared to fathers (Denham, Bassett, & Wyatt, 2010). Perhaps revealing the foundation of these propensities, parents attributed anger more to boys, and sadness and happiness to girls when presented with gender-neutral characters in emotion pictures (van der Pol et al., 2015). Interestingly, however, very recent meta-analytic findings suggest that mothers' frequency of emotion talk does *not* differ by child gender (Aznar & Tenenbaum, 2020).

Despite these meta-analytic findings, studies suggest that differences found in parents' emotion talk begin to show up in children's own emotion language very early (Fivush, 1989; Kuebli et al., 1995; Kuebli & Fivush, 1992, 1996). By 24 months, girls themselves referred to feeling states more often than did boys. By 3 years of age, girls were using substantially more emotion language, with the difference increasing across the preschool years (see also Cervantes & Callanan, 1998). Differences in the ways girls and boys discuss emotions with others can influence how they come to think about their emotional lives as they grow older (Kuebli & Fivush, 1992). Because parents use an interpersonal framework in discussing emotions with girls, girls think of emotions as something to share with others, whereas boys learn to express anger directly, but not to talk about it to others as much.

Mothers and fathers also often differ in their propensity to talk about emotions. In LaBounty et al. (2008), mothers and fathers used an equivalent amount of overall language in discussing an emotion-laden picture book, but mothers made more frequent references to emotions, particularly regarding causal language. Other research showed that mothers' emotion talk was more elaborative and engaged than fathers' (van der Pol et al., 2015; Zaman & Fivush, 2013). Further, although in our work mothers' and fathers' total emotion talk did not differ, mothers talked more than fathers about their own emotions, which I have posited here as an important teaching mechanism; they also reported that they valued teaching about emotions more than fathers (Denham, Bassett, et al., 2010).

What's more, mothers' and fathers' emotion talk may differentially predict children's emotion knowledge. For example, we found mothers', but not fathers', use of emotion terms during reminiscences to predict their children's later display rule knowledge (Denham, Bassett, et al., 2010). Thus the story is far from clear on mothers' and fathers' relative contributions to preschoolers' emotion knowledge; perhaps the important differences are qualitative rather than quantitative.

### SUMMARY: Teaching and Emotion Knowledge

Teaching works to increase emotion knowledge. Caregivers should be encouraged by the growing body of information on this aspect of emotional competence. Clearly, there are some moderating factors, including the type of emotion language used, its function, the way it is imparted, and the gender of the child to whom it is imparted or of the parent doing the imparting. Nonetheless, the major finding is that talking about emotions with young children is beneficial to their development. We need to know more about fathers', teachers', and siblings' contributions to this development, however.

## OVERALL POSITIVE PARENTING INFLUENCES ON EMOTION KNOWLEDGE

At the most molar level, the components of generally positive parenting contribute to emotion knowledge. At least two groups of researchers have addressed this molar level (Abraham et al., 1983; Denham, 1996b). Maternal and paternal reasoning and limit setting, as well as maternal intimacy with the child, were related—in complex, age-dependent ways—to young children's knowledge of emotional expressions and situations (Abraham et al., 1983).

More specifically, mothers' use of reason to help children learn acceptable behavior was related to emotion knowledge, regardless of child age (Abraham et al., 1983; Denham, 1996b). In fact, mothers who resorted to guilt induction in their reasoning, appealing to their children's connection to others in order to gain compliance, had children who spontaneously verbalized more causes of emotion (Denham, 1996b; Pavarini et al., 2013). Paternal reasoning guidance was related to younger, but not to older, preschoolers' emotion knowledge (Abraham et al., 1983).

More recent research alludes to other possible "active ingredients" of the use of reasoning. Maternal reflective functioning (i.e., appropriate understanding and explanation of others' emotions and behaviors; awareness of the nature of mental states, effort to understand the mental states underlying one's own and others' behaviors, recognition of the developmental aspects of mental states) may be the emotion-related foundation for reasoning's support of developing emotion knowledge (Jessee, 2020).

Turning to limit setting—including the consistency of setting and enforcing limits and the extent to which daily routines were defined—paternal limit setting was negatively related to younger preschoolers' emotion knowledge. Similarly, maternal limit setting was negatively related to older preschoolers' emotion knowledge (Abraham et al., 1983). As limit setting was endorsed more strongly—perhaps *too* strongly?—emotion knowledge was compromised.

I (Denham, 1996b) also found that mothers' inconsistent limit setting was positively related to children's knowledge of emotional expressions and situations,[3] as well as to the accuracy of emotion language when examining infant emotion photographs, in two samples. In contrast, indulgent mothers (those who were not necessarily inconsistently applying limits, but just not applying them at all) had children who demonstrated less knowledge of emotional situations, particularly ones requiring somewhat personalized inferences.

How can these results be explained? Parents who value order and rules may be less apt to address the world of emotion. Families in which disciplinary rules are less consistently followed may be more relaxed and open to both positive and negative emotional experiences, from which the children learn. Alternatively, when limit setting is inconsistent, children may need to become attuned to parental emotion by necessity: "Is Mom angry now, and does she 'mean business' this time?" In contrast, when there are few rules at all, there is little pressure to learn about social relations, including the emotional domain.

Additionally, maternal intimacy—mothers' openness in expression of physical affection for her children and others in the children's presence—was negatively related to younger preschoolers' knowledge of emotional situations. As with limit setting, emphasis on this aspect of parent–child relations, which is admittedly positive in an overall sense, may preclude more direct tutelage about emotions. Perhaps in this case, intimacy also is associated with a more overprotective shielding from emotions.

## SUMMARY: Overall Positive Parenting and Emotion Knowledge

Parents who self-report using most positive parenting techniques then create an emotional environment in which emotions are openly shown and discussed. As such, the home is a crucible for learning about emotions' expressions, situations, and causes. It is revealing, however, that some parenting techniques are generally positive for child development overall, but not quite as beneficial for the development of this specific component of emotional competence. Further, the age-specific and sometimes parent-specific associations of parenting techniques and emotion knowledge underscore the complexity of the picture.

## SUMMARY: Socialization of Emotion Knowledge

Much has been determined about the socialization of preschoolers' emotion knowledge, although questions always remain. In general, parental positivity, with a modicum of

[3] Fathers' inconsistency, on the other hand, was marginally negatively related to children's knowledge of emotional situations. This finding highlights the need to obtain information from both parents.

negative expressiveness for learning, promotes such knowledge. Supportive reactions from parents also give young children safe room in which to experience emotions, reflect on them, and learn about them. Particular methods of teaching about emotions are emerging as important, especially the elaborative conversational pattern, perhaps pertaining to parents' own emotions. General parenting styles embedded in the authoritative pattern also often support the development of emotion knowledge. Attention must also be given to age and gender differences in these findings. In short, there is much food for thought here for caregivers and for parents: their emotions, reactions, and conversations have lasting impact.

## SOCIALIZATION OF INDIVIDUAL DIFFERENCES IN PRESCHOOLERS' ER

Aspects of socialization also contribute to individual differences in young children's ER. Parents demonstrate ER templates for their children via their own emotional expressiveness and regulation. Their means of reacting to their children's emotions also can prompt preschoolers to utilize differing ER strategies. Finally, talking about emotion-laden experiences in daily life also can instruct preschoolers in how to regulate emotions.

### Parents' Own Emotional Expressiveness and Children's ER

The profiles of emotions displayed by parents can be very helpful in the socialization of children's ER; as mentioned in my discussion of supported ER in Chapter 6, socializers model ways of dealing with emotions. Some parents teach their children to hide or suppress their emotions, but others emphasize coping techniques such as direct problem solving or seeking social support (Eisenberg, Fabes, Carlo, et al., 1992; Roberts & Strayer, 1987).

In general, in a positive emotional environment, emotional demands on children are manageable and their models of emotional expressiveness are effective (Thompson, 2014). Thus Garner (1995) found that mothers who reported more positive emotion in their families had toddlers who were more capable of self-soothing when they were absent, a developmentally appropriate means of ER. And, if one possible endpoint of ER as product is an emotional profile with greater positive than negative emotionality, my work supports the hypothesis that parents model ER via their expressive patterns (Denham, 1989; Denham & Grout, 1992, 1993).

Other more recent research continues to support this connection between parental (usually mothers') expressiveness and children's ER. For example, in the context of an intervention to teach maltreating mothers to deal with emotional issues, positive family expressiveness predicted the children's ER 6 months later (Speidel, Wang, Cummings, & Valentino, 2020). Contrastingly, negative family expressiveness predicted the children's level of emotional lability (assessed via the ERC) 6 months later. The impact of parents' expressive patterns may be bolstered by their emotion beliefs:

Maternal positivity (supported by positive beliefs about children's emotions) also contributed to Korean children's ER (Cho & Lee, 2015).

Further, other recent investigations have shown that maternal positive expressiveness relates to children's specific ER strategy usage. For example, their positivity was related to 3- to 5-year-olds' use of cognitive reconstruction and problem-solving strategies and lack of venting; it also was associated with girls' ER via choosing an alternative activity (Chen, Wu, & Wang, 2018).

In a set of very complex findings, we found that mothers' observed balance of happiness over anger was negatively associated with their reports of preschoolers' use of avoidant strategies (e.g., distracting themselves, or leaving or ignoring emotional situations), but positively associated with teachers' reports of kindergartners' use of avoidant strategies (e.g., leaving the situation or distracting oneself, Denham, Bassett, et al., 2010; the same kindergarten finding held true for fathers' self-reported emotional balance).

We speculated that the maturing of ER between age 3 and kindergarten formed a possible explanation. That is, for younger preschoolers, when mothers are overall more emotionally positive, young children may have little need to leave when faced with emotionally difficult situations. In contrast, by the time children are mature kindergartners, their parents' positive emotional styles may have laid a foundation for the profitable use of distraction to maintain an even keel. Avoidance as a strategy may have changed in its predominant expression and meaning over time.

A negative emotional environment can provide a model for emotional *dys*regulation. Especially if directed at the child, frequent and intense negativity could promote preschoolers' ER difficulties (Thompson, 2014). For example, a cluster of toddlers' mothers defined in part by low positivity and high negativity (in this case, family conflict; Brophy-Herb, Martoccio, et al., 2013) reported that their 2-year-olds were less able to regulate their emotions.

Here too researchers have examined maternal negative expressiveness as it relates to children's specific ER strategy usage. For example, mothers' overall negative expressivity was related to 4-year-olds' more "negative" ER strategies, including passive reactions, venting, and self-comforting (Cheng, Wang, Zhao, & Wu, 2018). More negatively expressive parents also had 3- to 6-year-olds who used similarly maladaptive ER strategies (i.e., aggression, focus on a distressing object, venting, avoidance, and suppression; Mirabile [2014]).

> Colin's mother is often grumpy, abrupt, and displeased. Sometimes she yells. And then for a long time she shows no emotion. So it may not be surprising that when a playmate takes a toy from Colin, he doesn't talk about it; he hits.

As with emotion knowledge, it might be expected that exposure to nonhostile, safely expressed and managed "submissive" negative emotions (i.e., sadness, disappointment, rather than "dominant" negative emotions, e.g., anger) might allow the child to learn about ER. In one study, however, mothers' ratings of their own negative submissive emotions were positively related to their ratings of 3- to 8-year-olds' use of venting strategies (Goodvin et al., 2006). Although these results run counter to my hypothesis about "submissive" negative emotions, I consider that these connections have not been adequately tested yet.

Overall, in concert with the emotional environment hypothesis, it is likely that both emotional contagion and social learning are mechanisms for these findings. At the same time, a caveat should be highlighted—many of such studies' data emanate completely from maternal reports (e.g., Goodvin et al., 2006), again raising the issue of monorater bias. The general convergence of studies may largely obviate this problem, however.

At times maternal emotional expressiveness has been found to be especially related to daughters' ER. In one study, maternal negativity was related only to Chinese preschool girls' passive and venting strategies (Chen et al., 2018). We also found that preschoolers' mothers whom we observed to be *less* positively expressive (more happy than angry), but who self-reported *more* positivity, had daughters who used more constructive coping strategies. The self-report of expressiveness focused on several positive emotions (e.g., joy, gratitude, excitement, and affection), whereas we observed only happiness (Denham, Bassett, et al., 2010). Daughters who witness the wider range of positivity at home but also some negativity (e.g., the mild anger mothers were willing to express while being observed) may come up with constructive ER strategies, having a positive emotional substrate from which to work. Perhaps too daughters' close relationships with their mothers explains this unique relation, at least in part.

It also could be that parents' own ER (as modeled, regulated, or dysregulated emotion) is an important contributor to children's ER (Thompson, 2014). Thus parental dysregulation also contributes negatively to children's ER, often in concert with aspects of family emotional expressiveness (see also Milojevich, Machlin, & Sheridan, 2020; Ulrich & Petermann, 2017) or in conjunction with their less-supportive reactions to children's emotions (Price & Kiel, 2022). In contrast, parents' use of adaptive emotion regulatory strategies predicts better emergent ER in preschoolers (Davis, Suveg, & Shaffer, 2015b; Kao, Tuladhar, & Tarullo, 2020; see Zimmer-Gembeck, Rudolph, Kerin, & Bohadana-Brown, 2022, for meta-analytic results corroborating this relationship). Further, Are and Shaffer (2016) found that preschoolers' mothers who affirmed their own emotion dysregulation also reported less-positive family expressiveness and more negative expressiveness. Maternal dysregulation directly predicted children's overall ER, as well as more specifically their lability/negativity; it also indirectly predicted children's dysregulation via lack of positive expressiveness.

Another aspect of parents' ER that could be pertinent to their children's ER is lack of awareness of one's own emotions, which includes difficulties in both identifying and coping with emotions. Parents who are not aware of their emotions may have difficulty scaffolding children's ER in challenging situations and teach ER skills less ably. Thus, children witness parents' abilities to regulate emotions, so that parents' regulation or dysregulation, including their awareness of emotion, contribute to children's own ER. In support of these ideas, Brajsa-Zganec (2014) found that Croatian mothers' and fathers' awareness of their own and their preschooler's emotions were negatively related to the children's negativity (as an indirect index of their ER). Similarly, Crespo, Trentacosta, Aikins, and Wargo-Aikins (2017) found that mothers' lack of awareness of their own emotions predicted their children's difficulties with regulation.

## SUMMARY: Parents' Expressiveness and Children's ER

As following from emotion socialization theory, parental (again, usually mothers') positive expressiveness usually is associated with children's constructive ER, and their negative expressiveness follows the opposite pattern. However, the story is more complex, and some exposure to negative emotions, perhaps specifically for girls or boys, may be useful for the development of preschoolers' ER. Further, parents own ER is witnessed by young children as their parents dealing with their own expressiveness. Thus the contributions of parental dysregulation and general awareness of emotions are now being studied. Caregivers and parents could benefit from knowing how important their own emotions are to their preschoolers' ER.

## Parents' Reactions to Children's Emotions and Children's ER

Parents' responses when their children show emotions not only influence preschoolers' expressiveness and emotion knowledge; they also are very important to their developing ER, as well. Parents' positively expressed concern over children's need for ER fosters their awareness of and attention to their own emotions and subsequently their own ER. In contrast, negative, overbearing parental reactions to children's distress exacerbate child negativity and dysregulation, exemplifying punitive emotion socialization (see Eisenberg, Schaller, et al., 1988; Fabes, Eisenberg, & Miller, 1990; Grolnick et al., 1998). Overly strict sanctions about emotional expressiveness can motivate children to hide, not regulate, their emotions.

Several researchers have tested these possibilities even more specifically. Mothers reported on their means of responding to children's negative emotions (Eisenberg & Fabes, 1994; Fabes, Eisenberg, & Bernzweig, 1990). When they endorsed minimizing or punitive responses (e.g., "I tell my child that he is overreacting," or "I tell my child that if he starts crying, then he'll have to go to his room right away"), their children were more likely to try to escape anger situations, less likely to vent their emotions, and more likely to self-soothe and not to ask their mothers for assistance with ER. Perhaps they had learned only too well the price of showing or becoming involved in emotion. These outcomes of their mothers' reported reactions did not constitute optimal ER.

Mothers who evidenced distress about their children's negative emotionality (e.g., "I feel upset and uncomfortable because of my child's reaction") had children who were assertive when angry but did not vent their emotions and showed less-intense anger. These children shielded others from their difficult displays of feelings; they wanted to "deal with things" on their own.

The endorsement of problem-focused responses that encouraged the child's constructive action to deal with emotional challenges (e.g., "I help my child think of something else to do") were negatively associated with children's anger intensity, but positively associated with escape strategies. These children dealt with emotional issues in ways that defused their feelings, but relatively indirectly.

Mothers' emotion-focused reactions to children's negative emotions (e.g., "I comfort my child and try to make him or her feel better") were related to children's use of verbal objection as a means of coping with anger and were negatively related to the intensity both of anger and venting as a means of coping. The emotional needs of these children were met sufficiently, so that they "used their words" instead of ranting and raving.

Interestingly, the associations of most of these reactions to children's negative emotions with their ER strategies remained significant even when the contribution of child temperament was accounted for. Hence, mothers' socialization was important regardless of the children's own emotional reactivity. Supportive socialization in the form of emotion- and problem-focused reactions was most closely allied with children's adaptive coping.

More recent research has continued this line of investigation. In accord with earlier research, mothers' supportive reactions to children's negative emotions (e.g., encouraging emotions, focusing on the problem or emotion) positively relate to preschoolers' ER (Denham, Bassett, & Wyatt, 2010; McGee et al., 2022; Meyer et al., 2014; Spinrad, Stifter, Donelan-McCall, & Turner, 2004; Suh & Kang, 2020, found this linkage for girls only). More specifically, parents' supportive reactions predicted 6-year-olds' use of cognitive reappraisal a year later (Gunzenhauser, Fäsche, Friedlmeier, & von Suchodoletz, 2014). In contrast, parents who used unsupportive reactions to preschoolers' negative emotions (e.g., dismissing, punishing, and showing distress) are more likely to have children with compromised ER (Luebbe, Kiel, & Buss, 2011; Mirabile, 2014; Suh & Kang, 2020; Woods, Menna, & McAndrew, 2017), including their use of emotion suppression (Gunzenhauser et al., 2014). Recently, Mirabile (2015) also created a measure of parents' *ignoring* children's emotions; it was related to punitive and minimizing reactions and also to children's difficulties with ER.

Jeremy's mother is warm and approachable. When her son is upset because a classmate was mean to him (she shouted, "I'm not your friend!"), his mother listens and tells him, "That would upset me too," as she rubs his back that shakes with sobs. As he calms, she looks thoughtful. Then she says, "I have an idea. The next time she says a mean thing, maybe you could tell her, 'Stop talking like that' and go to another center to play." In one interaction, Jeremy's mother validates and comforts him, and gives him a problem-solving set of strategies. And next time his classmate is mean, Jeremy remembers and tries his mother's ideas, and he does come home feeling better. He has regulated his earlier emotions and succeeded in staying calm.

But Carrie's mother has a hard time tolerating her grouchiness that so often mushrooms into full-on tantrums. "Stop it! Be quiet!" she shouts when Carrie cries about being treated meanly by that same girl in preschool. When Carrie whines, "She called me names!!," her mother says, "Oh well. So what?" The next day Carrie gets very upset in preschool just at the sight of the mean friend. Her emotions are dysregulated.

Even more specifically looking at reactions to both positive and negative emotions, fathers who reported unsupportiveness to their 5-year-olds' negative emotions had children who they rated as having more trouble with ER (Shewark & Blandon, 2015). Especially when they were *less nonsupportive* of their children's positive emotion, their nonsupportiveness to negative emotions was related to the children's ER difficulties. These results highlight the importance of supportive reactions to children's positive, as well as negative, emotions. In this case, fathers' inconsistent contingent reactions may have amplified the contribution of nonsupportiveness to negative emotion: "Daddy only likes it when I smile. But I feel like crying right now and maybe he'll fuss at me."

We also found gender-differentiated contributions of parents' supportive and nonsupportive reactions to preschoolers' emotions. First, mothers' balance of observed reactions to their children's emotions (i.e., matching positive emotions + validating emotions + comforting + helping—responding with negative or passive emotions and behavior) was negatively associated with kindergarten teachers' ratings of children's venting (Denham, Bassett, et al., 2010). Mothers who more often showed the more supportive reactions to their children's emotions were good models of ER; they conveyed the sense that emotions were manageable. Second, the opposite relationship held true for fathers—their observed reaction balance was related to children's increased venting in kindergarten. Why this finding was confirmed was a bit of a puzzle. Perhaps again, the supportive style of fathers as playmates could reflect an "anything goes" attitude toward emotions, so that their children's later ER was compromised.

Earlier I considered that parents' modeling of their own ER is important for children's ER. In fact, the effect of parents' own approach to regulating emotions may be mediated by their reactions to their children's emotion, as well as their expressivity (Meyer et al., 2014). When positive reactions (i.e., problem- and emotion-focused reactions, encouragement of children's emotions) and positive expressivity were examined in conjunction with parents' attention to and regulation of their own emotions, mediation was indeed found: Children's constructive ER (attention–distraction, as well as problem- and emotion-focused strategies) was predicted by mothers' ER (attention to their own emotions and regulation of them) and the contribution of these emotional abilities was mediated by positive emotion socialization (positive reactions and expressivity). Thus again parents' ER is related to children's ER, but specifically as it promotes their positive emotion socialization practices. This study is unique in underscoring a path seen in Figure 7.1.

## SUMMARY: Contingent Reactions and Young Children's ER

Again based on emotion socialization theory, parental (and again, usually mothers') supportiveness often is associated with children's constructive ER, and their nonsupportiveness follows the opposite pattern; a recent meta-analysis corroborates this assertion (Zinsser et al., 2021). However, more work needs to address how parents react to positive emotions, as this area of inquiry generally has been neglected. Caregivers and parents could benefit from knowing how important their reactions are to their preschoolers' ER.

## Parents' Modeling of Specific ER Strategies

As I have noted for other aspects of emotional competence and socialization, parental reactions to children's emotions and their ER often are assessed by parent report. In studying children's ER, there again can be a problem of monorater bias (i.e., one person providing all the information in a report, thereby raising the issue of lack of independence of the construct's measures). Again, the convergence of studies helps somewhat in deflecting this problem.

It also is worth examining how parents teach children ER on their own. One intriguing report was unfortunately subject to monorater bias, although the problem was somewhat eased by its longitudinal nature. The study showed that parents' reports of their own ER strategies of reappraisal and suppression predicted 6-year-olds' use of the same strategies (Gunzenhauser et al., 2014). However, at least seven studies have carefully observed both aspects—parent emotion socialization and children's ER. In this case, the observed emotion socialization consists of naturalistically observed maternal strategies and children's subsequent ER.

Sometimes parents scaffold children's emotional experiences by demonstrating certain ER strategies that can assist children in regulating emotions themselves. For example, mothers used various strategies to aid the child when they and their toddlers (at 18 and 30 months) had to clean up toys and experienced having an ECG electrode placed on the child. These strategies were coded from their utterances following the child's positive *or* negative emotion, and included distraction, soothing, granting the child's wish, and bribery, as well as questioning and explaining the emotion. These strategies were related over 2 years later to children's own emotions and ER strategy usage during a disappointing gift task (Spinrad et al., 2004).

In this ecologically valid disappointment situation, in which children use display rules, the emotions and strategies shown were taken as markers of ER. Further, more display rule usage is expected when there is another, potentially evaluating, person present. Thus when mothers did not ignore their 30-month-olds and did provide strategies, their children later showed more positive emotion during the disappointment task, whether or not the experimenter was present, and less negative emotion in the experimenter's presence. The preschoolers were able to show positivity even in a potentially upsetting context and to inhibit negativity when it might be considered impolite.

However, focusing on specific strategies, when mothers had soothed their 30-month-olds, their 5-year-olds, apparently unable to muster any "front," or expecting to be soothed, showed less positive emotion when the experimenter was present. Similarly, preschoolers whose mothers had granted their wish at 18 months showed more negative emotion in either condition. Instead, when mothers asked questions about their 30- months-old's emotion, their 5-year-olds showed less negative emotion when the experimenter was absent. Such emotion conversations may have afforded children, over time, with greater knowledge of their emotions.

It is important to note here that the developmental appropriateness of some maternal strategies seemed to differ across the important 18- to 30-month period when so much ER and emotion knowledge development takes place. In this case, maternal strategies provided needed support for 18-month-olds, with resultant associations with children's ER at age 5. For example, when mothers had appropriately soothed 18-month-olds (as opposed to 30-month-olds), children were less likely to use *no* strategy during the disappointment task and more likely to use distraction. However, mothers' questioning of 18-month-olds (e.g., "Why are you crying?") may have been perceived as dismissive by children not yet old enough to have a good answer. Children of mothers who used such questioning showed a pattern opposite to that of young toddlers who had been soothed. In sum, this study offered some support for the view that mothers' ER strategy demonstration helped children to learn how to use independent strategies and remain emotionally positive when challenged later. Their strategies' effectiveness in terms of children's later independent ER also differed depending on when they were utilized.

Another study looked at mothers' demonstration of strategies with older children. When mothers used attention refocusing, cognitive reframing, and comforting strategies to aid their child during a disappointing gift task, their 4- to 7-year-old children did so as well. In addition, mothers' attention refocusing (especially with preschoolers) and joint attention refocusing, as well as cognitive reframing, were related to children's lessened sadness and anger (i.e., greater regulation) after their own strategy use (Morris et al., 2011). So the mothers' strategies helped in two ways: (1) as supported ER to help the children feel better and (2) as demonstrations of strategies that could (and did) work.

In another study that also examined the linkage between mothers' strategies and children's ER in real time, mothers and preschoolers experienced a challenging wait, in which mothers had to complete questionnaires and the child had only one boring toy to play with. Later, the children were presented with an attractive toy in a locked box but given the wrong key (Cole, Dennis, et al., 2009). When the mothers presented their children a strategy or other problem-focused reaction during the challenging wait, the children later managed the frustrating locked- box task less negatively and with less misbehavior. Also children whose mothers had provided them with strategies demonstrated less support seeking during the locked box task. In sum, in one short afternoon, mothers who provided supportiveness had children who regulated their emotions better when frustrated.

Longitudinal change in young children's ER can also be examined via naturalistic observation. Looking at a longer span of time within the larger study from which Cole, Dennis, et al.'s (2009) data was drawn, parental supportive responses to 18-month-olds' negative emotion, observed during a home visit, were related to growth in the children's use of distraction during the waiting task assessed from 18 months to 4 years (Ravindran, Genaro, & Cole, 2021). That is, parents' helping their toddlers to stay positive or persist in the face of frustration, assisting them in solving a problem, or otherwise aiding them in modulating their behavior predicted the children's growth in independent ER ability. More specifically, these supportive behaviors included (1) verbally helping the child understand the situation; (2) helping the child with attention—either sustaining it to solve the problem or, when necessary, shifting attention away; (3) helping the child delay a behavior or emotion; (4) helping the child work toward her or his goal; (5) acknowledging, explaining, or asking questions about their child's emotions.[4]

Another study utilized both maternal-report and observational measures of reactions to emotions across small time periods to examine dynamic changes in their support after their toddlers expressed negative emotions and disruptive behaviors during a snack delay (Ravindran, McElwain, Berry, & Kramer, 2018). Mothers reported on

---

[4]It should be pointed out that researchers' varying definitions of maternal strategies, although operationalized somewhat differently across studies, share essential commonalities.

their usual distress after the toddlers' negative emotions, and this propensity to feel distressed predicted declines in their observed support (defined as responding to the child's entreaties positively, providing explanations, praising, distracting, or validating the child's emotion) immediately after children's increases in either disruptive behavior or negative emotion. In other words, dispositional aspects of emotion socialization predicted moment-to-moment fluctuation in supportive reactions in the face of children's negativity. These generally more nonsupportive mothers struggled with giving supportive ER strategies to toddlers experiencing difficulty.

In an even more microanalytic examination of mothers' reactions to children's emotions, transactionality was again seen between mothers and their children (Chan, Feng, Inboden, Hooper, & Gerhardt, 2021). That is, when 5-year-olds and their mothers worked together on frustrating puzzles, children's lack of positivity predicted mothers' problem-solving responses 2 seconds later. When mothers showed approval of their children's actions and engaged in less problem solving, children were more positive 2 seconds later. The connection between maternal strategies and children's emotions was almost dialogic. This dialogic nature did not preclude inertia in specific responses, however; some continuity was found in maternal approval, problem solving, and comforting even given their dependence on child behavior; this inertia occurred most markedly for depressed mothers. Children's negativity also exhibited a level of inertia. The dialogue sometimes faltered.

Stepping back from these moment-by-moment within-dyad analyses, when children's aversive behavior was high in Ravindran et al. (2018), their mothers' supportive responses were associated with lower levels of between-group aversive behavior; the opposite was true for maternal self-reported dispositional distress to children's negative emotions. Thus again we see that examining moment-by-moment changes in ER is meaningful—in this case, watching maternal responses dynamically showed that supportiveness worked, especially when it was needed. But overall supportiveness was important too. Thus, the interplay of both dispositional and real-time supportive and nonsupportive reactions was related to toddlers' ER.

### SUMMARY: Parents' Modeling of ER Strategies

Parents demonstrate many ER strategies to their preschoolers—these behaviors are evident when they are summed across time and contexts, examined microanalytically in real time, or specified longitudinally. Reflection upon just what sort of ER strategies a parent or caregiver uses would be an important step if one wishes to influence a child's ER development. We do need to know more about these important and very specific types of reactions and more about differences related to the age or gender of the child or parent. Moreover, we need to learn about the important role of fathers in demonstrating and providing ER strategies.

## Parents' Teaching about Emotions and Children's ER

Parents' teaching about emotions may not be as direct a means of promoting ER as either expressivity or contingent reactions, but nonetheless could be important. For example, Thompson (1990) posited several ways in which parents' verbal discourse or conversations with children could contribute to ER. First, there are direct commands and instructions about emotions—the guiding and socializing language that my colleagues and I measure in examining children's and parents' naturally occurring discourse and reminiscing about emotions. Parents constantly try to aid their children in approximating cultural and family norms about the expression of emotions: "Stop that crying!" "We don't laugh at people like that when we beat them at games. It's mean!" Although it varies across families, this socialization pressure is always present to one degree or another and can be made explicit when parents talk about emotions.

Second, sometimes parents not only state the rules of expressiveness, but they also suggest clear ways of performing ER. As good coaches, they try to weigh the potential effect of stressful circumstances and then to think of solutions.

> Will the waiting-room time at a father's own doctor's office be just a bit too long for Carlos to tolerate? The father thinks it may be. He suggests that Carlos look at a book as a distraction: "We're waiting a long time. Let's look at a book so our wait will be happier."
>
> With her two children in tow, a mother remembers their last visit to her own mother as she pulls into the parking space in front of the house. Wisely, she not only tells Sophie and Sebastian, "You need to be kind to Grandma and not fuss about how you can't get good channels on her television," but also helps them redefine goals: "You might feel less frustrated if you don't even try to watch TV at Grandma's house. I'll bet it would be more fun to use her swing in the backyard."

Parents present their children with the full complement of ER strategies at one time or another, and often combine their exhortations with reference to the emotions children are experiencing.

Third, discussions about parents' own emotions affect children's ER by shaping their conceptions of emotion in general and of "big people's" ER strategies in particular. Is it normal to feel anger in a wide range of social interactions? In one of these situations, would it be perfectly okay to punch a hole in the wall? As already noted, preschoolers are keen observers of parental emotion; no doubt they also listen and glean much explicit and implicit information targeted at ER when parents talk about their feelings.

Fourth, a final way in which parents' teaching could contribute to ER is by managing what information is given to the child about potentially emotional events. Their attempts to lessen stress may include strategically omitting or deemphasizing information. For example, in foretelling the experience of camping in a tent, parents would not mention bears or even raccoons; when talking about learning to swim, they would not describe the "bottomless" feeling at the deep end of the swimming pool. An experience can also be redefined by parents, in a sort of preemptive ER: An injection will only "pinch, a tiny owie," or the feeling of a roller-coaster ride makes a person want to say "Wheeeeeeee! This is fun."

In fact, in one of our studies, mothers' reminiscing about positive emotions was associated with girls' less-frequent usage of avoidant ER strategies, and boys' less-frequent usage of venting (Denham, Bassett, et al., 2010). Similarly, maternal emotion language during a reminiscence task (i.e., total emotion words, coaching/elaborative questions and statements, validation) was negatively related to children's emotional lability (Ellis, Alisic, Reiss, Dishion, & Fisher, 2014). Beliefs about the importance of discussing emotions also can be related to preschoolers' ER. For example, beliefs such as "It is important to help my child find out what caused his or her anger" and "When my child is sad, I try to help him or her figure out why the feeling is there" were related to children's ER as assessed with the ERC, especially in conjunction with parental warmth (Yule, Murphy, & Grych, 2020).

However, some emotional experiences call for greater information in the service of ER, and some call for less. And some children feel more comfortable with more information, and some with less. Parents need to perform a delicate calibration so that this means of ER socialization by discourse does not backfire (Thompson, 1990). Recent support for this injunction, in which sensitive guidance in reminiscing about emotion was related to preschoolers' ER—both in terms of an initial level and of growth across an intervention for maltreating mothers (Speidel et al., 2020)—reminds us that sensitivity is always a watchword when living with growing preschoolers. In this case, mothers' sensitive guidance during reminiscences about emotions included (1) a focus on the task, (2) acceptance and tolerance, (3) involvement and reciprocity, (4) the resolution of negative feelings, (5) structuring, (6) adequacy of reminiscing, and (7) coherence of reminiscing.

### SUMMARY: Teaching and Children's ER

Parents' use of language does several things to promote preschoolers' ER: (1) state feeling rules and display rules; (2) suggest different ER strategies, and in particular strategies they themselves are using; and (3) manage the level of emotional situations they discuss with their children. These can be important teaching moments but also may require some finesse and emotional awareness on the part of parents so as not to overwhelm children. Much more work could be done in this important area to yield even more empirical results, and consider likely age and gender differences. Finally, this discussion of parents' emotional sensitivity leads to a broader discussion of overall positive parenting and ER.

## Overall "Positive Parenting" Influences on ER

The findings on generally positive parenting suggest that parents who are responsive, inductive, and warm—who are in close relationships with their preschoolers—have children who are emotionally well regulated and responsive themselves (Dereli, 2016). The structure and encouragement of autonomy implicit in authoritative parenting require and allow children to make ER attempts. More specifically, sympathetic parents help children cope effectively with their emotions when they are distressed. Accordingly, these children are less likely to become overaroused. Such parents are demonstrating supportive emotion socialization. On the other hand, conflict between parents and their children portends their preschoolers' ER difficulties (Dereli, 2016). In short, generally positive parenting pairs with more specific emotion socialization to promote preschoolers ER (Eisenberg, 2020); findings for both positive and negative parenting in fact extend to older children and adolescents (Goagoses et al., 2022).

### SUMMARY: Socialization of ER

All aspects of emotion socialization theory again are upheld for the socialization of ER. Parents' generally positive, rather than negative, expressiveness, and open display of their own ER strategies help give children exposure to the world of emotion, as well as convey the need to manage emotions for one's own and others' good. Supportive contingent responses are important here too, although more research on supportive and nonsupportive reactions to children's emotions and their effect on subsequent ER, especially in real time, could be useful. A particularly useful, new, and productive area of recent research, however, centers on parents' reactions to children's emotions that are actually modeled strategies that the children can use. Parents who discuss emotions often focus productively on ER in conversations and reminiscences. In general, further examination of age and gender differences could be useful here, as with other components of preschoolers' emotional competence. Overall, research on these means of emotion socialization is replete with possibilities that parents and caregivers can use.

## BETWEEN- AND WITHIN-PARENT CONSISTENCY AS SOCIALIZERS OF EMOTIONAL COMPETENCE

So far, although differences and similarities in mothers' and fathers' emotion socialization have been mentioned, especially in their contributions to preschoolers' emotional competence, my discussion has not gone as far as it might. Another important issue, especially in the socialization of reactions to emotions, is whether, and if so how, parents' emotion socialization works in concert. Perhaps having one parent who behaves supportively is "good enough" for positive child outcomes (Poon, Zeman, Miller-Slough, Sanders, & Crespo, 2017). Or having mothers and fathers who engage in a range of positive and negative emotion socialization practices, either singly or together, could promote optimal outcomes in children's emotional competence and behavior problems. These possibilities are uncovered at several developmental periods.

Differences between parents in emotion socialization has been found to be beneficial in one study. McElwain, Halberstadt, and Volling (2007) found that having one supportive and one nonsupportive parent was positively related to young children's emotion knowledge and lower peer conflict in boys. Greater support by both parents was associated with less-optimal functioning on these outcomes. Echoing arguments already suggested here, the authors speculated that high levels of supportiveness may shield children from emotionally challenging situations, hampering their ability to process emotional circumstances and learn about conflicts.

Colin's mother may be grumpy, but she does respond by suggesting solutions when he gets upset. He couldn't get his Legos to go together became very frustrated, throwing them around. She said, "My goodness, I believe you're very frustrated," gathered them up, and showed him one way to do it, which he then uses, calming surprisingly quickly. In contrast, when something similar happened when his dad was around, his dad said, "Hey, knock off that whining!!" Colin learned about the difference between frustration and whining from his parents' language but also by the way they reacted. Frustration can be tackled; whining is just not okay.

Although more studies are needed, it may be that such findings are restricted to Western cultures. That is, when mothers were less supportive and fathers were more supportive, Chinese preschoolers were rated as showing more internalizing emotions (Yu, Volling, & Niu, 2015), and when mothers were less controlling (i.e., less nonsupportive) and fathers were more controlling, children were rated as having more externalizing symptoms. These authors point out that fathers do the disciplining in China, so that their reactions are the most salient, especially when mothers' emotion socialization seems subdued. In any case, mixed emotion socialization messages, as noted for U.S. parents, do not appear salutary for young Chinese children.

These studies have focused on the differences between mothers' and fathers' approaches to emotion socialization. In contrast, Mirabile (2014) found that a slightly different type of within-parent inconsistency (i.e., negative expressiveness paired with punitive reactions to preschoolers' negative emotions—two seemingly contradictory manifestations of socialization, in that parents punished children for the very emotion that they modeled) was related to internalizing emotionality and maladaptive ER, but *also* to adaptive ER (self-directed speech, instrumental coping, information gathering, distraction, self-soothing, comfort- and support-seeking behavior). In this case, depending on the child, perceiving a parent who shows negative expressiveness and also punishes the child for negativity could overarouse *or* motivate efforts to comply with the parent's push for the child to control her or his emotions. Again, "mixed messages" may capture certain children's attention and, for some, promote emotional competence.

To sum up, much more work is needed to clarify these potential mechanisms and the boundary conditions under which differences between and within parents' emotion socialization are beneficial or detrimental.

## DIRECT CONTRIBUTIONS OF PARENTS' EMOTION-RELATED SOCIALIZATION TO SOCIAL COMPETENCE

Finally, the model of emotion socialization I have put forward in this book (shown in Figure 7.1) emphasizes that emotion socialization affects social competence indirectly via the mediation of children's emotional competence. But, of course, it is possible that the reassuring constellation of parenting strategies—positive expressiveness, supportive reactions, and teaching—makes a direct contribution to elements of young children's social competence. So, taking into account the influence of parent–child interaction on children's competence in the peer group, some researchers have examined the direct effects of emotion socialization techniques.

In one line of research, investigators have focused on parents' expressiveness as measured by specific emotions observed during interactions with their children. Not only should the children's expression of positive and negative emotion contribute to children's peer acceptance, but parents' expression of positive and negative emotion may also make a direct contribution (Butkovsky, 1991), presumably through the modeling of socially appropriate functioning in emotional situations.

In Butkovsky's (1991) study, mother–child and father–child dyads played a ball-toss game and a ring-toss game. Each child played four times, but the game was rigged: the child won the first and fourth trials but lost the middle two trials. Parents were given vague instructions requiring them to participate relatively passively in the experience. Nonetheless, their peak positive emotion was associated with their child's peer acceptance, especially for fathers and girls. The appropriateness of emotion was related to their child's peer acceptance, especially for sons and mothers. Thus, dimensions of parents' emotional competence—their positive and appropriate expressiveness—predicted their child's likability.

In another effort to study the direct contribution of family emotions to peer relations, Carson and Parke (1996) also utilized a game-playing context. Children ages 4 and 5, who had previously been identified as popular or rejected, and their parents played a "hand game." The object was for the first person to reach out and grab the other's hands before that person pulled their hands away. Popular and rejected preschoolers and their parents displayed different patterns of facial, vocal, and gestural emotions. Parents of rejected children showed more anger and more neutrality, whereas parents of popular children gave more emotion-laden guidance and apologized more.

Other researchers have focused on families' overall emotional environment in searching for direct links between family and peer systems. Kindergartners who varied in popularity were observed with their parents during dinner, and parents reported on emotional expressiveness in their families (Boyum & Parke, 1995). Results in this study were specific to fathers: Fathers who self-reported higher levels of expressiveness also showed more positive emotion and less negative emotion in the home. Fathers who reported more positive expressiveness overall and showed less negative emotion during dinner also had more popular children. So both specific expressed emotions and the overall emotional environment, particularly for fathers (who have been too often ignored in emotion socialization research), are important for young children's social competence.

Maternal and paternal expressiveness in the home and paternal emotions in a laboratory ring-toss game similarly predicted peer acceptance in yet another study (Cassidy, Parke, Butkovsky, & Braungart, 1992). An important addition to the general findings previously noted was that the children's overall emotion knowledge influenced this link between parental emotion and social competence. That is, statistically controlling for emotion knowledge in the prediction of peer status lessened the predictive strength of parental emotion. Although the total mediation effect predicted in Figure 1.2 was not upheld, the child's emotion knowledge buffered too-little or too-intense family emotion.

Parent–child emotional dialoguing also directly predicts social competence. In the Carson and Parke (1996) study, different sequences of child–parent emotions were revealed for popular and rejected children playing with same-gender parents. Rejected boys playing with fathers and popular girls playing with mothers showed more negative emotion reciprocity than their same-gender, opposite sociometric-status counterparts. The pattern for popular daughters and mothers is a bit difficult to explain (except to mothers of daughters!), but Carson and Parke noted that there were intensity differences in the negative emotion of the two dyad types. Popular girls, they reasoned, are learning assertion, as opposed to the aggression that rejected sons learn in interactions with their fathers.

Contingent reactions to children's emotions also directly predict social competence. Encouragement and support for children's emotions help them to express emotion acceptably and provide children with ways to deal with emotions *in the peer group*, which then influence evaluations of social competence. Punitive emotion socialization increases arousal and undermines the performance of socially competent interacting. In my own work, parents' self-reported and observed positive and negative emotions and positive reactions to their children's emotions predicted teacher-rated social competence even after the children's negative emotions in preschool and antisocial reactions to paternal emotions were accounted for (Denham, Mitchell-Copeland, et al., 1997). This set of findings suggests that not only parental expressiveness, but also parents' accepting reactions to their children's emotions predict social competence even when children's own emotional competence is taken into account.

Long-term outcomes have been reported by Hooven, Katz, and Gottman (1994). These researchers found that supportive, rewarding socializers of emotion had children who not only got along better with them, but also were better at handling their own emotions, were more popular, were more socially competent, and were even more physiologically relaxed. Amazingly, they also had higher mathematics and reading achievement scores by third grade. My interpretation of these findings is that emotional competence developed early gave these children a head start on the social aspects of schooling, so that they could focus on academics. As Goleman (1995) asserts, "the payoff for children whose parents are [rewarding socializers] is a surprising—almost astounding—range of advantages across, and beyond, the spectrum of emotional intelligence" (p. 192). In sum, these rewarding socialization techniques promote the integrated emotional organization of personality.

## SUMMARY: Direct Contributions of Emotion Socialization to Preschoolers' Social Competence

It is clear that emotion socialization techniques *may* directly influence social competence, without mediation by emotional competence (the direct contributions of various elements of parental coaching, such as their emotion language, have not yet been demonstrated). However, in the majority of these studies (with the exception of those by Cassidy and colleagues [1992] and by our group), there is no way of knowing whether emotional competence mediated the effects of parental emotion socialization. Elements of emotional competence in the preschool were not tested or rated.

But both direct and indirect mediated effects are possible, and they should continue to be explored. More explicit attention also should be given to *why* a parent's emotion socialization should directly predict the evaluation of another person's (the child's) social competence. Finally, an interactive approach also might be profitable—examining whether emotionally competent children of rewarding socializers are at the least risk for social competence problems (or vice versa; see Auerbach-Major, Kochanoff, & Queenan, 1997, for findings supportive of this proposition).

## OTHER SOCIALIZERS OF EMOTIONAL COMPETENCE: PEERS AND SIBLINGS

Usually we think of parents as socialization agents, with good reason. But the scanty research available suggests that researchers should also look at other aspects of social interaction, especially that with peers and siblings, to unearth other contributors to emotional expressiveness. It is clear that both peers and siblings exert modeling, coaching, and contingency influences on preschoolers' emotional expressiveness.

Interacting with other children is another important aspect of social experience that promotes the development of emotion understanding. A central tenet of Piagetian notions about emotion and intelligence is that socializing with others at one's level of development, in which negotiation and renegotiation are necessary, brings the young child to a new level of awareness (Piaget, 1977/1995). Peers' immaturity often leads children in the direction of punitive socialization; in peer situations, one's anger is often responded to in kind (Denham, 1986) and with escalated conflict.

> Jonathan's best friend is probably less patient than his parents about putting up with Jonathan's grousing about Donald. He tells Jonathan, "Be quiet!," and Jonathan learns more about the nuances of emotion—specifically, that complaining and fussing can stimulate answering annoyance.

Moreover, he learns that the social costs of such anger may include rejection by the peer group (Arsenio & Lover, 1997; Denham & McKinley, 1993; Denham, McKinley, Couchoud, & Holt, 1990; Lemerise & Dodge, 2008; see also Chapter 10). Children are likely to be gleaning unique socialization messages from their peers!

Another aspect of peer interaction is pertinent to socialization of emotional competence. Practice and experience in bouts of pretend play at 33 months (especially with siblings) was related to emotion knowledge at 40 months (Youngblade & Dunn, 1995). It is easy to imagine pretense, where one child acts the role of the crying baby and another responds as the comforting mother, as a stage on which a panoply of emotions is acted out. The participants feed each other's emotion knowledge. Intriguingly, more emotional children also engaged in more pretend play, which then stimulated their emotion knowledge. More positive mother–child and sibling–child relationships also were associated with a greater amount of pretend play.

Older siblings are particularly potent socializers of emotion knowledge, because their relationship with their younger brothers and sisters is characterized by power amid egalitarianism and love amid conflict. Strandberg-Sawyer and colleagues (2002) uncovered tantalizing indicators of this richness: When older siblings show a supportive socialization pattern, reacting positively to positive emotion, prosocially to negative emotion, and not ignoring either positive or negative emotion, their younger siblings demonstrate more proficient emotion knowledge. These younger siblings also were more prosocially responsive to their peers, were rated as more socially skilled by teachers, and were considered more likable by their peers (Sawyer et al., 1996). Similarly, cooperative interaction with older siblings is associated with preschoolers' contemporaneous use of more sophisticated emotion language and with their later ability to comprehend ambivalence (Brown, Donelan-McCall, & Dunn, 1996; Brown & Dunn, 1996).

Siblings teach each other about emotions via emotion language too. In Brown and Dunn's (1992) study, children's emotion language directed at siblings also was predicted by siblings' emotion language. So when the other member of a dyad uses emotion language, even a young preschooler is more likely to do so as well.

Another difference is that, in contrast to the complementarity seen in mother–child conversations even about mothers' own emotions, child–sibling conversations about feelings tend to be reciprocal, with each dyad member manifesting his or her own emotional point of view. This distinction is important. Coupled with evidence that preschoolers talk more about emotions with siblings and friends than with mothers (Brown et al., 1996), a transition can be seen from the "emotion language with mother" stage to the even more mature, social-competence-enhancing "emotion language with equals" stage. Hence the particular relationship between persons talking about emotion also makes a difference in the content of preschoolers' feeling-state conversations. Children learn about distinctive aspects of emotion from different conversation partners.

### SUMMARY: Peer and Sibling Emotion Socialization

Children's growing emotional expressiveness and emotion understanding are grounded in their own emotionality and in their own peer and sibling relationships: pretending, deceiving, teaching, joking, and comforting (Dunn, 1988, 1995). More research about these important socializers at the preschool level is needed.

## CULTURAL CONSIDERATIONS IN EMOTION SOCIALIZATION

Of note, culture, context, gender, and individual children's temperaments are obvious potential boundary conditions—does emotional competence "work" similarly for all children and groups, in all settings, and do notions of promoting it come as "one size fits all"? The answer is undoubtedly "no." For a deeper understanding, the reader is referred to Cole and Tan (2007), Friedlmeier, Çorapçı, and Benga (2013), von Salisch et al. (2022), and Trommsdorff and Cole (2011).

All beliefs and practices associated with emotions are created and interpreted within cultural and historical socially embedded contexts, such as the situational ecologies in which emotions and interactions actually occur, and how social–emotional events are evaluated (De Leersnyder et al., 2015). Thus, emotion socialization is situated within every culture's narrative regarding the child outcomes that are most valued, and the best ways to reach these outcomes.

Friedlmeier et al. (2011) have put forward clear descriptions of how and why preferred modes of emotion socialization differ across cultures that value either individualistic or collectivistic/relational emotional competence (whether based on nationality or ethnicity). The research described in this book most often emanates from Western, individualistic cultural values. These values permeate the very conceptions and expected outcomes of emotion socialization that already have been described here. Thus culture underlies the very notion that "optimal" emotion socialization includes being mostly emotionally positive; using care when expressing negative emotions; reacting supportively to children's emotions; discussing emotions; and being aware of children's emotions.

In contrast, within collectivistic/relational cultures, emotion socialization is often informed by the need to consider the interpersonal group and its needs, rather than those of the individual child. Such values may emphasize *not* encouraging emotional expressiveness—in fact, punishing it; negative expressiveness may be used more liberally to inform children of their need to refrain from their own expressiveness. Emotions may not be discussed because they need to be suppressed. Finally, child outcomes of such emotion socialization messages may be positive, although Western thinking would predict them to be negative. For any cultural narrative, it is imperative to understand *what matters*. What matters in any given culture may translate into similarly valued emotion socialization techniques, or it may translate into big differences, but it is imperative that we consider these issues.

## Expressiveness and Cultural Values for Emotion Socialization

At the same time, attention must be given to notions of culture, because this valuing of positive expressiveness over a relative excess of negative expressiveness may be distinctly Western, and encouraged in individualistic cultures where the focus is on the child's autonomous success in the environment. In contrast, non-Western, collectivistic/relational cultures may value an altogether less-expressive presentation of self, because of the goal of group harmony. In support of this possibility, Louie and colleagues (2015) found that for Korean and Asian American preschoolers, both their sadness and happiness expressivity were associated with negative peer or teacher outcomes. More value was perhaps placed on a calm demeanor for these children.

Regarding parents' modeling of expressiveness, American, Japanese, Hispanic, and Romanian parents described what could cause them to feel happy, sad, and angry. The four cultural groups showed a high level of consensus on how emotions are evoked by common events in young children's families (Denham, Caal, Bassett, Benga, & Geangu, 2004), and all the groups referred to both collectivistic/relational and individualistic issues. For example, happiness was usually evoked by children's endearing behavior or goal attainment and anger by difficult child behavior or marital issues.

However, Saarni (1998) urged caution regarding units of analysis in studying cultural issues, appreciating that similarities could mask differences in how parents elaborate on these themes. Thus looking more closely at why mothers said they would show emotions, American mothers' elaborations broadly fit a largely individualistic view, but Japanese mothers stressed common goals and the societal unacceptability of expressing (and even talking about) emotion, consistent with an overall collectivistic/relational view. For example, in discussing anger Japanese mothers noted, "We don't bring family problems outside . . . we avoid confrontation. . . ." These parents suppress certain emotions in the larger social context because of the need for peace and harmony, which may be interrupted by individual needs.

Hispanic parents also interpreted their emotions more relationally, but with more emphases on values within the family, including respect for others. Both Hispanic and Romanian parents mentioned hardship and injustice, with which they arguably have more experience. Further, underscoring Saarni's (1998) emphasis on viewing emotions in a social context, Hispanic and Romanian parents stressed expressing emotions differently with children and adults. Romanians referred to physical means of expressing happiness to children, but being more muted (e.g., smiling less) with adults. Hispanic parents described suppressing sadness around children.

In short, the parents of preschoolers in different cultural groups cite some similar antecedents for various emotions within the family but give different reasons for them and expressing them differently. Similarities in construing family emotions exist within larger societal culture in which specific expressive acts are nested. These broader variations capture where cultures stand on the collectivistic/relational and individualistic continua.

## Reactions to Child Emotions and Cultural Values for Emotion Socialization

Differences emerge between broadly collectivistic/relational and individualistic cultures when responding to child emotion. Chinese immigrant mothers endorsed supportive reactions to children's negative emotions that were equivalent to American mothers, but more often adopted reactions commonly considered nonsupportive (Yang, Song, Doan, & Wang, 2020). Similarly, Korean mothers suppressed emotion and shamed their preschoolers' emotions more than European Americans (Louie, Oh, & Lau, 2013).

Even supportiveness can vary across cultures (Çorapçı et al., 2018) when it serves different goals, such as helping children achieve individual goals or conform to social norms. However, despite these unique foci, parents in more collectivistic/relational cultures, like their individualistic counterparts, do sometimes also endorse reactions that are attuned to the child's individual needs. Although American, Turkish, and Romanian mothers reported many differences in their preferred modes of reacting to their toddlers' differing emotions (e.g., U.S. mothers endorsed discipline to cope with anger, whereas mothers from the more collectivistic/relational nations emphasized reasoning), all endorsed comforting their toddlers' fear and helping them solve problems related to anger (Çorapçı et al., 2018). Some goals regarding supporting children's emotions may be more universal.

## Teaching about Emotions and Cultural Values for Emotion Socialization

There also are cultural differences in teaching about emotions. European American mothers talked more about emotions than Chinese mothers while reading a wordless storybook with preschoolers (Doan & Wang, 2010). African American mothers' perception of racism predicted their use of emotion words while reading a storybook, perhaps preparing children for bias (Odom, Garrett-Peters, Vernon-Feagans, & Family Life Project Investigators, 2016).

## Relationship of Cultural Variations in Emotion Socialization to Preschoolers' Emotional Competence

Given these similarities and differences, how do cultural variations in emotion socialization relate to children's emotional competence? Despite numerous differences in how emotions are construed, valued, and expressed, collectivistic/relational and individualistic cultures' emotion socialization behaviors are often (but not always) similar in predicting children's emotional competence (Friedlmeier et al., 2011). For example, Chinese families' positive expressiveness predicted older children's ER (Gao & Han, 2016). Also supportiveness that was defined to include Chinese and Indian parents' valued collectivistic/relational practices, some of which are considered nonsupportive in individualistic cultures, was related to school age children's ER (Raval, Li, Deo, & Hu, 2018). In addition, mothers' nonsupportive reactions were negatively associated with European American primary grade schoolers' emotion knowledge and ER, but this association did not appear for the children of Chinese immigrant mothers (Yang et al., 2020).

Latina mothers' supportiveness also was associated with preschoolers' emotion knowledge, but nonsupportiveness also was (marginally) positively related (Pintar Breen et al., 2018). Thus, *non* supportiveness may have a different meaning in non-Anglo, individualistic cultures that emphasize obedience and proper demeanor within the context of warm parent–child relationships. The cultural value *respeto* emphasizes children's obedience and proper demeanor within an affectionate atmosphere. Given these findings, investigators suggested that what is generally termed *non* supportiveness may have a different meaning in this group (as with African American mothers previously discussed); that is, reflecting *respeto*, Latina mothers exhibit a mixture of warmth and control when responding to their children's emotions, and children, seeing this as normative, glean information about the nature of their emotions (see also Fiorilli, De Stasio, Di Chicchio, & Chan, 2015, who found that Chinese mothers demonstrated high scores on both teaching and dismissing approaches to children's emotions—somewhat similar values of emotional restraint within care and affection also may be operative).

Regarding teaching about emotions, Spanish parents' emotion labeling was related to preschoolers' emotion knowledge (Aznar & Tenenbaum, 2013). Similarly, European American and Chinese mothers' relative use of emotion language, despite cultural differences, related to children's emotion knowledge (Doan & Wang, 2010). Reactions to children's emotions may be more culturally specific in their nature and in their relationship to emotional competence, whereas talking about emotions may promote emotional competence in many if not all cultures.

Do cultural differences in emotion socialization impact the relationship between emotional competence skills with social and school success (see Chapters 10 and 11)? An approach to emotion socialization that is generally considered individualistic may be related to positive outcomes even in more collectivistic/relational cultures. First consider parental expressivity. For example, Chinese fathers' and mothers' positive and negative expressivity were associated with preschoolers' social competence in predicted directions (Liang, Zhang, Chen, & Zhang, 2012).

Contingent responding also bears examination. Latina mothers demonstrated more minimizing and ignoring of preschoolers' emotions than European American mothers (Lugo-Candelas, Harvey, & Breaux, 2015). Nonetheless, the association between supportive and nonsupportive reactions and behavior problems did not differ across groups. Chinese parents' supportiveness and nonsupportiveness were associated with older children's ER and dysregulation, respectively, which mediated relationships with behavior problems (Jin, Zhang, & Han, 2017). Further, in Yu et al. (2015), Chinese fathers' controlling responses to children's emotions were related to children's behavior problems. Thus, even when there are differences in aspects of emotion socialization, their association with social competence and behavior problems often can be similar across cultures.

Despite some similarity in emotion-related behaviors, and even though in several cases the outcomes of emotion socialization are similar in both individualistic and collectivistic/relational cultures, there do remain differences in both the endorsement of emotion socialization strategies and the concomitant outcomes. For example, Indian immigrant mothers were more likely than U.S. native mothers to endorse minimizing older children's emotions (probably because of their disruption to collective harmony). However, minimizing predicted only U.S. native children's negative outcomes (McCord & Raval, 2016). Perhaps it is considered so normative in Indian families that it does not motivate such outcomes.

Sometimes child outcomes are the opposite of those expected in more individualistic cultures (e.g., Louie et al., 2015). For example, Korean parents' controlling attitudes toward preschoolers' positive emotions were associated with fewer behavior problems and greater social competence (Lee, Eoh, Jeong, & Park, 2017). Collectivistic/relational emotion socialization prioritizes modesty; less exuberant, incurious children are viewed as more competent. As another example, Jin and colleagues (2017) found that *only* when mothers were more controlling regarding their preschoolers' positive emotions, was the children's emotion knowledge associated with lower behavior-problem and higher social competence scores. These investigators suggest that the Confucian heritage prioritizes collectivistic/relational emotion socialization, whereby children who embody modesty, and in this case also are more knowledgeable about emotions, are viewed as more competent.[5]

---

[5]See also the earlier material presented on African American families.

### SUMMARY: Culture and Emotion Socialization

Thus attention must be paid to make our conceptualization and measurement of emotion socialization culturally sensitive, informed by the entire corpus of belief that undergirds a culture's view of emotion. That is, conceptualizing what is optimal emotion socialization is to an extent culturally relative, such that care needs to be taken to know what are the goals for emotion socialization from a culture's perspective. Viewing the outcomes of emotion socialization across cultures also requires careful conceptualization and measurement, which needs to refer to emotional situations and parental reactions that make sense in a given culture. The promising work done so far needs to continue apace.

## OVERALL CONCLUSION ON EMOTION SOCIALIZATION AND A CALL FOR CONTINUED PROGRESS

Overall, there is much accumulating evidence pointing to various elements of parents' and other caregivers' modeling, coaching, and contingency contributions to the expressiveness patterns seen in young children. The emotions adults demonstrate, the ways they react to children's emotional experiences, and the ways they talk about emotions are valuable contributors to children's enduring patterns of emotional expressiveness. More research to flesh out the patterns of parental socialization more fully—in Tomkins' terminology, via not only parents' monopolistic emotional organization, but also their intrusive or competitive expressive profiles. Furthermore, fuller views clarifying the moderating influences of child age and gender, culture and ethnicity, and fathers' special contributions would be very useful. Even more work also needs to be done on the socialization of more complex emotions and display rule usage.

In addition, I would like to see more research on what lies behind all the correlational evidence that has accumulated. If maternal positivity predicts child positivity, for example, what actual cognitive, emotional, and social *processes* are at work to account for the association? Experimental paradigms, such as those discussed by Cummings (1995b), could be used advantageously.

# 9

# Teachers' Emotion Socialization of Preschoolers' Emotional Competence

## INTRODUCTION

Parents' substantial impact on young children's emotional competence was elucidated in Chapters 7 and 8. Given the contributions made by these adults who are so infinitely important in young children's lives, it follows that *teachers'* socialization of emotional competence will also promote social–emotional and even academic success in school. Preschool is rich in emotional experiences, and in this fertile context, young children learn about emotions through daily interactions with teachers (Bassett, Denham, Mohtasham, & Austin, 2020; Denham & Bassett, 2019; Denham, Ferrier, et al., 2020; Hyson, 1994). In addition, even when children are not directly involved in an interaction, they can learn about the emotional norms of their classroom through observing their teachers' socialization behaviors directed at others. Whether directly during interaction or indirectly via observation, preschoolers are experiencing teachers' expression and regulation of emotions, reactions to emotions, and teaching about emotions.

Considering the *overall* emotional support in preschool classrooms is not a new idea; for example, high levels of teacher emotional support and positive emotional tone in the classroom are related to better social–emotional outcomes for young children (Curby, Brock, & Hamre, 2013; Spivak & Farran, 2016). Examining broadly defined classroom emotional environments is very useful, but more research is warranted to flesh out more specific teacher contributions from an emotion socialization theoretical perspective: Preschool teachers clearly display emotions, react to children's emotions, and enact teaching about emotions (Ahn & Stifter, 2006; Ersay, 2015). Knowing about these emotion socialization behaviors and their contributions to preschoolers' emotional competence in more detail would be useful for teacher training and emotional competence programming.

In fact, early childhood educators in many nations do prefer to promote emotional competence via such incidental, implicit strategies (i.e., as opposed to programmatic curricula; Humphries, Williams, & May, 2018; Licardo & Purgaj, 2019; Loinaz, 2019). Teachers' emotions, reactions to children's emotions, and teaching about emotions, then, can be seen as important behavioral "kernels" of emotion socialization and the "essential ingredients" of promoting preschoolers' emotional competence, compared to the "brands" of curricula or the overall umbrella of classroom emotional support (Jones & Bouffard, 2012). Thus these more microanalytic emotion socialization behaviors, such as those I've discussed for parents, deserve to be studied.

The assertion that early childhood teachers are likely to engage in many of these more microanalytic emotion socialization behaviors previously observed in parents, and that these behaviors are important, derives from three circumstances. First, early childhood teachers spend significant amounts of time with children, performing emotion-laden caregiving tasks and providing individualized emotional support. Second, many teachers are trained to deal with emotionally charged events and, notwithstanding the importance of more microanalytic socialization behaviors, may have specific curricula supports that help them address the emotional development of their charges. Third, teachers categorize their own emotion socialization behaviors similarly to current theoretical models of emotion socialization and the empirical parent emotion socialization literature, suggesting that their role as emotional socializers may be compatible with these viewpoints (Denham, Bassett, & Miller, 2017).

So given the relative strength of the abundant literature on parents' roles in emotion socialization, as well as the similar roles that parents and teachers have as socializers and the increasing time children are spending in group settings, it might be assumed that there is a fundamental relationship between early childhood teachers' emotion socialization and young children's emotional competence. The relatively small amount of early childhood education research that exists on how teachers show emotions, react to children's emotions, and teach about emotions does in fact demonstrate that preschool teachers engage in a wide variety of discrete emotion socialization behaviors in the classroom that parallel those of parents (Ahn & Stifter, 2006; Ersay, 2007). Accordingly, teachers' emotion socialization behaviors, undergirded by their beliefs about emotions and their role as emotion socializers, are likely to send messages to children about specific emotions and emotion-related behaviors, contributing to children's emotional competence in some similar ways.

Thus preschool teachers are likely to be pivotal socializers of preschoolers' emotional competence (Denham, Bassett, & Zinsser, 2012). Supporting this idea, early childhood teachers in several nations consider emotional competence important and are aware of its foundations (Bridgeland, Bruce, & Hariharan, 2013; Ferreira, Reis-Jorge, & Batalha, 2021). They understand that emotion socialization consists of helping children feel comfortable expressing emotion within their social milieu, and that they want to create a warm, secure, comfortable environment where children's emotions are supported (Kiliç, 2015a). Further, they assert that their own emotional competence allows them to care for children and their emotions, and to use positive emotion socialization practices in the classroom, such as being good role models of emotional expression and regulation and supporting children's awareness and understanding of emotions (Türkmen & Ulutaş, 2018).

However, the contribution of early childhood educators' emotion socialization may sometimes vary from that of parents owing to several contextual differences. These differences point to potentially unique contributions of teacher emotion socialization—the sheer number of children in the classroom, for example, and the concomitant need for both structural and behavioral organization may dictate teachers' stricter reactions to emotions (Denham & Bassett, 2019). Teachers also may feel the need to project an emotionally calm demeanor in the classroom, despite the often-stressful nature of their work; they are subject to the "emotional labor" of displaying emotions that they may not feel (Brown, Vesely, Mahatmya, & Visconti, 2018; Shewark, Zinsser, & Denham, 2018). Such emotional labor may impact how they enact emotion socialization behaviors.

Other factors that could augur differences in how teachers socialize emotional competence, along with differential outcomes, include the following: (1) the differential amounts of time spent with children, (2) the special emotional tie between parents and children, and (3) teachers' need to assume an instructive role. That is, teachers' contributions to preschoolers' emotional competence might be less strong, less clear, or just different from their parents' contributions because children are exposed to the emotion socialization of teachers for smaller amounts of time or the teacher–child relationship is not as close as that between the parent and child.[1] Some early childhood educators also may not clearly endorse their role as emotion socializers, or they may feel that they need to emphasize other aspects of their job, such as promoting preacademic skills and/or maintaining an orderly classroom. So early childhood educators are likely emotion socializers, but their contributions to preschoolers' emotional competence may differ from parents at various points.

Even though teachers assert that emotional competence facilitates young children's development across many domains (Bridgeland et al., 2013), we still lack a thorough understanding of how early childhood educators can promote such competence in individual children via mechanisms of emotion socialization. That is, compared to the research on parents, very little has been published specifically about how early childhood educators promote emotional competence through the aforementioned emotion socialization behaviors. This assertion remains true even though the subject has attracted interest during the last 20 years (e.g., Ahn & Stifter, 2006; Bellas, 2009; Reimer, 1997), and despite an uptick in more recent investigations (e.g., Bassett et al., 2017; Denham & Bassett, 2019; Denham, Ferrier, et al., 2020).

What *do* we actually know about teacher emotion socialization? Despite the possible differences with parent emotion socialization, we can use the parent emotional socialization model and the empirical literature to make informed predictions about teachers' contributions to young children's emotional competence. Teachers do show

---

[1]Of course, these assertions may not always be the case; for example, children can develop very close attachment relationships with their teachers, which may even buffer them from the deleterious effects on their social competence as a result of insecure relationships with parents (Mitchell-Copeland, Denham, & DeMulder, 1997).

emotions, including both anger and joy (Fu, Lin, Syu, & Guo, 2010). They also encourage and discourage young children's emotional expression via a variety of behaviors, such as comforting, distraction, problem solving, punishment, or minimization, but they infrequently validate children's emotions (e.g., "It's okay to feel sad"; Ahn, 2005b; Ahn & Stifter, 2006; Ersay, 2007). Finally, they teach about emotions via their use of language (Ornaghi, Brockmeier, & Grazzani, 2011, 2014; Ornaghi, Conte, Agliati, & Gandellini, 2022; Ornaghi, Grazzani, Cherubin, Conte, & Piralli, 2015). I now review what we would expect in terms of outcomes for teacher emotion socialization, followed by the available evidence.

## TEACHERS' MODELING OF EMOTIONS

Teachers and children affect one another emotionally (Becker, Keller, Goetz, Frenzel, & Taxer, 2015; Curby, Downer, & Booren, 2014; Frenzel, Goetz, Ludtke, Pekrun, & Sutton, 2009), and teachers' emotions affect children's behavior in the classroom. In terms of predictions in this area, teachers' positive expressiveness would be positively related to preschoolers' positive expressiveness, emotion knowledge, and ER. Specifically, teachers' positive emotionality would help children express and experience calmer, more regulated positivity themselves, and render them receptive to learning about emotions in the new school environment. In contrast, intense teacher negativity would create an atmosphere where regulation and emotional learning is difficult. Occasional mild teacher negativity might help children learn about emotions, but inexpressive teachers would not provide a welcoming platform for such learning.

> The children in Ms. T's classroom see her emotions rather frequently. She gives a big smile when Jeremy comes into the room with his mother, and holds Sarah in her lap until she feels comfortable to enter activities for the morning. On the other hand, her "stern face," eyebrows down, and mouth a tight straight line, tells Joelle that she is NOT pleased when Joelle, fed up at last, hits Carrie. All the children recognize her sad face when she reads about a pet getting lost.
>
> In contrast, the children in Ms. A's classroom rarely see much at all in the way of overt feelings, because she firmly believes that a calm, unemotional mien makes for an environment more conducive to learning. At times, though, she yells when children misbehave, and once she starts, she might yell a lot. Her pupils really dread that.

There is probably a lot of variability in the emotions early childhood educators display, with likely differing impacts on children. Despite these predictions though, little research has yet targeted expressive modeling by teachers. In one of the first, still unpublished, studies, DeMorat (1998) examined a kindergarten teacher's emotions and four students' responses, over 3 months. The teacher most frequently showed emotions of pride and happiness; students matched her interest and happiness. She showed pride in acknowledging student achievements and used happiness to encourage their good behavior. Unfortunately, given the study's design, DeMorat (1998) did not note other child outcomes related to these teacher emotions.

Recent work has suggested that teachers' self-reported negative expressiveness was negatively related to older preschoolers' emotional positivity during peer interaction (Morris, Denham, Bassett, & Curby, 2013). Further, when Greek preschool teachers of 5- and 6-year-olds self-reported more positive expressiveness in the classroom, they rated their pupils lower on both anger and anxiety (Poulou, Garner, & Bassett, 2022). Moreover, their approach to behavior management interacted with their negative expressiveness, in that children had higher scores for anger when teachers reported both higher negative expressiveness and controlling, teacher-centered behavior management in the classroom. These authors speculated that teachers who showed more negative emotions and who believed that they should tightly control their behavior may more likely adopt other negative emotion socialization practices. In sum, older preschoolers' emotional expressiveness seems susceptible to their teachers' own expressiveness.

Results from observations of teachers' emotions with small groups of children go further; contemporaneous observations suggest that when teachers in the United States and Italy showed predominantly positive emotions in such interactions, so do the children (Denham, Mortari, & Silva, 2022); further, when children were sad, teachers reacted at the time with tenderness. Of course, the direction of effect is not necessarily from teacher to child; children's emotions can arouse teachers' emotions; notably, in one study, teachers' negative emotional expressions were more likely when children expressed negative emotions (Garner, Bolt, & Roth, 2019).

Some of our recent longitudinal findings have been specific to children living in different socioeconomic environments; for example, where teachers showed more tenderness while interacting in small groups of children, low-income children showed more verbally expressed ER with peers (i.e., talking about something that was upsetting) and exhibited more productive play (Denham & Bassett, 2019). In that study we found that teachers' *observed* affective balance (i.e., more happiness than anger) also was related to all children's emotion knowledge, but in another study, teachers' *self-reported* positivity was more strongly positively related to low-income children's emotion knowledge (Denham, Ferrier, et al., 2020). Children at socioeconomic risk also showed emotion knowledge difficulties that children not at risk did not; these children may have especially needed teachers' emotion socialization input, the support of their emotional positivity creating an emotionally open environment.

In contrast, several of our findings have run counter to those generally found with parents and may be unique to the classroom context (Denham & Bassett, 2019). For example, children displayed greater ER and involvement in play when teachers across all classrooms were less affectively balanced (i.e., less happy, angrier). These findings were most pronounced in low-risk classrooms; in fact, children in high-risk classrooms were emotionally regulated and productive where teachers were happier and *less* angry. Sadder teachers in low-risk classrooms also had more emotionally regulated, productive children. Most of these findings contrast with findings with parents, where maternal positivity is related to preschoolers' ER (Are & Shaffer, 2016; Cho & Lee, 2015).

Tamikka and Lorene were very mad at each other over a toy Lorene had brought to childcare. Lorene accused Tamikka of taking it and putting it in her own cubby, and Tamikka vigorously denied this. Squatting down, their teacher put an arm around each of them, listened to both sides, and tried to get them to discuss the problem. Much finger pointing ensued, with angry words not defusing the situation. The teacher sighed, looked downcast, and said a bit grumpily, "You two try my patience," as she stood up and stiffly walked away. Later, it turned out that the two had solved the problem and were playing amicably in the dress-up area. Their teacher had been tenderly supportive but also let them know that their fretting was not an acceptable outcome.

Why might angrier, less happy, and even sadder teachers spur some children's ER and productivity? In our observational system, we noted that both emotionally negative/dysregulated and emotionally regulated/productive behaviors originate with a frustrated, often angry child; in the case of the emotionally regulated/productive behavior, children are distressed but then calmly use words to feel better and continue with focused play. Teachers in classrooms where children show the negativity that spurs regulation may show their own negative emotion in response, without considering the aftermath of shared teacher–child negativity. Dealing with multiple emotional preschoolers at any one time—over weeks—is not easy. Young children, when faced with a somewhat frequently sad or angry teacher might feel "on their own" in emotional situations, but also become motivated to marshal personal resources to express fewer negative emotions and use words to modulate those they do express. Whether these contributions of aspects of emotion socialization, so often considered nonoptimal in the family literature, continue to have salutary effects would require longer-term longitudinal investigation.

### SUMMARY: Teachers' Expressiveness and Young Children's Emotional Competence

More research obviously is needed, but there are some empirical data suggesting that teachers' positive emotions (e.g., happiness, tenderness) are related to young children's emotional competence—for example, their own positive emotions and emotion knowledge. Some findings occur mostly when studying children living in poverty; perhaps teachers are especially potent emotions socializers for them. Further, other findings seem at odds with what is known of parents' emotion socialization. Finally, some of their negative emotions, especially where children in their classrooms were not at socioeconomic risk, seemed to motivate preschoolers to "buckle down," deal with their emotions, and get on with their play. Clearly replication and extension of these findings are needed.

## TEACHERS' REACTIONS TO PRESCHOOLERS' EMOTIONS

Young children absorb not only the content, but also the form and quality of teachers' emotional support (Dunn, 1994). They watch and learn. To examine just what sort of reactions to children's emotions teachers perform, Ahn (2005a) and Ahn and Stifter (2006) carefully described such contingent responding to children's emotions. In her work, teachers encouraged positive emotional expression and responded positively to it. In response to children's negative emotional expressions, teachers demonstrated positive responses, such as empathy, physical comfort, distraction, problem solving, and ignoring, and negative responses, such as restriction, threatening, ridicule, punishment, or minimization of children's expression.

Based on these descriptions, several predictions can be made about what to expect regarding early childhood educators' reactions to children's emotions (Kurki, Järvenoja, Järvelä, & Mykkänen, 2016). We expect that teachers' supportive reactions to children's emotions, such as validating them (e.g., "It's okay to feel sad"), helping to solve a problem, or comforting would be positively related to children's positive expressiveness, emotion knowledge, and ability to regulate emotions. Encouraging responses from teachers could assist children in both tolerating and regulating emotions, teaching them that emotions are okay to show and are moments for sharing, and that emotions are manageable and even useful. Finally, supportive reactions would help children to "stay in the moment," and to thereby learn more about emotions.

So some teachers are supportive in response to preschoolers' emotions.

> Sebi cries because other kids at the table are choosing some stickers and he can't reach them. His teacher comes over, sits by him, and looks through the stickers with him to find a nice one.
>
> Carrie is upset and frustrated because her leggings got wet while playing at the water table, crying "It's water! it's water!" Her teacher tries to dry her leggings with napkins, saying, "Water on your leg like this bothers you? It would bother me too!"
>
> Kara is jumping and singing, "Jumpy, jumpy." Her teacher smiles; and touches her head as she walks by.

As for the empirical results related to these predictions, we have found that teachers' supportive reactions to preschoolers' emotions contributed to children's positive expressiveness and social skills, negative expressiveness and aggression, and ER, in expected directions (Bassett et al., 2017). Further, although Ahn's work (Ahn, 2005a; Ahn & Stifter, 2006) demonstrated that early childhood teachers rarely validate that children's negative emotion are okay to feel and express—one of the major tenets of positive emotion socialization –when they do, observers report a greater prevalence of positive emotion and prosocial behaviors in the classroom (Bassett et al., 2017; Karalus, Herndon, Bassett, & Denham, 2016). Even more specifically, such positive emotion socialization techniques are related to the successful resolutions of tantrums (Shafer, Wanless, & Briggs, 2022). We also found that teachers' positive reactions to children's emotions were related to their emotion knowledge in socioeconomically high-risk classrooms (Denham, Ferrier, et al., 2020).

Punishing and minimizing children's emotional display would be deleterious to the development of emotional competence. For example, preschoolers would learn not to show emotion to avoid punishment or to feel bad about themselves when ridiculed, belittled, or ignored. Adaptive responses to children's emotions also would support their social competence and academic success; the converse would be true for their punishing or minimizing reactions.

Erica called, "Ms. Mary, Ms. Mary!!" She was smiling and trying to show or tell the teacher about what she was painting. Her teacher did not respond or even look her, and just kept walking. Joey looks downcast when his father leaves the classroom, and his teacher says, "Don't be such a baby! Do I need to tell Daddy what a baby his boy is?"

We found that teachers' dismissing reactions were negatively related to 4½- to 5-year-olds' positive expressivity and emotion knowledge (Morris et al., 2013). Similarly, a lack of nonsupportive reactions (e.g., minimizing or punishing children's emotions) facilitated development of children's emotional positivity, prosociality, and ER (see Berlin & Cassidy, 2003, and Luebbe et al., 2011, for similar findings with parents).

In another of our studies (Denham, Ferrier, et al., 2020), the lack of teachers' self-reported punitive reactions also facilitated the development of children's emotion knowledge (see also Perlman, Camras, & Pelphrey, 2008). Then when faced with a teacher who is regularly punitive about their own and others' emotions, preschoolers might be sufficiently aroused to mute their positivity, and as with parents their arousal also may render them somewhat avoidant of emotional information surrounding the expression or experience of emotion. It appears that punitive and dismissive responses to children's emotions, separately and cumulatively, can contribute to variability in preschoolers' positive, sympathetic emotions and emotion knowledge in ways we would expect from the parental emotion socialization literature.

However, again the pattern of findings for teachers' reactions to children's emotions may not always parallel parental emotion socialization findings in the literature. To pinpoint an already reported finding, when teachers were observed to show nonsupportive reactions (i.e., punitive and/or minimizing) to children's emotions, children were *less* emotionally negative/dysregulated when interacting with peers (Bassett et al., 2017; Denham & Bassett, 2019); in general, the opposite pattern is found for maternal nonsupportiveness (Berlin & Cassidy, 2003). Teachers dealing with multiple children in classrooms where children show such negative emotional behavior may use nonsupportive reactions to quell these emotional outbursts. Again, as with teachers' negative emotions, such reactions send a message: "Stop that behavior!" Teachers are applying socialization pressure for preschoolers to conform to group settings.

However, different nonsupportive reactions may have dissimilar effects. Thus, in contrast to the negative contributions of teachers' punitive responses to children's positive emotions, teachers' minimization seemed at times to convey a different message than that documented in the literature for parents (Denham, Ferrier, et al., 2020; cf. Denham, Mitchell-Copeland, et al., 1997). This message again appears unique to the classroom context: Specifically, children displayed greater emotion knowledge when teachers self-reported that they minimized children's negative emotions. Minimization (e.g., telling children that they are overreacting or behaving immaturely), unlike punitiveness, may focus children's attention on their own and others' emotions, with subsequent attentiveness to teachers' emotion socialization and consequent gains in emotion knowledge.

Perhaps when parents use minimization, preschoolers feel disparaged, but in a classroom where a premium is placed on behavioral regulation of the group, the message's meaning is different; it's less hurtful and more a reminder that "regulating your emotions in school is important." The contribution of teachers' minimizing reactions, as already noted, differs for toddlers, who may be unable to glean the message suggested here (King & La Paro, 2018). It may also be different for other aspects of social–emotional behavior such as prosocial behavior or compliance (Morris et al., 2013). Finally, such teacher emotion socialization might interact with the emotion socialization to which preschoolers are exposed at home. Obviously, a fuller picture is needed.

Of course, not all teachers' contingent responding to children's emotions is either supportive or nonsupportive (Kurki et al., 2016). Very often teachers may respond to children's emotions with verbal directives or information gathering, for example, both of which could be rather cut-and-dried means of expediently keeping classroom activities running smoothly rather than attending to children's emotional development.

## Moderators of Teachers' Contingent Reactions: Child Age, Gender, and Temperament

No doubt, an important first step is to know how teachers' supportive and nonsupportive reactions to children's emotions occur and that they make contributions to preschoolers' emotional competence that are both similar and justifiably dissimilar to those of their parents. It also should be noted that teacher responses to child emotions and the concomitant associations with children's emotional competence may differ by child age, gender, and temperament.

Accordingly, it has been noted that more socialization reactions are targeted at younger rather than at older preschoolers (Ahn, 2005a; Ahn & Stifter, 2006; Kiliç, 2015b; Silkenbeumer, Schiller, & Kärtner, 2018). Just entering the peer world and facing the demands of interacting in a group with peers and teachers are more emotionally demanding for these children whose emotional competence is less advanced. So, younger preschoolers' teachers were more encouraging, especially of positive emotions, and used affection, physical comfort, and distraction in response to children's negative emotions more often than older children's teachers, who relied more on verbal mediation.

However, teachers of younger preschoolers also more often minimized younger children's negative emotions (Kiliç, 2015a). In general, early childhood teachers appear very focused on having their students, especially the youngest, develop independent ER (Ahn, 2005a; Ahn & Stifter 2006; Karalus et al., 2016; Reimer, 1997). Their more frequent efforts to tailor specific reactions to children's emotions exemplify this goal. Productive techniques aimed at aiding preschoolers' ER also may be more generally rooted in the children's ER proficiency, with more meta-cognitive prompts given to preschoolers who could make use of them (Silkenbeumer et al., 2018).

But relying on minimizing language ("You're not sad" or "Stop that whining, you're a big girl!") to promote ER, especially with toddlers, seems less than productive in developing emotional competence. For example, minimizing language shown by toddlers' (12- to 36-month-olds) teachers was negatively related to the children's social–emotional competence (including empathy, prosocial behavior, and compliance; King & La Paro, 2018).

The gender of the child showing the emotion also may matter. Some supportive reactions from teachers may differ for girls as compared with boys. For example, in one study, teachers' reactions to children's emotions were observed while they were engaged in free play, group play, and outdoor play. After children's positive emotional displays, teachers showed more physical affection and comfort, as well as encouragement of both expressing positive emotion and showing empathy, to 4- to 6-year-old girls, compared to 4- to 6-year-old boys. They used verbal support after positive emotion displays (without emotion language) more with boys (Kiliç, 2015b).

Regarding children's negative emotional displays, teachers showed girls more physical affection and comfort. In contrast, they responded to boys' negative emotional displays with more empathy, problem-focused solutions, regulation assistance, and even encouragement to express negative emotions. Nonsupportive reactions may differ by child gender too; Kiliç (2015b) found that teachers matched girls' negative emotions more than boys', but minimized and ignored boys' emotions more (see also King, 2020, who found minimizing language directed especially at boys' sadness).

Responding positively to girls' positive emotions and disapprovingly to girls' negative emotions, even while showing them physical support, seem akin to socializing behavior (e.g., "being nice and not upset" and "helping people with emotions") being treated uniquely as a female attribute. In contrast, boys' negative emotions elicited more support and even encouragement (Kiliç, 2015b). As Ahn and Stifter (2006) suggested, boys may be more negatively emotionally volatile at these ages, seemingly requiring this combination of supportive reactions. Nonetheless, this set of reactions, too, seems to send a gendered message that boys' negative emotions are generally ok. But boys also may get mixed messages: Minimizing their negative emotions, according to King (2020) shows a very early gendering of negative emotionality. Moreover, this side of such a mixed message can have a negative impact on boys' social–emotional development.

Children's temperamental dispositions also must be considered, because these propensities may be related to variability in how children perceive their teachers' emotion socialization behaviors. So, some of our findings occurred particularly for children with low-surgent temperaments (Bassett et al., 2017). Specifically, more reticent children especially were less emotionally negative and/or aggressive with peers when teachers were observed to show more supportive reactions, and less emotionally regulated when teachers showed more nonsupportive reactions. We speculated that low-surgent children were more likely to be vigilant in observing their teacher and more sensitive to teachers' emotion socialization.

## SUMMARY: Teachers' Reactions to Children's Emotions and Preschoolers' Emotional Competence

Reactions to children's emotions are powerful socialization mechanisms; directly reacting (or even *not* reacting) are specific messages to children. Thus, many contributions of teachers' supportive and nonsupportive reactions resemble the parent literature. However, teachers' contributions to preschoolers' emotional competence don't always resemble the contributions made by parents—at times, their nonsupportiveness seems to convey a different message: for children to stop their negative behavior or regulate their emotions in general. This different message sometimes can have a positive rather than a deleterious effect on developing emotional competence. Moreover, it is important to consider that early childhood educators do show differential reactions to the emotions of younger and older preschoolers, girls and boys, and children of differing temperaments (being less tolerant of older children's and girls' emotions). These different patterns of response may explain the differential qualities of emotional competence in these groups. As usual though, much more research is needed on all these topics pertaining to teachers' contingent reactions to preschoolers' emotions.

## TEACHING ABOUT EMOTIONS

What would we expect in terms of how teachers talk about emotions? It is to be expected that teachers who discuss emotions, the way parents do, give children tools that can be used in expressing, regulating, and understanding emotions. Thus teachers who discuss emotions would help children feel better or figure out ways to do so, helping them in expressing and regulating their emotions. Through such direct tutelage that is neither misleading nor idiosyncratic, teachers also could help children learn much about emotions. In short, teachers' individual or even group emotion conversations with children are key parts of the emotional scaffolding that are a central, active ingredient in emotion socialization (Park, Tiwari, & Neumann, 2020). Consider an extended conversation between a rather emotionally competent little fellow and his helpful teacher.

> At resting time, Jeremy and his teacher are talking quietly about why he cried today when Kara Anne took his toy. This behavior was unusual, and his teacher wanted to explore it. "It seemed like you were so sad today when Kara Anne took your Power Ranger. You didn't use words to talk about how you felt." "I know [Jeremy's face puckers a little in recollection]." "Why do you think you were so sad?" "I don't know." "Maybe you feel kinda bad today because Daddy and Mommy are going on a trip tomorrow." [Jeremy sniffles and nods.] "It's okay to feel sad about that. But everything will be all right; I know your Nana and Papa will be with you, they love you. And I'm here at school too."

Empirical results that support these predictions about how early childhood educators teach children about emotions are emerging. First, they do use emotion language in the classroom, although they do so relatively infrequently (Ahn, 2005a; Yelinek & Grady, 2019). They explain and question during teacher-led activities and use socializing and guiding language during free play (e.g., "We smile when we say hello," "You can pound these blocks if you're mad"). Teachers' emotion-related discussions with preschoolers, more than with toddlers, help children infer the causes of their negative emotions and teach them constructive ways of expressing negative emotions (Ahn, 2005b). Moreover, Kolmodin (2007) found individual differences in teachers' propensity to talk about emotions with preschoolers, not unlike those of their parents.

Teachers' propensities to talk about emotions can translate into classroom practice. For example, book reading is a noteworthy outlet for emotion socialization, especially useful because children can identify with and share the story character's emotions, applying story characters' experiences to their own emotional challenges (Garner & Parker, 2018). So it is not surprising that when teachers read books that include an enriched emotional lexicon, and then talk about them, children show growth in emotion knowledge (Grazzani, Ornaghi, Agliati, & Brazzelli, 2016; see also Bergman

Deitcher, Aram, Khalaily-Shahadi, & Dwairy, 2020, for concordant cross-cultural results). An emphasis on the added value of discussing the emotional content of books is the focus of Grazzani and colleagues' (2016) research program; informal but elaborative conversations about the emotional content in books imparted added value. And, as noted in Chapters 7 and 8, discussing emotions with children who are not themselves particularly emotionally aroused—or optimally empathically aroused—can be a productive technique.

Expanding on these ideas, the *picture-book-storytelling* context may be a particularly rich one for the acquisition of emotional competence and should be made explicit in books for preschoolers and during the classroom day (Alvarenga, Zucker, Tambyraja, & Justice, 2020). Teachers can elicit both toddlers' and preschoolers' emotion language in such a setting, with beneficial effects on their social–emotional behavior and emotion knowledge; research with parents supports this position (Alvarenga et al., 2020; Drummond et al., 2014; Martin & Green, 2005).

Furthermore, in comparison with other settings, more elaborative discussion of emotion transpires during picture book reading—probably because the plot of even a wordless book, replete with illustrations of emotions (or perhaps *especially* a wordless book, where teachers' creativity can blossom), can allow adults to highlight emotions in a way most other contexts cannot. In fact, the freedom of storytelling rather than reading may lend itself to wider-ranging emotion discussions (Ziv, Smadja, & Aram, 2015). Further, reading emotion-laden picture books may increase preservice teachers' references to emotions, which could translate into a greater use of emotion language when they enter the classroom (Garner & Parker, 2018).

Talking about negative emotions during picture book reading has been shown to be particularly useful in promoting emotion knowledge for children living in poverty (Denham, Ferrier, et al., 2020). Explaining the importance of talking about negative emotions makes sense given the context of emotion knowledge development. That is, teachers' references to negative emotions during book reading thus may be especially useful to children living at socioeconomic risk, given their needs in the area of emotion knowledge and their exposure to negative emotion (Denham, Ferrier, et al., 2020; Garner, 2006; Raver, Blair, Garrett-Peters, & Family Life Project Key Investigators, 2015).

These teachers' linguistic focus on positive emotions and on clarifying emotions made sense given that the level of emotion knowledge in these children was lower, with teachers highlighting "easier" emotions and scaffolding the discussion more. Knowledge of positive emotions develops earlier than negative emotion knowledge, which continues to develop throughout preschool (Denham & Couchoud, 1990b).

In addition to examining the amount of positive and negative emotion talk and the discrete functions of emotion talk (e.g., clarifying), several picture-book-reading styles of preschool teachers also have been identified. Several such styles relate positively to children's growth in emotion knowledge (Bassett et al., 2017). For example, children whose teachers used more questions for explaining the causes and consequences of characters' emotions (e.g., "Do you think she is sad because the ball fell in the river?") showed greater growth in emotion knowledge than children whose teachers did not. Moreover, teachers' use of explanation in a nonquestion form (e.g., "She is sad because the ball fell in the river") did not relate to preschoolers' emotion knowledge.

So, as has been found with parents' emotion socialization, it appears that questions are more effective in engaging children's thinking about emotions. In addition, teachers' use of other specific strategies (e.g., connecting a story to children's life or brainstorming about a story-related concept) promoted growth in children's emotion knowledge.

A few age- and gender-related differences in how teachers teach about emotions were also identified by Kiliç (2015b). Teachers discussed their own positive emotions and labeled negative emotions more in response to 4-year-olds' emotions than to 5- and 6-year-olds' emotions. They labeled positive and negative emotions more in response to girls' rather than boys' emotions. Again, younger children probably require (and can make use of) emotion language, and by talking more to girls teachers are perpetuating the gendered message that emotions are the purview of females.

### SUMMARY: Teachers' Conversations about Emotions and Young Children's Emotional Competence

Teachers' conversations about emotions seem very powerful for preschoolers' emotional competence, especially for emotion knowledge. The storytelling and picture-book-reading contexts offer natural jumping-off points for language about emotions to emerge. Further, teachers' questions about emotions seem to engage children in the dialogue and promote growth in emotional competence. Finally, as is so often found, there are age and gender differences in early childhood educators' emotion talk, and this mechanism of the socialization of emotion has particular value for children living in poverty. Even more detailed research for how to promote this aspect of teachers' emotion socialization is warranted.

## TEACHERS' BELIEFS

What teachers *believe* about emotion socialization also can be revealing because beliefs can motivate behavior. Ahn (2005a) noted that her observations of Korean early childhood educators showed a congruence between their emotion-related beliefs and emotion socialization behaviors. As I noted for parents, then, teachers' emotion-related beliefs can be important foundations for specific emotion socialization behaviors. For example, accepting beliefs about children's emotions promoted teachers' supportive reactions to children's emotions (Swartz & McElwain, 2012). Specifically, teachers reporting more accepting beliefs about children's emotions exhibited more supportive responses to children's negative emotions, but only when they also reported high levels of reappraisal in their own approach to ER. In this study, teachers' beliefs *and* their own emotional competence, an important topic to which I return, worked together to inform their emotion socialization behaviors.[2]

In contrast, in one study, teachers' lack of belief that instruction and/or modeling about emotions is important and their belief that one needs to protect children from emotions were related to dismissing, nonsupportive reactions (Ornaghi, Agliati, Pepe,

[2] In ongoing work (Denham & Ferrier, under review), we are finding that preschool teachers' beliefs and emotional competence form a foundation for their self-reported emotion socialization behaviors.

& Gabola, 2020). So it appears that beliefs can underlie both supportive and nonsupportive reactions to children's emotions.

Early childhood educators' beliefs about children's emotions and educators' role regarding them also can contribute directly to preschoolers' emotional competence. In one of our early studies, preschool teachers who valued teaching children about emotions also had students who exhibited more adaptive ER (Denham, Grant, & Hamada, 2002). More recently, we have found some ways in which teachers' beliefs contribute to children's emotion knowledge, albeit in socioeconomically high-risk classrooms only: when teachers valued teaching about emotions, adopting "emotion coaching" beliefs (i.e., When a child is sad, I try to help the child explore what is making him or her sad"), children demonstrated greater emotion knowledge (Denham, Ferrier, et al., 2020).

### SUMMARY: Teachers' Beliefs about Emotions and Young Children's Emotional Competence

Much less research on preschool teachers' beliefs about emotions and emotion socialization has been performed. What is known suggests that, as is often the case, beliefs motivate behavior and may be related directly or indirectly to preschoolers' emotional competence. Exploring the importance of teachers' emotion-related beliefs could benefit understanding of their emotion socialization and its contribution to preschoolers' emotional competence.

## PROFESSIONAL CONSIDERATIONS FOR BETTER EARLY CHILDHOOD EMOTION SOCIALIZERS

Even though we clearly need to know much more about how early childhood educators socialize emotional competence, some suggestions can be made for optimizing preschool teacher training and practice that take into account the following issues: (1) the emotional labor and stress of being an early childhood educator; (2) in contrast, the factors promoting the resilience of early childhood educators and the satisfaction they can find in their job; and (3) specific aspects of training that may serve to maximize best practices to promote young children's emotional competence. After discussing these topics, I focus on two more intrapersonal aspects of being an emotion socializer in the early childhood classroom. First, much support and specific suggestions are offered for promoting teachers' own emotional competence; as found for parents (see Chapter 8), one is a better emotion socializer when one is emotionally competent oneself. Finally, it is crucial to acknowledge that what constitutes optimal emotion socialization varies for members of differing ethnicities.

### Teachers' Stress and Resilience Affect Their Ability to Be Emotion Socializers

Much has been written about how job stress is associated with negative emotions. Specifically, even though their profession is often fulfilling, early childhood educators also are often emotionally challenged and experience much stress (Kwon et al., 2022; Zinsser, Christensen, & Torres, 2016; Zinsser, Denham, Curby, & Chazan-Cohen, 2016). Teachers who are stressed by job demands provide less and inconsistent emotional support, as well as reacting negatively to children's emotions (Buettner, Jeon, Hur, & Garcia, 2016b; Denham et al., 2017; Zinsser, Denham, et al., 2016; Zinsser, Weissberg, & Dusenbury, 2013). Dealing effectively with stress is thus an important factor in helping early childhood educators be positive emotion socializers.

One clear source of stress for early childhood educators, already mentioned here, is emotional labor. The effort, planning, and control required to express appropriate emotions around young children are very taxing and can negatively affect the overall classroom environment, and likely the specific emotion socialization behaviors shown by teachers (Brown et al., 2018; Day & Hong, 2016; Schutz, Aultman, & Williams-Johnson, 2009). Even the caring relationships that early childhood educators create with children can engender emotional strain (Day & Hong, 2016).

Other sources of stress include high child–teacher ratios, demanding parents, and increased pressure for professional competence; these stress inducers also can coexist with a sense of isolation. Along with emotional labor, these further causes of stress can not only hamper emotional socialization, but even affect how teachers view the children in their care. Jeon, Buettner, Grant, and Lang (2019) found that early childhood educators' stress was related to less-positive evaluations of preschoolers' anger and anxiety, as well as their social competence. In short, early childhood teachers need support to combat stress. I consider possible pathways to ameliorating stress in a later section. It also is important to consider wellsprings of strength that coexist alongside sources of stress.

## Resilience

Early childhood teachers can also find sources of resilience in their jobs. Teachers reporting more job resources (e.g. knowing the work they are doing matters; knowing they are appreciated by the parents) were more likely to endorse positive emotion socialization; the converse also was unfortunately true (Denham, Bassett, & Miller, 2017). Teachers who feel supported in their job, and feel that their job is meaningful and fun, are likely to serve as positive forces in the growth of preschoolers' emotional competence. Further, creating relationships with parents, children, other teachers, and directors—*enjoying teaching*—are grounding strengths that allow one to approach emotion in the classroom more positively. These positive lenses for viewing their demanding job supports early childhood teachers' positive emotion socialization (Denham, Bassett, & Miller, 2017). Additionally, aspects of the organizational culture also can support teachers in fostering this sense of resilience (Stearns, Banerjee, Mickelson, & Miller, 2014; Zinsser & Zinsser, 2016). In sum, enjoying teaching and the feeling of making a difference are goals we should strive for, both specifically for emotion socialization and more generally for teachers' personal well-being.

Job satisfaction exemplifies this strength that teachers can find to assist them in being optimal emotion socializers. For example, Stremmel, Benson, and Powell (1993) found that satisfaction with working conditions and the work itself were related to lower emotional exhaustion. Moreover, education and experience in the field can also be sources of strengths for teachers as emotion socializers. In one of our studies, less-experienced, less-educated teachers endorsed more negative emotion socialization techniques (Denham, Bassett, & Miller, 2017). These findings support others' work (Jeon, Buettner, & Hur, 2016; Swartz & McElwain, 2012). Cross-national studies also corroborate these findings; more educated Italian preschool teachers adopted a more "emotion-coaching" emotion socialization style (e.g., "Children's sadness is an emotion worth exploring"; Ornaghi, Agliati, et al., 2020). Similarly, more experienced Chinese preschool teachers reported greater frequency of and confidence in using positive emotion socialization practices (Luo, Snyder, Huggins-Manley, Conroy, & Hong, 2021; see also Loinaz, 2019). However, sometimes these relations do not hold, suggesting that the contributions of education and experience can be very complex (Kwon et al., 2022; Ornaghi, Agliati, et al., 2020).

Sometimes, aspects of teachers' lives work together to bolster their potential ability to be positive emotion socializers. Specifically, teachers in different programs, such as Head Start, faith-based centers, university-affiliated childcare, and private preschool childcare may differ in not only education and level of experience, but also in other important ways that should be considered (Sedgwick, 2015). They include funding and regulatory control, along with cultural and pedagogical differences in approaches to early childhood, and teacher credentialing and pay discrepancies. For example, in the United States, the Head Start Reauthorization of 2007 required lead Head Start teachers nationally to have a bachelor's degree, and teacher assistants to have a Child Development Associate credential. Further, Head Start programs also often have the support of mental health coordinators. Teachers in other programs that may not have these requirements and benefits may suffer higher stress and subsequent turnover due to lower pay. Given these conditions, it is not surprising that we have found Head Start teachers to endorse positive emotion socialization behaviors, and teachers in other programs to be more likely to endorse negative socialization behaviors (Denham, Bassett, & Miller, 2017).

Unpacking the differences experienced by teachers in each program type, especially as the stress and resilience of teachers relates to the structure of their programs and their emotion socialization techniques is warranted. Teachers who note high levels of stress and endorse negative emotion socialization techniques deserve better, evidence-based support, and the experiences of teachers who support positive emotion socialization need to be identified. Knowledge about *how* program differences translate into differences in emotion socialization should be discovered and disseminated to maximize teacher strengths

## SUMMARY: Teachers' Stress and Resilience and Their Emotion Socialization

Accumulating research suggests that not only should we work to minimize the sources of stress in early childhood teachers' jobs if we are hoping for positive emotion socializers, but also we should maximize several aspects of teachers' lives. In particular, the markers of resilience and well-being already discussed here, and more, need to be supported. They include teachers' balance of job resources and demands, better wages, and perceptions of being able to pay for their basic expenses (Cassidy, King, Wang, Lower, & Kintner-Duffy, 2017; Denham, Bassett, & Miller, 2017; King et al., 2015).

Further, considering the importance of job satisfaction and years of experience, we need to retain positive emotion socializers in the classroom. Lack of resilience and well-being in the early childhood workplace is, not surprisingly, related to the very high levels of turnover (i.e., around one-third!), especially for teachers in childcare centers and those who teach the youngest children (Bassok, Markowitz, Bellows, & Sadowski, 2021; Grant, Jeon, & Buettner, 2019). In contrast, the sources of resilience already discussed (e.g., feeling supported and professional in one's job through having a sense of security, agency, comfort, and engagement) are negatively related to early childhood educators' job dissatisfaction, as well as their considerations of quitting their jobs or leaving field entirely (McMullen, Lee, McCormick, & Choi, 2020).

Better meeting these emotional needs of early-career teachers so that experienced teachers can be retained, could not only be beneficial for emotion socialization; even more, attending to stress and maximizing resources and resilience could benefit the teachers themselves (Schonert-Reichert, Kitil, & Hanson-Peterson, 2017). Additionally, student teachers in early childhood education need ample training in promoting emotional competence. Thus, emotion-specific training also is critical.

## Training

What sort of training is needed? Many early childhood teachers are aware of the characteristics of children's social–emotional competence, as well as the value of children's and their own emotions to learning and well-being; further, they want to attend to these issues in the classroom (Ferreira et al., 2021; Koludrović & Mrsić, 2021; Somerwil, Klieve, & Exley, 2020; Zembylas, 2007; Zinsser, Denham, Curby, & Shewark, 2015; Zinsser, Shewark, Denham, & Curby, 2014). However, this intuitive sense of the importance of preschoolers' emotional competence is not shared by all early childhood teachers, and there are marked differences in teachers' enactment of adaptive practices (Zembylas, 2007; Zinsser, Denham, et al., 2015; Zinsser, Shewark, et al., 2014). What's more, even when early childhood teachers do acknowledge the vital status of preschoolers' emotional competence, they often also report being very unprepared to promote it and use only a limited number of emotion socialization strategies in their classrooms, asserting the need for emotion-specific training (Ferreira et al., 2021; Somerwil et al., 2020; Türkmen & Ulutaş, 2018).

Specifically, preservice teachers report little training on promoting emotional competence or on managing their own internal feelings and external displays of emotion (Buettner, Hur, Jeon, & Andrews, 2016; Garner, 2010; Poulou, 2005; Schonert-Reichl et al., 2017), and relatively few schools of education are prepared to train teachers on these matters (Marlow & Inman, 2002; Schonert-Reichl et al., 2017), although encouraging research has suggested that emotional competence concepts can be successfully infused into an undergraduate course on curriculum and instruction (Waajid, Garner, & Owen, 2013).

Emotion socialization training is needed not only at the undergraduate level. Evidence-based practices for in-service training and professional development regarding emotion socialization also are required (Steed & Roach, 2017; Ulloa, Evans, & Jones, 2016), particularly because many early childhood educators do not have undergraduate degrees (Hale-Jinks, Knopf, & Kemple, 2006). Teachers and their supportive administrators, as well as preservice teachers in undergraduate preparation, could profit from attention to and training in this area (Ferreira et al., 2021; Garner, 2010; Waajid et al., 2013). The need is clear.

Broadly speaking, early childhood educators could benefit from a deeper knowledge of how to interpret the need for emotion or its regulation in the classroom, how to show emotions authentically, and why children show emotion and how to respond to it (Cole & Tan, 2007). More specifically, many professional development techniques could contribute to how early childhood educators understand the behavioral aspects of emotion socialization, advancing their modeling of emotions, contingent reactions, teaching about emotions, and positive beliefs about emotions. For example, regarding modeling, teacher training could focus on helping teachers to be willing to show emotions, to remain emotionally positive in the classroom despite challenges, and to modulate understandable negative emotions (Zinsser, Denham, et al., 2015; Zinsser, Shewark, et al., 2014). In all these considerations, the culturally and ethnically bound nature of emotion socialization must be addressed sensitively.

Teacher training also could focus on ways of assisting teachers in valuing their supportive role concerning children's emotions and give them specific strategies to use in reacting to children's more difficult emotions (e.g., anger, fear, sadness, even overexcitement). Stress reduction could help teachers maximize their expression of positive reactions to children's emotions.

Further, training could focus on ways of helping teachers to value teacher–child emotion conversations and to sustain interchanges about emotions in classroom activities and dialogues about ongoing classroom interactions. These values and propensities for emotion talk can translate into classroom and parenting practice.

Finally, training can promote positive beliefs about children's emotions and their socialization, as well as teachers' self-efficacy in being effective emotion socializers (Ornaghi, Agliati, et al., 2020). Specifically, courses on emotion socialization boosted preschool teachers' beliefs that teachers should openly express their emotions, should talk about and label their emotions, and should not protect children *from* emotions, as well as boosted their confidence about their abilities to socialize emotional competence. In fact, Ornaghi and colleagues (2020) consider that training at least partly accounted for a significant association between beliefs and self-reported emotion socialization styles.

## SUMMARY: Training for Early Childhood Teachers' Emotion Socialization

There is a pronounced need for training about emotion socialization in early childhood education, at both pre- and in-service levels. It has been shown that training can be accomplished, and I make suggestions that address specific needs in training teachers about the contributions of their emotions, their reactions to emotions, and emotion talk about their students' emotional competence. But another worthy area of need is supporting teachers in developing their own emotional competence.

## Teachers' Own Emotional Competence

Early childhood teaching can be an emotionally draining and unpredictable endeavor; teachers need support regarding emotional labor and in nurturing their own emotional competence (Jeon, Hur, & Buettner, 2016; Kremenitzer & Miller, 2008; Mortari, 2009, 2012; O'Connor, DeFeyter, Carr, Luo, & Romm, 2017). Such support puts a spotlight on teachers' own emotional competence as critical for promoting preschoolers' emotional competence (Ornaghi, Agliati, et al., 2020; Ulloa et al., 2016). What mechanisms fuel this connection? An emotionally competent teacher can be more comfortable addressing emotion with children (Garner, Parker, & Prigmore, 2019) and react to and utilize classroom emotional encounters more advantageously (Rivers, Tominey, O'Bryon, & Brackett, 2013b).

So, as well as being trained in classroom practices regarding emotion socialization, promoting teachers' own emotional competence would contribute to their abilities to (1) become aware of and accurately recognize their own and others' emotions; (2) understand why these emotions occur; (3) label and discuss them; and, finally (4) express and manage them (Brackett & Katulak, 2006; Emde, 2009; Zinsser, Denham, et al., 2015; Zinsser, Shewark, et al., 2014).

Why would such training be useful? The ways in which teachers deal with their own emotional lives contribute to their socialization of pupils' emotional competence (Brackett & Katulak, 2006; Swartz & McElwain, 2012). Awareness of one's own emotions is the first step to recognizing them accurately; this aspect of preschool teachers' emotional competence is related to their reactions to children's emotions (Ulloa et al., 2016). In Ersay's work (2015), preschool teachers with low awareness of their own emotions were less likely to self-report that they would help children label and regulate their emotions or to try to help solve the problem. Teachers low on emotional awareness more often ignored children's emotions and less often comforted children's negative emotions or mirrored their positive emotions (Ersay, 2007). Further, teachers' lack of attention to their own emotions was related to their greater minimization of children's emotions.

Promoting teachers' ability to perceive emotions accurately enables them to talk about emotions more usefully with children. Also, teachers' ability to regulate their emotions during the daily stress of early childhood education is related to their positive emotion socialization (Buettner, Jeon, et al., 2016). Thus helping teachers learn to regulate their emotions productively—allowing themselves to express emotions in the classroom, but to monitor their intensity—also would help them be more positive emotion socializers. Teachers who can regulate emotions tend to be emotionally positive in the classroom (and coincidentally demonstrate higher job satisfaction; Jones & Bouffard, 2012). They are better equipped to treat even challenging students sensitively, and children can model their emotions and management of them.

For example, where teachers implement the useful cognitive reappraisal strategy to regulate emotions, their students show less negative emotion with peers (Sahin Asi, Ocak Karabay, & Guzeldere Aydin, 2016) Conversely, when teachers are not good at regulating their emotions, their emotion socialization can be more negative; for example, teachers' reports of their own negative emotional intensity were associated with their punishing of children's emotions (Ersay, 2007), and their use of emotion suppression as a regulation strategy is related to preschoolers decreased positive emotions with peers (Sahin Asi et al., 2016).

Several methods can promote teachers' emotional competence (Jennings & Greenberg, 2009). First, mindfulness training could assist teachers in maintaining positivity, in being willing to accurately express emotions, and in modulating their understandable negative emotions. Mindful attention and awareness could be helpful in responding successfully to the stress involved with juggling the needs of children, colleagues, supervisors, and parents (Jennings, 2015; Kemeny et al., 2012; Shewark et al., 2018; Zinsser, Denham, et al., 2015; Zinsser, Shewark, et al., 2014). In fact, Kemeny et al. (2012) have shown that mindfulness training is effective in promoting teachers' own emotional competence, with lasting effect.

Second, in reflective supervision, teachers reflect on their classroom practice, share challenges, and brainstorm potential solutions with their supervisors—in short, they tend together to teachers' emotional competence and emotional self-efficacy (Lang, Jeon, Sproat, Brothers, & Buettner, 2020; Mortari, 2009, 2012; Ornaghi et al., 2021). These techniques can be very useful in helping early childhood teachers become aware of and understand their own emotions, as well as in gaining access to a broader emotion vocabulary (Gilkerson, 2004; Jennings, 2015; Ulloa et al., 2016). These outcomes could increase their ease of discussing feelings with children, among other positive emotion socialization techniques.

Third, as already noted, stress reduction is vital for teachers' own well-being and for reacting optimally to children's emotions (Buettner, Jeon, et al., 2016). Practice recommendations for reducing stress also could include concrete steps, such as training in physical relaxation, gratitude, and cognitive reappraisal. Physical activity also can buffer early childhood educators from emotional exhaustion (Baumgartner, Carson, Apavaloaie, & Tsouloupas, 2009; Carson, Baumgartner, Matthews, & Tsouloupas, 2010).

### SUMMARY: Early Childhood Teachers' Own Emotional Competence and Their Emotion Socialization

Maximizing teachers' own emotional capacities could aid in creating better social–emotional learning environments and could serve to improve their well-being (Buettner, Jeon, et al., 2016; Zinsser, Weissberg, et al., 2013). Learning ER strategies especially could be useful in their often-stressful profession. Mindfulness techniques, reflective supervision, and other stress reduction techniques could improve not only their professional practice, but also their personal lives.

## Considering Teacher Ethnicity

A final, important professional and research consideration is to be mindful of how different cultures and ethnicities value and envision emotion socialization. As already noted, in my research we sometimes find significant teacher contributions to children's emotional competence for high-risk classrooms only. Why might these positive emotion socialization techniques be especially salutary for children who are at socioeconomic risk? Arguably, these children could benefit most from teachers' emotion socialization (see also Garner & Parker, 2018), and in fact low-income children are especially sensitive to quality social–emotional programming, which advantageously promotes their emotional competence (Fishbein et al., 2016; Nix, Bierman, Domitrovich, & Gill, 2013). Knowing this, we argue that teacher emotion socialization may be especially important for children living in poverty. So these findings are important.

At the same time, considering that both the children and teachers in the high-risk classrooms I have studied are more likely to be African American than in the low-risk classrooms, an examination of teacher emotion socialization from the perspective of ethnicity and culture is warranted. Emotion socialization has been most often studied with European American families and teachers so that a deeper understanding of its workings in other groups is called for.

Focusing on ethnicity in our work, we showed that African American teachers, in comparison with their European American counterparts, more highly endorsed their own self-reported positive emotion socialization techniques, including positive expressiveness, teaching about emotions, and reacting supportively (e.g., comforting, Denham, Bassett, & Miller, 2017; cf. Parker et al., 2012). Moreover, they also less highly endorsed one aspect of nonsupportive reactions, laissez-faire or ineffective reactions. What might underlie such differences?

First, what are the particular strengths that African American teachers bring to the classroom? Compared to teachers of other ethnicities, African American teachers often see their students in a more positive light (Mashburn, Hamre, Downer, & Pianta, 2006). They may be especially open to the world of emotions, putting emotion socialization in the forefront of their implicit classroom agenda (Parker et al., 2012). Such positive views may facilitate the endorsement of the positive emotion socialization techniques that we have identified (Denham, Bassett, & Miller, 2017).

Second, most African American teachers in our sample worked in Head Start centers; Head Start teachers have a strong service ethic coupled with access to training and report high levels of satisfaction, efficacy, and confidence (Bullough, Hall-Kenyon, & MacKay, 2012). African American teachers reported having more job resources than did European Americans educators (Denham, Bassett, & Miller, 2017; Stearns et al., 2014). These considerations suggest multiple determinations of African American teachers' endorsement of positive emotion socialization.

I have already discussed how sometimes teachers', predominantly African-Americans', observed emotion socialization behaviors in these high-risk classrooms made some contributions to variability in children's emotional competence that run counter to findings with parents and European American teachers (Denham & Bassett, 2019). To reiterate, although African American teachers' emotional balance (i.e., more happy than angry) and observed tenderness did contribute to children's emotionally regulated/productive behavior, tenderness also was related to their pupils' observed emotionally negative/dysregulated behavior. Tenderness here seemed to serve a dual function in these high-risk classrooms— creating a comforting milieu, but perhaps in a cultural context, *too* comforting. This interpretation was supported by the counterintuitive finding that, African American teachers' observed supportive behavior reactions to children's emotions also were predictive of their emotionally negative/dysregulated behavior. Similarly, emotion knowledge was predicted by teachers' positive emotional responsiveness (i.e., smiling back at a smiling child) in high-risk classrooms, but *also* by their nonsupportive behavioral reactions (i.e., punishing, minimizing) to the children's emotions. Further, although such teacher-reported punitive reactions to children's emotions were associated with lower emotion knowledge in low-risk classrooms, these reactions were not deleterious for the emotion knowledge of children in high-risk classrooms (Denham, Ferrier, et al., 2020). In fact, the "nonsupportive" reaction aggregate was positively associated with end-of-year emotion knowledge for children in high-risk classrooms.

Parallels are rather clear between African American teachers' and African American parents' emotion socialization, as noted in Chapter 7. Although some of the "positive" socialization techniques endorsed by the teachers did not match those reported in the literature for mothers (e.g., Nelson et al., 2012; Nelson, Leerkes, et al., 2013), there were some similarities in the two groups' emotion socialization behavior. For example, African American teachers endorsed comforting children and showing them positive expressiveness, such as tenderness, but like African American mothers, also made use of "nonsupportive" reactions to children's emotions in practice to promote social–emotional competence.

Thus, these results with African American teachers, similar to those with African American mothers described in Chapter 7, paint a picture of warmth and demandingness as the most salutary aspects of children's emotional environment (Bondy & Ross, 2008). African American teachers focus on emotions, but their behavior may require a more nuanced view of adaptive emotion socialization (Labella, 2018; Morelen & Thomassin, 2013), in which "celebration and restriction of children's emotion coexist closely . . . , perhaps reflecting the joint influences of traditional Afro-cultural values and the historical context of slavery and discrimination" (Labella, 2018, p. 1).

Given these considerations, a very complex picture can be painted of these African American teachers valuing of positive emotion socialization, but also performing some unique behaviors necessary and useful in their specific context. Children in these socioeconomically high-risk classrooms are receiving a complex message about emotions, one that includes both punitive and minimizing reactions to their emotions, as well as the "supportive" reactions and emotionally warm practices already mentioned. This message may be something like this: "I am cared for. Emotions are okay—I can show them and learn about them, but I'd better regulate them, too."

## SUMMARY: Early Childhood Teachers' Ethnicity and Their Emotion Socialization

We have found that largely African American teachers in high-risk classrooms reacted behaviorally to children's emotions in ways that historically have been considered *both* "supportive" and "nonsupportive" of the development of emotional competence, with both making positive contributions to children's observed positive social–emotional behaviors in this context (Denham & Bassett, 2019; Denham, Ferrier, et al., 2020). Taken together, these dovetailing findings from both studies suggest that the meaning of reactions traditionally termed "nonsupportive" may have differed in a racially and culturally divergent context.

More broadly, adaptive emotion socialization practices may look different for different racial, ethnic, cultural, and/or income groups. Given these more fine-grained considerations, considering a unified model of ethnic and emotion socialization is warranted in future research (Dunbar, Leerkes, Coard, Supple, & Calkins, 2017). As we have found, adaptive emotion socialization may include both "supportive" and "nonsupportive" behaviors, such that children learn not only emotional competence skills, but also when *not* to show negative emotions. Thus, "positive" and "negative" or "supportive" and "nonsupportive" emotion socialization can be considered ethnically bound terms, not universally applicable to individuals from differing ethnic and socioeconomic backgrounds. Value-laden terminology, such as "supportive" and "nonsupportive" reactions, should be renamed, perhaps as "adaptive" and "nonadaptive," with definitions varying by context (e.g., including race). It behooves researchers of emotion socialization to consider their terminology and the logic models underlying their predictions carefully; along with early childhood educators, we too must become culturally competent.

## CONCLUSION

What needs to be done? Much more research is absolutely needed, but the path is set. We have given examples from our own past and ongoing work, and others are beginning to take up the endeavor of studying emotion socialization in the preschool classroom. More about all three mechanisms of emotion socialization—modeling, reacting, and talking— employed by teachers is becoming known. Professional questions of importance involving teachers' stress, resilience, and training, and promotion of teachers' own emotional competence merit further attention. Finally, further research, for both basic and applied purposes, could observe how early childhood teachers in different cultures and of differing ethnicities enact their endorsement of positive emotion socialization. All these issues, along with teachers' emotional interactional behaviors with children, need much more scrutiny.

# 10

# Contributions of Emotional Expressiveness, Emotion Knowledge, and Emotion Regulation to Preschoolers' Social Competence

## INTRODUCTION

So far, I have discussed in much detail the elements of emotional competence—expressiveness, knowledge, and ER—and how they are promoted by parents and teachers during early childhood. But why do I deem them so important? The model put forward in Chapter 1 (see Figure 1.2) reserves a central position for the contributions of emotional competence to the daily lives of young children as they interact with others. Children who can understand emotion, express a wide range of emotions in appropriate settings, and regulate their own and cope with others' emotions are more likely to be seen as competent social partners by parents, teachers, and peers. Joey, the young "pirate" described at the beginning of Chapter 1, is likely to be sought after as a play companion, commended by his teacher, and viewed as demonstrating effective social–emotional behaviors by anyone who knows him. These positive outcomes occur at least in part because he so readily understands the interplay of his partners' and his own emotions, reacts accordingly, and vividly expresses a variety of predominantly positive feelings himself, knowing when to down- or up-regulate his experience and expression of emotion. To move forward in detailing the contributions of each of these aspects of emotional competence to preschool social competence, I must first define this construct.

## DEFINING OUTCOMES OF PRESCHOOL EMOTIONAL COMPETENCE

Social competence can be broadly conceived of as effectiveness in interaction (Rose-Krasnor & Denham, 2008), as evaluated by peers, parents, or teachers who have seen the child in question interact with others over time or by observers examining a child's specific social behaviors relating to initiating and maintaining interaction. Traditionally, social competence has been operationalized through the examination of four factors: (1) social skills (e.g., sharing, cooperation, caring, and respecting peer norms while remaining assertive); (2) peer status (e.g., popularity, acceptance, and rejection); (3) successful relationships with teachers and peers; and (4) social information processing (e.g., positive social goals). Such early childhood markers of successful interactions with others often involve an emotional underpinning (Denham, Blair, et al., 2003). Thus the extant literature often depicts aspects of emotional competence as precursors and/or supports for social competence (Denham, Blair, et al., 2003; Denham, Brown, et al., 2010; Denham & Grout, 1993; Denham & Weissberg, 2004; Garner & Estep, 2001; Izard, Fine, et al., 2001; Junge, Valkenburg, Deković, & Branje, 2020). Most often social competence is operationalized in their reports as peer status, teacher ratings, or observed social interactions.

Accordingly, evidence for the importance of emotional competence is clear in many aspects of social competence. For example, expressing and regulating emotions can be integral parts of preschoolers' success in their social world.

Darryl, whose absence was remarked upon sadly by friends in Chapter 1, gets mad at Takisha while playing in the dramatic play area—she is hogging the blocks– and hits her with one of them. Takisha acts hurt, and Darryl yells, "I need some blocks!! Give me!!," and Takisha yells back, "Don't hit! There's more over here!" Somehow, even though their interaction didn't begin so well, through their assertively and clearly conveyed anger and their words they seem to resolve the conflict. Each appears to understand that the other was angry, and why, and regulates his or her own emotion so that their relationship is safeguarded. They move on, sharing the blocks that provoked their original conflict and cooperating to build a very tall tower.

Darryl shows clear emotions while asserting himself; it is obvious that Takisha knows he's mad (Field & Walden, 1982). At the same time though, he regulates his emotions when they threaten his interaction (and maybe even his friendship) with Takisha. His understanding of his own and others' emotions may be part of the reason people miss him when he's not around——his peer status is very positive despite being a pretty emotional boy!

As with Darryl's understanding of Takisha, sometimes knowledge of one's own or others' emotions can facilitate interaction.

Andy hits Mohammed, who calls for Ben to help. Ben sternly tells Andy, the instigator, to go away, and squats down to put his arm around Mo. He leads him over to the book corner, where they share their favorite book. Ben's understanding of emotions helps him respond prosocially to his friend. He understands Mo's hurt and is motivated by his own empathic concern. This ability to show empathic concern in the sometimes-riotous preschool classroom may be one reason that his peer relationships are generally positive. He also is assertive when necessary, backing up his assertion to Andy with clear emotion, but no aggression. Peers and his teacher all see the "whole package" that he presents—his emotional competence at understanding Mo's pain, his ability to express empathic concern, and his regulation of his own anger supports his relationships with others.

Three-year-old Miranda understands that Tiffany is only playacting being sad, as the baby in the house corner (Serrat Sellabonna et al., 2020). Miranda gives Tiffany very solicitous care rather than becoming personally distressed. She even explains to others that this is a posed emotion: "Tiffy's just pretending; she's the baby. Waaaa!!" Some specific aspects of emotion knowledge make one a more sophisticated play partner.

Sometimes the ability to regulate emotions is the key factor in maximizing a preschooler's social competence. For example, when children must wait for a turn at play, they may become disruptive if they do not have the ability to regulate their disappointment. Peers' quarrels can be frequent, but preschool friends become able to moderate the intensity of their emotion because they know each other well and want to maintain the friendship (Hyson, 1994).

John really doesn't like it when Pei Lin runs her tricycle right through his sandcastle. He's worked so hard! "Hey!" he yells, and he can feel his skin getting all hot and tingly. He's about to hit one of his very best friends. Instead of hitting though, he shouts, "You shouldn't wreck it!" Pei Lin comes back over and screeches the trike to a halt. "I'm sorry, Johnny!" They begin to work on rebuilding the castle together. If John hadn't regulated his justifiable anger, the interaction might have escalated, damaging their relationship. But he did regulate his anger, using assertive language, and this ability not only protected his feelings, but also allowed him to use his social skill of cooperation. It is clear that emotional and social competencies worked together for him.

The complex relationship between emotional and social competence may be summarized this way: More spontaneously expressive children may be seen as better play partners and more fun to be with, especially if they can regulate their negative emotions—and even sometimes their positive ones—when the situation calls for it. Similarly, children who can understand the emotions experienced by playmates are at an advantage when responding to others' emotions during play. Because of this asset, they also may be able to use their social skills in a targeted way and become better liked. In fact, children who are more expressive actually may have a better chance of comprehending others' emotional situations because they have "been there."

Having defined what is meant by both emotional and social competence, I now examine how patterns of emotional expressiveness, emotion knowledge, and regulating one's own, and coping with others', emotions contribute to early childhood social competence. I also consider how difficulties with emotional competence may contribute to externalizing and internalizing behavior problems. In terms of behavior problems, I refer to externalizing ones (i.e., physical or verbal aggression, tantrums, disobedience, agitation and hyperactivity, inattention, failure to comply, and other disruptive behaviors) and internalizing ones (i.e., sadness and unhappiness, behavioral inhibition, and withdrawal or overly constrained behavior in social situations and play).

## CONTRIBUTIONS OF EMOTIONAL EXPRESSIVENESS TO SOCIAL COMPETENCE

As suggested in the previous examples, emotional expressiveness makes varied and specific contributions to social interaction. In the broadest sense, emotions are useful social signals that can facilitate interaction. When one child smiles at another while approaching their play area, the signal is "I like you. Want to play?"

> In contrast, imagine Antonio's thoughts when Jared screams at him to get away from his Lego construction. It is clear to Antonio and to all onlookers that Jared is very mad and about to attack. Antonio begins to holler, but then, thinking better of this plan, backs off, going to play elsewhere. After Jared is calmer, Antonio returns and offers to help rebuild the Legos. Jared's emotions offer Antonio immediate, easily processed feedback regarding his own behavior, as well as information about Jared's intentions.

Expressed emotions also can facilitate the understanding of verbal cues. One child's ambiguous statement to another— "Come here"—can take on very different meanings, depending on whether it is accompanied by happiness, sadness, anger, or some other emotion. In short, both verbal and nonverbal signals provided by emotional expressiveness can influence whether the beginning of a social interaction, the course of any given interchange, and communication within it are successful or unsuccessful, and will culminate in friendship or enmity.

Not only do young children's specific emotional interactions, but also their overall emotional styles, contribute to their overall success in interacting with their peers. Thus, emotional expressiveness is important even more generally than suggested by the previous example on the communicative value of Jared's anger. An often sad or angry child is less able to notice and understand, let alone respond to, others' emotional needs, lacking internal resources, and unready to use any social skills. Given these inabilities, a child's interactions may be less than effective; the child's emotions are hampering her or his social competence. It is no wonder when a child's peers flatly assert, "She hits. She bites. She kicked me this morning. I *don't like* her." Conversely, a generally happier preschooler may better afford to respond positively, socially effectively, to another's overtures. If Leah approaches usually sunny Chelsea to play, she knows the odds of a positive interaction are high. In sum, enduring patterns of preschoolers' emotional expressiveness become potent intrapersonal supports for, or roadblocks to, interacting with age-mates.

Many investigations of emotional competence highlight such connections between preschoolers' observed emotional expressiveness and various indices of social competence. In my work, preschoolers' expressions of specific emotions, as observed during free play in their classrooms, are often associated with ratings of their sociometric likability and/or teachers' evaluations of their social competence (Denham, Bassett, Mincic, et al., 2012; Denham, Blair, et al., 2002, 2003; Denham & Burger, 1991; Denham, McKinley, et al., 1990). These social outcomes depend on whether the emotions expressed during interactions are positive or negative.

### Positive Emotion and Social Competence

As already suggested, positive affect has great appeal, promoting social interaction and its continuation. People like to be with others who show joy, and young children are no exception to this rule. Even more specifically, emotional positivity helps children initiate and regulate social exchanges (Sroufe, Schork, Motti, Lawroski, & LaFreniere, 1984). Duration of cooperation episodes also is longer when there is more frequent happy affect within dyads (Marcus, 1987). More recently, Garner and Waajid (2012) found that preschoolers' positive expressiveness during peer play was positively related to social competence (see also Denham, Bassett, Mincic, et al., 2012; Denham, Blair, et al., 2003).

> Four-year-olds Jamal and LaToya are both playing in the house corner. LaToya is making pretend soup and humming. Jamal approaches and begins to sweep the area with a child-size broom. Suddenly, LaToya twirls around and smiles, saying, "Want some soup?" Jamal smiles, too. "Yes, I do. Mmmm . . . that's good." LaToya beams at his praise. She then suggests with a grin, "I'm going to work. I need you to vacuum this floor." Jamal gets the toy vacuum, and pretty soon they choose clothes from the dress-up box for their roles of executive mom and stay-at-home dad, giggling together. When Jamal drops the plastic vacuum on LaToya's foot, he flashes a tiny smile, as if to say, "I didn't mean to," so LaToya doesn't get mad. Later, Jamal and LaToya walk to circle time hand in hand and sit next to each other, still smiling. They are seen together on an everyday basis.

Jamal and LaToya's enjoyment of each other and of their shared activities illustrates how especially vital positive affect is in initiating, regulating, and maintaining social communication during socially directed acts, and in forming friendships. Clearly their play was of a high quality, without disruption or disconnection (Kwon & Min, 2021).

Positive emotion is important in the moment, but it also has a more far-reaching influence. Because patterns of expressiveness are becoming more stable during the preschool years, enduring individual differences in expressiveness influence how children view each other and how teachers see them. Happier children are at an advantage here.

> Layne is often cheery, with smiles of greeting to teachers and peers alike. She smiles when the teacher announces what song they will be singing in circle time, and the other children join her. She also often expects the other children to follow her lead and will sternly tell them to do what she wants if they overlook her suggestions. Despite her grouchiness when crossed, they like her, and her teacher sees her as a friendly, though assertive, person.

Layne's social reputation, based largely on her positivity, thus becomes established. In particular, preschoolers' ability to balance their happy emotional displays over angry ones are seen as more socially competent: Preschoolers like Layne who show more positive than negative emotions respond more attentively and prosocially to their peers' emotions and are seen by teachers and peers as more likable, friendly, assertive, less aggressive, and less sad (e.g., Denham, Blair, et al., 2003; Denham, McKinley, et al., 1990; see also Eisenberg, Fabes, Bernzweig, et al., 1993).

These outcomes of preschoolers' emotional expressiveness patterns continue to garner empirical support, corroborating and extending earlier findings. As I would hypothesize, more frequent or prevalent positive emotional expressiveness during dyadic play was related to several indices of social competence, including peer acceptance, initiating peer interaction, receiving peers' attention, and teachers' ratings (Shin et al., 2011; see also Garner & Waajid, 2008). These relationships are not restricted to the earlier preschool years; the positive emotions of both interest and happiness were associated with first and second graders' peer status (Schultz, Izard, Stapleton, Buckingham-Howes, & Bear, 2009).

Lindsey (2017, 2019b) extended these findings even further, demonstrating that preschoolers who were observed sharing more *mutual* positive emotions with peers, like LaToya and Jamal, were better liked and even considered more socially competent and less aggressive by teachers 1 year later (see Lindsey, 2019a, and Sallquist, DiDonato, Hanish, Martin, & Fabes, 2012, for similar concurrent findings, including cooperation and prosocial behavior). Adding further longitudinal results, Morgan, Izard, and Hyde (2014) found that observed happiness and engagement in a happy task (blowing bubbles) predicted children's positive social behavior six months later.

## *Moderators of Positive Expressiveness Outcomes*

In sum, there is much accumulating evidence on the beneficial and often very specific contributions of positive expressiveness to preschoolers' social competence. But does this contribution hold true for everyone? Are there moderators of this relation?

### GENDER

Sometimes the effects of positive expressiveness are particularly pronounced for boys; for example, in Denham, Blair, et al. (2003), boys who were more emotionally positive at age 3 were rated as more socially competent by their kindergarten teachers. Indeed, boys who were observed to show more positive expressiveness with peers, and who also were able to use words to regulate their emotional distress during peer conflicts, were seen by teachers as more socially competent with peers and in better relationships with the teachers themselves (Herndon et al., 2013). In contrast, there also is some evidence that overintense positivity is more pronounced for boys; the association between overall frequency of happiness and peer competence was not found for intensely happy boys (Lindsey, 2019b). Well-regulated positivity may stand boys in good stead when peers and teachers alike consider their social interactions.

### INTENSITY

Further, overall intensity of expressiveness (not just positive) may be important in its own right—or only as moderated by gender, and possibly by the specific emotion or valence of expressiveness (Eisenberg, Fabes, Bernzweig, et al., 1993; Eisenberg, Fabes, Murphy, et al., 1995; Eisenberg, Fabes, Nyman, et al., 1994). In Eisenberg and colleagues' work, adults rated 5-year-olds' emotional intensity ("This child responds very emotionally to things around him or her"). Mothers' reports of boys' low emotional intensity were associated with teachers' ratings of boys' positive social functioning, but teachers' reports of girls' low emotional intensity were *negatively* related to their ratings of girls' social competence.

In these cases, the message conveyed by boys' low-intensity emotion seemed to be one of calmness, allowing for positive interactions, whereas girls' lower intensity might have signaled a more apathetic message to teachers. How boys and girls send emotional messages may be important, as well as how others interpret them. Of course, the valence of the girls' and boys' emotions was not considered in these analyses, but nevertheless, in this case it seems important to consider gender norms for boys' and girls' emotionality. Are girls *expected to show more emotion, more clearly and intensely?* Are boys' intense emotions *seen as typically disruptive?* Taken together, these results suggest that the social competence outcomes of expressiveness patterns may differ by intensity, especially for boys and girls, and this is a theme to which I return.

### SUMMARY: Positive Emotion and Social Competence

Over three decades of research support the importance of positive expressiveness to successful social interactions and growing social reputations, with both peers and teachers, even across time. That is, it is beneficial in the moment, easing interactions as they proceed, and it also impacts long-term evaluations of social competence by others as emotional reputations are built. Moreover, recent research has supported and elaborated on the assertion that positive expressiveness specifically during peer play is positively related to social competence. Sharing positive affect may further facilitate the formation of friendships and renders social contact satisfying for all concerned, adding to children's likability, even at this early age.

Finally, there do appear to be some moderators of the contribution of positive emotionality, which seems more advantageous for boys, particularly at moderate intensity. A consideration of the *message conveyed by* expressing particular emotions, which differs for boys and girls and alters others' evaluations, is imperative.

## Negative Emotions and Social Competence

In contrast, negative emotions, especially anger, have aversive and disruptive effects on both ongoing interaction and even social information processing about that interaction (Lemerise & Dodge, 2008; Rubin & Clark, 1983; Rubin & Daniels-Byrness, 1983). Like positive emotions, then, negative emotions have effects both in terms of social-behavioral and/or social-cognitive processes and in terms of social reputation. More negatively expressive children experience more difficult social interactions with peers, understand their social interactions less adaptively, and are evaluated by others as more difficult to deal with.

Accordingly, negative emotionality contributes to the quality of social relationships even during toddlerhood; by 30 months of age, toddler emotional negativity was related to aspects of mother–child conflict, especially its resolution (Laible, Panfile, & Makariev, 2008). Thus, it is not difficult to imagine that, as children start interacting with their peers, these difficulties involving negative emotionality continue within these new relationships. Preschoolers showing more negative emotions have more difficulties with disrupted and disconnected play (Kwon & Min, 2021). Consider the negative social behaviors arising from Carrie's emotions while she plays, which make her social life very challenging.

> As already noted, 3-year-old Carrie has trouble with emotions. Today she is having a very bad day. Her negative emotions, mostly anger but also considerable sadness, involve her over and over in difficult interactions. She has trouble initiating social exchanges, maintaining them once begun, communicating without fussing, and nurturing friendships. She cries so piteously when her friend Eve uses the "wrong" pretend food in the house corner that a teacher must comfort her for some time. Then, just after she begins her pretend play again, she yells at Noah when he approaches and unknowingly sits in "her" chair while playing Birthday Party. Sounding quite irritable, she yells to explain, "I have a cold!!" Noah looks thoroughly nonplussed. Later, she screams when she is inadvertently jostled at the play sink. By the end of one 3-hour morning session, neither teachers nor peers want to have anything to do with Carrie. No doubt her screeches are still ringing in their ears.

Overall individual differences in anger expression also make a difference in the schemas children have for each other. Information about enduring anger may reside at the core of their notions about one another.

> Connor is often inexplicably grumpy when he comes into the classroom, and he also flares up when crossed. He snarls, "Don't talk to me," and pushes angrily at Jessie when she tries to sit close to him at circle time. Although he often gets his way in such interchanges, his classmates consider him less likable than Layne (even though she can be bossy), and his teachers see him as far more aggressive and definitely less friendly.

Connor's expressions of unhappiness are more "out of balance" than Layne's, tipped more toward an overall angry demeanor. In line with this example, preschoolers who show larger proportions of negative affect are often seen by teachers and peers alike as troublesome and difficult (Denham, Blair, et al., 2002, 2003; Denham & Burger, 1991; Denham, McKinley, et al., 1990; see also Denham, Bassett, Mincic, et al., 2012 for similar findings specifically for children living at academic risk who demonstrate high negative emotion along with other emotional competence deficits). Schultz, Izard, et al. (2009) even found out that, for children in the early primary grades, negative emotions attenuated the salutary relation between children's positive emotions and peer status.

Thus, negative emotion (particularly anger) often indexes concurrent social difficulty. In recent work, kindergartners' observed frequency of negative emotions was related to lower levels of peer acceptance and greater conflict with teachers (Hernández et al., 2017b[1]; see also Arsenio et al., 2000, for similar earlier findings). Furthermore, the intensity of negative emotion also was related to more conflict and less closeness with teachers (see also Diaz et al., 2017). However, although anger with mutual friends was more frequent than with acquaintances, it also was less intense and was resolved more often (Lindsey, 2019a). To predict the effects of preschoolers' anger and other negative emotions, then, it may be important to know the relationship status of peers who show anger to one another.

Like the salutary effects of positive expressiveness, the considerably deleterious outcomes of anger, in particular, can extend across time. For example, toddlers' observed and reported anger indirectly negatively predicted early grade school social competence, via its dampening effect on ego resiliency (i.e., the ability to bounce back after encountering difficulty; Taylor, Eisenberg, Van Schyndel, Eggum-Wilkins, & Spinrad, 2014). Such findings support the idea that experiencing and expressing anger limits the emotional, self-regulatory, and behavioral resources that children have to move on from negativity to the equanimity that allows them to learn, practice, and solidify how to interact positively.

Other longitudinal findings support the prediction of diminished social competence from earlier anger. For example, more intense observed anger during preschool was related to lower scores on measures of peer social competence a year later (Denham & Burger, 1991; Lindsey, 2019b). Slightly older children's anger also was negatively related to their later social competence (i.e., assertion, cooperation, and self-control; Chang, Shelleby, Cheong, & Shaw, 2012; see also Hernández et al., 2022, for an extension of their earlier findings). Negative reactivity at age 6 also predicted lower levels of helping at age 7 (Laible et al., 2017). The sum of all these findings confirms the problematic outcomes of preschoolers' negative emotions. But there may be important boundary conditions of these relationships that should be considered.

### *Moderators of Anger Outcomes: Gender*

Gender differences again seem necessary to consider. There may be specific risks involving negative emotions not only for boys, but also for girls. For example, boys who exhibited more frequent anger with acquaintances were rated by teachers as less prosocial and more aggressive (Lindsey, 2019a; see also Diener & Kim, 2004; Eisenberg, Fabes, Bernzweig, et al., 1993; Eisenberg, Fabes, Nyman, et al., 1994, for more general results connecting young boys' anger especially, and its intensity, to negative peer and teacher evaluations). Perhaps emotional expressiveness is more vital to boys' social relations because their often more intense, more externalizing negativity has a greater impact on their interactions and peers' memory of them.

Or again, expectations about their negative emotionality may lead others to exaggerate these emotions' damage to relationships. In particular, such unbridled negativity also is likely to especially impact teachers' views of boys' social competence. Although

[1]It should be noted that Hernández et al. (2015, 2017a, 2017b, 2022) and Diaz et al. (2017) observationally measure negative emotions as a whole (e.g., anger, frustration, sadness, and for Diaz et al. [2015], including fear as well).

teacher biases are lessening (Sette, Baldwin, Zava, Baumgartner, & Coplan, 2019), teachers may *expect* boys to be angrier and more aggressive, and their negative ratings of such behaviors may be based as much on reputation or other factors as they are on direct observation.

Conversely, when teachers do witness anger and antisocial reactions to peer emotions in girls, they may factor them into their social competence ratings more directly, without the cloud of reputation and expectation hanging over their evaluations. A clearer picture of these associations results when indices of emotion are assessed independently of ratings of social competence, and not by the same rater. When this suggestion is followed, the picture for girls' negative emotions' relationship to their social competence becomes more comprehensible.

For example, Hernández et al. (2017a) corroborated the general finding regarding the negative contribution of observed negative emotion to teacher ratings of peer acceptance, but with some gender differences. That is, they noted that especially kindergarten girls' negative emotions were related to lessened peer acceptance. At first this finding seems to contradict those I reported earlier, with such results found especially for boys. Given that Hernández et al.'s (2017a) measure of negative emotion included sadness, however, these findings may make more sense, especially in conjunction with the results found by Walter and LaFreniere (2000). In their study, girls' sadness was negatively related to peer acceptance, whereas both anger and sadness for boys were positively related to peer rejection. In contrast, girls' peer rejection was *negatively* related to their infrequent anger—bringing to mind Layne's bursts of bossiness that seemed to "work" in terms of her prominence in the peer group. So, girls' sadness may render them difficult to interact with, whereas the way they show anger often may differ from boys in its effect on others.

## Other Negative Emotions and Social Competence: Sadness and Shyness

Thus, anger is not the only negative emotion that contributes to the picture of social competence or incompetence. Preschoolers' sadness, whether observed in the classroom or in interaction with their mothers, was related to teachers' ratings of social withdrawal and "miserableness," even when child gender and age are accounted for (Denham & Burger, 1991; Denham, Renwick, & Holt, 1991; see also Eisenberg, Sadovsky, Spinrad, Fabes, et al., 2005, and Lindsey, 2019b, for more global negative social competence outcomes of sadness).

As seen for both positive and overall negative expressiveness and anger, some moderation by gender has been identified. For example, in Denham, Renwick, et al. (1991), boys were particularly at risk for the link between their sadness in interactions with their mothers and teachers' views of their classroom misery. Perhaps again the meaning of sadness differed for boys and girls, especially when teachers' views were considered. In this case boys' sadness with their mothers, rather than with their peers, as in Hernández et al. (2017a) and Walter and LaFreniere (2000), generalized to the classroom context in ways that were noted specifically by teachers and, unlike girls' sadness, were not necessarily noted by peers. My thought here, given the measurement differences in these studies, is that teachers saw the kind of sadness in boys that was demonstrated by social withdrawal, whereas peers in earlier studies saw, and judged, girls' sadness *during interaction*.

> Thomas shows sadness when observed in the preschool classroom, as well as when visiting the laboratory with his mother. His facial demeanor is forlorn, and his expressiveness is muted. He also often sits alone in school, head down, and is loath to play with others. His social exchange with peers is usually limited to single words. Watching Thomas over time, his teachers clearly see him as miserable, isolated, not interacting with others. His social competence skills do not seem to be developing.

Peers are not oblivious to such emotional expressiveness either. As already noted, boys showing sadness during in Walter and LaFreniere (2000) were seen more negatively by peers. Even more specifically, when asked to name classmates who were sad, afraid, and worried or cried a lot, first graders readily completed the task, and their ratings were related to teachers' lower ratings of the target children's social competence (especially for "afraid" and "cry a lot"; Perry-Parrish, Waasdrop, & Bradshaw, 2012). In this case, a range of more "submissive" negative emotions were noticed by classmates, and their problematic outcomes were confirmed by teachers.

Other negative emotions need to be considered as well. For example, the emotional picture of shyness includes wariness and reticence toward people in both familiar and, especially, unfamiliar situations (see Chapter 3); as such it constitutes a component of behavior inhibition. Because children who are shy may experience anxious, uncomfortable emotional arousal in social situations and can be hesitant and inhibited in approaching others (see Chapter 6), this emotion can be particularly relevant for social competence. Teachers may see these children as cooperative because they are inhibited (and nondisruptive) in class, but also as less assertive. But such inhibition and lack of assertion could take a toll on effective social interaction with peers (Rudasill & Konold, 2008; Séguin & McDonald, 2018). In fact, longitudinal trajectories from shyness (or more broadly, behavioral inhibition) in toddlerhood to social reticence at age 4 have been found (Rubin, Burgess, & Hastings, 2002), especially when mothers behaved intrusively and derisively about their children's shyness. Lack of support made it even harder for behaviorally inhibited, shy children to enter the world of peers in an age-appropriate manner.

In support of these ideas about the negative outcomes of shyness, Sette and colleagues (Sette, Baldwin, et al., 2019; Sette, Baumgartner, Laghi, & Coplan, 2016, Sette, Baumgartner, & Schneider, 2014; see also Armer, 2004) found that shy preschoolers experienced more peer rejection and other peer difficulties than nonshy peers (see also Zhu et al., 2019; further, Zhang, Eggum-Wilkens, Eisenberg, & Spinrad, 2017, found this effect also with 6- and 7-year-olds). Xiao, Spinrad, and Eisenberg (2019) found such children to be less prosocial as well (see also MacGowan & Schmidt, 2021). Multiple examinations of shyness suggest that it dampens the probability of children's positive peer relationships and positive social behavior.

Again when broadening the construct to examine preschooler's behavioral inhibition (e.g., not only shyness, but also a low approach to novelty and risk taking and greater caution), children temperamentally characterized by such behavior were less socially integrated, less dominant, and less involved in aggressive encounters (Tarullo, Mliner, & Gunnar, 2011). In contrast, highly exuberant children exhibited anger more often and had more conflictual friendships (Tarullo et al., 2011); experiencing stable high exuberance since infancy was related to their behavior problems, but at the same time their lack of reticence (Degnan et al., 2011).

It is important to acknowledge the potential pain of children experiencing shyness or its broader cousin, behavior inhibition. In fact, Eggum and colleagues (2009) have found that 18-month-olds' fearfulness predicts their shyness at 30 months; it is likely that they measured more fearful or "negative" shyness. Thus Leah, who was fearful when reciting a nursery rhyme in Chapter 2, is probably also feeling shyness, and it's no fun at all. In the preschool classroom, Leah's shyness makes it hard to join play, and her classmates see her as standoffish and hard to understand and like—why won't she play? Indeed, Diener and Kim (2004) found that girls' mothers' ratings of their shyness were related to teacher-rated social withdrawal. So, both teachers and peers may find Leah's behavior troubling, and she may experience continuing difficulties approaching and engaging with others.

However, elements of Leah's experience may be more frequently observed in boys. That is, again there exist potential gender differences; it has been more common in the literature to see deleterious outcomes of shyness for boys, perhaps because gender norms suggest a greater cost of social withdrawal for them—"boys should be brave and assertive!" Thus, some studies have, in comparison to Diener and Kim (2004), found that boys' shyness is related to negative peer status. In one such study, kindergartners' through second graders' shyness was negatively predictive of peer status 2 years later, as well as positively related to lack of positive emotionality and internalizing problems contemporaneously and/or predictively, but more for boys than for girls (Eisenberg, Shepard, et al., 1998). Boys' shyness also was related to their asocial behavior (Coplan & Armer, 2005).

More recent work, however, has not as frequently found evidence of such gender differences in how shyness is related to social competence and behavior problem outcomes (Sette et al., 2019), again suggesting that especially early childhood teachers' experiences and training are reducing gender bias, even though preschoolers themselves may still be prone to consider boys' social withdrawal as less acceptable (Sette, Colasante, Zava, Baumgartner, & Malti, 2018). It will be interesting to see what future research holds in terms of gender differences in the contribution of emotional expressiveness to social competence. Untangling sometimes-conflicting gender differences in how emotional expressiveness relates to social competence is important, and as noted earlier, may depend strongly on the context in which expressiveness is measured and on the person who is evaluating social competence as well.

Possible buffers for the negative outcomes of shyness also should be mentioned; the picture is not bleak for all shy preschoolers. For instance, peer preference may moderate the contribution of shyness to social difficulties. If preschoolers are able to achieve peer acceptance despite their shyness, they are not as likely to prefer solitary play and behave unsociably (Sette, Zava, Baumgartner, Baiocco, & Coplan, 2017). Perhaps having a well-accepted "buddy" can help shy children enter the peer group and succeed there, although this possibility has not been tested.

Amplifying these results, being able to talk to peers can be a strength that mitigates shyness. Shy children with lower vocabulary scores were rated as more asocial and needing more teacher attention, and self-reported lower perceived competence (Coplan & Armer, 2005; Zhu et al., 2019; see also Buss's (1986) theorizing about shy children's inhibited speech with peers). Being literally less able to talk to one's peers, *and being shy*, is a double whammy.

Another buffering factor may be having a positive relationship with one's teacher. In Sette, Baumgartner, et al. (2014), shy children's lack of a close relationship with the teacher was negatively related to teacher-reported social competence and positively related to teacher-reported peer rejection. Similarly, shy preschoolers without a close relationship with their teacher were less able to participate independently in classroom activities (Wu et al., 2015). At high levels of dependence with the teacher, shyness and social competence also were negatively related (see also Wu et al., 2015, for findings specifically focused on preschoolers' cooperation). In contrast, in Sette et al.'s (2014) study, having a close, nonconflictual relationship with one's teacher was related to social competence whether children were shy or not. All these findings are suggestive of the protective role a positive child–teacher relationship may play in enabling shy children to avoid social difficulties—perhaps especially in a country like Italy, where most preschoolers remain with the same teacher for 3 years. Being able to interact with a trusted teacher, who can coach peer interactions, supports the shy child.

Finally, it is important to consider the cultural evaluations of shyness. Early behavioral inhibition does not necessarily predict long-term difficulties (Chen et al., 2020), especially in cultural contexts where such behaviors are not sanctioned, perhaps even valued.

## SUMMARY: Negative Emotion and Social Competence

In short, enduring negative expressiveness—whether involving anger, sadness, shyness, or an undifferentiated mix—can set about a cascade of equally negative social outcomes, just as positive expressiveness often sets a child up for both contemporaneous and later positive social outcomes. These robust cross-time relationships underscore the highly salient contribution of young children's emotional expressiveness to evaluations of social competence made by significant social partners.

Are these cross-time relationships for both positive and negative expressiveness primarily driven by a continuity in children's emotional expressiveness, as addressed in Chapter 2? Or did children very early develop persistent reputations, based on their emotionality, as particularly pleasant or nasty social partners? Either way (or both!), the strong emotional expressiveness component of interacting with others is already well established by the preschool period and figures prominently in success in the social world. Increasingly stable patterns of expressiveness contribute to increasingly stable evaluations of social competence (Denham & Holt, 1993; Denham, McKinley, et al., 1990). Negative emotion is especially problematic, sometimes especially for boys, but establishing positive relationships with peers or teachers can assuage some of its damaging outcomes.

## CONTRIBUTIONS OF EMOTIONAL EXPRESSIVENESS TO BEHAVIOR PROBLEMS

### Negative Emotion and Behavior Problems

Behavior problems (e.g., aggression, social withdrawal, and anxiety) impact social competence in a negative manner. Such problems often are related to a preponderance of negative expressiveness, especially when it is frequent or long lasting, dysregulated (e.g., overly intense), or contextually inappropriate (Kim et al., 2012; Locke, Davidson, Kalin, & Goldsmith, 2009). For example, for children whose levels of anger remain high from infancy to early elementary school, both externalizing and internalizing behavior problems are more frequent (Liu, Moore, et al., 2018; Perra, Paine, & Hay, 2021). Other work by Lipscomb et al. (2012) confirms the contribution of early negativity to externalizing problems at age 3. Similar results were found from infant negativity to first-grade aggression, mediated by both parents' stress (Bernier, Marquis-Brideau, Dusablon, Lemelin, & Sirois, 2021). Thus anger shown as early as infancy and toddlerhood can show continuity across a long time period, and this continuity does contribute to behavior problems.

As already suggested in my discussion of positive expressiveness, temporal and intensive aspects of anger also are important: kindergartners' overall observed anger frequency positively predicted parent- and teacher-reported externalizing symptoms, whereas anger intensity positively predicted both observed externalizing and parent-reported internalizing symptoms (Hernández et al., 2015; see also Nwadinobi & Gagne, 2020). Similarly, prekindergarten and kindergarten children who showed dysregulated anger when receiving an unwanted prize were rated by teachers, both concurrently and predictively, as exhibiting more externalizing behavior problems (Morris, Silk, Steinberg, Terranova, & Kithakye, 2010). Additionally, 4-year-olds' reports on their *own* anger and its regulation showed that less-regulated anger was related to caregiver ratings of both their reactive and proactive aggression (Jambon, Colasante, Peplak, & Malti, 2019).

In all these studies, anger was observed or self-reported, and its vivid expression—frequent and/or intense and dysregulated—signaled behavioral difficulties. Thus the anger shown by Carrie and Connor in the earlier examples is seen by both teachers and classmates as problematic and is often tied to aggressive behavior. Their frequent outbursts, at the very least, seriously disrupt social interaction and are definite warning signs of incipient behavior problems, especially if they persist over time.

The longitudinal trajectory from anger to disruptive behavior problems may be complex: Kim and Kochanska (2021) found that toddlers' unmanageable temperament, which included anger and low levels of self-regulation, predicted parents' power-assertive, punitive control of the children at 4 to 5 years old, which then predicted children's disruptive behavior problems in early elementary school. This unfortunate pathway was especially acute when family risk was high. This set of findings highlights the need to consider toddlers' and preschoolers' anger within the family context. Certainly angry, dysregulated toddlers can elicit negative disciplinary tactics from parents trying to manage their behavior. Children with anger problems are immersed in both classroom and family systems, with children affecting adults and vice versa.

Experts' reports also have demonstrated the deleterious effects of anger, in this case across large time spans and focusing on very negative outcomes: diagnoses of psychiatric disorders (Vogel, Jackson, Barch, Tillman, & Luby, 2019). Irritability (i.e., tantrums, frustration, and anger) in children already at risk for psychiatric diagnoses, assessed during preschool via psychiatric interviews with parents, predicted later global functioning, depression, and oppositional defiant disorder through age 19, even with baseline diagnoses, demographic factors, social adversity, and maternal psychiatric status accounted for. Anger may be a potent sign of continuing severe problems for young children who are already experiencing serious behavioral difficulties.

Again, however, as with social competence, anger is not the only negative emotion whose expression can be associated with such behavioral difficulty. First-grade peer nominations of a combination of negative emotions (i.e., sadness, worry, fear, and crying) were also related to teacher ratings of externalizing behavior problems (Perry-Parrish et al., 2012).

Fear can be important here. As already noted, Lindsey (2019a) uniquely differentiated preschoolers' emotions directed at friends and acquaintances. Fear shown to acquaintances, perhaps similar to shyness, was related to teachers' ratings of children's withdrawal; similarly, but without the friend/acquaintance distinction, Turkish preschoolers' fearfulness was related to their internalizing problems (with externalizing problems taken into account; Melis Yavuz, Selcuk, Çorapçı, & Aksan, 2017). In fact, Rydell, Berlin, and Bohlin (2003) found that children exhibiting high-level, dysregulated fear late in the preschool period evidenced internalizing problem behavior at 8 years. Going even further, Buss and colleagues (2013, 2021) have found that dysregulated fear (e.g., fear when there is little or no threat) at age 2 predicted social anxiety at the end of preschool, in the early school years, and into adolescence even with prior social anxiety accounted for. Such clear longitudinal pathways between early fearfulness and later social anxiety suggest the need for concerned adults' support.

Delving into negative emotions' expression further, shyness also was related to teachers' ratings of Italian children's withdrawal and anxiety (Sette et al., 2016), as well as to broader externalizing behavior problems (Sette et al., 2019; see also Han, Wu, Yu, Xia, & Gao, 2016). In fact, it was related to internalizing problems or social anxiety in multiple populations and cultures, including both Western and Asian (Colonnesi et al., 2017; Sanson et al., 1996; Sette et al., 2014; Zhu et al., 2019).

Despite these overall findings, several important distinctions should be made regarding the shyness/behavior problem connection. As mentioned in Chapter 3, the *type* of shyness may be important. For example, children who displayed any negative shyness during a performance task (i.e., the number of *negative* facial expressions co-occurring with aversions of gaze, the head, or both) were more socially anxious compared to children who showed only positive shyness (i.e., the number of *positive* facial expressions co-occurring with aversions of gaze, the head, or both) or displayed no shyness (Colonnesi et al., 2017). Expressing positive shyness was negatively related to both expressions of negative shyness and social anxiety. Coy positive shyness does not communicate the same negative emotional experience as does negative shyness.

Further, the ability to create a close relationship with one's preschool teacher, as shown in Sette et al.'s (2014) findings related to the lack of social competence, may buffer the shy child from demonstrating behavior problems (Arbeau, Coplan, & Weeks, 2010). That is, when children had close relationships with their teachers, shyness was actually *negatively* related to school avoidance, anxiety with peers, and asocial behavior with peers. Again the pattern of results suggested a protective role for close teacher–child relationships for shy children's adjustment. Lack of a closer teacher–child relationship also puts the child at risk for aggression problems (Han et al., 2016) and dislike of school (Wu et al., 2015). Leah's teacher is extremely skilled at connecting with the children in her classroom, and Leah's positive relationship with her will help assuage any difficulties that result from Leah's shyness.

Thus the predominance and intensity of all the negative emotions do not augur well for preventing children's behavioral problems. Searching for some sort of mechanism for buffering these deleterious outcomes may center on the relationships children experience, especially with supportive adults.

Moreover, neurobiological differences among children exhibiting negative emotions may be important to monitor. For example, frontal brain EEG asymmetry is related to outcomes for shy, fearful, and angry children, with right frontal asymmetry and either shyness or fear related to internalizing problems and left frontal asymmetry and anger related to externalizing problems (Fox, Schmidt, Calkins, Rubin, & Coplan, 1996; Liu, Calkins, & Bell, 2021). In contrast, exuberance in children with left frontal symmetry is positively related to their social competence (Degnan et al., 2011). These patterns reflect upon children's abilities to regulate their emotional arousal and are useful markers that could support emotional competence programming.

## Positive Emotions and Behavior Problems

Along with the problematic nature of negative expressiveness, the *lack* of positive emotion (both the observed frequency and, in this case, the intensity) also becomes a problem; it has predicted both parent- and teacher-rated internalizing symptoms (Hernández et al., 2015; see Lindsey, 2019a, for similar but more narrowband findings on teacher ratings of aggression). Examining longitudinal contributions, Ghassabian and colleagues (2014) found that the lack of positive emotions observed at age 3 predicted age-6 internalizing via lower attention shifting at age 4. The authors suggested that the originally less emotionally positive children may have acquired a self-regulatory inflexibility that contributed to social withdrawal at school entry. In any case, the inability to show enjoyment is a sign of difficulties and should alert adults to the child's predicament. Thomas, whose sadness was discussed in an earlier example, also very rarely shows positive emotion. His teachers and parents are trying to help him.

At the same time, very intense positive emotional expressiveness can make a negative contribution to evaluations of young children's social competence. Because positive expressiveness is usually seen as an undiluted advantage, an important point here is to differentiate between the frequency or prevalence and the intensity of emotional expressiveness. Frequency or prevalence can be indicative, as suggested in Chapter 1, of aggregated emotional reactions to events that are experienced and overtly expressed

(Lindsey, 2019b). I generally take such a viewpoint in discussing emotional expressiveness and its correlates.

In contrast, emotional intensity more specifically denotes the strength and regulation of expression, dependent on the context in which children interact, and their past experience (Lindsey, 2019b). From a functionalist perspective, the information gleaned from the valence or type and frequency or prevalence of emotional expressiveness is different from that obtained by an emotional expression's intensity. A mild but clear smile tells the recipient something very different from loud, prolonged laughter—in the first case, a playmate may want to join whatever the child is doing, but in the second, a more cautious approach may be called for—what is going on here? It is important to consider the intensity of specific emotions, even the positive ones I am now discussing.

> One afternoon on the playground Mike gets Joey and the other boys to have races. They are smiling, laughing, and running fast, faster, faster! Rounding a corner by the swings, one of them clips Caroline as he passes by. She falls down and starts to cry. They then run through the sandbox, ruining the elaborate highway system Pei Lin is constructing (she likes building in the sand, just like her friend John). They are still laughing hard and running, running, running! Finally, they run headlong into their teacher, who scolds them and instructs them to settle down and come inside. Both classmates and teacher were left with racing hearts and negative impressions of what just happened. Pei Lin and Caroline in particular and their teacher may form opinions that Mike especially has problems.

Thus consistent high-intensity happiness and glee just may be too much of a good thing. For example, frequent intense positive emotion and exuberance rated by parents of preschoolers was related to parents' and teachers' ratings of externalizing behavior problems, both concurrently and over approximately 3 years; similarly, such emotionality was negatively related to preschool teacher ratings of prosocial behaviors (Rydell et al., 2003). Sallquist, Eisenberg, Spinrad, Eggum, and Gaertner (2009) also found that preschoolers rated as demonstrating high-positive emotional intensity (as well as high-negative expressiveness and overall expressivity) declined in social skills across a 6-year period. Moreover, excitability (i.e., poorly regulated and intense positivity) in 3- to 5-year-olds at risk for psychiatric problems predicted diagnoses of mania and externalizing problems from the end of preschool through age 19, even with social adversity and maternal psychiatric history accounted for (Vogel et al., 2019).

However, like the contrasting ways that exuberant positive emotions seem to be interpreted by social partners, this evidence of difficulties are not universal. Walter and LaFreniere (2000) found that peers' nominations of acceptance and impact were related to children's high-level observed positivity. However, in their study a broad smile accompanied by joyful verbalizations defined strong positive emotion; this definition may not index as strong an emotion as the difficult-to-calm positivity in the other findings cited here. Further, the difference between ratings, which examine emotionality across time and context, and observations of specific contexts can be telling. In the case of Walter and LaFreniere's findings, then, both their operational definition and their mode of data collection may have changed the meaning of strong positivity. It is clear that evaluation of this literature must be done with care.

### SUMMARY: Expressiveness and Behavior Problems

As with social competence, profiles of both negative and positive expressiveness are related to behavior problems. In this case, a preponderance of negative emotions, especially anger that is easily elicited and intense, is a key indicator of many diagnosable behavior problems. Children with more frequent and intense anger can be on a negative trajectory as early as toddlerhood. Characteristic patterns of sadness, worry, fear, and negative shyness also can be warnings of behavior problems. Even a lack of positive emotion and too-intense positive emotions also are problematic. There is some indication that some of these difficult outcomes can be ameliorated by a good relationship with a teacher. This silver lining, like that for expressiveness and social competence, suggests to me that varying relationship factors could buffer children who have difficult emotions from experiencing the harmful trajectory to serious behavior problems; increased research in the area could prove profitable.

## CONTEXTS OF EMOTIONAL EXPRESSIVENESS

Sometimes other dimensions of emotional expressiveness need to be considered when examining the contribution of preschoolers' emotionality to their social competence and behavior problems. The context of emotional expressiveness and the meaning of the message it conveys are extremely important, particularly the contextual appropriateness of both anger and happiness.

Thus negative emotion may not invariably lead to equally negative evaluations of social competence or the presence of behavior problems. Even though being angry much of the time is a real problem, anger during conflict is pretty much expected, and does not predict either peer acceptance or teachers' ratings of social competence (Arsenio et al., 1997).

Further, anger observed in children sometimes *positively* predicts teachers' ratings of the children's assertiveness (Denham & Burger, 1991), which may reflect the context in which the anger is observed, as well as the gender of the child. Thus, expressing anger can be associated with teachers' perceptions of a sometimes unfriendly and aggressive, sometimes bossy, but nonetheless socially successful child. Layne comes to mind when considering this nuance of emotional expressiveness—she sometimes shows annoyance when telling her classmates what to do during play, but this does not seem to diminish her appeal. The meaning of her emotional message in the house corner seems to be "Let's get organized and do this right!"

As another example, being angry when exposed to unfairness is not unhelpful. In fact, preschoolers who showed this type of anger, especially those not highly shy, 1 year later were more prosocial to an experimenter's simulated distress than those who showed more troubling dispositional (i.e., "day in, day out") anger (Xiao et al., 2019).

But, on the other hand, contextually *in*appropriate anger does not portend well for preschoolers' social competence; a greater proportion of anger shown in *non*aggressive encounters was related to negative peer status and the initiation of aggression (Arsenio et al., 2000). Why should anger be shown when interacting nonaggressively?

Anger that is contextually inappropriate in other ways also is related to parent/teacher ratings of externalizing behavior problems, peer assessments of *un*likeability, and even self-reports of problems, sometimes especially for boys. For example, showing anger when witnessing positive stimuli was especially related to preschoolers' self-reported loneliness and negative peer nominations, usually with the expression of anger when witnessing negative stimuli accounted for (Locke, Miller, Seifer, & Heinze, 2015).

Regarding the context of happiness, being happy during a conflict is quite a different matter from expressing happiness in general everyday interaction. As already amply noted here, having a generally happy demeanor is inviting and an advantage to the development of friendship. But smiling while hitting another child is seen as very mean; for example, Arsenio et al. (1997) have found that children who show such contextually "misplaced" happiness are less well accepted by their peers. In fact, Arsenio and colleagues (2000) found that expressing happiness during aggression was related to the initiation of aggression, which subsequently predicted negative peer status. Moreover, Miller and Olson (2000) observed what they termed "gleeful taunting" in preschool boys, and such behavior early in the school year predicted later negative peer status and teacher ratings of disruptive behavior. Finally, preschool-age boys who showed anger *and* "disharmonious happiness" while playing a game with their parents, were rated as higher in externalizing problem behavior in early elementary school; this combination of emotions depicted the boys' intense competitiveness and rather unpleasant satisfaction in besting their parent (Chaplin et al., 2005). Happiness in such contexts is not part of emotionally competent expressiveness.

> At 4, Michael has real trouble controlling his behavior. He is unpredictably aggressive, can't seem to follow class rules, and wanders during circle time. His large size for his age adds to the threatening nature of his aggression, but most eerie is his frequent smiling when a classmate is writhing on the floor after Michael hits or kicks him. Michael's teachers worried about him a lot when his parents suddenly withdrew him from childcare.

Another important contextual matter to consider is whether the child is immersed in a more collectivistic/relational culture, where expressiveness often may be valued differently than it is in a more individualistic culture. For example, Korean children's sadness *and* happiness during "I'm not sharing" and "Bubbles" emotion-eliciting laboratory tasks were related to teachers' evaluations of them as antisocial. In contrast, these relationships were either reversed or nonsignificant for European American preschoolers (Louie et al., 2015). Asian American children's anger also was related to teacher evaluations of diminished peer acceptance and prosocial behavior. Thus expressivity in general was seen as a detriment to social competence for children living in a generally collectivistic system. As noted in Chapter 2, emotions in these contexts were likely seen as conflicting with the goals of group harmony.

## SUMMARY: Context of Emotions

It matters when and where emotions are shown in considering how they relate to social competence and behavior problems, even as early as preschool. In some contexts, anger is not as much of a problem as when it is predominant in a preschooler's emotional profile; similarly, happiness in specific contexts can herald real difficulty. As can be seen for other issues related to emotional competence or its lack, sometimes these issues are particularly important for boys' development.

## THE SPECIAL ROLE OF EMPATHIC CONCERN AND OTHER SOCIAL AND SELF-EVALUATIVE EMOTIONS

### Sympathy/Empathic Concern and Social Competence/Behavior Problems

Sympathetic emotional responsiveness is another specific aspect of emotional expressiveness that supports preschoolers' social competence, especially prosocial behavior. As theory has long suggested (e.g., Eisenberg, Schaller, et al., 1988; Lennon & Eisenberg, 1987a), children who respond to the emotional needs of others, reacting sympathetically to others' distress, are more likely to exhibit prosocial behavior, an important component of success in the challenging world of preschool peer interaction (Ross, 2017; Saarni, 1990; Sroufe et al., 1984). In fact, this relationship has held true across both Western and Southeast Asian cultures (Trommsdorff et al., 2007).

However, this connection between empathic concern and prosocial behavior may begin even earlier. As noted in Chapter 2, the connection between empathic concern and prosocial behavior has been examined beginning in infancy and toddlerhood. Researchers studying these earliest manifestations and relationships found that prosocial behavior was rare in the first year but increased substantially during the second year of life. Importantly, individual differences in empathic concern assessed in the first year, amazingly as early as 3 to 6 months, predicted different levels of prosocial behavior observed in the second year (Davidov et al., 2020; Roth-Hanania et al., 2011; Young et al., 1999). Further, increases in empathic concern from 3 to 18 months were related to teachers' evaluations of social competence at 36 months (Paz, Davidov, Orlitsky, Roth-Hanania, & Zahn-Waxler, 2021).

Moreover, these early indications of empathic concern protected against increases in externalizing problems from 18 to 36 months; infants and toddlers classified as "high-empathy" remained stable in externalizing problems from 18 to 36 months, whereas the "low-empathy" group experienced an increase. Additionally, for toddlers whose empathic concern increased, teachers reported more positive peer relationships compared to those of "low-empathy" toddlers. More specifically, boys' earliest indicators of empathy (as early as 3 months) were related to a lack of externalizing problems at 18 and 36 months, but the opposite trend was often found for girls, especially at the younger age (Paz, Orlitsky, et al., 2021). It may be that at this age externalizing measures are more likely to capture girls' arousal levels and assertiveness, rather than problematic behavior.

Other studies have focused on the period from toddlerhood to preschool age, and much early theorizing concentrated on this age span. Early work suggested that children's facial and gestural sympathy to another's distress are particularly related to their unrequested prosocial behavior. These spontaneously prosocial behaviors constitute a more mature form of prosocial responsiveness, as compared to requested prosocial behavior, which is associated with "wimpiness" (Lennon, Eisenberg, & Carroll, 1986; see also Eisenberg, McCreath, et al., 1988). Preschoolers who react both sympathetically and prosocially to their peers' emotions are also seen as more socially competent by both teachers and peers (Braza et al., 2009; Denham & Burger, 1991; Denham & Holt, 1993; Marcus, 1980). Thus, both sympathy and prosocial behavior continue after toddlerhood to form intricately related aspects of preschool social success.

Longitudinal research also has upheld the prediction that toddlers' and preschoolers' empathic concern specifically supports their prosocial behavior. For example, 30- and 42-month-olds' empathic concern (via concerned facial expressions and hypothesis testing when an experimenter feigned injury) was related to at least one index of prosocial behavior (i.e., observed, parent rated, or experimenter rated; Edwards et al., 2015). Moreover, sympathy in 30-month-olds significantly predicted ratings of prosocial behavior at 42 months in an analysis controlling for prior levels of prosocial behavior.

Also examining empathy and prosocial responses longitudinally during both the toddler and preschool age period, the mothers in Taylor, Eisenberg, Spinrad, Eggum, and Sulik (2013) rated their children's empathy (including both sympathy and personal distress, e.g., "is aware of other people's feelings," "is worried or upset when someone is hurt") five times between the ages of 24 months and 54 months. The initial levels and growth of sympathy positively predicted prosocial behavior rated by teachers at 72 to 84 months. The story of empathy promoting both prosocial behavior, and even its growth is supported by these two studies.

Other research has focused more specifically on how older preschool children's and early primary school-age children's empathic concern, both contemporaneously and longitudinally, predicts prosocial behavior. Varying methods were used to assess both empathic concern and prosocial behavior. For example, among 5-year-olds, Strayer and Roberts (2004) found that empathic concern, as assessed via both child interviews and parent/teacher ratings, was contemporaneously related to observed prosocial behavior, as well as to diminished anger and aggression. Regarding exclusively nonparental adult reporters, preschool teacher-rated empathic concern also was related to their assignment of prosocial roles to their preschool students in a class play methodology (Belacchi & Farina, 2012; see also a replication by Farina & Belacchi, 2014, who found that Albanian preschoolers' empathic concern also was negatively related to hostile, victim, and outsider roles assigned by teachers).

In the longitudinal findings, the multi-informant ratings of 6-year-olds' sympathy were related to the level and change in children's helping and cooperation across the next 6 years (Malti, Gummerum, Keller, & Buchmann, 2009; Song, Colasante, & Malti, 2018; see also Eggum et al., 2011, where maternal ratings of children's sympathy predicted prosocial orientation longitudinally from 45 to 72 months). These time spans are impressive. The ability to respond with empathic concern forms a foundation for positive behavior and positive thinking.

Moreover, along with observing children and asking the important people in their lives how they are doing, it is worth asking the children themselves what they are thinking and feeling when they witness another's distress (as noted by Strayer & Roberts,

2004). Preschool through grade-school children's sympathetic story completions about their own emotional responsiveness to others were related to their actual prosocial behaviors (Chapman, Zahn-Waxler, Cooperman, & Iannotti, 1987). Their observed helping of a kitten, an adult experimenter, and a mother with an infant were also associated with the positive affect that the children attributed to the act of helping itself, and with their guilt over the story protagonist's distress. Thus the meaning which children attribute to their own emotional arousal when confronted by others' distress and the accompanying sense of responsibility for the other person's plight are important ingredients of empathic responsiveness to others—itself so critical in social relationships. The propensity to cope with others' emotions by expressing sympathy, by feeling guilty, and by being pleased about one's helping adds to young children's prosocial development. These other complex emotions (e.g., guilt and pride) are considered later.

Since Chapman et al.'s (1987) work, several investigators have collected young children's own evaluation of their level of sympathy and found that these reports positively related to prosocial behavior (e.g., Malti et al., 2009; Song et al., 2018; Zava, Sette, Baumgartner, & Coplan, 2020). Malti and colleagues' work already has been mentioned, but Ongley and Malti (2014) also found that even 4-year-olds' self-reported sympathy predicted their sharing during a dictator game. Further, in Jambon et al. (2019) a *lack* of self-reported sympathy was related to reactive and proactive aggression in both 4- and 8-year-olds. It bears emphasizing that preschoolers were able to provide relatively consistent answers to questions such as "When I see someone being picked on, I feel sorry for them," when asked whether the statements described them, and if so, how much. Obtaining reliable information about sympathy and broader empathic concern from children this young is important both methodologically and theoretically.

Along with research that examines feeling concern for others' distress, recent work also has conceptualized *positive empathy*—responding with happiness to others' positive emotion. Sallquist and colleagues (2009) asked mothers to report on how their children reacted when others were happy (e.g., another child getting a gift or good news or appearing excited) and rated the children's happiness when an experimenter showed happiness at receiving a gift. This "positive empathy" was positively related to observation of the child's happiness during a bubble-blowing task, as well as parent or caregiver ratings of the child's positivity. Mothers also rated their children's positive empathy, and these reports were positively related to observed and parent or caregiver ratings of positive emotionality, prosocial behavior, and overall social competence, both concurrently and 1 year later. Thus, as noted in my earlier discussion (Lindsey, 2017, 2019a, 2019b), sharing positive affect can be foundational to other positive social outcomes. This new research development seems very auspicious to me—I have long considered the sharing of positive emotion to be crucial to attachment and to other positive relationships (Denham & Burton, 2003).

## SUMMARY: Empathic Concern Outcomes

The relationship between variously operationalized empathic concern and social competence, especially prosocial behavior, is identified early. This connection is seen both contemporaneously and across longitudinal periods, from late infancy to the primary grades. Informants have included parents, teachers, and even the children themselves. The theoretically predicted association between concern for others' distress and prosocial responding has garnered much support. More recently, studies of "positive empathy"—feeling positive with another person—have been conducted.

## Factors That Influence the Empathic Concern/Prosocial Behavior Connection

### *Attachment*

Attachment security also may be an important factor in the empathic concern/prosocial behavior connection in very young children. For example, similar to earlier reported studies, 3-year-olds' empathic concern, as rated by their mothers, was related to their prosocial behavior in a laboratory analogue situation in which an experimenter "lost" her baby's pacifier (Panfile & Laible, 2012). In a more complex analysis within this study, children's secure attachment to their mothers predicted their ER, which then predicted empathic concern. These findings fit theoretical predictions that security of attachment promotes ER, which then allows the child to respond with empathic concern rather than personal distress, supporting prosocial responding (Stern & Cassidy, 2018). The relation between attachment and empathic concern is indirect, via ER.

Empathic concern can be related to attachment in even more complicated ways (Kim & Kochanska, 2017). For example, toddlers' empathic concern to mothers' or fathers' portrayals of pain (e.g., "Spontaneously comforts, apologizes, kisses the hurt finger") was related to later preschool ratings of prosocial behavior, as in the studies already reviewed here. Feelings of security with mothers were also related to the empathic concern that was shown to the children. However, empathic concern shown to both mothers and fathers was related to later prosociality with peers, specifically for children who had been insecure toddlers; without at least moderate levels of empathic concern, their prosociality was very low. Still, nonempathic preschoolers who has been insecure toddlers were less prosocial than their equally nonempathic, but secure, peers. Conversely, at high levels of empathy, both insecure and secure children were seen as prosocial in preschool.

Put another way, if children were capable of reacting empathically despite their insecure attachment status, they also were later able to respond prosocially to peers. Their emotional responding to their parents' distress, that they believed they had caused, buffered any deleterious effect of insecure attachment. It is important to note that this study, like that of Taylor et al. (2013), combined both empathic concern and personal distress for one empathy score, so that the empathy/prosocial behavior trajectory may have been fueled by the personal distress aspect of insecure children's empathy. Nonetheless, empathy, considered overall as responding to another's distress, facilitated their prosocial behavior across time.

So, although these two studies differed in the way in which attachment was hypothesized to relate to empathy and subsequent prosocial behavior, and in their somewhat complex results, it is clear that there are important ways in which attachment can affect the trajectory from empathic concern to prosocial behavior in the toddler to preschool age group.

## *Gender*

The path from empathic concern to evaluations of social competence also may differ for boys and girls, at least in terms of the focus of peers' evaluations. In one study (Carreras et al., 2014), teachers rated children's empathic concern (e.g., "Comforts others when they are sad," "Understands when a partner feels bad"). Kindergartners rated each other on same-gender peers' overall social preference, as well as rating aspects of same-gender peers' social conflicts (i.e., regarding physical, verbal, and indirect aggression; constructive conflict resolution; assisting others in their conflicts; and withdrawal from conflict). Boys' empathic concern contributed to peers' evaluations of their positive social preference via lessened physical aggression within social conflicts. Girls' empathic concern contributed to their positive social preference via increasing assistance to others within conflicts. In other words, empathically responsive boys were seen as likable via the cessation of a gendered negative behavior (aggression), whereas girls who showed such responsiveness were liked via a somewhat differently gendered, but positive, behavior (see also Braza et al., 2009, who found teacher-rated empathic concern to be more highly related to peer acceptance for boys than for girls, despite an overall positive relation).

## *Other Emotions*

One's other emotions may be important to consider in their interaction with empathic concern to better understand its relation with prosocial behavior. That is, the prevalence of certain other emotions may facilitate or hinder action emanating from empathic concern. More specifically, in Zava et al. (2020) older preschoolers provided self-reports of sympathetic feelings toward others. Results revealed interaction effects between their reports of empathic feelings and parents' reports of their shyness in the prediction of outcome variables. Among children with lower levels of parent-rated shyness, sympathy rated by the children themselves was positively related to prosocial behavior. At higher levels of shyness, these connections were attenuated. Thus, although shy children may not differ from their more sociable counterparts in experiencing sympathy toward others, they seem to be less likely to act on it.

Another emotion that may impact the relationship between empathic concern and prosocial behavior is one's *own* sadness. To feel sympathy and act upon that feeling, one's own distress needs to be dealt with first. Underlying negativity, even sadness, may fuel the distress that blocks sympathetic responsiveness. In Song et al. (2018), sympathy was indexed by child and caregiver report, whereas sadness regulation and prosocial behavior were solely caregiver reported. Higher sympathy was associated with greater prosocial behavior, but children's ability to regulate their own sadness contributed to their sympathy. Recent research corroborates this linkage and extends to anger regulation: 4-year-olds who self-reported better regulation of both sadness and anger (and the interaction of both) self-reported greater sympathy (i.e., "When I see another child who is hurt or upset, I feel sorry for him or her"; Galarneau, Colasante, Speidel, & Malti, 2022).

> Leah feels sad when she sees Antonio cry when his mother leaves the preschool in the morning—she knows how he feels. It can be really hard when Mommy says goodbye. But she also is very sorry for him, and stands watching him, feeling sorrier and sorrier. So not feeling shy because she's known him since they were babies, she goes over and offers him a coveted toy, patting him on the back. He looks surprised, takes the toy (Leah's cherished fidget spinner!), and a tiny smile appears through his tears.

Cross-time linkages between underlying negativity, sympathy, and prosocial behavior also deserve further study, especially given their complexity. Specifically, longitudinal connections among sadness, sympathy, and prosocial behavior are important; as already noted in Chapter 2, Edwards et al. (2015) considered how toddlers' and preschoolers' own overall sadness contributed to their ability to show empathic concern and prosocial behavior. Parent-rated dispositional sadness was negatively related to reported prosocial behavior at 18 months, but positively related to sympathy at 30 months. Then, once the ability to feel sympathy was well in place by 30 months, it facilitated prosocial behavior at 45 months. Leah, at age 4, was able to put aside any momentary sadness or shyness and act upon her feelings of sympathy.

### *Social-Cognitive Abilities*

Along with an awareness of one's own emotional reactions to others' distress and one's other emotions (especially sadness), aspects of social cognition are important in the sympathy–prosocial connection. Sympathy requires especially focusing on others' negative emotion. Understanding and "taking in" the other's distress is key; empathy can be considered to involve not only children's emotional reaction to another's emotion, but also their cognitive attributions about that distress (Strayer, 1993; Strayer & Roberts, 2004). Thus when preschoolers anticipated higher levels of sadness for the withdrawn, excluded peers they heard about in vignettes, they also were rated higher in sympathy and, in turn, higher in prosocial behavior. Attributing high levels of sadness to these peers, who portrayed relatively heightened need, may be an early social cognitive characteristic of children who are more sympathetic and more likely to channel other-oriented concerns into prosocial actions (Sette et al., 2018). This awareness involves emotion knowledge, obviously, but also aspects of more cognitively advanced perspective taking. Together, Song et al. (2018), Edwards et al. (2015), and Sette et al. (2018) show the importance of a social cognitive focus on the other's sadness, as well as the ability to deal with one's own.

It also could be worthwhile to examine even further the social cognitive foundations of empathic concern. Parents' ratings of kindergartners' and first graders' sympathy were related to the children's more frequent prosocial, as well as fewer aggressive and socially withdrawn, responses to social vignettes involving prosocial, aggressive, or shy peers (Findlay, Girardi, & Coplan, 2006). Importantly, these researchers concluded that young, more sympathetic children showed a greater understanding of shyness and aggression than less-empathic peers—their social sensitivity in terms of social understanding *and* social behavior were evident. Thus understanding others' sadness, shyness, and the reasons for these feelings are also crucial in discerning the nature of sympathetic concern and its links with prosocial behavior.

## SUMMARY: Factors Influencing the Empathic Concern/Social Competence Linkage

There are several factors that should be considered when trying to predict when children's empathic concern supports various aspects of their social competence. These prominently include (1) children's attachment status (although findings here can be rather complex); (2) gender; (3) the impact of other emotions (e.g., sadness and shyness) as they interact with empathic concern; and (4) social cognitive abilities undergirding cognitive empathy, such as perspective taking. A fuller story of the workings of empathic concern in the context of social relationships can be told by considering these factors.

## Relationship of Other Social and Self-Evaluative Emotions with Social Competence and Behavior Problems

Regarding preschoolers' other social and self-evaluative emotions, several studies have recently looked beyond empathy to examine how guilt, shame, and pride relate to young children's prosocial behavior, more general social competence, or behavior problems. One candidate for promoting social competence might be guilt; as noted in Chapter 3, the experience of guilt highlights one's responsibility in a transgression, such that reparation could be an outcome. In fact, Vaish (2018) found that the experience of guilt motivated reparative behavior in 2- and 3-year-olds (see also Colasante et al., 2014, who found that caregivers' reports of both children's guilt and sympathy were related to their reports of children's reparations for transgressions). Also observing toddlers, Drummond et al. (2017) led children to believe they had broken an experimenter's prized possession. Toddlers who attempted to repair the toy or confessed, as opposed to those showing a more shame-related response pattern of avoiding the adult and *not* confessing or attempting to repair, were quicker to help the adult in later tasks where the experimenter feigned being cold or being sad. Likewise, when older preschoolers showed shame-related avoidance in a similar mishap situation, their parents reported their greater aggression and less empathy toward a young sibling (Kolak & Volling, 2022).

Guilt and its relation to positive social behavior also has been studied with preschoolers. Four-year-olds who had self-reported low levels of sympathy, but who also said they'd feel guilty, sad, or bad in vignettes in which the protagonist was not prosocial given the chance (e.g., "Imagine that you and another boy are both making sandcastles. The other boy asks you to help him finish his big sandcastle, and you say 'no' "; Ongley & Malti, 2014, p. 1151), shared more in a dictator game. So feelings of guilt, rather than necessarily sympathy, also seemed to motivate these older children's prosocial behavior. Widening the context to evaluations of positive social behavior and lack of behavior problems, when children believed that they had broken the experimenter's treasured object, their signs of guilt, in terms of shortened latency for trying to fix the object and confessing, were positively related to parent-rated adaptive social functioning and negatively to emotional and behavior problems (Bafunno & Camodeca, 2013; see also Chapter 3).

Looking at prosocial responses and several self-conscious emotions within one paradigm, 3- and 4-year-olds were given opportunities to spontaneously help the experimenter retrieve a dropped crayon as well as to make amends by attempting to fix a broken toy (Ross, 2017; see Chapter 3 for details). Making amends for the broken toy was predicted by sympathy (e.g., furrowed brows and/or sad expressions) and achievement pride, and negatively by achievement shame. Help was predicted by a different pattern—by both moral and achievement pride, marginally by guilt, and negatively by achievement shame. Interestingly, children's pride may have indexed a sense of agency that facilitated both making amends and helping.

Focusing in on behavior problems, making reparations after feeling guilty was related to children's *lack* of disruptive behavior or depression diagnoses (Luby et al., 2009). Similarly, Ferguson and colleagues (1999) found that "shame-free" guilt was adaptive—at least for boys, for whom such guilt was associated with fewer behavior problems. These authors cogently noted, "Even when a person fails to resist temptation . . . or unwittingly does harm, guilt acts to restore severed relational bonds by reaffirming one's commitment to considerate behavior" (p. 355). Cumulatively, results reviewed so far underscore my earlier suggestion, that guilt and other self-conscious emotions may be related to prosocial responding, especially in situations where preschoolers feel some personal responsibility.

Patterns of association again may differ by children's gender, however. The mechanism whereby shame-free guilt motivates prosocial responding may not be as operative for girls as it is for boys, however, because of their possible *overinvolvement* in others' distress at their transgressions. In this case, guilt may hinder rather than enable prosocial behavior. Further, as already noted, girls are subjected to socialization pressure to be kind, helpful, and not hurt others, so it may not be surprising that in Ferguson et al. (1999) girls' guilt was related to internalizing problems. Feeling that one had done wrong motivated girls not as much to reparative behavior as to feeling sad and anxious about the larger transgression against what "nice little girls" do. Because not every study has found such an effect of gender, however, more study and consideration of the roots of the effect is required.

In contrast, shame-related responses (e.g., bodily tension, gaze aversion, avoidance, reticence to interact, or themes in children's story-stem completions) were related to negative outcomes (Bafunno & Camodeca, 2013; Drummond et al., 2017; Luby et al., 2009; Ross, 2017). In fact, 5- to 12-year-old children's shame responses on a scenario-based self-report measure were related to psychological symptoms (with no particular age differences), as well as to self-blame and attempts to minimize painful feelings (Ferguson et al., 1999).

### SUMMARY: Self-Conscious Emotions' Outcomes

Thus all the social and self-conscious emotions can play a role in predicting positive social behavior as well as behavior problems—either as observed in the moment or as rated by important adults. Along with empathic concern, guilt and pride seem conducive to prosocial behavior and other indices of social competence or lack of behavior problems. Again, however, the negative effect of shame is apparent. The functions of social and self-evaluative emotions are important and require further study.

## SELF-REGULATION AND THE RELATIONSHIP OF EXPRESSIVENESS WITH SOCIAL COMPETENCE OR BEHAVIOR PROBLEMS

I have mentioned self-regulation repeatedly as contributory to aspects of emotional competence; it also can modify the outcomes of emotional expressiveness in early childhood. First, relative level of self-regulation may moderate contributions of positive expressiveness. For example, preschoolers' positivity was especially predictive of peer acceptance for children who exhibited deficits in self-regulation (i.e., attention and inhibitory control; Hernández et al., 2017a, 2017b). That is, positive expressiveness was very important for more impulsive children in terms of peers' evaluations of them as playmates; it served a protective function. For example, even though sometimes it's hard to predict Mike's behavior—recall the ruckus he raised on the playground and his difficulty calming in the earlier example—his general positivity disarms peers and teachers alike. They find him charming.

In the case of positivity, emotion moderated the contribution of self-regulation problems to social outcomes. Self-regulation also can moderate the contribution of emotion. That is, self-regulation can alter the outcomes of negative expressiveness, buffering or exacerbating difficulties. For example, when children showed anxiety, concern, and/or embarrassment during self-regulation tasks, those who were still able to do the tasks well were rated higher on social competence by their teachers (Pecora, Sette, Baumgartner, Laghi, & Spinrad, 2016). Even more specifically, children whose teachers indicated were high in negative expressiveness, but who could nimbly shift their attention during a task involving depictions of different emotions, were rated as less likely to show externalizing behavior and more likely to cooperate in social situations (Wilson et al., 2021). As another example, children rated by mothers as more fearful but assessed as higher in delay ability (a component of self-regulation) were rated as showing fewer externalizing problems (Moran, Lengua, & Zalewski, 2013; see also Morris et al., 2014). In these cases, more skilled self-regulation buffered the effects of negative emotions.

Self-regulation and emotions also can have additive effects. For example, children who could self-regulate relatively well through their attention and self-control, and were low or moderate in negative expressiveness, were rated as the most prosocial and cooperative by parents and teachers (Laible, Carlo, Murphy, Augustine, & Roesch, 2014). These children's self-regulatory abilities helped them to prevent any negativity from "getting in the way" of social functioning.

Conversely, self-regulation difficulties in combination with higher-level negative emotions are facilitative of behavior problems. For example, Hughes, White, Sharpen, and Dunn (2000) found that "hard to manage" preschoolers showed more anger *and* poorer self-regulation. Also examining negative emotion and self-regulation together, children's negative emotional expressiveness (anger, sadness, and fear) was related to their behavior problems and lack of cooperation and prosocial behavior, particularly for children with lower self-regulation (see also Diener & Kim, 2004). As another example, children observed as more fearful or frustration prone and lower in self-regulation were rated by their mothers as showing more externalizing problems. Cumulatively, these results suggest that dealing with intense, difficult emotions may be especially problematic for children with less-developed self-regulation, exacerbating or actually reflecting aspects of their behavior problems (Diaz et al., 2017; see also Eisenberg, Sadovsky, Spinrad, Fabes, et al., 2005).

Along with *moderation*, longitudinal *mediation* of preschoolers' negative emotionality, leading to self-regulation difficulties, may extend to adolescence. Thus ratings of preschoolers' overly high positive or angry emotions were related to adolescents' adjustment problems, via age-7 difficulties with self-regulation. In contrast, low-intensity positive emotions predicted age-7 self-regulation, and hence more positive adolescent adjustment (Dollar et al., 2022).

These general trends also may be seen in non-Western cultures; for example, Chinese 6-year-old children's anger and self-regulation interacted to predict different behavior problems, depending on the reporting source. Mothers' reports on anger and lack of self-regulation were each directly related to their views of their children's internalizing problems, whereas teachers' reports on the children's self-regulation instead moderated the effect of anger on their and peer's views of externalizing problems (Eisenberg, Ma, et al., 2007). For those reporters, as with U.S. research reported on here, higher-level anger accompanied by less-effective self-regulation constituted a risk for young children's behavior problems.

## SUMMARY: Self-Regulation and Expressiveness

Taken together with findings predicting social competence, it is clear that ability to regulate one's behavior in emotional situations is an important moderator of the contributions of expressiveness to indices of social competence and behavior problems. For both anger and fear especially, and across some cultures, children's ultimate behavioral strengths or difficulties may depend in part on their abilities to inhibit action and focus their attention.

It is not hard to imagine how being able to inhibit one's behavior and focus on something other than that which is upsetting might aid preschoolers in dealing with their negative emotions. But the converse also could be true. In the example of Connor, it comes as no surprise, then, that he has trouble paying attention when playing a matching game and can't play Simon Says too well. His self-regulation difficulties and negativity may be operating together, promoting subsequent behavior problems that important people in his life—parents, teachers, and peers—note with regret.

### SUMMARY: Expressiveness as a Whole

The expression of emotions is a core component of social interchange. The valence and readability of the emotions that predominate during preschoolers' interactions with others are central to the impression others gain about their skillfulness and attractiveness as play partners. Sadder or angrier children, or those who send mixed, murky emotional messages, are involved in enough problematic exchanges that their developmentally appropriate social relations are compromised. Happier children who more readily show empathic concern fare much better. Although the paths from emotional expressiveness to social competence sometimes differ for girls and boys, and many qualifiers such as the context of the emotion, relationships with adults, and self-regulation have been identified, the main outlines of this overarching picture hold true. Moreover, the contributions of shyness, empathy, guilt, and shame also have important links with social competence and behavior problems. Adults in children's lives could support them in acquiring optimal patterns of expressiveness to support their social competence and protect them from debilitating behavior problems.

## CONTRIBUTIONS OF EMOTION KNOWLEDGE TO SOCIAL COMPETENCE

Accurate interpretation of others' emotions provides critical information about social situations. The facial expressions of others provide valuable clues to the qualitative meaning of interpersonal exchanges—information that can otherwise be disguised by verbal content. Consider a preschool boy who says, "I am *not* scared of dogs." If he utters these words while chewing on his finger, looking down with a wary expression, a peer understanding his expressive message may feel sympathy that motivates positive, prosocial reactions (Eisenberg, 1986), such as showing the other child how to pet a puppy. Alternatively, a peer who sees this boy tightening his brow and hears him using his gruff tones while making the same statement may take the expedient action of leaving with the puppy and coming back to play later, when the prognosis is more favorable! A third possibility is that accurate interpretation of a peer's subtle cues of pleasure while saying the same thing will allow the preschooler to enter into positive interaction. Children who strategically apply emotion knowledge in highly charged positive and negative situations succeed more often in peer interactions. I assert that children who have acquired developmentally appropriate emotion knowledge are at a distinct advantage at many crucial moments during play.

### General Emotion Knowledge and Social Competence

Such understanding of emotions does correlate with a variety of indices of social competence—beginning as early the 1980s and 1990s, it was becoming clear that preschoolers' emotion knowledge is related to a range of positive social outcomes, such as positive peer status; teachers' ratings of friendliness and lack of aggression; parents' ratings of social competence; children's positive, prosocial reactions to the emotions of others; and even children's own positive perception of their own peer experiences (Denham, 1986; Denham & Couchoud, 1991; Denham, McKinley, et al., 1990; Field & Walden, 1982; Gnepp, 1989b; Goldman, Corsini, & de Urioste, 1980; Philoppot & Feldman, 1990; Strayer, 1980). Various components of emotion knowledge are represented in these investigators' reports.

Several points are useful to make here. First, studies may use different direct assessments of children's emotion knowledge, although most use the AKT (e.g., Denham, Bassett, Brown, et al., 2015; Denham & Couchoud, 1990a, 1990b, and see also Chapter 4), the Test of Emotion Comprehension (TEC; Pons et al., 2004), the Assessment of Children's Emotion Skills (Schultz & Izard, 1998), Izard's Emotion Matching Test (Morgan, Izard, & King, 2010), or vignettes drawn from Lewis and Michalson's (1983) work (Garner & Toney, 2020). The differing theoretical views on the structure and development of emotion knowledge that I mentioned in Chapter 4 are important here, for their relationship to differing assessments of preschoolers' emotion knowledge.

First, one theoretical issue impacting all such methodology is determining which aspects of emotion knowledge should be focused on. For example, in the early Field and Walden (1982) study, accurate discriminators of emotional expressions were rated as more extroverted, more popular, and more affectively positive by their teachers; knowledge of emotional expressions was the aspect of emotion knowledge in which the authors were interested. Other early investigators found positive associations between knowledge of only basic emotion situations and differing indices of social competence. My colleagues and I have generally utilized an aggregate of comprehension of emotional expressions, both expressive and receptive labels, and both equivocal and unequivocal situations, from the AKT. Others, such as Gnepp (1989b), have examined the link between more sophisticated, personalized emotion knowledge and social competence (see Chapter 5 and Pons et al., 2004). Thus many aspects of emotion knowledge contribute to various ways of measuring social competence. These multi-faceted constructs seem deeply intertwined.

Second, another way to consider how emotion knowledge relates to social competence involves how young children *mis*understand emotions (Bullock & Russell, 1984, 1985). Thus specific types of emotion knowledge errors made by young children can also predict deficits in social competence. We can easily envision how particular weaknesses may engender difficulties in the social arena and lead a child to behave in an unpopular way; for example, mistaking a peer's displeasure for pleasure may be particularly dangerous, because the child may continue disliked behaviors. And in fact, we found that confusing happy and sad expressions and situations was negatively related to peer ratings of likability, elaborating overall findings that emotion situation knowledge was related to peer status (Denham, McKinley, et al., 1990). Not understanding happy expressions and situations is unusual even for young preschoolers. Other types of errors, on the other hand, would be more developmentally appropriate, and even logically expected, in the preschool age range: Children at this age often confuse sadness and anger (see also Chapter 4), and such an error was not found to be associated with peer ratings (but see Acland, Jambon, & Malti, 2021). Error analyses are, however, not common in recent literature.

More recent research has corroborated and greatly expanded earlier work, though, particularly in how emotion knowledge relates to aspects of social competence. First, research after the 1980s has highlighted further that although there are developmental progressions in the various aspects of emotion knowledge, there also are marked individual differences in these developments that figure very strongly in young children's social success. Specifically, this new research confirms that preschoolers who apply their more substantial emotion knowledge in emotionally charged situations have contemporaneous and later advantages in social competence (variously measured by parent or teacher report, but sometimes including peer assessments or observations of social–emotional behavior) (Alonso-Alberca, Vergara, Fernández-Berrocal, Johnson, & Izard, 2012; Alwaely, Yousif, & Mikhaylov, 2020; Deneault & Ricard, 2013; Denham, Bassett, Zinsser, et al., 2014; Denham, Blair, et al., 2003; Dunsmore & Karn, 2004; Ensor, Spencer, & Hughes, 2011; Farrant, Devine, Maybery, & Fletcher, 2012; Garner & Estep, 2001; Garner & Toney, 2020; Garner & Waajid, 2012; Izard et al., 2001; Klein et al., 2018; Parker, Mathis, & Kupersmidt, 2013; Sette et al., 2015; Thompson et al., 2020; Vernon & Teglasi, 2018). In fact, when 3-year-olds had greater early emotion knowledge, they self-reported more positive perceptions of their peer experiences (Dunn, 1995). The sheer numerosity of these studies emphasizes the ubiquity of these findings. Further, even very young children's emotion knowledge is important; toddler's understanding of emotion predicted observed free play quality and helping behavior as early as 2 years old (Conte et al., 2018; see also Ensor et al., 2011). Several of the just-cited studies also show cross-cultural validity of the link between emotion knowledge and social competence.

At age 3, Leah and Carrie play together a lot. Emotionally, they seem a rather mismatched pair; however, they've known each other since infancy, and somehow the friendship works. Carrie understands that Leah is sometimes shy. Being the assertive and sometimes negative little person that she is, when she sees signs of Leah's sadness, annoyance, or shyness, she may go into protective action. For example, she may determinedly tell someone urging Leah to relinquish an object or act according to a play script (e.g., giving the scrambled eggs to Dad in the house corner), "Just wait a minute!!" or "Stop that!" At the same time, Leah also knows the signs of Carrie's impending sadness and annoyance, and since she is sympathetic, may offer a helping hand when there aren't enough baby dolls to play with.

Although all these studies support the notion that emotion knowledge contributes to social competence, there are details that distinguish some of the reports. Some work showed concurrent relationships (e.g., Deneault & Ricard, 2013; Denham, Bassett, Brown, et al., 2015; Denham, Bassett, Zinsser, et al., 2014; Garner & Toney, 2020; Sette et al., 2015). For example, Garner and Toney (2020) found that children who could furnish the correct emotions for different situations of happiness, sadness, anger, and surprise were rated as more socially competent by teachers (see also Garner & Waajid, 2012), and Denham et al. (2015) found that a concurrent connection between an aggregate of expressive, receptive, and situation knowledge and teacher-rated social competence was significant even with preschoolers' self-regulation accounted for.

More detailed aspects of social competence also have been shown to be related to preschoolers' emotion knowledge. For example, teachers' reports of preschoolers' prosocial roles during conflict (i.e., as defender, consoler, and mediator; Belacchi & Farina, 2010) were related to the children's emotion knowledge. Denham, Bassett, Zinsser, et al. (2014) also went further, showing that emotion knowledge was related to observed emotionally regulated, prosocial behavior in the classroom. Adding to these findings, Deneault and Ricard (2013) found that preschoolers' knowledge of the *consequences* of emotions was concurrently related to several aspects of social competence, such as security, autonomy, and integration within the peer group. Thus, multiple aspects of social competence, evaluated by differing methodologies, are related concurrently to several different assessments of emotion knowledge during preschool.

Other reports noted the longitudinal effects of emotion knowledge on indices of social competence. For example, in a short-term (fall to spring) longitudinal design, preschoolers' emotion situation knowledge predicted teacher-rated social competence (Bassett et al., 2012; see also Denham, Bassett, Way, et al., 2012). Emotion knowledge at 3½ years old also predicted children's prosocial orientation when they were 4½ (Eggum et al., 2011). Deficits in emotion knowledge also predicted early primary school peer nominations of children's anger by the spring, with age, gender, verbal ability, and attentional control accounted for by the fall (Trentacosta, Izard, Mostow, & Fine, 2006). With slightly older children, first and second graders' understanding of emotional expressions, behaviors, and situations in the fall predicted teacher-rated social skills in the spring (Mostow, Izard, Fine, & Trentacosta, 2002). Again, across short time spans emotion knowledge predicted differing indices of social competence, sometimes with potential confounding information accounted for.

Over a longer period, early emotion knowledge at age 2½ years predicted observed prosocial behavior at age 4 years, even with verbal ability, age, gender, and mother–child mutuality accounted for (Ensor et al., 2011). Similarly, age-3 emotion knowledge predicted concurrent, but also social competence by kindergarten (including teacher ratings of cooperation/sensitivity and lack of isolation/withdrawal and aggression, as well as positive peer status; Denham, Blair, et al., 2003). Examining a more discrete index of social–emotional success, emotion knowledge predicted ratings of children's sympathy from 3½ to 6 years old (Eggum et al., 2011). Finally, 5-year-olds' emotion expression recognition and labeling, even with verbal ability and aspects of temperament accounted for, predicted 9-year-olds' teacher-rated assertion, cooperation, and internalizing (negatively) (Izard et al., 2001). So across and beyond the preschool period, developmentally appropriate assessment of emotion knowledge predicted even *later* aspects of social competence.

At 5 years old, Juan, as already noted, is usually genuinely emotionally positive, and such equanimity, along with a keenly observing eye, may have helped him to learn a lot about emotions in preschool. He can understand, for example, that some people might be sad to come to school (even though he's always happy to be there), and some people might get mad if their brother yells, whereas he'd be mostly sad. These understandings make it easier to comprehend his classmates' behaviors—for example, Roberto might still be mad from yesterday when he was jostled in line coming in from the playground, so treating him kindly might be the way to make play go smoothly. By the time Juan is in the third grade, his earlier wide-ranging emotion knowledge has helped make his school transition smooth enough that he can build a collection of social skills satisfying himself and others and helping him to continue to feel positive about life.

## SUMMARY: General Emotion Knowledge and Social Competence

The linkage between general and developmentally appropriate emotion knowledge—assessed using various measures—and parents', teachers', and even young children's, evaluations of social competence is routinely found. The contribution of this aspect of emotional competence is both contemporaneously and longitudinally strong and can buffer preschoolers from the inception of behavior problems. This is an aspect of emotional competence that can be taught by teachers and parents (see Chapter 13), and such training could be very fruitful.

### General Emotion Knowledge and Behavior Problems

So far it looks like emotion knowledge certainly is a positive facilitator of various aspects of social competence during preschool and early primary grades. Conversely, deficits in aspects of emotion knowledge put the preschooler at risk for oppositional behavior and aggression (Denham, Blair, et al., 2002; Denham, Caverly, et al., 2002; Di Maggio et al., 2016; Garner et al., 2008; Parker et al., 2013; Ren, Wyver, Xu Rattanasone, & Demuth, 2016); overall externalizing problems (Alonso-Alberca et al., 2012); peer rejection (Denham, Blair, et al., 2002; Miller et al., 2005; Schultz, Izard, & Ackerman, 2000; Schultz et al., 2001; Thompson et al., 2020); and internalizing issues, such as shyness, loneliness, and peer victimization (Di Maggio et al., 2016; Fine, Izard, Mostow, Trentacosta, & Ackerman, 2003; Garner & Toney, 2020; Heinze, Miller, Seifer, Dickstein, & Locke, 2015; Kujawa et al., 2014; Miller et al., 2005; Schuberth et al., 2019; Schultz et al., 2001; Sette et al., 2016; Thompson et al., 2020). The sheer amount of this converging multicultural evidence again underscores the importance of emotion knowledge, as early as the preschool period. Emotion knowledge may buffer the emergence of behavior problems because it allows children to know the emotional meaning of their various experiences, allowing them to learn more about adaptive responses and strategies. Given this foundation, children may be better able to both overcome their mothers' minimizing, punitive reactions to their emotions (Song, Smiley, & Doan, 2022), as well as to deal with negative experiences, and not resort to problematic behavior (Doan & Wang, 2018).

Colin had a hard time learning about emotions during preschool. When a classmate's emotion was somewhat ambiguous—when he slipped on the unfortunately wet floor by the water and knocked Pei Lin's boat out of her hand, she looked sad, startled, and a little confused. But he didn't understand her complex expression and figured she was mad, so then he bumped hard into her on purpose.

Some of these findings are longitudinal. For example, Schuberth and colleagues (2019) found that children with less-advanced emotion knowledge at age 5 experienced linear increases in aggression and that these increases were related to the emergence of callous-unemotional features through age 8 (see Chapter 12). Insensitivity to negative emotions (e.g., considering a sad face neutral) or misspecification (e.g., considering a sad face angry) was related in even more detail to 4- and 8-year-olds' concurrent aggression (Acland et al., 2021). Further, and in contrast, 3-year-olds' emotion knowledge protected them from having their anger proneness contribute later to hostile attribution bias (Wong, Chen, & McElwain, 2019). In the first case, particular errors in emotion knowledge were a risk factor for aggression, as in the previous example of Colin. For the second case, growth in aggression and negative thinking was buffered by emotion knowledge.

Regarding internalizing problems, Fine et al. (2003) found that first graders' emotion knowledge was negatively related to such difficulties; even more, their first-grade emotion knowledge predicted less self-reported internalizing problems in fifth grade. Regarding peer negative nominations, Miller et al. (2005) found longitudinal contributions of emotion recognition knowledge deficits to not only peer negative nominations, but also self-reports of victimization/rejection, even after the earlier behavior problem scores were accounted for. Deficits in early emotion knowledge may have made the social world a confusing, unwelcoming place, so that problematic levels of sadness and anxiety were more likely, snowballing over time.

Other researchers have noted a connection between deficits in early emotion knowledge and attention problems or attention-deficit/hyperactivity disorder (ADHD) diagnoses (Chronaki et al., 2015; Lugo-Candelas, Flegenheimer, McDermott, & Harvey, 2017; Rodrigo-Ruiz, Perez-Gonzalez, & Cejudo, 2017; von Salisch et al., 2016). Importantly, the connections between such behavior problems and emotion knowledge are likely to be bidirectional. In one study, early hyperactivity contributed to emotion recognition problems, which then contributed to internalizing behavior problems (Castro, Cooke, Halberstadt, & Garrett-Peters, 2018; see also Strand, Barbosa-Leiker, Arellano Piedra, & Downs, 2016; Székely et al., 2014). The confirmation of a cascading relationship over time between emotion knowledge difficulties and differing aspects of behavior problems is worthy of notice and further study.

Although there is some robust cross-cultural support for the importance of emotion knowledge in developing behavior problems, most of the significant associations found are in various Western, individualistic cultures. The function of emotion knowledge in Eastern, collectivistic cultures may be quite different. For example, Doan and Wang (2018) have found important differences in the trajectory from emotion knowledge to internalizing problems in European American and immigrant Chinese children. Emotion knowledge at 3½ years old predicted less incidence of internalizing problems for European American children, as expected, at age 7. However, the opposite pattern was found for the Chinese children. Doan and Wang (2018) suggest that for Chinese children, a focus on inner subjective experiences like emotions runs counter to the cultural norms of focusing on the functioning of the social group. In fact, greater emotion knowledge may allow Chinese children more access and sensitivity to the criticism and social shaming prevalent in their enculturation (Doan & Wang, 2018; see also Chapter 8), rendering them more susceptible to internalizing problems.

Given these unique findings, it is recommended that emotion knowledge research be expanded to include a greater emphasis on nonindividualistic cultures.

## SUMMARY: General Emotion Knowledge and Behavior Problems

Just as with the strong association between emotion knowledge and aspects of social competence, the negative linkage between preschoolers' behavior problems and emotion knowledge has been found repeatedly, and with varying sorts of behavior problems—externalizing, internalizing, and more narrow band behavior problems, such as aggression or ADHD, or even peer reports of rejection and self-reports of victimization. As part of a plan to prevent or ameliorate behavior problems, programming for emotion knowledge is important (see Chapter 13). At the same time, cultural interpretations of the association between emotion knowledge and behavior problems deserve closer scrutiny.

## Moderators of the Emotion Knowledge/ Social Competence–Behavior Problem Linkages

Moderators of these central findings should be examined. Gender again looms large on the list of possibilities. There are very mixed gender-related findings for the contribution of emotion knowledge to social competence. For example, Kuhnert, Begeer, Fink, and de Rosnay (2017) found that emotion knowledge predicted later prosocial behavior only for girls ages 5 to 7 years old, and Dunsmore, Noguchi, Garner, Casey, and Bhullar (2008) also found emotion knowledge to be uniquely related to young girls' popularity. More research has, however, targeted emotion knowledge as especially important for aspects of boys' social competence, such as for their friendships (Dunsmore et al., 2008) and teacher-rated social skills (Parker et al., 2013). Denham, Bassett, Way, et al. (2012) found that school success (as noted in Chapter 1, including classroom adjustment and learning behaviors as well as social competence) in kindergarten was greater for boys who at age 3 were more skilled at recognizing emotional expressions. Thus positive social outcomes related to emotion knowledge have been found for just girls or just boys, and the exact origin and import of these differing findings are not yet clear.

By contrast, boys are somewhat more clearly predominant in the picture in which emotion knowledge buffers behavior problems. For example, Heinze and colleagues (2015) found that 5-year-old boys who recognized or named emotional expressions better self-reported less loneliness; girls who were better at naming expressions and understanding emotional situations were reported as showing fewer internalizing problems by parents. Examining gender moderation of emotion knowledge's contributions from the perspective of externalizing behavior problems, the emotion knowledge of 3- and 4-year-old boys was negatively related to kindergarten teacher-rated anger and aggression (Denham, Caverly, et al., 2002). More specifically, misattributing anger was related to boys' aggression (Schultz et al., 2000; but see also Garner & Lemerise, 2007, for relations between anger misattribution and physical victimization, unmodified by gender). In the earlier example of Colin and Pei Lin, Colin's misattribution of anger led to his aggression. But again, although boys may be more frequently implicated in this misperception, the jury is far from out on the matter.

In other cases, there is moderation by preexisting emotions, such as shyness (Sette et al., 2016). For Sette et al., shy children who were not proficient at recognizing emotions were especially at risk for both anxiety–withdrawal and for rejection by peers. Such outcomes of shyness were attenuated at higher levels of emotion recognition.

### SUMMARY: Moderation of Emotion Knowledge Contributions

Thus, although replication and consideration of the meaning of gender moderation are required for the association between emotion knowledge and social competence or behavior problems, it again appears that deficits in emotional competence can render boys vulnerable to difficulties.

Further, the experience of specific emotions again may interact with another aspect of emotional competence, in this case emotion knowledge. Evidence of this proposition has been found for shyness. Understanding emotions may have given these shy children the information they needed to be less anxious in social situations—with less mystery involved—and thus allowed them to join in play more readily and become more accepted.

## SELF-REGULATION AND ITS ROLE IN THE RELATIONSHIP WITH EMOTION KNOWLEDGE AND SOCIAL COMPETENCE OR BEHAVIOR PROBLEMS

As with emotional expressiveness, self-regulation supports emotion knowledge. Self-regulation predicted aspects of emotion knowledge both concurrently and predictively in one study in which emotion knowledge also predicted later school success (including social competence and classroom adjustment; Denham, Bassett, Way, et al., 2012). Children, especially those in families at low socioeconomic risk, who could concentrate and inhibit irrelevant actions, demonstrated greater emotion knowledge. Their emotion knowledge, supported by self-regulation, then predicted end-of-year school success.

Taking this topic one step further in terms of longitudinal analysis and zeroing in on social competence, Klein et al. (2018) found that emotion knowledge longitudinally mediated the association between self-regulation and teacher-rated social competence. These authors suggested that emotion knowledge is one mechanism through which self-regulation contributes to social competence; paying attention to others, inhibiting action when it is wiser to wait, and remembering how different peers usually feel could promote the later emotion knowledge that facilitated even later social competence.

Similarly, but looking at the conjunction of emotion knowledge and self-regulation in a different way, with more specific observed behaviors as outcomes, Gal-Szabo, Spinrad, Eisenberg, and Sulik (2019) found that emotion situation knowledge acted as a moderator. It predicted social play when self-regulation (attention shifting, attention focusing, and inhibitory control) was high, but negatively predicted reticent play at lower levels of self-regulation. In these rather complicated findings, children possessing higher-level emotion knowledge *together with* self-regulation were best equipped to join others in play. For children lacking in self-regulatory abilities, emotion knowledge served as a buffer in the pathway to social competence.

> Jimmy understands emotions at an age-appropriate level, and he is good at paying attention, refraining from impulsive behavior, and changing activities when necessary—doesn't he sound like a great playmate? Billy also understands emotions; but without such understanding—is Amanda smiling at me in welcome or is that a funny scowl?—his more limited self-regulation might make it harder for him to figure out how to join in the play. He might not be able to decide what emotional message Amanda was sending, and not be patient enough to wait and figure it out. He would hover and hang back instead, or alternatively perform some off-putting behavior in his attempt to play. Either way his social goals would not be met. His emotion knowledge really supports him in making social choices.

Finally, the buffering ability of emotion knowledge also was examined in a longitudinal study. Poor self-regulation but higher emotion knowledge set 3-year-olds on a trajectory on which their severe behavior problems decreased by the time they reached 10 years old (Ip et al., 2019). Emotion knowledge appeared to ease the worrisome path the children seemed to be on.

## SUMMARY: Self-Regulation and Emotion Knowledge

Taking all these studies together, emotion knowledge may operate as a mediator of the effects of self-regulation, or in fact act as a moderator, buffering early self-regulation difficulties. In either case, it is important to know that these two aspects of development work together, as suggested in Chapter 5. Promoting each may bolster the other, particularly in their association with social competence and behavior problems.

## Specialized Emotion Knowledge and Social Competence/Behavior Problem Outcomes: Understanding of One's Own Emotions

One of the most robust and differentiated relationships between emotion knowledge and social competence involves peer status. Usually when emotion knowledge is measured, however, it involves vignettes in which another person's emotions are portrayed. An investigation by Parke et al. (1992) extended this measurement specifically to include an understanding of one's own emotions. Children were interviewed extensively about their understanding of their own emotions. This understanding was assessed across a range of domains: (1) identification of happiness, sadness, anger, and fear; (2) one's own experience of each emotion; (3) circumstances leading to one's own emotion; (4) the expression of one's own emotions; and (5) behavioral and emotional reactions to the display of one's own emotions by mothers, fathers, and peers.

Children who had more positive peer status showed more extensive emotion knowledge in every domain except in the experience of one's own emotion (Cassidy et al., 1992; Parke et al., 1992). Moreover, total knowledge scores for each separate emotion also predicted peer status as rated by both teachers and peers, especially in ratings of overall peer acceptance, shyness, and prosocial behavior. Strengthening these findings, emotion knowledge added to the prediction of peer acceptance even when contributions of maternal and paternal expressiveness in both the home and laboratory were taken into account (Cassidy et al., 1992). Thus, emotion knowledge, most of which referred to the self, "mediate[d] the link between family and peer systems" (Parke et al., 1992, p. 123), just as asserted in the model in Figure 1.2 (see Chapter 1).

Visiting Joey's family, one is struck by the positive emotions shown—joy, gratitude, and intense interest. When Joey's pet kitten knocked over a side table, though, his mother's facial and vocal expressiveness clearly let her annoyance be known. When Joey has a rare bad day at preschool, he and his father talked about how this felt. So there is a firm foundation for Joey to understand emotions in general and his own in particular. When Mike got everyone to create that ruckus on the playground, Joey knew that he, for one, ended up feeling a little exhilarated, but also tired and a little embarrassed that his teacher was upset with them. He didn't know the words for all those feelings, but he was learning.

Since Parke et al. (1992), little research has examined preschoolers' self-report of their emotions (see Chapters 2 and 4). Denham (1997) examined how children expected parents to respond to their emotions, and these responses were appropriately related to the child's imagined emotions, but knowledge of the child's actual feelings was not assessed; the child's emotion was a given in the procedure. However, children's clear conceptions of how their parents would react to their specific emotions (e.g., comforting or discussing emotions with them) were related to teachers' ratings of peer relations, cooperativeness, and empathy. Further, children were very involved in this play measure, using dollhouse and dolls. When induced to consider parental reactions to *their own emotions* within the procedure, these preschoolers could demonstrate a coherent narrative.

Even more closely related to children's conceptions of their own emotions, Warren and Stifter (2008) devised a procedure to ask preschoolers what emotions they were experiencing in real time. Although the results were promising for the assessment itself, the investigators did not associate this emotional self-awareness knowledge with social competence or behavior problems. However, this means of obtaining information on their feelings from young children could be used in a more extended inquiry regarding their understanding of their own emotions.

In another measure, children were asked to choose how they themselves would feel, not in real time, but *if they were involved in* a challenging emotional situation (e.g., having a toy taken away, not being invited to a birthday party; Denham, Way, et al., 2013). Those who indicated that they would feel happy were rated lower on our aggregate of school success. Asserting that one would feel happy in such situations reflected a lack of understanding. In comparison, those who said they'd be sad, a reasonable reaction to the social difficulties depicted, were rated higher on this aggregate.

## SUMMARY: Understanding One's Own Emotions

Despite these efforts, it is admittedly not easy to ask young children about their own emotions in a direct assessment. Nonetheless, Parke et al.'s (1992) and Cassidy et al.'s (1992) results, my (1997; Denham, Way, et al., 2013) and Warren and Stifter's (2008) methods, and children's own often self-referent emotion language would suggest that this area is fruitful for new exploration. The corpus of evidence noting a relationship between self-understanding of emotion and social competence or behavior problems is still quite small.

## Specialized Emotion Knowledge and Social Competence/Behavior Problem Outcomes: Less Global Indices of Understanding of Emotion

There is growing evidence that more discrete elements of emotion knowledge also contribute to both particular and molar indices of social competence. For example, the use of emotion language—a special demonstration of emotion knowledge—enhances preschoolers' attempts at regulating interpersonal relationships (Kopp, 1989). Knowing how to talk about feelings can help preschoolers convey their needs, get their way, or demonstrate an understanding of others. Children learn to use emotion language to influence others' emotional states, as in comforting or asking for comfort, teasing, negotiating, and joking (Dunn, Brown, et al., 1991). In my work, preschoolers who used more emotion language with their mothers when looking at baby photos and used more emotion language to explain how they felt when their mothers simulated sadness and anger, were rated as more likable by peers up to 9 months later (Denham, Cook, et al., 1992).

More recent work has highlighted that children's ability to verbally explain emotions may be particularly important in enhancing their social relationships. Garner and Estep (2001) found that children who explained the emotions they observed while "reading" a picture book with their mother made more social initiations in the classroom and were more often the recipient of such initiations. These findings were extended by Garner and colleagues (2008), who observed children in their preschool in a triadic social interaction situation, involving free play, as well as in cooperative maze and drawing tasks. Again, in this study, children who explained emotions in the picture book were observed as more prosocial in triadic play; they showed more spontaneous and requested acts of helping, sharing, and comforting. Children who can use emotion language in flexible ways to attain social goals are more skilled with peers and better liked. Sometimes emotion language is central to social success.

> Todd has already been branded by both his childcare providers and his classmates as a difficult guy to be around. After learning a good deal of emotion language from his teacher though, he is heard taking part in a very heated discussion, replete with feeling terms, while negotiating a struggle over an object with a friend. The boys' smiles at the end of their argument testify to the power of emotion language to contribute to Todd's newfound social success.

An understanding of family emotion also is a special form of emotion knowledge. Unlike the quantitative measures of emotion knowledge that predict peer status and teacher-rated social competence, however, more qualitative parameters of children's conceptions of their parents' emotions are the important predictors. Children who more frequently depicted parents as tenderly comforting or as matching their positive emotions were seen by teachers as more skilled with peers, more cooperative, and more empathic (Denham, 1997). In contrast, children who more frequently depicted parents as matching negative emotions were seen as less cooperative. Children who more frequently depicted their parents as discussing emotions were seen as more empathic. In sum, these coherent and complete conceptions about family emotion predicted aspects of social competence. They also paralleled affect sharing and distress relief, which as I have previously noted, are important components of young children's internal working models of emotional security (Denham, 1997; Thompson, 1990).

Further, preschoolers who were able to describe the causes, the typical expression, and the resolution of their parents' emotions were rated as more socially competent overall by their teachers (Denham, 1996a). Hence, preschoolers' interpretations of family emotions are essential reflections of their notions about emotional reality. Children with richer, more complete, but also more emotionally secure conceptions of their families' affective environment are more able to succeed with their friends and school routine.

Finally, one last specific aspect of preschoolers' emotion knowledge—knowledge of display rules—is associated with later social competence (Jones et al., 1998). Knowing when and when not to show emotions is intimately tied to the success of ongoing social interaction. Thus, it is not surprising that those preschoolers who are better at this developmentally advanced skill are seen as more socially adept.

### SUMMARY: Less Global Indices of Emotion Knowledge

An ability to use emotion language, an understanding family emotion, and a knowledge of display rules are ways to operationalize emotion knowledge aside from the emotional expression and situation knowledge that are routinely assessed. It can be important to know how children fare on these aspects of emotion knowledge as well. In particular, emotion language is a powerful tool and can be trained (see Chapter 13).

## Emotion Knowledge and Less Global Indices of Social Competence

Emotion knowledge (sometimes more generally, sometimes particular facets) also is related to more particular components of social competence, such as taking care of others, creating a moral sensibility, or dealing with conflict. One particular aspect of emotion knowledge contributed to young children's responsiveness to the emotional needs of others: Emotional role taking, the ability to be open to and recognize the unique cues generated by the individual in a particular situation, predicted preschoolers' caregiving toward their younger siblings during a modified 4-minute Strange Situation (Garner, Jones, & Palmer, 1994). Older siblings with a greater emotional role-taking ability showed more concern and caring behavior, such as comforting their crying sibling; those without such emotion knowledge more often performed unhelpful behavior, like singing loudly to cover the noisy crying. In another study, both emotion situation knowledge and emotional role taking, which together permit children to understand both unequivocal and more equivocal situational sources of emotion, contributed to preschoolers' ability to remain positive in a disappointing circumstance (Garner & Power, 1996). The connection here is that emotion knowledge gave preschoolers a boost in their ability to deal constructively with a problem situation.

> Joelle is understandably disappointed about her parents' divorce, but she knows that she is sad. She knows that's the feeling that hurts and seeks out Benjie because he's been so kind to her. Playing with him makes her feel better.

Moral development may be facilitated by emotion knowledge as well. Dunn, Brown, and Maguire (1995; see also Dunn, 1995) first administered the AKT when children were 40 months old, and then Gordis et al.'s (1989; see also Chapter 5) measure of understanding of simultaneous, ambivalent emotions when the children entered kindergarten. Kindergarten and first-grade children also responded to a narrative measure of feelings about moral transgressions, such as cheating: "How would you feel? Why? What would you feel if no one found out (and why)? What will happen next?"

Young children's early understanding of emotion buttressed their moral sensibility. Their ability to identify emotional expressions and situations, as indexed by the AKT earlier in the preschool period, was related to a more empathic moral orientation and more reparative story completions in kindergarten. Those who scored higher in kindergarten on understanding of emotional ambivalence also showed more empathic moral orientation and more intense discomfort on the story completion measure in first grade. A developmentally appropriate understanding of emotion formed a foundation for these young children's morality, over and above intelligence and verbal ability. Children witness emotions, think about emotion–event links, and use these emotion-related social cognitions to contribute to their moral reasoning and behavior (Arsenio & Lover, 1995).

In more recent investigations of other specialized indices of social competence, young children's overall ability to recognize emotions was associated with their tendency to predict that story characters would reconcile after episodes of overt and relational aggression (Liao, Li, & Su, 2014). Moreover, these children's affective perspective taking (here defined as identifying the victim's emotion and showing empathy toward the victim) was related to their prediction of the characters' reconciliation, but only in overt aggression stories. Finally, these children's affective perspective taking in overt aggression conflict scenarios was associated with teacher reports of children's prosocial behaviors toward their peers. The investigators suggested that an ability to recognize emotions in the stories allowed for empathic concern and the motivation to propose reconciliation; these abilities translated to classroom social behaviors seen by teachers. Relatedly, preschoolers' emotion knowledge was associated with peer nominations of their taking a defender role in conflict (Camodeca & Coppola, 2016). In both these studies, emotion knowledge figured prominently in children's prosocial reasoning about—and behavior within—conflictual encounters, as well as how socially successful both teachers and peers found them.

As another example of the linkage between emotion knowledge and empathic concern, preschoolers who could accurately describe the causes of emotion also attested to greater cognitive and affective empathy on the Strayer Empathy Continuum, and described more prosocial themes (e.g., "Please wait, I will play with you later") on the MacArthur Story Stem Battery (Schapira & Aram, 2020). Also examining empathic concern, Ekerim-Akbulut, Şen, Beşiroğlu, and Selçuk (2020) found that understanding sadness from the AKT predicted preschoolers' empathy specifically for demonstrated pain and that such empathy was related to less evidence of disruptive behavior. Although more research is necessary, extant studies are very suggestive as to the pivotal role of emotion knowledge in children's empathic concern and moral/prosocial reasoning. These results also corroborate the importance of social cognitive abilities as a support for empathic concern, as discussed earlier in this chapter. More prospective longitudinal research on these linkages would be useful.

## SUMMARY: Emotion Knowledge and Less Global Indices of Social Competence

Findings with more specific aspects of social competence and emotion knowledge thus range from sibling caregiving, to moral sensibility, to conflict resolution, to empathic concern. The scope of emotion knowledge is wide in its implications for young children's successful social lives. Adults would do well to internalize the wide reach of emotion knowledge in young children's development and work to augment it.

## SUMMARY: Emotion Knowledge and Social Competence/Behavior Problems

In the last four decades, more researchers, instead of studying only the normative social–cognitive attainment of the toddler-to-preschool period, have begun to entertain the notion that young children exhibit important individual differences in emotion knowledge. Exploring these individual differences has shown that variations in emotion knowledge are contributors to social competence and behavior problems as reported by a wide range of raters and observers, with both outcomes and emotion knowledge operationalized in a number of ways. At the same time, important moderators of these associations have been found. The role of self-regulation also has been given more attention, and issues of culture have come to light.

But, even given this newly discovered information, why is this general link found so robustly across decades of study? The power of emotion knowledge appears substantial. It allows a preschooler to react appropriately to others, whether calmly or sympathetically, thereby bolstering social relationships. Moreover, children with greater emotion knowledge skills can communicate and engage with others more effectively, in part because they can talk about negative emotions. Thus, interactions with an emotionally knowledgeable age-mate would likely be viewed as satisfying, rendering one more likable; for instance, emotion knowledge may allow the preschooler to interact more successfully when a friend gets angry, and talking about one's own emotions can facilitate negotiating disputes with friends. Similarly, teachers are likely attuned to behavioral evidence of emotion knowledge, such as the use of emotion language and the sympathetic reaction, and to evaluate it positively. In contrast, deficits in age-appropriate emotion knowledge may make the social tasks of preschool more difficult. Not understanding when others are happy, sad, or angry makes learning to engage in social relationships with other children and adults challenging.

Overall, Trentacosta and Fine's (2010) meta-analysis emphasized these connections of emotion knowledge to both social competence and externalizing/internalizing behavior problems. In terms of its connection to social competence, the findings were consistent across nonclinical and clinical samples, in ages 3 to 11 years, and across ethnicities, socioeconomic status, emotion knowledge measures, social competence sources/reporters, and concurrent or longitudinal associations. A more recent meta-analysis corroborates Trentacosta and Fine's (2010) work concerning peer acceptance (Voltmer & von Salisch, 2017).

Regarding externalizing and internalizing problems, Trentacosta and Fine's (2010) findings were largely consistent across similar potential moderators; emotion knowledge was negatively related to these behavior problems. Such effects also are found cross-nationally (e.g., Lee et al., 2017). These strong findings suggest that teaching emotion knowledge to toddlers and preschoolers could be an effective intervention, a topic I return to in Chapter 13 (Grazzani, Ornaghi, Agliati, et al., 2016; Ornaghi, Brazzelli, Grazzani, Agliati, & Lucarelli, 2017; Ornaghi et al., 2014, 2015).

## CONTRIBUTIONS OF ER AND EMOTION DYSREGULATION TO SOCIAL COMPETENCE AND BEHAVIOR PROBLEMS

### Emotion Regulation

Expressiveness itself is, as amply shown already in this chapter, an important part of skilled social interaction and a predictor of the assessments made by people in the child's social world. But sometimes emotions need to be regulated (see Chapter 6). So not only is the relative profile of the child's expression of positive and negative emotions important; the child's ability to deal with these emotions, or ER, also is vital.

In my earlier book, I unfortunately had to report that little research had been done on this linkage. Most early research had been performed by Eisenberg, Fabes, Bernzweig, et al. (1993), Eisenberg, Fabes, Nyman, et al. (1994), and Eisenberg, Fabes, Murphy, et al. (1995). In this body of work, teachers and mothers captured children's coping techniques. At the time I took the coping construct as an index of the trait-like "product" of ER; however, in the ensuing years I and others have come to view these coping techniques as ER strategies, which is the term I'll use now.[2]

Thus I first discuss Eisenberg et al.'s still-relevant early findings and one set of my own, using the same measures of emotion regulatory strategies (Denham, Blair, et al.,

---

[2] Given that these "coping" strategies are rated over time and in different contexts by parents and teachers, in some sense they *are* trait-like.

2002, 2003). Then, I examine more contemporary research focusing on emotion strategies used by young children; most reports of ER and social competence or behavior problems view ER as strategy usage.

Accordingly, in the Eisenberg research, teachers and mothers rated the likelihood that each child would *ever* engage in a range of ER strategies: instrumental coping, crying to elicit help, instrumental aggression, behavioral avoidance, distraction, venting, emotional aggression, cognitive restructuring, seeking emotional support, cognitive avoidance, instrumental intervention, seeking instrumental support, and denial. Second, they also rated the child's likelihood of using these strategies in specific everyday conflict scenarios. For each operationalization, these scales were finally collapsed into aggregates of constructive, acting out, and avoidance strategies.

Many of Eisenberg et al.'s (1994, 1995) findings were moderated by child gender. Teachers' ratings of boys' constructive ER strategies were positively related to social competence, as rated by teachers, and to sociometric status (see also Denham, Blair, et al., 2003, for similar findings not differentiated by gender). Mothers' reports of boys' support-seeking strategies also were associated with the boys' positive social functioning. A picture emerges then of the socially competent boys using a flexible assortment of ER strategies to deal with strong feelings that erupted during their interactions, and using problem solving and looking for help when this was not possible. These connections held true both contemporaneously and over a 2-year period. Boys' passivity or avoidance in emotional situations seemed to be a particularly ineffective, debilitating means of regulating emotions for them: Teachers saw such boys as actually showing *more* anger 1 year later (see also Denham, Blair, et al., 2002).

In contrast, girls' rated social skills were positively related to avoidant regulation strategies, but no other significant relations were reported (again, see Denham, Blair, et al., 2002, for findings not differentiated by gender). Girls seen as socially competent were those who tended to deal less actively with difficult situations. It is likely that girls in general are already socialized into more uniformly "nice," controlled, and culturally approved and competent social behavior. For them, the important determinants of sociometric preference and being seen as competent by their teachers was perhaps less determined by this aspect of emotional competence, and more so by other facets of their social interaction and personality (e.g., their cooperativeness). Further, passively avoiding emotionally distressing circumstances as a means of ER could have been seen as the "right" thing for a little girl to do.

In sum, these early findings showed that the ability to regulate emotions makes important contributions to social competence. However, one criticism of Eisenberg and colleagues' work is that core findings centered on teachers' ratings of both ER and social competence (as I've mentioned repeatedly, monorater bias is a complaint that still could be made about a lot of research today). Hence, an alternative interpretation is that a shared method variance accounts for the association between ER strategy usage and social competence. The complex pattern of findings partially forestalls this problem.

To avert such alternative explanations, and to extend their findings, Eisenberg, Fabes, Nyman, et al. (1994) evaluated the associations between the ratings of the 5-year-olds' social competence and *observed* their means of dealing with anger. Peer acceptance and teacher ratings of social competence were related to young children's observed use of verbal objections when angry, a relatively socially competent tactic ("using their words"), even when contributions of gender and age were accounted for. Again though some intriguing findings were gender specific in this study. The observed venting in girls when angry was negatively related to teacher ratings of social competence, whereas the use of escape tactics was positively related. The socially competent preschool girls again used more avoidant ER strategies, and their venting outbursts were censured.

Even early research gave way to new ideas about how more clearly differentiated ER strategies could contribute to social competence and behavior problems (see Chapter 6). For example, Losoya and colleagues (1998) found that teacher ratings of 4- to 6-year-olds' cognitive restructuring or instrumental problem solving, as well as support seeking, were related to both their teacher-rated popularity and socially appropriate behavior (i.e., social skills plus aggression and disruptive behavior reversed). Avoidant strategies were related positively to socially appropriate behavior for both genders (it may be useful to retreat from the fray). In contrast, use of aggressive strategies (either verbal or physical to solve the problem or "let off steam") were negatively related to both aspects of social functioning. Doing nothing was negatively related to prosocial behavior/popularity, and venting (here defined, e.g., as crying to release frustration) was negatively related to socially appropriate behavior.

These relationships were found across time as well, again obviating the monorater bias because children had different teachers in different years. In that case, the ratings of socially appropriate behavior when children were 6 to 8 years old were at least marginally positively correlated with support-seeking and avoidant strategy ratings that were made when they were 4 to 6 years old and negatively correlated with aggressive strategies. Popularity/prosocial behavior at age 6 to 8 was related to age 4 to 6 support-seeking and instrumental strategies. Both concurrently and longitudinally, then, the ER strategies that teachers saw preschoolers performing were related to important aspects of social functioning.

Several major means of evaluating ER have been developed since the earlier research to predict social competence as well as behavior problems: questionnaires, observations, analogue laboratory tasks, and interviews. First, the strategies questionnaires already referenced were still being adapted and used (e.g., Denham, Blair, et al., 2002). Most simply, Blair and colleagues (2004) showed that mothers' reports of venting strategy use were negatively related to teacher ratings of social competence (and positively to their reports of externalizing problems). The use of constructive strategies was related to the lack of internalizing problems; more recently, an ability to use the constructive strategy of active distraction showed a similar pattern (Feng et al., 2011). In Blair and colleagues (2004) work, the *lack* of passive/avoidant strategy use was related to girls' social competence. This last finding seems to contradict Eisenberg, Fabes, Bernzweig, et al. (e.g., 1993), but participants in that study were close to a year older than in the Blair et al. (2004) study; it may be that behavioral and cognitive avoidance, distracting oneself, leaving, or even denying the problem is seen as helpful when a girl is older and has been exposed to socialization pressures for a longer period.

Maternal and teacher reports of effective ER also are often obtained via the ERC (Shields & Cicchetti, 1997; see Chapter 6). These are associated with success with peers and overall social effectiveness during the preschool years (Di Maggio et al., 2016; Hamaidi, Mattar, & Arouri, 2021; Orta et al., 2013; Ren et al., 2016; Son & Chang, 2018; Spritz, Sandberg, Maher, & Zajdel, 2010), For example, in Miller, Fine, et al.'s (2006) study, the ER scale of the ERC was positively related to teacher ratings of social skills, even controlling for verbal ability, age, emotion knowledge, and negative emotion expression. In contrast, the lability scale of the ERC was negatively related to teacher-rated social skills, even with the same covariates. It also should be noted that these findings are markedly cross-national.

Looking more specifically at how ER can protect preschoolers from exhibiting noticeable behavior problems, Kao et al. (2020) found that ER, assessed by the ERC, was negatively related to emotional symptoms, conduct problems, hyperactivity–inattention, and peer problems (see also Graziano et al., 2007). In another example related specifically to aggression, Ersan (2020) found that ER assessed by the ERC was negatively related to teachers' ratings of both physical and relational aggression in a large sample of Turkish preschoolers (see also Orta et al., 2013).[3] Further, ER, in its negative connection with anger, mediated the path from anger to both forms of aggression (see similar relations with overall aggression in a large sample of Chinese kindergarteners, Chang, Schwartz, Dodge, & McBride-Chang, 2003). If Colin could control his anger, he might be less likely to hit.

In many of these studies, the means of evaluating social competence also was via questionnaire, so that often here too there was the threat of monorater bias (i.e., one rater rated both ER and social competence). Orta et al. (2013) mention this issue but suggest that differential associations with social competence and behavior problems may bolster the trustworthiness of the findings. I also think that the repetition of similar results across so many investigations is helpful but continue to remind the reader to be careful consumers of research.

Not only has ER been operationalized in various ways. Examining social competence outcomes in a different way, Camodeca and Coppola (2019) found that ER assessed by the ERC was related to the child's social preference as well as to greater closeness and less conflict with the child's teacher (see also Graziano et al., 2007; Kam et al., 2011), and being assigned by peers to a defending role in bullying situations. But it also was positively related to *bullying* in hierarchical linear modeling! It could be that being calmly regulated also contributes to being a successful bully. Further, Kao and colleagues (2020) found that ER assessed by the ERC was related to observed instrumental helping when an experimenter had difficulty staying warm or getting a clip for her messy hair. Introducing a new means of assessing social competence adds to the evidence base for its association with ER during these early years.

Although most of these investigations using the ERC have been contemporaneous, there are some longitudinal studies using the ERC, some of which have been short term. In one such study that spanned a school year, 3½- to 5½-year-olds' ER emerged as an important predictor of later social skills and positive relationships with teachers (Spritz et al., 2010). Similarly, Cohen and Mendez (2009) found that ER was related

---

[3]Arslan, Durmuşoğlu-Saltali, and Yilmaz (2011) also found relationships between Turkish preschoolers' ER, measured another way, and their interpersonal skill.

to more adaptive play patterns concurrently and across the preschool year in predominantly African American students from low-income families.

Using a different questionnaire measure (Mirabile's 2014 Emotion Regulation Skills Questionnaire, which focuses on strategies to regulate fear and anger), Hipson and colleagues (2019) completed a short-term longitudinal study predicting prosocial, anxious, and withdrawn behavior. Active regulation (i.e., self-directed speech, information gathering, and constructive coping, assessed by parents in the fall) was related to both prosocial and withdrawn behaviors rated by teachers in the spring, in expected directions. In fact, active regulation also moderated the connection between shyness and subsequent prosocial and socially withdrawn behavior; when shy children were able to use such ER, they were more likely to be rated as prosocial, and shy boys were less likely to be rated as withdrawn. This finding is a hopeful one for adults wanting to help shy children.

This longitudinal association between ER and adaptive functioning also has been studied with slightly older children. With first-grade teachers as reporters, ER-related questions (i.e., whether children can calm down, think before acting, express feelings appropriately, and control temper in disagreements), formed a coherent latent variable that predicted peer preference in the second grade (Kam et al., 2011). Research involving much larger time spans ending in elementary school also conveys intriguing results. For example, Streit, Carlo, Ispa, and Palermo (2017) gathered information on ER when children were 24 months old, using the Bayley Scales of Infant Development regulation ratings of the toddlers' handling of frustration during the testing session. Remarkably, these ratings predicted lower levels of aggression and delinquency, as well as higher levels of prosocial behavior and compliance with their teacher, for children in fifth grade.

Cascading and reciprocal connections between ER via the ERC and aspects of social competence also emerge in such long-term longitudinal investigations. For example, age-5 ER predicted age-7 social competence and peer acceptance, which then predicted age-10-peer acceptance and friendship quality (Blair et al., 2015). Others have found a cascade effect from early (age-4) ER and decreases in subsequent levels of externalizing behavior at ages 5 and 7, even controlling for earlier levels of externalizing (Blandon et al., 2010).

Along with using questionnaires to assess the use of ER strategies, there has been a focus on assessing ER strategy usage via observing expressiveness and behavior in several investigations. Multiple informants and sometimes observation of child social competence in the classroom were utilized as well. In a first series of studies, we focused on the ER strategy of venting. Thus Denham, Blair, et al. (2002) created a variable called "dysregulated anger" by multiplying the observed prevalence of anger by mother-rated venting; 3- and 4-year-olds' dysregulated anger predicted a lack of social competence as evaluated by kindergarten teachers and peers. In another study (Denham, Blair, et al., 2003), a latent variable was created, composed of negatively weighted mother-rated venting and observed "venting" reactions to peers' emotions (i.e., matching negative emotion, opposite affect matching, and volitionally exacerbating a peers' emotional difficulty). This "nonventing" ER variable was contemporaneously related to a latent variable for social competence that included teacher reports and peer evaluations.

"Nonventing" ER also was related to kindergarten social competence, but especially for angrier children. Thus conceptualizing ER in a more complex way, in terms of how it is executed during peer interaction in the preschool, and examining it observationally, yielded several robust findings.

We also have observed 3-year-old children who were able to talk about their feelings when angry (as a proxy for ER); it forms a latent variable with prosocial behavior that then predicts both contemporaneous and kindergarten school success (i.e., teacher-rated social competence, learning behaviors, and getting along with classroom routines; Denham, Bassett, Zinsser, et al., 2014; see also Herndon et al., 2013). In contrast, observed negative emotion and aggression, together making an index of emotion dysregulation, showed opposite effects. Other than these efforts, however, ER has not often been examined observationally in the classroom.

Preschoolers' ER also has been measured observationally in the laboratory, sometimes across longitudinal periods. When 5-year-olds were faced with a disappointing gift, their use of active (e.g., trying to fix the problem, asking for the correct toy), rather than passive (e.g., just tolerating the problem) or disruptive ER strategies, predicted their age-7 socially competent peer play (e.g., initiations of play, responses to initiations, and level of play; Penela et al., 2015). Similar contemporaneous findings have been obtained with ER during disappointing gift or negative affect induction procedures predicting older preschoolers' peer status (Nakamichi, 2017).

As amply described in Chapter 6, another paradigm that has been used to observe young children's ER strategies uses some form of a delay—for example, waiting for a cookie. Three-year-olds who did not focus on the delay and showed lower peak anger as well as lower total time angry during the delay showed greater social competence at home compared with 5-year-olds and at school compared with 6-year-olds (as indexed by cooperation, self-control, assertion, and responsibility; Chang et al., 2012). A dynamic examination of ER strategies observed when children waited to open a gift (Cole et al., 2017) showed that less-effective strategies were, in contrast, related to externalizing problems. Further, another analogue task sometimes used to observe preschoolers' ER in the laboratory is the locked box task, in which an attractive toy is placed in a locked box, but the child is given the wrong key—obviously it is very frustrating! Dollar and Stifter (2012) used this task to mark children's ER during a laboratory visit, and also observed and rated children's temperament across two visits, one of which was a visit with an unfamiliar peer. The ER strategies they noted included goal-directed behavior, social support seeking, distraction, and self-soothing. Mothers also rated their children's aggression (e.g., "My child starts fights with peers") and social competence with peers (e.g., "My child gets along with peers").

In this study, Dollar and Stifter (2012) were the most interested in children's temperamental surgency (i.e., in this case operationalized as social responsiveness, shyness/fearfulness reversed, activity level, and positive affect) and its interaction with ER in predicting social competence. Given their focus, they found that high-surgent children, who also showed high levels of social support seeking, were less likely to be rated by their mothers as high in aggression than high-surgent children who did not seek social support. Furthermore, results revealed that low-surgent children who showed high levels of distraction and/or self-soothing were more likely to show behavioral wariness around unfamiliar peers, whereas high-surgent children who used more distraction and/or self-soothing behaviors were rated by their mothers as lower in social competence.

Temperamental dispositions, then, can interact with ER in influencing the development of social competence. High-surgent children can be something of a "handful," but their ability to ask for support during a frustrating experience indexed their more socially acceptable disposition. In contrast, children's tendencies not to be very active or emotionally positive, and perhaps shy, may only exacerbate their social difficulties by resorting to distraction and self-soothing ER strategies that did not help solve the locked box problem.

Continuing the theme of biological predispositions, examining preschoolers' behavioral and physiological ER together also has been profitable, especially regarding vagal activity. As already noted in Chapter 6, meta-analytical results showed that greater levels of RSA withdrawal—that is, more mobilization to deal with emotions—were related to fewer externalizing and internalizing problems, especially in nonclinical groups (Graziano & Derefinko, 2013). In a study examining both heart activity and ER strategies, negative emotion and disengagement in a distress task predicted negative social behavior 6 months later, and marginally negatively predicted positive social behavior (Morgan et al., 2014). However, the results of importance in this work included physiological markers. That is, greater heart *reactivity* during the distress task was related to more negative social behavior, but greater *recovery from* the distress task was related to more positive social behavior. In contrast, greater physiological recovery from an exuberance task predicted less positive social behavior. The authors suggested that effective regulation at this age may consist of maintaining positive emotions and decreasing negative arousal; the valence of the experience matters.

However, recent investigations also have pointed out the context- and age-dependent relations of RSA reactivity, both withdrawal and recovery, with ER strategy usage (Kahle, Miller, Troxel, & Hastings, 2021). These authors' complex pattern of findings suggests that, in the moment, using distraction as an ER strategy is associated with physiological calming, but there may be a developmental process by which earlier ER behaviors shape later physiological responses, with different short-term and long-term results. Further elucidation of these complex findings is required.

Along with completing questionnaires, observing preschoolers at play, setting up analogue laboratory situations in which to observe ER, and considering physiological indicators of ER, asking the children themselves about ER strategies has proven fruitful. Dennis and Kelemen (2009) asked 3- and 4-year-olds what strategies might work to change emotions, using puppets. Those who saw venting as an effective way to change sad, angry, and fearful emotions were seen by their mothers as less socially skilled (i.e., cooperation, self-control, assertion, and responsibility). In other studies where young children were asked about ER strategies, even the sheer number of ER strategies comprehended and generated predicted coping with peer pressure, social preference, and lack of aggression (Gust et al., 2014; Ogelman & Fetihi, 2020). And the diversity of ER strategies generated also was negatively related to later problems with hyperactivity (Thomsen & Lessing, 2020). Thus, even preschoolers can articulate views of ER that are related to their functioning in the social world.

## SUMMARY: ER

Both contemporaneous and longitudinal results using (1) parent/teacher questionnaires (including the ERC and strategy questionnaires); (2) observations in the preschool classroom and laboratory; (3) asking children themselves about ER; and (4) accessing biological data suggest that preschool ER predicts adaptive social functioning across short and larger time spans. In addition, important evidence that levels of ER can begin a cascade toward positive or negative functioning in the elementary classroom is emerging. Programming for ER is crucial (see Chapter 13).

## Emotion Dysregulation

Despite the growth demonstrated in ER, emotion regulatory failure still occurs throughout the preschool period. Children are still prone to lapses in their emerging ER (especially, as seen in Chapter 6, when other aspects of their self-regulation falter). Such emotion dysregulation or lack of positive emotion regulatory strategy usage is often associated with young children's concurrent or later difficulties with aggression, as well as with other externalizing and internalizing behaviors (Chang et al., 2003, 2012; Crespo et al., 2017; Di Maggio et al., 2016; Ersan, 2020; Ersan & Tok, 2020; Graziano et al., 2007; Helmsen, Koglin, & Petermann, 2012; Kao et al. 2020; Leerkes et al., 2008; Miller et al., 2004; Miller, Fine, et al., 2006; Ren et al., 2016; Woods et al., 2017). For example, the lability/negativity scale of the ERC was positively related to teacher-rated aggression and anxiety, with controls as noted earlier; in contrast, ER assessed by the ERC was related negatively to anxiety (Miller, Fine, et al., 2006). Emotional lability was a significant predictor of student–teacher conflict and negative peer status. In fact, emotional lability mediated the negative relation between student–teacher conflict and peer likability (Spritz et al., 2010). Ersan and Tok (2020) also found that preschoolers' ERC lability was positively related to both physical and relational aggression, even with positive connection of aggression with anger and the negative connection with sadness accounted for.

More specifically, the use of maladaptive emotion regulatory strategies can be associated with behavioral difficulties. For example, in our already cited study, venting strategies were related to externalizing, and more passive, nonconstructive strategies with internalizing behavior problems (Blair et al., 2004). Blair et al. found some outcomes of maternal/teacher ratings of ER strategies moderated by gender and temperament. Passive strategies in this study, which included avoiding the situation or even thinking about it, were detrimental for girls' internalizing problems, especially if the girls were temperamentally highly irritable. For boys who were temperamentally irritable, passive strategies were related to externalizing, but for low-irritable boys, they were related to internalizing. Highly sad/fearful boys showed less externalizing problems when they used passive strategies, but the opposite was true for low sad or fearful boys. Thus, the biologically based predispositions toward differing patterns of emotionality interacted with ER strategy usage, sometimes specifically for girls or boys. However, Zimmer-Gembeck et al. (2022) found a significant meta-analytic effect size linking emotion dysregulation with internalizing behavior, irrespective of child gender, so more investigation may be useful.

In another study, preschoolers rated as anxious by their parents were reported as using more venting strategies both generally and in emotionally difficult situations, and young children with ADHD symptoms evidenced difficulties using regulation strategies during a frustration task (Lugo-Candelas et al., 2017; Yeo, Frydenberg, Northam, & Deans, 2014). Dysregulation and more specific internalizing and externalizing symptomatology also seem to go hand in hand.

Rather than focusing on specific strategies, it may be better to have a good repertoire of strategies to choose from, in the varying emotionally difficult situations that a preschooler with these disorders may experience. In fact, Thomsen and Lessing (2020) found that symptoms of preschool hyperactivity were negatively related to the size of early primary children's repertoire of ER strategies (as directly assessed). Further, the diversity of their ER strategy repertoire in preschool was negatively related to later hyperactivity—attention problems. So overall young children with symptoms of hyperactivity seem to have impoverished ER strategies.

Emotion dysregulation was measured in most of the above-cited work via the ERC or strategy questionnaires, but Miller et al. (2004) observed emotional *dys*regulation in the classroom. In this case observed classroom dysregulation included children (1) overwhelmed by negative emotions, such as hysterical sobs, thrashing, temper tantrums, or so sad, upset, or angry that emotions disorganize behavior, as well as those (2) whose emotionally neutral or positive behavior included out-of-control running, yelling, bumping into peers, shoving furniture, and finally those (3) who exhibited aggression. Children who showed classroom dysregulation were also observed to engage in more conflict and antagonism, and were rated by teachers as more aggressive, anxious, hyperactive, emotionally labile, and less regulated (via the ERC) and less cooperative. Observations of dysregulation and its correlates fit with theoretical predictions.

Moreover, some dysregulation has been observed in laboratory tasks, and findings have again been longitudinal. For example, toddlers' emotional and/or behavioral undercontrol (including anger at their inability to get at a toy car and an inability to wait to use crayons when asked in two different laboratory situations, as well as in maternal ratings of anger and approach tendencies) predicted 4-year-olds' mothers' ratings of their externalizing behavior, especially for those high on earlier maternal ratings of anger and approach tendencies (Rubin, Burgess, Dwyer, & Hastings, 2003). As theoretically expected and discussed here in other contexts, emotional expressiveness and ER work together in this case toward an unfortunate outcome.

Across an even longer longitudinal period, Halligan et al. (2013) found that 12- to 18- month dysregulation, based on observing children during testing, was correlated with concurrent externalizing problems and predicted them by age 5. These findings were robust, even with gender, psychosocial risk status (i.e., young maternal age, single parenthood or relationship instability, unemployment, limited income, unstable/unsatisfactory living conditions, smoking during pregnancy, maternal depression/anxiety; see Chapter 12), and, for the age-5 analyses, earlier behavior problems accounted for.

Regarding the contributions of psychosocial risk across time, Halligan found that children in high-risk families, as just defined, showed more dysregulation at each time of assessment. Specifically examining the risk factor of low socioeconomic status, Cohen and Mendez (2009) found that for low-SES African American preschoolers, emotional lability in the fall of an academic year was associated with consistently maladaptive behavior and declining social competence later in the year. As might be expected, then, children living under such stress may be exposed to less-than-optimal emotion socialization and emotional stressors, multiply determining emotional dysregulation and its route to behavior problems.

Asking about important peer relationships in the classroom also has shown promise for viewing the outcomes of dysregulated ER. As already noted, in Camodeca and Coppola (2019), peers nominated children to various roles in the classroom, such as bully, defender, and bystander. The authors also used the ERC; its teacher-rated lability/negativity scale was related to children's nominations of peers as bullies and "outsiders" (especially for those whose teachers were also rated as high on teacher–student conflict), as well as overall low social preference. Dysregulation is not only seen as troublesome by adults, but also by children's playmates.

### SUMMARY: Emotion Dysregulation

Clearly emotional dysregulation, variously considered, already constitutes a risk factor by the preschool period. As I have found for other aspects of emotional competence in their relationship with social competence and behavior problems, these findings appear both contemporaneously and across even relatively lengthy longitudinal periods.

## CONCLUSION

Recent explorations confirm that the central elements of preschool emotional competence posited here are indeed related to success in the preschool and day care environment. Children who are relatively positively expressive and clear in their expressiveness, who know how to regulate especially negative emotions when these do occur, and who understand their own and others' emotions are liked by peers and considered friendly, cooperative, assertive, prosocial, and nonaggressive by their teachers and independent observers. They experience fewer behavior problems. Because early peer experience is pivotal to later social and cognitive attainments, and behavior problems tend to be persistent once experienced, even more attention should be paid to these specific issues (Parker, Rubin, Erath, Wojslawowicz, & Buskirk, 2006; Rose, Rose, & Feldman, 1989). Careful multisetting, multimethod work needs to continue, and more specific areas of social competence also need to be considered, such as they have been in the study of moral sensibility and emotion knowledge (Dunn, Brown, et al., 1995).

# Contributions of Emotional Expressiveness, Emotion Knowledge, and Emotion Regulation to Early School Success

## INTRODUCTION

Preschoolers are learning more than their ABCs; emotions and evidence of emotional competence are ubiquitous in early childhood classrooms. To learn alongside and in collaboration with teachers and peers, young children must utilize their emotional competencies to facilitate learning—expressing healthy emotions and regulating them and understanding the emotions of the self and others (Denham, Brown, et al., 2010). In fact, according to Izard's emotion utilization model, the components of emotional competence work together to help young children recognize emotionally arousing situations and guide their arousal into constructive thought and action (Izard, 2002; Ursache et al., 2020). Emotional experiences can be accompanied by techniques and strategies that motivate adaptive cognition and action, such as when children use both emotion knowledge and regulation to direct their angry arousal into assertion rather than into a physical response such as hitting (Izard, Stark, Trentacosta, & Schultz, 2008). Concomitant with such emotion utilization is the social competence I discussed in Chapter 10, but also early school success; "dealing with" or utilizing emotions allows children to focus on learning and adapting to the new school environment. Thus a growing literature pinpoints just how emotional competence skills contribute to early school success (Denham, Bassett, Mincic, et al., 2012; Zins, Bloodworth, Weissberg, & Walberg, 2007).

But it is not just researchers who are aware of the importance of emotional competence during early childhood. Educators and parents are becoming ever more aware of the importance of emotional competence and related issues, especially regarding early school success (Blewitt, Fuller-Tyszkiewicz, et al., 2018; Bridgeland et al., 2013; Piotrkowski, Botsko, & Matthews, 2000). Teachers especially view children's "readiness to learn" and "teachability" as marked by positive emotional expressiveness and the ability to regulate emotions and behaviors (Rimm-Kaufman, Pianta, & Cox, 2000), as well as by emotional competence-related social strengths (Lin, Lawrence, & Gorrell, 2003). Head Start programs cite emotional–behavioral issues among their top needs for training and technical assistance (Buettner, Hur, et al., 2016; Zinsser et al., 2014).

Clearly, the important adults in children's lives realize that to succeed in school, children need the tools of emotional competence *from the beginning*. Thus there have been many calls for early childhood educators to help young children to acquire just such competencies, while they model genuine, appropriate emotions and responses to emotions, discuss emotions with children, and use positive emotions to support learning (e.g., Hyson, 2002; see Chapters 9 and 13).

Moreover, children's emotional competence is being recognized as important within the educational policy area. Most U.S. states have early childhood standards that include social and emotional competencies, albeit less systematically and with fewer indicators than cognitive skills (Barnett, Epstein, Friedman, Sansanelli, & Hustedt, 2009; Dusenbury et al., 2015; Dusenbury, Zadrazil, Mart, & Weissberg, 2011; Scott-Little, Kagan, & Frelow, 2006; Zinsser et al., 2013). The integration of social–emotional competencies into U.S. state standards has increased the examination of these outcomes at the classroom level.

Such standards occur less systematically in other nations (e.g., see the "end of key stage statements" that help teachers assess progress in the United Kingdom; Torrente, Alimchandani, & Aber, 2015). But times are changing. For example, the ERASMUS project recently called for member European states to create early childhood social–emotional competence standards and curricula (Cefai, Bartolo, Cavioni, & Downes, 2018); in particular, Cefai et al. cite Italy as having clear preschool social–emotional curriculum standards. An entire volume on social–emotional learning in Asian Pacific countries also recently articulated early childhood social–emotional standards across the region (Frydenberg, Marin, & Collie, 2017). It is evident that the importance of early childhood emotional competence to educational success is receiving increasing international attention.

Additionally, recent U. S. national legislation authorizing the allocation of funds for technical assistance, training, and programming related to emotional competence, including the Every Student Succeeds Act, and several other bills specifically referring to social–emotional learning (Collaborative for Academic, Social, and Emotional Learning, 2018; O'Connor et al., 2017), have been proposed. Although as yet unfunded, this proposed legislation appears to have staying power, to be put forward again.

Thus emotional competencies are identified by early childhood researchers, parents, educators, and policy makers as among the most important abilities supporting early school success and the growth of even later academic competence (Denham, Bassett, Mincic, et al., 2012; Jennings & DiPrete, 2010; Romano et al., 2010). But how should early school success be defined?

In my view, and as suggested in reported findings earlier in this book, early school success includes both classroom adjustment and academic readiness as crucial outcomes for children's successful introduction to schooling. Classroom adjustment can be defined as young children's behaviors and attitudes associated with learning in the classroom environment, such as showing a motivation to learn, persisting and paying attention, participating positively in classroom activities, and enjoying school. Young children's *pre*academic readiness is defined as having mastery of certain basic skills, such as literacy, numeracy, and general knowledge, which help ensure success in the new formal learning environment. In this chapter, I use the term *academic success* in referring to such outcomes later in schooling; I use the term *school success* in discussing both classroom adjustment and either preacademic or academic success, or refer to each term separately. At times I use other researchers' specific terms and define them.

Overall, as already mentioned in Chapter 1, emotionally competent young children have advantages when they enter school—they get along with peers and teachers, participate in classroom activities, and achieve at higher levels throughout their early years in school. In contrast, a lack of these emotional competencies often destines children to peer rejection, less-supportive relationships with teachers, less enjoyment of school, a risk for behavior problems and school difficulties, and finally, lower levels of achievement. A comprehensive longitudinal study from preschool to grade 3 confirmed this last pathway: children who in preschool could experience, recognize, and regulate emotions obtained better grades in third grade (Shala, 2013). In short, emotional competence facilitates early school success, with potentially long-lasting effects. In fact, again as already noted in Chapter 1, a major longitudinal study has shown that aspects of children's emotional competence in kindergarten predicted young adult success in education, independent of child, family, and contextual factors (Jones et al., 2015).

So, what is the state of research about just how emotional competence skills support early school success? In this chapter, I review recent research that has contributed to knowledge in this area, discussing how emotional expressiveness, emotion knowledge, ER, and their interrelations, contribute to school success. Within this review, I give my thoughts about what emotional competence *processes* may assist children as they enter the primary grades.

## PRESCHOOLERS' EMOTIONAL EXPRESSIVENESS AND SCHOOL SUCCESS

Attention is being given to the contribution of emotional expressiveness styles to school success. Positive emotion (e.g., interest, pleasure) may, for example, support and direct attention, facilitate information processing, and enhance both motivation and resilience (Izard, 2002; Pekrun & Linnenbrink-Garcia, 2012). As already discussed, emotional expressiveness styles (often conceptualized as temperament) begin as early as infancy. Even infants described by mothers and observed in the laboratory as demonstrating positive affectivity and/or surgency had higher scores in preacademic success as 4-year-olds on color, letter, and number skills (even with age, gender, other demographic variables, and other temperament dimensions accounted for; Gartstein et al., 2016). It may be that these early demonstrations of enjoying and approaching novelty may be manifestations of a later motivation to learn, reflected in later preacademic success.

In alignment with this assertion, emotionally positive engagement with an examiner was related to literacy outcomes (Denham, Bassett, Sirotkin, & Zinsser, 2013). This positive emotional experience and expressiveness with adults signaled enjoyment and motivation to learn to the self and others. Elaborating on contexts where young children display positive emotions, Hernández et al. (2016) examined patterns of kindergartners' emotional expressiveness during fall classroom free play as well as during lunch and recess; positive emotions were positively related to spring school success (i.e., literacy and numeracy skills rated by teachers, achievement tests, and/or school engagement), either directly or via relationships with teachers and peers, even with verbal ability accounted for. Again emotional positivity grounded children for learning.

More specifically, some relationships were context specific in this study (Hernández et al., 2016)—I have already considered in this book that knowing *when* to express various emotions is key in determining their outcome even for children as young as preschoolers. Thus Hernández et al. (2016) found that expressing positive emotions specifically when in class, presumably while interacting with teachers and peers and completing academic tasks, positively predicted academic skills. The evidence of positive emotion *during classroom activities* likely indicates the presence of both enriching social relationships and enjoyment of the academic tasks children encounter, pleasure at success, and enthusiasm to keep learning.

Joey likes numbers, and he also enjoys working together with Layne because she likes numbers too and can help him when he gets a bit confused. When Layne came over to the numbers table, he smiled because he was glad she was joining him. Together, they laid out buttons in a muffin tin with paper liners numbered 1 to 12. They took turns and said the numbers when they put the buttons in. After he put in number 7, he said, "Seven is heaven!" and started to laugh. Layne laughed too, and they continued the activity amicably.

In contrast, when Hernández et al. (2016) observed positive emotion expressed at lunch or recess, direct associations with academic skills were negative. Recall the negative associations of overly intense positive emotions and social competence depicted in Chapter 10—it seems likely that similar difficulties might be operative here. Perhaps children who became overexuberant in the freer lunch and recess contexts, often but not always the children who also expressed positive emotions in the classroom, had trouble "buckling down" in the classroom.

After their wild, gleeful rumpus on the playground, Mike was actually a little tired for a few minutes, a little chagrined over annoying the teacher and wrecking Pei Lin's highway. He was feeling guilty too and just sat staring into space for several minutes while his teacher was reading a book to the whole class and asking questions about letter sounds.

Moreover, this study verified that the impact of positive emotion on social relationships is important in the trajectory toward school success (Hernández et al., 2016). Specifically, positive emotion expressed in the classroom was an indirect predictor of what these authors termed "school engagement" (i.e., observed and also rated by teachers as liking school and cooperating in class), as well as academic skills, via its association with greater peer acceptance. That is, positive emotions in the classroom predicted peer acceptance, which then predicted both academic skills and school engagement.

Further, in contrast with its direct association, positive emotion expressed at lunch and/or recess *in*directly predicted school success (both academic competence and school engagement) via both peer acceptance and decreased teacher-rated teacher–student conflict. That is, in this case, positive emotion expressed during these times not only predicted greater peer acceptance, but also less student–teacher conflict. Peer acceptance predicted school engagement and academic skills, and teacher–student conflict was a negative predictor of school engagement and both academic skills and achievement in the indirect analysis. Thus, although its direct association with academic skills was negative, positive emotion at lunch and/or recess made a positive contribution to social relationships that facilitated school success. More likable kindergartners could have experiences that helped them succeed in school-related domains.

> The fact that Joey has lots of classmates who like him because of his sunny demeanor is important—he can learn from his friends. When he and Layne were putting the buttons in the muffin tin, he said "10" instead of "9" when it was his turn, and Layne told him, with a smile, "No, that's 9, silly-willy," and they both laughed. He has lots of encounters with friends that bolster his learning and his zest for it.
>
> Even though the teacher takes a rather dim view of Mike's happily instigating mayhem on the playground, she does appreciate his consistently sunny approach to lunch and recess, where so many of her students have difficulties getting along. Once she gets over the "wild rumpus," she resumes her calm and rather affectionate relationship with him. In general, she feels like he's getting along well in the classroom (except for that day, right after the playground incident!) and supports him in his learning.

As opposed to the normally salutary contributions of positive emotion, Herndon et al. (2013) found that preschoolers' observed *negative* emotionality (especially when dysregulated) was negatively associated with later aspects of preschool classroom adjustment: (1) positive classroom behavior (a factor including the lack of anger or conflict with a teacher, cooperative participation and a positive attitude toward learning, attention and persistence, and liking school); and (2) independent motivation to learn (a factor including competence motivation, self-directedness, and lower levels of anxiety and dependency on the teacher). This finding held true, especially for boys. Similarly, my research group also has shown that patterns of preschoolers' observed negative expressiveness (predominantly dysregulated anger) were related to lower levels of both current and kindergarten classroom adjustment, as well as kindergarten academic success, with age, gender, socioeconomic risk status, and, for kindergarten classroom adjustment, earlier ratings, accounted for (Denham, Bassett, Thayer, et al., 2012; Denham, Bassett, Zinsser, et al. 2014; see also Diaz et al., 2017; Hernández et al., 2016).

In Hernández et al. (2016), negative emotions in both the classroom and at lunch and/or recess predicted lower academic achievement test performance, and as with positive emotion, indirectly predicted school success via conflict with the teacher. In this case, demonstrating negative emotions contributed to teachers' assessment of conflict with the student, which predicted lesser school engagement and academic success. Being less able to "connect" with the teacher can make the task of immersing oneself in academic activities harder, especially when the tendency to feel bad also is so prominent.

Even by kindergarten, Carrie still has trouble regulating her negative emotions, and everyone knows it. Although her teacher is sympathetic, she does admit that Carrie is often angry even with her, with her negative emotions making for long and difficult days. Moreover, she considers that that they seem to struggle a lot with each other, and that Carrie drains her energy. Having that negative "edge" between herself and Carrie brings some tension to her learning environment, and she's correct in thinking that Carrie at times has trouble being engaged in academic tasks, a problem also noted by classroom observers.

For her part, Carrie does have difficulty connecting with the more academic aspects of the day—it can take her a long time to calm down after a meltdown, and because of this she's lost time working in activities involving numbers and letters. Sometimes she misses out altogether, standing biting her lips and looking sad while she settles down.

Some specific emotions may be especially important in navigating the early learning environment. Studying kindergartners in a short-term longitudinal study, Valiente, Lemery-Chalfant, and Swanson (2010) found that adults' ratings of preschoolers' sadness, anger, and shyness were negatively related to academic success (letter–word and passage comprehension and applied problems subtests from the Woodcock–Johnson tests of achievement).

These negative emotions, which parents considered to be characteristic of their child, blocked the child's ability to focus on academic activities and enter relationships that support such participation. Extending my analysis, Valiente and colleagues (2010) go further to suggest that anger, sadness, and shyness disrupt effort and motivation, interfering with numerous school-related behaviors and outcomes, such as concentration; reflective planning and problem solving; and problems with health, attendance, and test performance.

Accordingly, as was noted regarding the association between emotional expressiveness and social competence (see Chapter 10), the outcomes of negative emotions were often moderated by aspects of self-regulation. For example, when anger or sadness were rated at lower levels, children high in self-regulation performed best on the achievement test (Valiente et al., 2010). Children who were less likely to experience negative emotions and more able to focus their attention on their academic activities while inhibiting distracting behaviors (e.g., not leaving an academic activity to get a toy) learned more.

In contrast, all children who had high levels of these negative emotions, irrespective of their self-regulation abilities, performed equally poorly (Valiente et al., 2010). Furthermore, as noted in Chapters 2 and 6 and already noted here, anger especially disrupts relationships, as noted in Hernández et al. (2016); during early childhood education in particular, relationships with teachers and peers are key to successful learning. These results in both self-regulation and in social relationships underscore the unfortunate power of negative emotions.

From the perspective of Izard's (2002) emotion utilization framework, dealing with negative emotion leaves the young child with fewer resources for cognitive tasks and less able to use flexible strategies to complete them. For example, sad children may focus on the difficulty of academic tasks and goals, envision failure, and then disengage and withdraw from interactions and tasks. These emotions also leave children more "on their own" owing to their relative lack of positive social relationships, rendering their attainment of school success more difficult.

Shy children also are prone to academic difficulties (Valiente et al., 2010; see also Curby, Brown, Bassett, & Denham, 2015, who found that anxious, withdrawn preschoolers performed less well on measures of print and phonological awareness). Preschoolers' shyness was related to their lower vocabulary and phonological awareness scores, as well as to less first-grade verbal fluency (Spere & Evans, 2009); shyness also has been found negatively related to more general academic behavior (Séguin & MacDonald, 2018). In terms of even later outcomes, Valiente, Doane, Clifford, Grimm, and Lemery-Chalfant (2021) found that shy 8-year-olds have difficulty with both reading and mathematics, and that these children's shyness made it hard for them to live up to their preacademic promise in reading.

What mechanisms may explain these relationships between shyness and academic success? A partial explanation may stem from viewing shyness as self-conscious (Schmidt & Poole, 2019). For one thing, shy children's hesitancy to participate verbally in classroom activities, and their difficulty in regulating their shyness once it is activated, may make it harder for them to learn or even show what they *have* learned (Coplan & Evans, 2009). For example, performing within the social context of reading groups may be particularly uncomfortable for shy children, thus limiting their accomplishments in that area. Teachers may interpret such behaviors as evidence of lack of *competence*, when it may be a lack of *performance* (Crozier & Hostettler, 2003; see also Hughes & Coplan, 2010, for results indicating that shyness was related to a lack of school engagement, which led to lower elementary-school teacher ratings of achievement).

In support of the competence–performance dichotomy and its effect on shy children, primary-school shy children performed worse on individual, face-to-face academic assessments—where they would feel exposed—than in peer group assessments (Crozier & Hostettler, 2003). Their self-conscious pain may be eased in the more anonymous group setting. Considering this distinction points to the need to help shy children work through their emotions, and also to recognize their sensitivities and duly adjust their learning environment.

However, the difficulties faced by shy or anxious children may not always be a competence–performance issue. The fearful type of shyness, which can coexist with the self-conscious type, may render it difficult for them to create social relationships. These shy children are less accepted by their peers and shy about approaching their teacher. In the primary school classroom, as in the early childhood context, relationships are paramount supports for learning, and these disadvantages can make learning harder for them (Zhang et al., 2017). Academic success itself can be seen as a social construct (Curby et al., 2015). If children are not *able* to be part of a group, because they are separated by their internally experienced emotions and rejected by peers (Sette et al., 2016, 2019), they may miss out on learning experiences.

Further bolstering this interpretation, shy Chinese children were less likely to have the benefit of a close relationship with their teachers and disliked and avoided school (Wu et al., 2015). Their lack of closeness with teachers in particular predicted low levels of school liking and less teacher-rated independent participation. Some relationship difficulties' association with shyness depended on child gender: Shy girls were rated as liking school less and avoiding school when they didn't have a closer relationship with their teacher; shy boys' lack of school liking was related to their highly dependent relationship with teachers. In short, as amplified by Spere and Evans (2009), shy children, especially extremely shy children, may not experience the same degree of stimulation and practice with academic tasks because their relationships with teachers and peers suffer, resulting in their dislike and avoidance of school. As noted, however, positive relationships with teachers can buffer this problem.

At the same time, issues of culture are also important to consider regarding all emotional expressiveness and early school success. Valuing positive expressiveness over a relative excess of negative expressiveness may be distinctly Western in individualistic cultures where the focus is on the child's autonomous success in the environment. In contrast, non-Western, collectivistic/relational cultures may value an altogether less expressive presentation of self, because of the goal of group harmony. In support of this possibility, Louie and colleagues (2015) found that for Korean and Asian American preschoolers, both their sadness and happiness expressivity were both associated with negative peer or teacher outcomes. More value was perhaps placed on a calm demeanor for these children, and one might expect any type of overt expressiveness ultimately to be deleterious to school success. However, Wu et al.'s (2015) findings regarding the deleterious outcomes of shyness ran counter to earlier suggestions that shyness might be valued in collectivistic/relational societies (Rubin et al., 2009). Advancing cultural change may diminish some of these differences, and it is clear that more work needs to be done to understand the relationship between emotional expressiveness and early school success across cultures.

## **SUMMARY:** Expressiveness and Early School Success

Consideration of children's patterns of expressiveness yields many important links with early school success. Harkening back to Izard's (2002) emotion utilization theory again is useful here. In general, showing positive emotion in the classroom denotes enjoyment of learning and fosters the social relationships that are so key, especially in early childhood. Children who show positive emotions (except perhaps at lunch and recess where things may get out of hand!) build a foundation for continued positivity, enjoying attentive engagement in their academic activities and learning more easily the literacy and numeracy skills that are appropriate for their age. Their positivity also supports the beneficial relationships with others that support school success.

However, negative emotion can block these pathways. It leaves the child with far fewer internal and relational resources for success in such tasks. Furthermore, disrupted relationships with teachers and peers make learning more difficult in the early childhood educational environment. It is important to identify the protective factors for these negative children as preschoolers, whether they are predominantly angry, sad, or shy, because the early childhood period is so critical for the transition to primary school—socially and academically.

## PRESCHOOLERS' SCHOOL SUCCESS AND EMOTION KNOWLEDGE

Increasingly, researchers are also confirming a link between early academic success and young children's emotion knowledge (Bierman, Domitrovich, et al., 2008; Blankson et al., 2017; Garner & Waajid, 2008, 2012; Izard et al., 2001; Leerkes et al., 2008; Torres, Domitrovich, & Bierman, 2015; Ursache et al., 2020). For example, emotion knowledge—but not ER—was related to preschoolers' preacademic achievement in several studies (Leerkes et al., 2008; see also Garner & Waajid, 2008). Cross-cultural evidence is emerging. My work with colleagues also showed that emotion knowledge predicts later preschool and kindergarten school adjustment and academic success, both directly and indirectly (Bassett et al., 2012; Curby et al., 2015; Denham, Bassett, Thayer, et al., 2012). Importantly, *growth* in emotion knowledge predicted kindergarten reading achievement and engagement in school (Nix et al., 2013; see also Torres et al., 2015). As with emotional expressiveness, cognitive resources are freed up when preschoolers and early primary students understand their own and others' emotions while taking part in collaborative, engaged learning within the so-important small groups of peers (Ursache et al., 2020).

Some of these findings regarding the relationship between emotion knowledge and school success were concurrent. For example, Bierman, Domitrovich, et al. (2008) found that emotion identification and recognition were related to vocabulary, grammatical understanding, sentence imitation, sound blending and elision, and print awareness. In Curby and colleagues' (2015) study, emotion knowledge was associated with preliteracy skills, above and beyond child gender, age, attention abilities, maternal education, and classroom emotional support.

> Jeremy knows Carrie well. They've been in preschool together for 2 (long) years. He can tell when she's angry, as can most everyone else. But he can also tell when she's just sad or tired (like when she had a cold on that "no good, terrible, very bad day"). He also knows what works to defuse her anger, at least sometimes. So when he was sitting at the writing table, working on the letters in his name (*J* is pretty easy, but *y* is not), and Carrie came up and started fussing at him, he correctly deduced that she was cranky today, not sad and needing his help. He sighed, and refocused on his writing. Getting the y correct was his goal!

It's likely that Jeremy's emotion knowledge helps to bolster his preacademic skills. He was able to disconnect from an emotional situation and continue attending to learning. His great relationship with his teacher was no doubt also a factor in his ability to utilize his emotion knowledge in this way; he felt safe to carry on, knowing his teacher would help him or Carrie should they require it.

To elaborate on these ideas, Garner and Waajid's studies (2008, 2012) are good examples. Their outcome measures included concept knowledge and language skills (e.g., knowing the concepts of big–little; knowing body parts, colors, letters, and numbers; using nouns and verbs in expressing oneself; and answering, "What would you do if . . . ?" questions). Teachers also rated children on the teacher–child relationship and on classroom adjustment (e.g., in this case including a positive attitude toward school and learning, following directions, complying with limits, and adapting to school routines). Emotion knowledge was assessed via 10 vignettes for happy, sad, angry, afraid, and surprise emotions, for which the child picked a face to show how the character felt.

Emotion knowledge in their 2008 study mediated the relationship between closeness with teachers and classroom adjustment. Children who had warmer relationships with their teachers had greater emotion knowledge (see Chapter 9), and using this knowledge helped them to feel great about learning while adapting to classroom routines. What's more, emotion knowledge also contributed to variance in concept knowledge and language skills, even with age, gender, income level, and classroom adjustment accounted for (Garner & Waajid, 2008). In their 2012 study, Garner and Waajid found very similar results. Not only did emotion knowledge facilitate classroom adjustment, but it also uniquely contributed to preacademic skill; Jeremy's skills no doubt benefitted from both these aspects of school success.

These authors do remind us of the connection between emotion knowledge and language ability (see Chapter 5 and von Salisch et al., 2013), which may have accounted for some of their findings. Although this caveat is important to consider, it seems to me that these relationships with school success prove robust given Garner and Waajid's (2008) and others' work (see Voltmer & von Salisch's [2017] meta-analysis).

Preschool emotion knowledge's contribution to school success extend even further in time in longitudinal studies. For example, in Bassett et al. (2012), emotion situation knowledge in the fall of the preschool year predicted spring classroom adjustment (i.e., in attention/persistence, competence motivation, attitudes toward learning). As already noted in Chapter 10, Denham, Bassett, Way, et al. (2012) found fall emotion knowledge to predict spring classroom adjustment (including attention/persistence, competence motivation, and attitudes toward learning, but also cooperative participation, self-directedness, school liking, comfort with teachers, and social competence).

Some studies extended the examination of this linkage from preschool into kindergarten. In Denham, Bassett, Way, et al. (2012), emotion knowledge in the fall of the preschool year predicted both classroom adjustment and academic success (i.e., language and literacy, general knowledge, and mathematical thinking) in kindergarten. Similarly, focusing even more specifically on children of color, Ursache et al. (2020) found that emotion knowledge at the end of preschool predicted higher math and reading achievement test scores in both kindergarten and second grade, despite accounting for preacademic skills, other social–emotional skills, and demographic information. These strong findings are critical for adding value to early childhood education for children of color—attending to emotion knowledge reaps benefits (see Chapter 13).

Finally, preschoolers' emotion knowledge specifically predicted kindergarten mathematical ability (Cavadini et al., 2021). In fact, it partially mediated a path from locomotor to mathematics abilities. These authors postulated that being motorically active not only aids in the development of the brain regions key to cognitive processes, but also boosts the social interaction that can fuel preschoolers' emotion knowledge. They noted that locomotor play allows children to interact while chasing, running, jumping, climbing, or engaging in rough-and-tumble or pretend play, and that such experiences would be rife with opportunities to experience and witness emotions.

Findings on both the teacher–child relationship and locomotor play with others, which both facilitate emotion knowledge, add value to the notion of school success as a social construct (Cavadini et al., 2021; Garner & Waajid, 2008). As another example, positive relationships with both teachers and peers indeed predicted gains in emotion knowledge across the preschool year, and these gains in emotion knowledge mediated the relationship between positive interpersonal relationships and kindergarten academic success, controlling for preschool preacademic success (Torres et al., 2015). Again, relationships with teachers and peers are important to emotion knowledge and its subsequent link with early school success.

Self-regulatory ability also plays a role in how children become academically able and may work in concert with emotion knowledge. With findings extending into the primary grades, Rhoades et al. (2011) also found, studying an economically disadvantaged urban population, that preschool emotion knowledge predicted first-grade academic achievement, this time mediated by kindergarten attentional abilities, even after accounting for the effects of maternal education, family income, and children's age, gender, and receptive vocabulary skills. Similarly, Trentacosta and colleagues (2006), in a short-term longitudinal study of rural, low-income first and second graders, found an association between emotion knowledge and teacher-rated academic attentional skills (e.g., staying on task, paying attention) over a year, even accounting for age, gender, verbal ability, and attentional skills at the beginning of the year. In both these cases, it should be noted that emotion knowledge appeared specifically to facilitate attentional focus. Greater emotion knowledge may have supported and been supported by social interaction to such an extent that attentional abilities were strengthened.

> Jeremy's emotion knowledge was supported by his relationships with his teacher and allowed him to coexist peacefully with Carrie. With both of these relationships in play, he was free to concentrate solely on that letter *y*.

The connection of emotion knowledge with academic progress remains important even after first grade. Izard (2002) and Izard and colleagues (2001) found evidence of a link between emotion knowledge and even later academic success in elementary school. To go into more detail on their work, Trentacosta and Izard (2007) assessed urban kindergartners' emotion knowledge of facial expressions, emotions in social situations, and emotions in social behaviors. They found that this measure of emotion knowledge predicted grade-1 academic success (i.e., direct assessment of reading, numerical operations, and spelling, plus teacher ratings), even accounting for age, gender, verbal ability, ER, and attentional ability at the beginning of the year.

Looking across an even longer time period, Izard et al. (2001) assessed economically disadvantaged 5-year-olds' emotion knowledge (recognition and labeling of expressions). Emotion knowledge predicted 9-year-olds' academic success and an element of classroom adjustment (ratings for reading, arithmetic, and motivation to succeed), even with verbal ability and temperament accounted for. It also mediated the contribution of verbal ability to academic success. In fact, in both this study and Trentacosta and Izard (2007), emotion knowledge appeared to be a mechanism through which children's verbal ability translated into school success. Thus verbal ability contributes to the development of emotion knowledge (see Chapter 5), and its contribution facilitates school success well into the elementary years.

## SUMMARY: Emotion Knowledge and Early School Success

Thus, children's ability to understand emotions, especially in context, plays an important role in their concurrent and later academic success. In fact, a recent series of meta-analyses (Voltmer & von Salisch, 2017) show that emotion knowledge in preschoolers *and* grade schoolers is related to academic achievement, school adjustment, and peer acceptance. Further, the age range of the participants in the studies included in the meta-analysis did not moderate the relation with academic success.

Like the link with social competence, emotion knowledge's link with school success bears consideration. Why would emotion knowledge contribute to school success? As already noted, classroom adjustment—being able to attend to instruction and cooperate, feeling good about school, remaining nonaggressive, focusing and succeeding on tasks—is carried out in a very social world. Highlighted in this analysis yet again then is the importance of interpersonal relationships with teachers and peers in the development and sequelae of emotional competence during early childhood (Ursache et al., 2020). Accordingly, as with emotional expressiveness, relationships loom large, specifically in trajectories from emotion knowledge to school success. In this case, in contrast with Hernández et al. (2016), research has shown that a path leads *from* relationships *to* emotional competence, rather than the reverse. It is not difficult to see that positive relationships allow for the exploration of and learning about emotions. Considering Torres et al. (2015) and again accessing the emotional utilization framework, positive interactions with others facilitate the growth of emotion knowledge, perhaps via experiencing others' emotions in a safe setting, and this very emotion knowledge provides children with increased abilities to maximize their focus on preacademic activities.

But how does emotion knowledge then support early school success? Along with the contribution of social relationships to its development, the subsequent path from emotion knowledge to school success may be mediated by smooth social interactions and satisfying relationships with teachers and peers. Understanding the potential barrage of one's own and others' emotions in the preschool classroom can make these social interactions smoother, so that more personal resources are left to focus on more cognitive aspects of the tasks.

More specifically, the role of emotion knowledge in facilitating early school success is likely via its easing of academic-related social interactions. Young children with more advanced emotion knowledge also may be better able to engage in the collaborative learning activities that characterize preschool and kindergarten classrooms because their emotion knowledge helps them understand socially complex interactions. That is, preschoolers who can understand peers' emotions and talk about their own can better communicate and engage with their social partners during academic activities (see, e.g., Denham, Bassett, Zinsser, et al., 2014). Because they can communicate more effectively with teachers, they also may elicit supportive behavior from them and establish a rapport that facilitates instruction.

These abilities, supported by emotion knowledge as a foundation, also may allow for more frequent, prolonged, and stimulating small-group exchanges with both teachers and peers. As a result, the classroom may become more predictable and controllable. Emotion knowledge may provide children with the satisfactory peer and teacher interactions that foster and allow for achievement motivation and attention to academic tasks so that they can "live up to" their general cognitive ability. Due consideration of this pathway requires further study (Ursache, Dawson-McClure, Siegel, & Brotman, 2019; cf. Trentacosta et al., 2006).

Further, another process should be considered in theorizing how emotion knowledge supports early school success. Consonant with the emotion utilization framework, emotion knowledge facilitates children's abilities to recognize their own emotional arousal and act upon it constructively, thus releasing resources that can be focused on academic activity (Izard et al., 2008; Rhoades et al., 2011; Schultz et al., 2001; Trentacosta & Izard, 2007). In particular, for children with emotion knowledge deficits, classrooms may be overwhelming and confusing environments, so that their attention is diverted to navigating this possibly threatening landscape to the detriment of attending to academic activities (von Salisch et al., 2016). Thus, emotion knowledge is key, not only for providing the social foundations for learning, but also for supporting the very personal abilities (e.g., attention) that allow for successful learning.

It should also be noted that the relationships between emotion knowledge and theory of mind and self-regulation also are important to how emotion knowledge may indirectly contribute to school success (see Chapter 5). Theory of mind facilitates knowing about *others'* thoughts, and self-regulation (especially inhibitory control and attention shifting) helps children control their attention and behavior. Both skills help children plan goal-directed actions that support academic activity.

Finally, we note in concluding that the bulk of the research reported here, especially the longitudinal work, suggests that emotion knowledge is a protective factor for both school success and social competence (see Chapter 10). Participants in many of the studies described here (e.g., Curby et al., 2015; Rhoades et al., 2011; Torres et al., 2015; Trentacosta et al., 2006; Ursache et al., 2020) focus on children from low-income communities, and their findings have implications for promoting such children's early school success. Social–emotional interventions targeting emotion knowledge should be promoted even more widely (Torres et al., 2015; see Chapter 13). It also seems that more interventions should include an emphasis on teacher and peer relationships (Denham & Burton, 2003), and, as noted by Rhoades et al. (2011), even more early childhood research is needed to examine school success as an outcome of such interventions (Durlak, Weissberg, Dymnicki, Taylor, & Schellinger, 2011, showed the relationship between social–emotional interventions and academic outcomes, but for older children).

## PRESCHOOLERS' SCHOOL SUCCESS AND EMOTION REGULATION

As already noted, the demands of the new preschool environment can also be emotionally challenging and call for ER. Thus, ER also is related to classroom adjustment, academic success, and other indices of school readiness (Bierman et al., 2014; Bisharat,

Mattar, & Jehan, 2020; Brophy-Herb, Zajicek-Farber, et al., 2013; Mattar, Hamaidi, & Anati, 2018). As with emotional expressiveness, children less able to deal with negative emotions may not have personal resources to focus on learning, whereas those who can maintain a positive emotional tone might be able to remain positively engaged with classroom tasks (Denham, Bassett, Sirotkin, et al., 2013; Graziano et al., 2007; Herndon et al., 2013; Miller, Seifer, Stroud, Sheinkopf, & Dickstein, 2006; Shields et al., 2001; Trentacosta & Izard, 2007). Again there is emerging cross-cultural evidence linking this aspect of emotional competence with school readiness.

> Erica doesn't have the ER problems that Carrie does. In fact, she is able to use self-talk to feel better, as seen in Chapter 6, and she can even "rethink" a situation to keep reasonable emotional control. She was utterly absorbed in using different lengths of construction sticks to create a really cool house for which her teacher had provided a model—needing to figure what lengths could go together to make the shapes properly. But at one point she pushed them together too hard and the whole structure fell apart. She yelped—once. She stared at the mess of sticks on the counting table and sighed deeply. Then she looked up at her teacher and said, "Well, I guess I can't push so hard. . . . Maybe I shouldn't have tried that last stick, I'll do it again different." Using both cognitive problem solving and reappraisal, she was able to stay connected with the preacademic task at hand. ER helped her stay engaged (part of classroom adjustment) and attain more skills too.

Concurrent results have highlighted the importance of both ER and dysregulation to early school success. For example, Bierman et al. (2014) found that kindergarten social competence ratings (including items on ER) were related to several academic skills: vocabulary, letter–word knowledge, phonemic decoding, sight-word reading, and learning behavior, as well as negatively related to attention problems in the classroom. Regarding emotion *dys*regulation, Miller, Seifer, et al. (2006) observed Head Start 4-year-olds' emotional dysregulation in their classroom, which was negatively related to teacher ratings of persistence (e.g., sticks to an activity as long as can be expected), and learning attitude (e.g., willing to accept help).

> Unlike Erica, Connor isn't adept at ER. Trying the same task, he too had difficulty replicating the model of a house that the teacher had taped to the counting table. He tried and tried. He kept having trouble getting the sticks to connect and repeatedly picked ones of incorrect lengths. Finally, he yelled—LOUD—and waved both arms, flinging sticks all over the place. By using the ineffective ER strategy of venting, letting his dysregulated anger get the better of him, he had lost control of a learning opportunity.

In another study with racially and ethnically diverse kindergarteners, who were oversampled to identify children with behavior problems (Graziano et al., 2007), results indicated that ER measured by the ERC was directly and positively associated with teacher reports of children's academic success and productivity in the classroom, as well as standardized early literacy and math achievement scores, even after accounting for IQ, behavior problems, and the quality of the teacher–child relationship. In short, better ER skills facilitated children's ability to independently attend to and learn new information presented by their teachers.

Longitudinal studies strengthen the assertion that ER contributes to school success and also reveal some important mediating factors. Thus even toddlers' ER has been examined as predictive of preacademic abilities. In Brophy-Herb, Zajicek-Farber, et al. (2013), toddlers' ER was assessed at 14, 24, and 36 months, via examiner ratings of their ability to tolerate changing test materials and tasks, as well as their negative affect and frustration during the assessment. Both the initial level at each age and the slope between the ages of these ER ratings predicted letter–word knowledge and applied mathematical problems subtests that formed a "cognitive school readiness" latent variable across the 22-month period. These authors asserted that ER allows children to better perform whatever task is put before them.

In a short-term longitudinal study with older children, Shields et al. (2001) studied 3- to 5-year-olds attending Head Start. Teachers completed the ERC near the beginning of the school year. They also rated the children's classroom adjustment/preacademic success (i.e., reading readiness, numbers/counting, language/communication, as well as adjustment to routines, ability to comply with directions and rules, and quality of relationships while participating in structured activities, which all loaded on a single factor) and the closeness or conflict in the relationship with each child at the end of the school year. The ERC regulation scale was related to closeness with the teacher and classroom adjustment, and negatively related to conflict with the teacher and the ERC lability/negativity scale, with the age of child accounted for.

Some moderating factors impact the relationship between ER and early school success. Relationships with teachers, as well as the quality of the entire classroom milieu, again require consideration. For example, older children in Shields et al. (2001), with whom teachers are considered to have a less close relationship, were at risk for lability and/or negativity and thence its deleterious effect on classroom adjustment and/or preacademic success.

Another study also highlighted the importance of the classroom environment created by the teacher for the relationship between ER and early school success (Bailey et al., 2016). Each child's ER was rated after each subtask of the Preschool Self-Regulation Assessment (i.e., being on an even keel and not defiant or passively noncompliant during the challenges of the assessment). This index of ER was correlated with children's positive classroom engagement and independent motivation to learn (already described for Herndon et al., 2013). But more than this, if emotional support or organizational support (i.e., the environment created by the teacher) were inadequate in quality, ER functioned as a buffer via its particular positive association with both positive classroom engagement and independent motivation to learn. In other words, preschoolers' ER was especially important for their school success if classroom quality was less than optimal.

Thus a conclusion can be reached in these two studies: It is crucial, when studying young children's ER and its contributions to early school success, to consider the relational and interactional milieus in which the child is feeling emotions and learning. Both the Shields et al. (2001) and the Bailey et al. (2016) studies are important for early childhood education, in which teachers can be seen as coaching the development of emotional competence (see Chapter 9).

In another moderation analysis, boys were again found to be at special risk for the effects of ER deficits. That is, Herndon et al. (2013) found that boys' emotional *dys*regulation (anger and associated aggression) was associated with lower levels of teachers' later reports on positive classroom engagement and independent motivation to learn. Boys' vulnerability for this and other aspects of emotional competence and its sequelae require urgent attention.

In addition to moderation, mediation pathways also should be considered in examining the ER–school success linkage. Also crucial to mention then are studies in which attentional abilities or behavior regulation mediated the contribution of ER to school success. Regarding attention, preschool ERC scores in the fall (in this case retaining items from both the ER and lability/negativity subscales, reversed) predicted school readiness in kindergarten, via attention regulation (e.g., being able to concentrate, pay attention, not be distracted, and stay on task; Shields et al., 2001). That is, children with more productive ER were better able to pay attention during various tasks, and this attentional advantage predicted school readiness. Similarly, first-graders' teacher-rated attention for academic tasks mediated the relationship between kindergarten ERC emotion regulation scores and an aggregate of first-grade achievement test scores and teacher ratings of academic success (Trentacosta & Izard, 2007). As with emotion knowledge, ER's contribution to attention is a major positive outcome leading to school success.

Examining a slightly different but not entirely unrelated construct, behavioral self-regulation, Howse, Calkins, Anastopoulos, Keane, and Shelton (2003) found that preschool parent-rated ERC emotion regulation contributed to variance in kindergarten literacy, mathematics, and listening comprehension achievement test scores, even accounting for maternal education and IQ, via kindergarten behavioral self-regulation. Behavior regulation was rated by teachers, and included the following items (some obviously weighted negatively): "is impulsive and careless in tasks and activities," "has difficulty planning and carrying out activities that have several steps," "finishes tasks and activities," "concentrates well and is not easily distractible when doing a task," "actively uses resources for help and information," "is not a self-starter," "does not readily ask questions," and "likes to do challenging tasks." Preschoolers who have difficulty regulating their emotions may become kindergartners who have difficulty regulating their learning in these ways during classroom activities, which ultimately could lead to difficulties in academic endeavors.

## SUMMARY: Emotion Regulation and Early School Success

A relatively small body of promising research points out strongly that ER supports early school success and that emotional dysregulation makes attaining both elements of classroom adjustment and preacademic and academic skills that much harder. ER is tightly bound with emotional expressiveness (even in the ERC scale), and we should consider how to support both of them.

For example, the importance of fostering excellent teacher–child relationships again surfaces—having a close relationship could make it easier for a teacher to react to a child's expressiveness and lack of regulation with appropriate emotion socialization. Further, the overall quality of the classroom environment also is likely to be crucial; feeling safe in a clearly organized environment can support preschool ER and its contribution to school success. As well, ER can facilitate preschoolers' ability to pay attention, leading to better classroom adjustment, and it can be a key contributor to the behavioral regulation—academic success pathway. Many of these issues would benefit greatly from further research.

## INTERRELATIONSHIPS OF COMPONENTS OF EMOTIONAL COMPETENCE AND RESULTANT SCHOOL SUCCESS

So far, I have reviewed evidence for how the components of early childhood emotional competence, one by one, support early school success. However, these components are only studied artificially if they are considered separately. In fact, all aspects of emotional competence work together to promote children's school success (Denham, Bassett, Mincic, et al., 2012). As briefly mentioned in Chapter 1, this study corroborated all these assertions in person-centered analyses: 4-year-olds with more positive profiles of emotional expressiveness, ER, and emotion knowledge (along with more positive self-regulation and social problem solving) did indeed show greater classroom adjustment as evaluated later that school year (i.e., competence motivation, attention/persistence, attitudes toward learning) and in both classroom adjustment and academic success (i.e., language and literacy, general knowledge, and mathematical thinking) in kindergarten. The children with lower emotion knowledge, as well as less-positive emotional expressiveness and ER abilities, were at risk for deficits in these indices. This most at-risk group comprised more boys and children living in poverty than the other two groups. Knowing person-centered views of emotional competence can be useful in determining the need to address these interconnected abilities in the classroom.

Indirect, mediational pathways also are possible; emotional competencies considered more foundational might have, along with their direct effects, indirect contributions to classroom adjustment and academic readiness via more overt behaviors. In one of the few studies examining how aspects of emotional competence may mediate one another in contributing to early school success, Denham, Bassett, Zinsser, et al. (2014) found that emotionally negative and/or aggressive behavior mediated the association between aspects of emotion knowledge and both concurrent and later classroom adjustment; in addition, emotion knowledge was related to observed ER and thence to classroom adjustment (see also the indirect relation of emotion knowledge deficits to teacher-reported anger/aggression in Di Maggio et al., 2016).

### SUMMARY: Interrelationship of Emotional Competence Components and Early School Success

Looking at how *all* components of emotional competence contribute to early school success expands our understanding of these phenomena and processes. Greater clarity on the synergy present among the components of emotional competence can help shape the means of promoting emotional competence, social competence, and school success (see Chapter 13).

## CONCLUSION

After decades of pinning down exactly what comprises the components of early childhood emotional competence, and then exploding into examination of its relationship with social competence and how parents support it, attention eventually turned to how preschoolers' emotional competence can facilitate school success, in terms of classroom adjustment and preacademic skills, and later academic success. There now is much empirical support for the outcomes that emotional competence theory suggests: a significant contribution to all aspects of school success.

Several interpersonal and intrapersonal factors are worth considering in analyzing these contributions, so that we can proceed to apply these findings. Relationships and interactions with teachers especially, but also with peers, must be considered as both precursors and outcomes of emotional competence that lead to school success. On the intrapersonal side, children's attentional abilities, as supported by emotional competence, must be included in any plans to apply these findings; emotional competence's impact on attention is another path to school success that must be considered. I am hopeful that these findings can lead to a serious consideration of how to promote emotional competence, and not only for social competence outcomes. However, I also urge much more research in this area, especially a careful examination of ER's role.

# 12

# Disruptions in the Development of Emotional Competence

## INTRODUCTION

Many factors in children or in their environment can compromise their developing emotional competence. Some preschoolers' emotional competence is at risk because of intrapersonal factors.

Jeff has been diagnosed with pervasive developmental disorder. He appears rather emotionally flat most of the time, but he sometimes erupts in contextually confusing laughter or rage that his parents, teacher, and peers don't understand. He seems oblivious to the emotional output of his developmentally delayed and nondelayed classmates.

Other preschoolers' emotional competence is at risk because of interpersonal factors.

Carla's mother suffers from major depressive disorder. When they are together—if she is awake—she is loving, but in a clingy, whining way that makes her, not 2-year-old Carla, seem the "baby" who needs caring for. She talks with great exhaustion about how to just make it through the day, and her monologue is laced with references to her need for Carla to be a "good girl." No wonder Carla is rather unemotional but very, very compliant when observed in her preschool class. Her play is restricted, but when other children cry hard, she looks pained and often intervenes in some way. Nonetheless, she performs less well than expected for her age on emotion knowledge assessments.

The development of preschoolers' emotional expressiveness, emotion knowledge, and ER does not always go smoothly. Thus, in this chapter I address three major issues.

First, I give examples of emotional competence disruptions that are consonant with conditions existing within the child. Next, I consider examples of disruptions in which environmental contributors are prominent, and finally, present disruptions that have a mix of contributors—part intrapersonal and part interpersonal.

## INTRAPERSONAL CONTRIBUTIONS TO DIFFICULTIES IN EMOTIONAL COMPETENCE

Two exemplary cases of intrapersonal contributions to emotional competence deficits are autism and Down syndrome. Autism is characterized by extensive deficits in both cognitive and social–emotional domains. Specific emotional competence features of autistic disorder can include the following: lack of awareness of the feelings of others, little or no facial expressiveness in communicating, distress over what others would consider trivial changes in the environment, and extreme comfort seeking when under distress (see also Cole, Michel, et al., 1994). Thus, an autistic child's lack of social responsiveness is reflected in an absence of emotional expressiveness, and autism's characteristic cognitive and social–emotional deficits are accompanied by deficits in understanding and in regulating emotions. These children's emotional competence often is impoverished.

In contrast, the emotional competence deficits associated with Down syndrome are more clearly due to cognitive or intellectual delay, especially in the areas of emotion knowledge and ER. Down syndrome also is accompanied by hypotonicity of the facial muscles which can cause differences in children's patterns of emotional expressiveness.

### Children with Autism and Emotional Competence

Even though I just articulated some potential concerns regarding young autistic children's emotional competence, there are important caveats to consider when evaluating emotional competence research with young autistic children. Research results can vary, probably for many reasons, including the methodologies used and the specific participants and focus of the studies (e.g., Are developmentally disabled or typically developing children, or both, the comparison participants? Are the autistic participants low or high functioning, or both?). Further, an autistic diagnosis is an umbrella term, such that research participants could vary in terms of the severity of a multitude of characteristics, including (1) sensory issues; (2) restricted/repetitive behavior; (3) lack of social communication; (4) difficulties in self-regulation and joint attention; and (5) language delays. These children's emotional competence also is impacted by these diagnostic features, which may or may not be controlled or even measured in research (Cibralic, Kohlhoff, Wallace, McMahon, & Eapen, 2019; Nuske et al., 2017; Zantige, Rijn, Stockmann, & Swaab, 2017). The influence of these factors on emotional competence is considerable and is not often taken into account in interpretations of emotional competence research with autistic children. Thus in what follows I am attempting to share converging evidence across studies and to include additional detail related to these potentially confounding issues given where available.

Regarding emotional expressiveness, autistic preschoolers display happy, sad, angry, and neutral facial expressions at a frequency like that of age-matched, typically developing children (Begeer, Koot, Rieffe, Terwogt, & Stegge, 2008; McGee, Feldman, & Chernin, 1991). But they are sometimes more likely to display these emotions during contextually incongruent situations (McGee et al., 1991; cf. Macari et al.'s, 2018, contradictory findings). This intriguing finding reminds us that the expression of various emotions has biological bases—*all* children show emotions. However, autistic children's deficits in joint attention, sensory integration, and language may make it difficult for them to learn *when* and *how* to show specific emotions. And they may be less able to receive and assimilate socialization messages about what emotions to show in varying situations.

So autistic children show emotions, but sometimes less frequent expressions of lower quality in inappropriate contexts (e.g., Keating & Cook, 2020). For example, compared to nondiagnosed children they smile or show other positive emotion less during peer or mother–child interaction, and in these settings, they are less likely to coordinate their emotional displays with eye contact (Dawson, Hill, Spencer, Galpert, & Watson, 1990; Lord & Magill-Evans, 1995; Mundy, Kasari, & Sigman, 1992; Snow, Hertzig, & Shapiro, 1987). They also show more flat or neutral emotion, as well as incongruous blends of emotions (e.g., joy and sadness; Yirmiya, Kasari, Sigman, & Mundy, 1989).

Other specific differences in autistic preschoolers' emotional expressiveness exist when compared to the expressiveness of typically developing children. For example, differences are seen in the intensity of autistic children's negative emotions: They demonstrated more intense fear than both typically developing and developmentally delayed matched controls and more intense anger than developmentally delayed children in naturalistic situations probing for emotions (e.g., exposure to a toy spider and dinosaur and increasingly scary masks for fear, and having to get into a car seat or having one's arm restrained for anger; Macari et al., 2018). Mothers also have rated their autistic children as showing greater negativity and lability on the ERC (Jahromi, Kirkman, Friedman, & Nunnally, 2021; see also Nuske et al., 2017).

Regarding positive emotion, Macari et al. (2018) observed these children to show, in nonsocial situations like blowing bubbles or watching a puppet show, equivalent positive emotions to both typically developing and developmentally delayed counterparts. However, it is important to note that their level of joy was negatively related to the severity of their autistic symptoms. In short, autistic preschoolers' expressiveness not only can be situationally less than appropriate and different from typically developing preschoolers in terms of contextual and intensive characteristics, but also show specificity at the individual emotion level. Again, these expressive characteristics are detriments to social interaction with adults and other children alike.

Regarding the expression of self-conscious and social emotions, children with autism smile when they complete difficult tasks such as puzzles, but do not look up to others or draw attention to their accomplishments (Kasari, Sigman, Baumgartner, & Stipek, 1993); although they may be considered to be experiencing pride, they do not display the constellation of expressions and behavior that is usually considered definitional for this emotion.

In terms of empathic concern, these children's attention, as well as their behavioral and emotional reactions, to adult displays of pain and fear differed from those of nonautistic children (Sigman, Kasari, Kwon, & Yirmiya, 1992). They spent significantly *less* time looking at a distressed or fearful adult than did matched groups of children with either typical development or developmental delay. The autistic children showed a different pattern—a different notion of what was important—in situations where an adult sustained an injury or was accosted by a strange robot. They looked at, for example, the pounding toys that resulted in the adult's self-injury. Although they also were rated as less concerned than the other two groups, the autistic children did seem influenced by the adult's demonstration of fear. Even though they did not attend visually to the adult's display of fear, their latency to approach the robot was greater and their play with it less extensive than when fear was not displayed. Thus these children somehow made use of emotional information to guide their own behavior in the service of regulating their own emotion, but in an atypically detached way.

In sum, autistic preschool children demonstrate an impaired ability to modify their emotions appropriately in response to others, showing heterogeneous responses to others' emotions, ranging from flat affect to heightened, inappropriate expressiveness (Sivaratham, Newman, Tonge, & Rinehart, 2015). They show more intense negative emotions and show contextual differences in positive, self-conscious, and social emotions. Taken together, these findings show that the expressiveness of autistic children is distinguished by differences that contribute to their social difficulties (Keating & Cook, 2020). As Kasari and Sigman (1996, p. 115) have stated, "A brief expression that appears odd and does not fit the tone of [an] interaction may significantly disrupt the flow of the interaction." Further adding to the problem, typically developing and autistic children each have trouble recognizing the others' emotional expressions. Moreover, these socially important differences are lasting: There is significant stability in autistic children's emotional responses over a 5-year period (Dissanayake, Sigman, & Kasari, 1996).

Autistic preschoolers also have some difficulties regarding developing emotion knowledge, but the parameters of their delay sometimes vary across studies. In one early study, causal understanding of typical emotional situations, along with emotions elicited by specific desires or beliefs, was tested in autistic children (Baron-Cohen, 1991). They did not differ from developmentally disabled, nonautistic children in their understanding of unequivocal situations that cause emotions (e.g., going to the zoo makes everyone happy; see also Begeer et al., 2008, for a review of both low- and high-functioning autistic children's emotion knowledge). However, both groups in Baron-Cohen's (1991) study performed less well than nondiagnosed children. Autistic children demonstrated even more severe deficits in comprehension of emotion caused by beliefs (e.g., a girl is sad because she thinks she is about to lose her toy forever when her brother takes it). Thus belief—a specific element of autistic children's theory of mind—was particularly difficult for them to utilize, especially in conjunction with emotional information.

Other aspects of an emotion-relevant theory of mind, such as desire, also are difficult for autistic children. For example, autistic children have a special difficulty with a task in which their own desire would differ from the story protagonist's (e.g., whether one feels happy or scared as a big dog approaches; Jahromi et al., 2021), or in equivocal situations in which two protagonists' desire-based emotions differed (e.g., one person would be delighted to get milk at snack time, but another would be annoyed at getting milk; Phillips, Baron-Cohen, & Rutter, 1995). In the work of Phillips et al., even though the autistic children had a verbal mental age of around 6 years, they performed on a par with typically developing 4-year-olds. Thus the skills of emotion knowledge that autistic children can perform well seem restricted generally to more basic emotions (i.e., "external," to use Pons et al.'s [2004] terminology for understanding unequivocal emotion situations involving basic emotions).

Considering other ways of assessing emotion knowledge, autistic children have had varying difficulties recognizing emotions from faces, voices, bodily posture, or contextually rich social exemplars, especially for emotions like disappointment, frustration, pride, or shame (Fridenson-Hayo et al., 2016). Finally, verbally describing emotions also is difficult for autistic preschoolers, who performed less well than typically developing counterparts in defining and giving examples of situations for 16 emotions (Gev, Avital, Rosenan, Aronson, & Golan, 2021). So, it seems that autistic children demonstrate deficits that may depend on what facet of emotion knowledge is studied and on how it is measured. Their difficulties seem to occur particularly for emotions considered more advanced conceptually or requiring a more sophisticated theory of mind or verbal production.

Thus, even though autistic children do show more attention to emotional faces than neutral ones, evidence suggests that it is a different sort of attention. Along with delays in theory of mind especially, the foundation of their difficulty with emotion knowledge also may emanate from their unique method of face recognition. Autistic children demonstrate atypical facial scanning patterns (e.g., spending less time looking at core facial features of emotion, not adapting their looking patterns to the social context, more briefly focusing with the eyes darting from one fixation to another; Vacas, Antolí, Sánchez-Raya, & Pérez-Dueñas, 2022). Some of these perceptual differences are more pronounced with greater symptom severity. Not perceiving important aspects of facial cues of emotion, especially in tandem with a diminished theory of mind, makes it difficult for autistic children to understand emotions well enough to react appropriately to a person expressing emotion, or even to their own emotions, for that matter.

Finally, Keating and Cook (2020) have surmised that difficulties in both emotional expressiveness and emotion knowledge in these children may be due to alexithymia, a subclinical inability to identify and describe one's own emotions. Bolstering the alexithymia hypothesis, others (e.g., Begeer et al., 2008) point out that autistic children seem to accrue emotion knowledge mostly from verbal and conceptual information, even if limited, rather than from personal experience with actual emotions.

These accumulated propensities seem to multiply determine emotion expressiveness and knowledge problems for autistic children. There may be some reason for hope, however. For example, attempts have been made to improve young autistic children's emotion knowledge (Romero, 2017; Ros-Demarize & Graziano, 2021). These programs took very different approaches—one using a DVD presentation of material, the other (Ros-Demarize & Graziano, 2021) employing a multifaceted intervention, including behavior training and specific lessons on emotion knowledge and ER, both of which improved during a summer school period. More efforts to create and evaluate such programming would be useful.

Regarding autistic children's ER, difficulties have been uncovered via both parent report and observation (Gev et al. 2021; Jahromi, Bryce, & Swanson, 2013; Jahromi, Meek, & Ober-Reynolds, 2012; Jahromi et al., 2021; see Cibralic et al., 2019, for a review). Both symptom severity and self-regulation abilities are related to the efficiency of autistic children's ER (Cibralic et al., 2019; Fenning, Baker, & Moffitt, 2018). The characteristics of young autistic children's ER include stability over 1 year (Berkovits, Eisenhower, & Blacher, 2017).

The quality of autistic children's usage of specific ER strategies is relatively immature and inefficient as well. For example, during peer interactions, autistic preschoolers differ from their typically developing counterparts in their increased use of aggressive venting, and less-frequent support-seeking, cognitive-restructuring, and instrumental strategies (i.e., working to solve the problem; Jahromi et al., 2021). Similarly, when they were frustrated during lockbox and unsolvable puzzle tasks, autistic children appeared more resigned than nondiagnosed children, made more negative and fewer positive or neutral vocalizations, and utilized more venting and avoidance strategies, rather than constructive or complex ER strategies (see also Gev et al., 2021; Hirschler-Guttenberg, Golan, Ostfeld-Etzion, & Feldman, 2015; Zantinge et al., 2017).

Further, ER strategy usage did not function for autistic children as it did for typically developing children: Asking for social support (via orientation or verbalizations to the examiner) strategies did not lead to decreases in their resignation, and their venting and distraction did not lead to as big a decrease in facial and bodily negativity as it did for typically developing children.

These findings suggest that when faced with a frustrating situation, autistic children employ different ER strategies than nonautistic children, and that the strategies they do employ are less effective at regulating emotions. One positive note is that their parents seem to scaffold their ER by appropriately avoiding more complicated strategies while coregulating with their children. In fact, when mothers of autistic children engaged in an intervention targeting joint engagement, their children showed a decrease in emotional negativity and avoidant ER strategies (Gulsrud, Jahromi, & Kasari, 2010); learning to better calibrate their participation in their children's needed coregulation was emotionally helpful to their children.

As with emotional expressiveness, these difficulties with ER prove problematic for autistic children's social competence outcomes, including prosocial development (Jahromi et al., 2021) as well as school and peer engagement (Berkovits et al., 2017; Cibralic et al., 2019; Gev et al., 2021). For example, Gev and colleagues (2021) observed autistic children in adult-mediated peer interaction and play, finding them to be more emotionally dysregulated in these social settings, even though they did not differ from their typically developing peers in actual frequency of observed positive or negative emotion. They were similarly emotional with their peers, but did not successfully regulate emotions when needed. Not surprisingly, their emotional dysregulation and lack of ER predicted behavior problems over a 1-year time span (Berkovits et al., 2017). One recent optimistic report, however, suggested that when mothers and their autistic children had more frequent conversations about emotions, their children's ER was more positive (Beaudoin, Poirier, & Nader-Grosbois, 2021).

### SUMMARY: Young Children with Autism and Emotional Competence

The *social* side of emotional competence—for instance, displaying emotions in "appropriate" situations, attending accurately to others' emotions to respond socially, and refraining from emotionally dysregulated behavior—is lacking or delayed in children with this pervasive developmental disability. Their abilities and predispositions in emotional expressiveness, emotion knowledge, and ER are compromised and affect their ability to interact successfully with others, self-regulate, and avoid behavior problems.

## Children with Down Syndrome and Emotional Competence

In some ways, children with Down syndrome are emotionally very similar to their typically developing counterparts; in others, they are quite different. Like nondelayed children, those with Down syndrome show stable expressive styles in the emotion-related components of temperament (although such stability is greater for typically developing children; Vaughn et al., 1993). In contrast, there are mean differences in these stable attributes of emotionality across groups: Down syndrome children, compared with nondelayed children, are generally hard to arouse emotionally and rather placid. Once aroused though, they have more difficulty with ER. Some of this apparent composure is undoubtedly due to the poor muscle tone common to this syndrome; these children show briefer, less intense expressions that do not involve the entire face (Kasari, Mundy, Yirmiya, & Sigman, 1990).

Nonetheless, these are rather subtle differences, which functionally may be relatively unimportant. For example, like nondiagnosed children, Down syndrome children show pride—positive emotional expression and social orientation at task completion (Hughes & Kasari, 2000). On some dimensions, then, expressive differences are not large between Down syndrome and nondisabled children; in these areas, the development of expressiveness follows a common path in the two groups. Down syndrome children do communicate their feelings and have their own unique "emotional styles."

Down syndrome children evidence markers of empathic concern as well (Kasari, Freeman, & Bass, 2003). In a standard empathy task in which an experimenter "hurt" her knee, a Down syndrome child looked at her more, and offered her more comfort via touching, patting, or other support, compared with both typically developing children and those with nonspecific developmental disabilities (see also Kasari et al., 1990). They did not look distressed like children with nonspecific developmental disabilities, nor did they ask for information to understand the situation like the typically developing children, and in fact they showed little positive *or* negative emotion. So even though aspects of cognitive and emotional empathy were missing, nonetheless, they did show empathic concern via their behavior.

In contrast, in this same Kasari et al. (1990) study, they could not endorse as their own the emotions shown by protagonist puppets (e.g., in answer to the question "how does this make you feel?" with the emotion the puppet felt: happy because of a birthday; sad because a pet runs away; angry when a peer takes a toy; scared when a big dog comes up). It seems that these Down syndrome children *showed* empathic behavior in real life but could not "get the hang of" the higher-level thinking required to feel the same as the puppet. I think it is easy to see that "the point" of this task might have been hard for Down syndrome children to discern (I even have some trouble with it, from the distance of almost 40 years since creating such a measure!). For them, other aspects of the task (e.g., the puppets, the puppeteer) might have been distractingly interesting. But when confronted with someone in pain, Down syndrome children acted.

In contrast, emotion knowledge can be compromised in Down syndrome children. Varying methodologies have shown some mixed results, which I attempt to integrate. It should be noted, however, that almost all the studies examined the emotion knowledge abilities of Down syndrome children at about a mental age of 3 to 5 years, and all matched the typically developing children on this attribute.

First, Kasari, Freeman, and Hughes (2001) examined Down syndrome children's emotion knowledge with my puppet measure (the AKT; see Chapter 4) across three studies. On this measure, which requires almost no verbalization (but does require receptive language), Down syndrome children with a developmental age of about 3½ years performed as well as developmental-age-matched nondisabled children. They could label and recognize expressions and identify situations as happy, sad, angry, and fearful as well as the matched typically developing children. For all the children, as I've noted in Chapter 4, correctly identifying happiness and sadness, across tasks, was easier than identifying anger and fear. Further, the Down syndrome children's abilities were correlated with their mental, but not chronological, age. This point suggested that the source of their abilities was tied more to their cognitive, perceptual, and linguistic progress developmentally than to their experience in observing others' emotions. Their emotion knowledge proficiency does not unfold separately from these other developmental domains (Cebula, Wishart, Willis, & Pitcairn, 2017).

Although Down syndrome children's emotion knowledge was understandably developmentally delayed, it showed only one actual anomaly. Most of the Down syndrome children's errors were in saying the puppet was happy when it was not (a positive bias). And although they had some trouble with negative emotions, they did not confuse them as typically developing children do (see Chapter 4).

However, a year later, when the Down syndrome children's mental ages were about 4 years, they could still recognize emotional expressions as well as the typically developing children, but they were less able to verbally label expressions and give the correct emotions for situations compared to the other children. It did not appear that these deficits were due to language issues, because the groups were matched on vocabulary. The typically developing children had expanded their conceptual understanding of emotions during the passing year, whereas the Down syndrome children had not.

This likely explanation was addressed more directly in Kasari et al.'s (2001) third study, in which an actual change in emotion knowledge over a 1-year period was examined. In this third study, the Down syndrome children did not improve in their emotion knowledge between their average mental age of approximately 3½ years and 4½ years; it stabilized even though their cognitive and language abilities improved.

What could account for this lack of change? Kasari et al. (2001) made several suggestions. First, it may be difficult for these children to focus on cognition and language *plus* emotion knowledge; as Piaget (1977/1995) famously asserted, domains of development do not necessarily advance together. Second, socializers in the Down syndrome children's environment may not be focusing on emotion in conversing with them: Kasari et al. (2001) cite research suggesting that the mothers of Down syndrome children talk to them less about emotions than do mothers of typically developing children and also refer less often to more complex or negative emotions. Third, the Down syndrome children's bias to consider emotions "happy" (as in Study 1's error analysis) should be considered: Socializers may be focusing on these children's perceived happy dispositions, and not reflecting on the more complex emotional world with them because they see no need, and their children therefore may remain "happily fixated" on happy emotions. Fourth, even though the groups in Kasari et al. (2001) were matched on language ability, auditory processing can be difficult for Down syndrome children. To conclude, these studies suggest that early in the preschool mental age range, Down syndrome children perform as well on emotion knowledge tasks as their nondelayed counterparts do, but that as they get older, they may start to lag in understanding. More research on Kasari et al.'s (2001) ideas about emotion socialization should be implemented.

In another study in which three emotion knowledge measures were administered (i.e., recognition of expressions, matching of expressions, and a situation task where contextual details were provided), Down syndrome children also had relative trouble identifying emotional expressions and situations (Barisnikov et al., 2022). Also, their identification of faces in general didn't seem to be a prerequisite support for situation knowledge, as it did for typically developing children. The authors conjectured that the self-regulatory abilities needed for dealing with the complex visual stimuli in their situation knowledge task, coupled with emotion processing difficulties, rendered this task especially challenging for these children. In addition, whereas general facial recognition comes "online" early because it is related to the early development of the fusiform gyrus in the brain, assigning emotions to faces may depend more on the growth in the amygdala and its functional connection with the fusiform gyrus, a development that may be delayed in Down syndrome children. These intriguing possibilities require further study.

As with autistic children, Down syndrome children have shown difficulties understanding some specific emotions (e.g., fear, disgust, surprise; Barisnikov, Thomasson, Stutzmann, & Lejeune, 2020; Cebula et al., 2017; de Santana, Souza, & Feitosa, 2014); these emotions, as noted in Chapter 4, are developmentally more difficult for typically developing children to understand as well.

At the same time, Cebula et al. (2017) note that sometimes specific expressions are difficult to discern because of nonlinguistic issues; as seen with autistic children's different face-scanning patterns, these difficulties may be exacerbated for Down syndrome children. In the case of fear, for example, Down syndrome children may have difficulty utilizing both parts of the face in their comprehension of the expression. As noted by Barisnikov and colleagues (2020, 2022) in both their studies, Down syndrome children are likely using a more piecemeal "local-processing" approach to discern emotional expressions rather than the more successful configural processing that typically developing children begin to use (e.g., using information on how the different facial features "go together" for different emotions).

However, other research indicates that Down syndrome children, matched on IQ, vocabulary, or developmental age with their typically developing counterparts, could understand emotions depicted via vocalizations (Pochon & Declercq, 2013), static or dynamic expressions (Channell, Conners, & Barth, 2014), or labels (Barisnikov, Thomasson et al., 2020). In fact, Channell et al. (2014) found that both Down syndrome and typically developing children showed similar developmental trajectories of emotion knowledge. The Channell et al. study is potentially important because they created a measure of emotion knowledge that required virtually no expressive or even receptive language; neither auditory processing nor linguistic ability could be considered an issue. Children were asked to point to the correct emotion after seeing very brief video clips of faces only, emotional contexts only, or emotions in context (both congruent, as in a happy cause for a happy expression, or incongruent, where the cause and expression did not match). Further, they had already practiced pointing to the faces of emotions on cards, and received corrections, so that both the pointing response and emotion choices were clear before beginning the actual tasks.

Given these methodological modifications, the Down syndrome children from the mental ages of 3 to 7 years were as accurate as their nondelayed participants on all the subtests. In fact, given the tutorial and experience with the dynamic subtests, they even performed as well as the comparison group on static photographs shown at the very end of the procedure (this part of the task also had been a relative strength in the studies by Barisnikov, Thomasson, et al., 2020, and Kasari et al., 2001). In a second study, Channell et al. (2014) examined how the Down syndrome and nondiagnosed participants' total scores varied across their mental ages and found that the trajectories of growth in emotion knowledge did not differ between the groups.

In sum, Down syndrome children often show deficits in emotion knowledge, although some of their problems may be due to methodology, as tentatively demonstrated by Channell et al. (2014). Taken together, these often-complex results suggest that Down syndrome children are sometimes, but not always, different from nondisabled children in certain aspects of both expressiveness and emotion knowledge. The various potential causal factors for any delays, such as the choice of methodology or problems with self-regulation, child personality, brain development, and emotion socialization, urgently require further study.

ER has not been extensively studied, as far as I can tell, in Down syndrome children. However, one could surmise, as I've already noted, that dealing with emotions once aroused might be difficult for them, given a potentially lessened ability to use productive ER strategies. This possibility was at least partly confirmed in Jahromi, Gulsrud, and Kasari (2008). Even though Down syndrome children are often seen by others as sociable and emotionally positive, they can have difficulties with their emotions and behavior when circumstances are very frustrating.

Given two unsolvable puzzles, Down syndrome children with a mental age of around 4 years showed more facial, bodily, and vocal negativity than typically developing children, and their negativity was more intense (Jahromi et al., 2008). In terms of ER strategies, unlike typically developing children, they tended to orient more toward the experimenter, but without asking for help. In contrast, the typically developing children used more goal-directed strategies, such as assistance seeking and cognitive and/or verbal self-soothing (including reappraisals). So, Down syndrome children used a limited repertoire of more social ER strategies, perhaps building on the successful use of social support in other settings. But ineffectively overrelying on others (i.e., not actually asking for assistance) in this specific setting was in fact unproductive: It did not lead to reduced negativity. Jahromi and colleagues (2008) surmise that Down syndrome children have more failure experiences as they age, and dysregulation, compounded by a lack of effective ER strategies, may occur more frequently. These children could benefit from practice in overcoming negative arousal, perhaps by involvement in programming described in Chapter 13.

### SUMMARY: Children with Down Syndrome and Emotional Competence

Down syndrome children have an uneven emotional competence profile. They show some subtle expressiveness differences from typically developing children, some of which may be attributed to facial hypotonicity; they also show empathic concern, but in a different manner than seen in typically developing children. They seem to plateau in the development of emotion knowledge, but this effect may be at least in part due to research methodology. Finally, their ER shows some unique patterns of strategy usage and strategy effectiveness. All of these issues necessitate not only more-focused research, but also the consideration of programming to ameliorate these difficulties.

### OVERALL SUMMARY: Intrapersonal Contributions to Emotional Competence

Conditions arising mainly "within" children, such as autism and Down syndrome, clearly can contribute to difficulties in young children's emotional competence. There are not merely unarticulated delays in all areas, however; delays for each group fit logically with the nature of their diagnoses. Despite what is known so far, more research is needed to give a more complete picture of all the components of emotional competence in autistic and Down syndrome children.

## ENVIRONMENTAL CONTRIBUTIONS TO DIFFICULTIES IN EMOTIONAL COMPETENCE

The emphasis I place on socialization of emotion points to the potentially extremely detrimental contributions of socializers, especially parents, to young children's delays in emotional competence (see Chapters 7 through 9). One foremost exemplar of the environmental disruption of emotional competence development is child maltreatment; another is parental affective disturbance. In families for whom either of these problems exist, the environment is emotionally, if not physically, punishing and unpredictable. Aberrant modeling of emotional displays, nonsupportive contingent reactions to children's emotions, and less teaching about emotions are all quite possible in such settings. I consider these contributors to deficits in young children's emotional competence in turn.

## Maltreatment and Emotional Competence

First, young children's expression and experience of emotion are altered substantially by unpredictable, harsh treatment from the very persons who are also their caregivers. Maltreatment exerts a far-ranging, deleterious effect on children's emotional expressiveness (Rogosch, Cicchetti, & Aber, 1995; Shields, Cicchetti, & Ryan, 1994). Regarding emotional expressiveness, maltreated children as young as 2 years old exhibit more anger and more situationally inappropriate, nonadaptively intense, and inflexible emotions, when compared to nonmaltreated children (Erickson, Egeland, & Pianta, 1989; Shields et al., 1994). Overall their emotions are more emotionally negative and less positive than the emotions of nonmaltreated preschoolers (Lavi, Katz, Ozer, & Gross, 2019; Robinson et al., 2009; Smith & Walden, 1999). Their profile of expressiveness and especially their dysregulated, intense anger during interactions with their parents, was associated with the children's internalizing problems (Robinson et al., 2009). Maltreating parents mirrored these expressiveness differences as compared to nonmaltreating parents, and their anger intensity especially was related to their children's, suggesting a breeding ground for the children's emotional difficulties.

Not surprisingly given their history of victimization, however, maltreated preschoolers express fear when hurt by a peer, rather than the more appropriate "righteous anger." They are also more emotionally labile, and they demonstrate depression, anxiety, and shame (Alessandri & Lewis, 1996; Bennett, Sullivan, & Lewis, 2005; Rogosch et al., 1995; Toth, Manly, & Cicchetti, 1992). The shame they demonstrate when evaluated as wanting coexists with increased anger and behavioral difficulties (Bennett et al., 2005). Finally, maltreated children's expressive patterns are less readable for their social partners (Camras, Ribordy, & Hill, 1988).

Nonempathic reactions to others' emotions are well documented for toddlers living in circumstances of maltreatment and neglect. Instead of expressing empathy or sympathy, maltreated toddlers were found to demonstrate more "abusive" emotional patterns in response to peers' distress, including intense anger or fear (Main & George, 1985; see also George & Main, 1979). In these early studies, not one maltreated toddler showed concern in response to a peer's distress. Toddlers from families in which there was stress, but no maltreatment, showed no such anomalous behavior; instead, they showed interest, sympathy, or sadness, as would be expected developmentally.

Maltreated preschoolers show similar, perhaps even more pervasive, distortions in their emotional expressiveness contingent upon peers' emotions. Howes and Eldredge (1985) observed maltreated, neglected, and nonmaltreated preschoolers in structured and free-play settings; the groups were matched on developmental status, age, height, weight, demographic factors, and time in child care (see also Klimes-Dougan & Kistner, 1990). These observations, in contrast to those of the toddlers just cited, extended to the preschoolers' reactions not only to peers' distress, but also to their anger and happiness.

Maltreated preschoolers, like toddlers, responded to peers' distress inappropriately, with angry aggression or sad withdrawal. These deficits in maltreated preschoolers' empathic concern even extend to self-report procedures (Straker & Jacobson, 1981). Further, when faced with angry, aggressive peers, maltreated preschoolers respond in kind more often than nonmaltreated children. Finally, only maltreated children routinely resisted peers' emotionally positive overtures during play.

Overall, then, maltreated toddlers' and preschoolers' reactions to others' emotions are atypical—alternately unconcerned, fearful, or punitive. In peer settings, maltreated youngsters are relatively unable to share others' positive emotions, relieve their distress, or defuse their anger. When opportunities for prosocial emotional responsiveness arise during interactions with peers, young maltreated children do not rise to the occasion.

In sum, the life situation of maltreated children unsurprisingly elicits negative emotions and promotes the development of these nonoptimal expressiveness patterns. It is understandable that expecting anger from others and not having distress relieved could disrupt young children's own emotionality. Because of their own difficult circumstances, these children feel justifiable fear when confronted with *anyone's* anger, see a need for self-defense where none exists, consider anger an automatic response to many social challenges, and learn nonempathic responses to others' distress. Understandably, they are easily overwhelmed by common emotional experiences, and they project their own experience onto the canvas of any emotional topic (Sachs-Alter, 1993). The emotional expression and experience of maltreated children thus become difficult to tolerate, from both their own and other people's perspectives. This set of expressive patterns can be seen not only as an outcome of their history of maltreatment, but also as a contributor to continued difficulty with the maltreating parents, other caregivers, and peers.

The principle of functional adaptation, in which seemingly maladaptive behavior patterns develop in children and persist over time (Malatesta, 1990), also helps explain these expressiveness patterns. Returning to a functional analysis of emotions shows the expressiveness of maltreated preschoolers in a different light: Their developing expressive patterns meet the unique goals emerging from their life circumstances. "The fear reactions of [maltreated] children, with the submissive content that fear postures convey, may help [maltreating mothers] keep hostile impulses in check" (Malatesta, 1990, p. 35). Furthermore, it is not surprising that these children show frequent anger—an emotion mobilized to overcome obstructions to goals and to notify social partners of one's frustration. Positive emotion promotes potentially dangerous social bonding, so that its relative absence also makes sense.

The development of emotion knowledge, both of expressions and situations, also is hindered in maltreated children (Harden, Morrison, & Clyman, 2014; Luke & Banerjee, 2013; Perlman, Kalish, & Pollak, 2008; Pollak, Cicchetti, Hornung, & Reed, 2000; Pollak & Sinha, 2002; Pollak & Tolley-Schell, 2003). In comparisons of maltreated and nonmaltreated children, for example, nonmaltreated 4- and 5-year-olds were better able to recognize both "pure" and "masked" emotions, such as happiness, sadness, anger, fear, surprise, and disgust, when compared to maltreated children matched on demographics and intelligence (Camras et al., 1988; Camras et al., 1990; During & McMahon, 1991). Moreover, maltreated children were less able to demonstrate the more-complex emotion knowledge skills discussed in Chapter 5, including processing multiple pieces of conflicting facial and situational emotional information, using personalized information, and integrating complex emotion messages (Camras, Sachs-Alter, & Ribordy, 1996; Sachs-Alter, 1993).

Another aspect of young children's emotion knowledge, emotion language, is adversely affected by maltreatment. As early as 30 months of age, maltreated toddlers use fewer internal state words, especially words referring to negative emotions (Beeghly & Cicchetti, 1994). In the service of maintaining their own equilibrium, they suppress any reference to the intense negative emotions they witness. Even when they do talk about emotions, they less often discuss their mothers' internal states or refer back to them after their occurrence; such a strategy is probably the safest one. These deficiencies in ongoing conversation make sense, given the hostile emotional environment of these youngsters. Compared to nonmaltreated children's intense interest in, and learning from, their mothers' emotions, it is obvious that the opportunity for maltreated children to develop emotion knowledge is lost.

Unfortunately, however, the precise proximal environmental source of disruption in emotion knowledge was not uncovered in Camras et al.'s (1988, 1990) early investigations because maltreating and nonmaltreating mothers did not differ in facial expressions. That is, both groups of mothers were similar in the expression and modeling of their own emotions, *when observed*. Theoretically, then, both groups could foster equivalent emotion knowledge by allowing their children to observe similar expression–situation linkages.

What, then, explains the differences in emotion knowledge between the two groups of children? Maltreating mothers do differ in their expressiveness during rarely observed, but frequent and extremely salient, emotional events (e.g., when their children misbehave; Wilson, Rack, Shi, & Norris, 2008). Their emotional behavior in these more naturalistic settings is much more aversive and negative than that of nonmaltreating mothers. Maltreating mothers clearly differ in another important area of socialization of emotion—in their reactions to their children's emotions, particularly in the deliberate expressions produced in reaction to their children's emotions. Nonmaltreating mothers show negative expressions and reactions to stress the seriousness of their instructions to children, but usually not in response to the children specifically. In contrast, maltreating mothers are more punitive and less validating in their specific behavioral reactions to children's emotions (Sachs-Alter, 1989; Shipman et al., 2007); their intense focus specifically on the child's emotions is pernicious. Maltreating mothers also are unlikely to show positive expressions in response to their children's positive emotion, instead showing negative expressions in a wide range of child-centered situations. The beneficial effects of sharing positive emotion—for all aspects of preschoolers' emotional competence—are missing. Instead, these children experience all the disadvantages of nonsupportive reactions to their emotions.

Maltreating mothers may also show uniquely skewed or idiosyncratic reactions to their children's emotions, so that the children themselves learn nonnormative conceptions of emotion. They also may exhibit more maladaptive teaching about emotions, focusing on anger or giving mixed or garbled messages about emotions. All these possibilities could partly explain Camras and colleagues' (1988, 1990) results. Others also have conjectured that maltreating mothers present emotions that are so extreme, inconsistent, and unpredictable that maltreated children consider positive, negative, or equivocal events as equally plausible causes of sadness and anger (Perlman, Kalish, et al., 2008).

These parental reactions of constant negativity and dissatisfaction, along with emotional unpredictability and punitive reactions, may encourage children to either perseverate about their mothers' emotional messages, becoming very vigilant and sensitized to them (Thompson, 2019), or to shut down regarding experiencing (and thus understanding) emotions altogether. Although the former strategy is very common, the latter strategy also can make good intuitive sense: one 3-year-old daughter of a maltreating mother, when witnessing our puppet's expressions of anger, turned her back and emphatically stated, "I will play when her is not mad no more."

At the same time, maltreated children may be neither vigilant nor inattentive to all emotions; it is important to consider their inaccurate interpretations of specific emotions. Often maltreated preschoolers begin to exhibit a functionally distinct and potentially important pattern of mistaken emotional awareness that extends into later childhood—a bias toward viewing emotional faces, even with relatively little perceptual input, as angry (Pollak et al., 2000; Pollak & Sinha, 2002; Pollak & Tolley-Schell, 2003; Shackman, Shackman, & Pollak, 2007). Thus errors are made, but in favor of more quickly perceiving anger more often in facial expressions than it actually occurs. In their threatening home environment, attunement to anger accrues some benefits.

Further, not all experiences of maltreatment are the same. Important distinctions can and should be made between the conditions of threat (e.g., physical maltreatment) and deprivation (e.g., neglect), and these experiences are related to maltreated children's attention to and knowledge of emotions. In fact, corroborating the possibility that some maltreated children can pay exquisite attention to maternal emotions, at least two studies have found physically maltreated children to perform as well as or better than nonmaltreated children on certain aspects of emotion knowledge. Pollak et al. (2000) found physically maltreated preschoolers as accurate at detecting anger as nonmaltreated children (perhaps not surprising, given their bias favoring angry faces), and that physically neglected children show a heightened sensitivity to sadness expressions within a generally poorer comprehension of emotional expressions.

In addition, accounting for age, vocabulary, and, most important, the level of deprivation, Carrera, Jiménez-Morago, Román, and León (2020) actually found that threat exposure predicted higher-level emotion knowledge overall. Isolating the effects of differing types of maltreatment revealed some unique contributions that the conditions of threat made to emotion knowledge. In contrast, in corroboration of Pollak et al. (2000), Carrera and colleagues (2020) found that deprivation predicted emotion knowledge deficits, probably because the child lacked situations in which to learn about emotion from caregivers (see also Sullivan, Carmody, & Lewis, 2010).

Although we must differentiate the effects of conditions of threat on maltreated children from the effects of deprivation on these children (which can, of course, coexist), the importance of maltreated preschoolers' deficits and biases in emotion knowledge cannot be underestimated. Even though vigilance for threat and danger poses a short-term advantage in allowing children to anticipate and prepare for difficult interactions with adults who previously have harmed them, the long-term consequences, particularly of the bias toward anger, obviously are negative (Thompson, 2019). An early inability to understand negative emotions accurately can mediate both the relationship between maltreatment and later dysregulated behavior in a peer setting and the effect of maltreatment on later rejection by peers (Rogosch et al., 1995). In other words, children who are maltreated (due to either threat or deprivation) often experience a delay or bias in their early knowledge of negative emotions, and this deficit predicts later maladaptive behavior with peers and consequent rejection. The pathway from emotional to social competence is compromised for these children.

Even more alarming, the emotional effects of maltreatment have clear biological roots. Neurobiological vigilance associated with maltreatment is apparent as early as age 1, and maltreated children show complicated patterns of stress reactivity. Thus the experience of maltreatment and children's concomitant efforts to adapt to chronic threat affect not only their behavior, but also their biology (Thompson, 2019). Coupling these potential biological changes with maltreated children's life experiences seems tailor made for ER difficulties (Shipman et al., 2007). For example, maltreated children who remain with their parents, rather than living in foster care, were observed to be less able to maintain positive emotion, cope with frustration, and persist and remain enthusiastic when frustrated at not meeting a goal. They also showed more dysregulated anger (Labella, Lind, Sellers, Roben, & Dozier, 2020). A recent meta-analysis concurred, in that maltreatment was related to both greater negativity and dysregulation (Lavi et al., 2019). In fact, Speidel et al. (2020) corroborated that maltreatment status was negatively related to preschoolers' growth in ER over a 6-month period and positively related to baseline levels of lability/negativity on the ERC. Vigilance and chronic stress contribute to dysregulation.

As important as the biological roots of maltreatment's emotional effects are, emotion socialization also contributes to maltreated children's ER. Maltreatment's effect on young children's ER can exert its influence via the mothers' lack of sensitive guidance during emotion reminiscences. Thus not only the experience of maltreatment, but associated suboptimal emotion socialization, resulted in deficits in preschoolers' ER (Speidel et al., 2020). Corroborating findings show that maltreating mothers' emotion socialization includes less validating and more invalidating of emotions and less teaching about emotions (Shipman et al., 2007), and that these emotion socialization tendencies of maltreating mothers lead to their elementary-age children's difficulties with ER.

What maltreated children learn about ER also differs from what nonmaltreated children learn. Thus the ER strategies that maltreated children use differ from those of nonmaltreated children (Smith & Walden, 1999). Maltreated preschoolers were rated high on emotional support seeking at school, but low on support seeking as well as on several other ER strategies at home. Home especially was a place where ER strategies were viewed as lacking. It is true that mothers, likely the originators of maltreatment, rated their children's home-based ER strategies, but it is indeed telling that these children were rated comparatively high on seeking support at school, with the opposite pattern being true at home. For these children, asking for support at home could be dangerous.

Moreover, it is not always dysregulation in a highly emotional sense that defines the ER of maltreated preschoolers. Maughan and Cicchetti (2002) found two patterns of dysregulation in response to interadult anger that were more than twice as often seen in maltreated children compared to nonmaltreated children: (1) undercontrolled/ambivalent and (2) overcontrolled/unresponsive. Either pattern could be useful perhaps in the short run, given the environment these children live in, but the undercontrolled pattern was related to maternal reports of children's behavior problems and in fact mediated the link between maltreatment and children's anxious and/or depressed symptomatology. At the same time, the overcontrolled pattern was related to depression in these children.

Jody's parents are being adjudicated for maltreatment. He is being well taken care of in his foster home, but one night his foster mother and father had a disagreement. It wasn't really even an argument, but their expressions definitely looked mad to Jody. What to do? Jody was scared and hid under the kitchen table until they left. Much later, when everyone in the family was watching TV and he was sitting in his foster father's lap, Jody suddenly turned around and punched his tummy.

## SUMMARY: Maltreatment and Young Children's Emotional Competence

Thus young children are at a definite risk for emotional competence deficits when they experience maltreatment. Not surprisingly given their home environment, their own patterns of expressiveness are more negative; in various contexts, they exhibit more anger, sadness, and fear than nonmaltreated children. They show atypical patterns of emotion knowledge and empathic responsiveness to the emotions of others, as well as pronounced emotion dysregulation. Exposure to a parent's overwhelming negative emotion, which is accompanied by equally negative behavior, can alter the child's emotional competence via the routes suggested. These major problem areas make much sense when we reflect on the likely life experience of the young, maltreated child. The more severe these emotion competence difficulties are or the longer they persist, children's later social competence will also suffer, and behavior problems are more likely (see Chapter 10).

Maltreated youngsters need the benefit of interventions focused on the development of emotional competence. Some encouraging evidence is emerging from randomized trials. For example, a brief intervention focused on helping maltreating mothers give sensitive guidance, while reminiscing about emotions, resulted in preschoolers' increased ER, both rated and measured physiologically via diurnal cortisol levels (Speidel et al., 2020; Valentino, Hibel, Speidel, Fondren, & Ugarte, 2020). Aspects of sensitive guidance that buffered the effects of witnessing interadult aggression (another form of maltreatment; Kitzmann, Gaylord, Holt, & Kenny, 2003) on preschoolers' ER included (1) caregivers' sensitivity to children's emotions during play, (2) listening effectively to children's expression of sadness, and (3) caregivers' own ER (Caiozzo, Yule, & Grych, 2018). A similar intervention also helped maltreating mothers to learn sensitive guidance, resulting in increases in their preschoolers' emotion knowledge (Valentino et al., 2019). Another 10-session intervention that focused on helping maltreating parents to behave in nurturing, dialoguing, and nonfrightening ways resulted in lower levels of toddlers' negative emotions during a challenging tool task (i.e., retrieving a toy in a Plexiglas container with a tool; Lind, Bernard, Ross, & Dozier, 2014). Along with the emotion reminiscence techniques involving open-ended questions and causal statements that Speidel et al. (2020) taught maltreating mothers, all of these behaviors are worthy of study. These children deserve such care.

## Parental Affective Disturbance and Emotional Competence

Parental affective disturbance is another conceivable disrupter of the typical course of emotional development. In particular, maternal depression has been much studied. The main characteristics of these emotional environments are the sadness, hopelessness, and inappropriate role reversal to which young children are exposed, along with critical and hostile behavior. Mothers' examination of photographs of emotionally expressive infants with their children and simulations of their own sadness highlight important aspects of this emotional environment (Zahn-Waxler, Ridgeway, et al., 1993). In this early study, depressed mothers focused on their own sorrow, often pointing to their children as the cause; in fact, some mothers got so caught up in the simulation that they were unable to bring the episode to resolution. Immersion in such distress on a chronic basis, characterized by enmeshment and the child's sense of responsibility, can obviously affect growing preschoolers' developing emotional competence (Thompson, 2019).

In terms of patterns of emotional expressiveness, these children's atypical overinvolvement and enmeshment in their mothers' sadness, and their feeling responsible to ameliorate it, are conducive to the development of many enduring negative emotions, including potentially incapacitating guilt (Zahn-Waxler & Kochanska, 1990). Toddlers are already absorbing their depressed mothers' explicit and implicit coaching about emotions, contingent reactions to their emotions, and modeling of the negative emotion in which the mothers are immersed. Imagine this double bind: "I am sad, just like Mommy. But if I show my sadness, I upset her. I have to take care of her, because she is sooo sad. Maybe it is my fault if I act sad."

Mothers' conflicting emotional demands can render their children very vigilant and attentive to their emotional state (Zahn-Waxler & Kochanska, 1990). Children of depressed mothers, especially daughters of preschool age and all children by late middle childhood, have attention biases for sadness (Gibb, Pollak, Hajcak, & Owens, 2016; Kujawa et al., 2011). In fact, the older children show evidence of increased attention to angry and happy emotions as well (Gibb et al., 2016). It is important, especially for preschool daughters, to mentally keep track of depressed mothers' emotions, to stay emotionally safe. Along with these daughters' emotion biases, their greater heritability of maternal depression means these daughters especially need our care.

Again this sort of attention may confer a short-term advantage in long-term negative consequences: Later in the preschool period, 5-year-olds of depressed mothers showed more overt behavioral difficulties associated with emotional competence deficits—a preponderance of anger and aggression, as well as a relative inability to interact with peers (Denham, Zahn-Waxler, Cummings, & Iannotti, 1991; Gagne, Spann, & Prater, 2013; Wu, Hooper, Feng, Gerhardt, & Ku, 2019; Zahn-Waxler, Mayfield, et al., 1988). At the same time, preschoolers also may project their careful way of dealing with mothers onto their relationships with others, attentive to and potentially dysregulated by emotions of social partners.

Regarding empathy, preschoolers observed their mothers engaged in a (staged) telephone call that included happy, sad, and angry sequences (Tully & Donohue, 2017). Their emotional empathic responses, both negative (for the sad and angry conversational segments) and positive (for the happy conversational segment), as well as their cognitive empathy (i.e., information seeking), were coded during the telephone call. Importantly, all three types of empathic concern predicted depressed mothers' ratings of children's depression, anxiety, and inhibition, when mothers' depression duration was 36 months or more during the child's lifetime (and the children were only 4 years old!). Sharing positive emotion (i.e., positive empathy) was salutary for children of nondepressed mothers, but actually was related to depression, worry, and inhibition for offspring of depressed mothers. Living with depressed mothers had deleterious effects on how preschoolers' reacted to their mothers' emotions and the sequelae of these reactions.

The duration of maternal depression also predicted mothers' views of children's depression, anxiety, and inhibition in this study. The longer the mothers had been depressed, the more likely they were to rate their child as having emotional problems; even accounting for the potential effects of being depressed on rating one's child, this finding stands out—living with maternal depression can render a young child depressed and anxious about doing the right thing, perhaps frozen in inhibited behavior.

Other, self-conscious motions are also affected by parental depression. At the end of the early childhood period, children of depressed fathers, who were led by an experimenter to tear an accomplice's "favorite" photograph, showed clear signs of how living with a depressed parent can lead to a hyperfocus on one's responsibility for transgressions (Parisette-Sparks, Bufferd, & Klein, 2017). These preschoolers made more verbal, facial, and bodily expressions of guilt and shame about tearing the photograph, compared to children whose fathers had no history of depression, perhaps because of their fathers' difficulties in expressing positive emotions and responding adaptively to their children's transgressions. The children showed negative emotion related to their unrealistic feelings of responsibility.

These results are consistent with a theoretical model stating that chronic exposure to parents' negative emotion, plus genetic propensities toward negative thinking (e.g., "It's all my fault") and empathic personal distress ("I'm so upset to see her like this") can increase children's risk of depression, anxiety, inhibition, and even maladaptive guilt and shame (Tone & Tully, 2014). Although empathy emanating from heightened sensitivity to the emotional environment could be a protective regulatory strategy for children of depressed parents, it is a "double-edged sword" (Thompson & Calkins, 1996; Tone & Tully, 2014); being sympathetic to one's depressed mother does not always lead one down a positive path.

Toma's mother is burdened by low income at a job where her schedule is always shifting. She is a single parent and lives with Toma in a chaotic extended family household. She is very depressed at times, and no wonder. Toma shows much empathic concern when she lies on the sofa crying, patting her, hugging her, and telling her, "It's gonna be okay. . . ." However, he is showing his own signs of sadness, distress, and withdrawal in his preschool classroom. He cares for his mother but pays a price.

Not only are patterns of expressiveness impacted by parents' affective disorder, young children's emotion knowledge too can be compromised. In a family in which the emotional environment is so predominantly negative, as can be the case with a depressed parent, the acquisition of emotion knowledge can be skewed. The very conceptual basis of differing emotions may have content that is not typical—what are the attributes of happiness in such a family, for example? These children also may have less exposure to varied emotions that can fuel their emotion knowledge. At the same time, children in families in which a parent is depressed also may have so much trouble regulating their own emotions that it is difficult for them to even concentrate on the emotional world. It is not surprising, then, that maternal depression symptoms related negatively to their 4½-year-olds' emotion knowledge (Thompson et al., 2020).

Further, the emotional characteristics of maternal depression may intensify the deleterious effects of negative parenting, particularly parental intrusiveness and hostility (anger at, frustration with, and criticism of the child during learning tasks), on the development of emotion knowledge (Kujawa et al., 2014). In this case, any potentially positive attributes of emotion socialization via modeling are in a sense "hijacked" by the parent's depressive affect and subsequent dysfunctional parenting. The possible usefulness of mild parental negative emotions, where emotion knowledge is concerned, can be swamped by the intensity and frequency of such negativity in a household where depression takes hold.

Young children who live in an environment of depression also have difficulties in regulating their own emotional expressiveness. These obstacles can take several forms. During an emotionally charged situation in one early study, 2-year-olds of depressed mothers regulated their emotions differently than children of nondepressed mothers. When confronted with escalating episodes of argument, conflict, and distress between experimenters, the depressed mothers' toddlers were unusually well behaved. They almost overused peacekeeping, comforting, and appeasement as ER strategies, but also were significantly more preoccupied and upset than the children of nondepressed mothers. In other procedures, they acted polite in the face of frustration and demonstrated less aggression than the children of nondepressed mothers (Cummings et al., 1985; Denham, Zahn-Waxler, et al., 1991; Zahn-Waxler, McKnew, Cummings, Davenport, & Radke-Yarrow, 1984). Thus they seemed to suppress negative emotions, but they also had trouble regulating them once they were expressed.

By the time preschoolers are 4 years old, few of either depressed *or* nondepressed mothers behave in an overcontrolled manner when witnessing scripted anger between their mothers and an experimenter (Maughan, Cicchetti, Toth, & Rogosch, 2007). During this procedure, over half of the participants in Maughan et al.'s (2007) study showed emotion dysregulation in the form of greater (1) emotional reactivity, including enduring high distress, fear, or active concern; (2) support seeking; and (3) verbal regulation of distress (i.e., talking about the witnessed angry exchange). In fact, these patterns of observed regulation persisted even after the angry interaction, through a neutral period with the experimenter absent and into a period of reconciliation between the adults. Notably, membership in this dysregulated group was associated with the mothers' previous diagnosis of depression when the children were 21 months old (but, interestingly, not current or recurrent depression). These findings show not only the

ER difficulties demonstrated by the children of depressed mothers, but also suggest that infancy and toddlerhood may be vulnerable periods for the long-term effects of maternal depression on ER.

But older preschoolers' ER is not immune from the effects of mothers' concurrent depression. In fact, mothers' symptomatology when their daughters were 3 years old predicted the girls' faster transition into sadness when they were frustrated in a lockbox task (Yan, Feng, Shoppe-Sullivan, Gerhardt, & Wu, 2021; see also Silk, Shaw, Forbes, Lane, & Kovacs's [2006] findings on daughters' greater likelihood to engage in passive waiting for a toy). During this frustrating task, there were no significant effects of maternal depression for sons or for children's transition into anger. At least for preschool-age daughters, having experienced the environment of depression left them less able to cope constructively with frustration. Pairing this conclusion with the earlier finding of preschool girls' pronounced attention to sadness suggests a true risk for young daughters of depressed mothers.

Further, teachers' ratings of early elementary school-age children's ER extended these findings, albeit without dynamic analyses or gender moderation, into the beginning of children's elementary school years (Kam et al., 2011; see Chapter 10): All teacher ratings of ER loaded onto one latent ER variable that was negatively related to mothers' concurrent depression symptoms. The mothers' inability to interact warmly and supportively during play was negatively related to their depressive symptoms, and in some analyses mediated the symptoms' association with children's ER. In short, depression contributed unfortunately to the mothers' lessened ability to parent positively and thence to children's diminished ER.

Other studies have amplified the understanding of the link between maternal depression and young children's dysregulation by studying mothers who have experienced depressive bouts occurring as early as their own childhood (child-onset depression [COD]). When experiencing a disappointment situation similar to that described earlier in this book—in which ER is an important marker of successfully negotiating the experience—4-year-old children of mothers with COD tended to have a difficult time of demonstrating active ER strategies, such as playing with and/or exploring the broken object or attempting to change the situation and maintaining a positive emotion (Feng et al., 2008). It is likely that the models that they had witnessed were inconducive to the emergence of active ER in the face of disappointment; irrespective of whether mothers were experiencing current depression, mothers with COD may have lacked the adequate skills to provide optimal emotion socialization regarding such issues.

Children's own emotional makeup also is important in understanding the contribution of child-onset maternal depression to preschoolers' emotional dysregulation. Learning to regulate emotions independently seemed especially difficult for 2- and 3-year-old behaviorally inhibited children of depressed mothers (i.e., those who showed a lack of approach to toys or showed anxious, wary expressions or behaviors or wary hesitance toward a stranger). Specifically, behaviorally inhibited children of mothers with COD showed more passive tolerance of the disappointment (i.e., sitting quietly or just staring at the broken toy without showing any overt activity) than less inhibited children of mothers with COD. This finding is concerning because such passive ER is no longer developmentally optimal or even effective by age 4 (Feng et al., 2008).

Children contribute to their own ER difficulties, which are magnified by maternal affective disturbance.

There was, however, a silver lining in these implications of children's own contribution to their nonoptimal ER. When these inhibited children's mothers, despite their COD, exhibited positivity (i.e., positive emotion, warmth, supportiveness, and involvement while playing with their children), the children also managed more active, emotionally positive ER during the disappointment task (Feng et al., 2008). As I've already noted, children who are at risk because of maternal depression are particularly sensitive to their mothers' moods, and are susceptible to the parents' own ER difficulties. But attention to their mothers' emotional positivity has benefits. Thus, the good news is that when mothers can be more emotionally positive, their inhibited children may be protected from the effects of maternal depression. It is a hopeful sign that children doubly at risk from both their own temperamental makeup and their mothers' history of depression benefit when mothers can "rise above" their history, especially given that mothers with COD are generally less responsive to their children's, particularly boys', distress (Shaw et al., 2006).

At the same time, children of depressed mothers may themselves play a similar role in their own emotional outcomes. In parallel with the finding regarding COD mothers' positivity, COD mothers' 4- to 7-year-olds who could manage their own positive anticipation during their boring wait to play with a toy demonstrated fewer internalizing problems (Silk et al., 2006). For both COD mothers and their children, then, the ability to generate positivity is a protective aspect of ER.

Children's "emotional reputation" with their mothers also may even more specifically promote or constrain depressed mothers' emotion socialization behaviors (Wu, Hooper, et al., 2019). For example, when children of depressed mothers were reported or observed as less angry at age 3, their mothers reported less nonsupportiveness to their anger at age 4 (contemporaneous results stood in contrast; at 3 years old, children's greater anger was associated with their mothers' more nonsupportive responses). Depressed mothers' responses to their children's sadness and fear also differed depending on their views of the children's earlier emotionality; when mothers had reported that their child expressed such "submissive" negative emotions more intensely at age 3, they reported more supportiveness to such emotion at age 4. However, they reported less-supportive responses for children whom they had considered less sad and fearful a year earlier. Thus they reported more-supportive reactions to the children they had seen earlier as needing it most. These authors did add a cautionary note to these interpretations: Could being less nonsupportive to one's less-angry child also mean less involvement for depressed mothers? Depressed mothers' children may need to pass a threshold of emotionality to inspire a response from their sad, withdrawn mothers. Overall, preschoolers' own earlier emotionality may be part of their own developing emotional competence, especially because depressed mothers may be very sensitive to their children's emotions.

Also children may make differential use of maternal emotion socialization when mothers are depressed versus when they are not. For example, both depressed and nondepressed mothers and their 3-year-olds engaged in an emotion reminiscence task, discussing recent happy, sad, angry, and frightening events; 1 year later the children were challenged by both a disappointment procedure and a lockbox task (Wu, Feng, Yan, et al., 2020). Mothers' reminiscences were coded as "low elaborative" when they described or explained the children's emotional experiences (i.e., labeling, acknowledging, or validating; explaining causes or consequences; providing coping strategies and/or teaching about emotions) and as "high elaborative" when they used open-ended questions about emotional experiences, their causes and consequences, and/or probing about problem solving. Note that in Chapters 7 through 9, I reported on research in which this "low-elaborative" teaching about emotions was quite salutary; of course, "high-elaborative," open-ended discussion of emotion, getting the child actively involved, also is a useful technique.

These researchers found several complex three-way interactions between both styles of elaboration and mothers' depression status. First, when depressed mothers of 3-year-olds *didn't* use much high-elaborative reminiscing about sadness, the low-elaborative conversational style about emotions was in fact helpful: it was negatively related to 4-year-olds' focus on distress and negative emotion in the disappointment situation. These complicated findings suggest that low-elaborative styles can help the children of depressed mothers learn to appropriately express and regulate disappointed emotion, but only in the absence of anything "better" (i.e., the high-elaborative style). In any other circumstance, it doesn't seem to be productive for their children.

Highly elaborative reminiscence styles might be what's "better" because they prompt children of depressed mothers to be active partners in socialization, especially given the passive stance these children sometime take in their ER (Feng et al., 2008). Questioning is, of course, a useful conversational style in emotion reminiscences, but perhaps children of nondepressed mothers do not require it as much.

In contrast, when depressed mothers used *both* a highly elaborative style about sadness or anger *and* low elaborativeness, their children focused more on distress in the disappointment and showed more negative emotion in the lockbox task, a full year later. Using both techniques frequently during the reminiscence task may be a marker of depressed mothers' intrusiveness and lack of responsiveness to children's emotional cues (Shaw et al., 2006). Talking about emotions with little cessation can backfire.

Overall, maternal depression places strains on both the enactment and the outcome of normally positive emotion socialization—like the "low"-elaborative reminiscence styles that we have seen are useful techniques when used by nondepressed mothers. Further, the enmeshment between depressed mothers and their young children underscores the relationship between parenting and child development (Kujawa et al., 2014). Thus the picture becomes one of mothers and children struggling emotionally together. Because of this possibility, more nuanced approaches are necessary to study how these families' emotion socialization—modeling, contingency, and coaching—promotes or inhibits the development of emotional competence.

## SUMMARY: Maternal Depressive Disorder and Young Children's Emotional Competence

Living in an affectively disordered family environment is very likely to engender disturbances in all aspects of preschoolers' developing emotional competence (see, e.g.,

Thompson, 1994; Thompson & Calkins, 1996). Difficulties in expressiveness emerge given the atypical emotional environment in which the children live. Specific sensitivity to maternal emotions skews their emotion knowledge, and many emotion socialization patterns lead them to less optimal ER. Daughters may be at special risk. Despite what has already been uncovered, the accumulating body of evidence has plenty of gaps, especially in what is known about the emotion knowledge of these children. More work needs to be done in that realm, as well as pursuing emotional competence-focused interventions for these children and their mothers.

## MIXED CONTRIBUTIONS TO DIFFICULTIES IN EMOTIONAL COMPETENCE

At times it is not clear whether intrapersonal contributions, environmental contributions, or both have provoked observed deficits in emotional competence. Even when clearly defined factors such as autism, developmental disability, maltreatment, or parental affective disturbance are not present, children can be clearly at risk for delays in emotional competence. One example of such risk is early evidence of precursors to disruptive behavior disorders. A second example is being subject to adverse childhood experiences (ACEs) more broadly.

### Disruptive Behavior Disorders

Diagnosed behavior disorders that emerge during early childhood often persist (Campbell & Ewing, 1990; Egeland, Kalkoske, Gottesman, & Erickson, 1990). They are in part defined by compromised emotional competence, and in turn constitute a definite threat to the further development of emotional competence. The environment of behaviorally disordered children often is emotionally atypical, with more negative emotion witnessed and experienced in both family and peer environments (Patterson, Reid, & Dishion, 1992). Such coercive home environments are characterized by bidirectional, escalating negativity between parents and children and put young children at special risk for difficulties in emotional competence and on a trajectory for oppositional behavior, aggression, and eventually conduct disorders (Thompson, 2019). I have discussed the impact of such parental anger and punitive reactions to their preschoolers' emotions in Chapters 7 and 8. Now it is necessary to expand upon what I've already discussed about the sequelae of such emotion socialization.

Hence, it is reasonable to expect that for children with disruptive behavior disorders, all three components of emotional competence—emotional expressiveness, emotion knowledge, and ER—will be aberrant. Patterns of emotional *in*competence in fact would be reflected in the very diagnoses of oppositional defiant disorder (ODD) and early onset conduct disorder. That is, the diagnostic criteria for and characteristics of these disorders include evidence of emotional incompetence, especially in terms of emotional expressiveness and ER, such as (1) lack of concern for others' feelings; (2) lack of guilt or remorse; (3) irritability and temper outbursts—especially problematic frequency, intensity, and/or contextual inappropriateness of anger; (4) low frustration tolerance and emotion dysregulation; (5) lack of positive emotion or too intense positive emotion; and frequently (6) comorbid anxiety and depression (see also Cole, Michel, et al., 1994; Martin, Boekamp, McConville, & Wheeler, 2010). Aspects of comorbid anxiety also suggest compromised emotional competence: an unrealistic persistence of worry and fear as well as marked timidity and tension. Bear in mind that deficits in emotionality and ER may be related to some but not all forms of externalizing behavior, so it is important to examine these issues in more fine-grained detail (Mullin & Hinshaw, 2007).

More detailed investigations of how emotional expressiveness is related to behavior disorders have been performed (Cole & Zahn-Waxler, 1988; Cole, Zahn-Waxler, et al., 1994). In Cole and colleagues' work, preschool-age children at risk for conduct disorder, as well as those not at risk, were observed while a disappointing gift was given to them. The boys who were at risk for conduct disorder showed more negative emotion in the experimenter's presence than the low-risk boys did. Their negative emotions (particularly anger) were associated with their disruptiveness during the paradigm, as well as with their overall symptomatology.

In contrast, high-risk preschool girls differed from low-risk preschool girls after the experimenter left; they actually displayed *less* negative emotion at this point. Their minimization of negative emotion predicted symptoms of ADHD and conduct disorder—overactivity, difficulty concentrating, immaturity, lying, and destructiveness. The authors hypothesized that these girls overregulated their expression of negative emotion, because of the undesirability of negative emotion in girls. This overregulation absorbed their attentional resources and behavioral control.

In essence, then, young boys at risk for conduct disorder differed from their low-risk peers in the anger they showed in the presence of the person who caused it. In contrast, young girls at risk for conduct disorder differed from their low-risk counterparts in their overregulation. Both showed exaggerated, nonadaptive patterns of gender-stereotyped emotional expressiveness. Similarly, children in this investigation who were either inexpressive or highly expressive during a negative mood induction showed more externalizing symptoms (Cole, Zahn-Waxler, Fox, Usher, & Welsh, 1996).

Examining longitudinal diagnostic data from the same project, my colleagues and I (Denham, Workman, et al., 2000) found that mothers' ratings of preschoolers' temperamental qualities of emotional intensity and negativity predicted both externalizing and internalizing problems 1 year later. Overall, the expressiveness patterns and ability to regulate emotions differ for preschoolers who already exhibit behavior problems commensurate with an ultimate diagnosis of conduct disorder and can predict later diagnoses as well.

Moreover, the characteristics of behavior-disordered children also suggest compromised emotion knowledge. Behaviorally disordered children spend less time scanning their social environment and hence do not pick up on emotion information emanating from other people. They may also have social–cognitive biases that prevent them from processing emotional cues accurately (see Dodge, 2006; Dodge & Frame, 1982). These biased social cognitions make these children think that other people mean them harm. As both the prototype and functional analyses of emotion suggest, such a lens for viewing the world primes them for anger and thus hampers their social interactions.

In fact, young children with behavioral difficulties do tend to see others' behavior with a hostile attribution bias; as with older individuals, this bias can prompt misplaced anger based on misunderstood emotion, beginning a chain of disturbed interactions and aggressive reactions (De Castro, Veerman, Koops, Bosch, & Monshouwer, 2002). Even nondiagnosed preschoolers with such biases fare more poorly in their peer setting (Barth & Bastiani, 1997). In contrast, compared to anger perception bias, recent evidence pointed to inaccuracy in identifying sadness as being more predictive of externalizing behavior in preschoolers involved in psychiatric day treatment (Martin et al., 2010, 2015). Obviously, more research needs to be performed examining both sadness and anger biases in young children.

Examining the implications of behavior disorder for emotion knowledge in a more fine-grained fashion, recent investigations have focused on callous–emotional traits within the constellation of behaviors potentially attributed to ODD and conduct disorders (Thomson, Centifanti, & Lemerise, 2017). A number of studies have noted that problems recognizing happy, sad, angry, and fearful faces are related to greater evidence of such callous–unemotional traits (Bedford et al., 2017; Martin et al., 2015; Rehder, Mills-Koonce, Willoughby, Garrett-Peters, & Wagner, 2017; White et al., 2016). Further, lower teacher ratings of young children's emotion knowledge and/or empathy (e.g., "Reacts with concern when another cries") also were related to the level of callous–unemotional traits (Zumbach, Rademacher, & Koglin, 2021).

When ODD coexisted with high levels of callous–unemotional traits, boys also had difficulties with emotion knowledge tasks involving perspective taking and ambivalent emotions, especially tasks involving conceptualizing *others'* emotions (O'Kearney, Salmon, Liwag, Fortune, & Dawel, 2017).[1] Other aspects of emotion knowledge also are compromised for children with ODD. In one study, 4- to 8-year-olds diagnosed with ODD demonstrated lesser emotion knowledge than nondiagnosed children only on giving causes for emotions (O'Kearney et al., 2017).

Why might the particular presence of callous–unemotional traits within behavior disorders be related to deficits in young children's emotion knowledge? First, mothers of children displaying callous, unemotional traits demonstrate more prevalent nonsupportive, dismissive emotion socialization (Pasalich, Waschbusch, Dadds, & Hawes, 2014); such socialization was shown to negatively impact preschoolers' emotion knowledge (see Chapter 8). Second, extending findings that children with behavior disorders in general take in emotional information in inefficient ways, it has been suggested that children with both conduct problems and callous–unemotional traits may pay less attention especially to a person's eyes, leading to deficits in emotion recognition (Cooper, Hobson, & van Goozen, 2020). Third, callous–unemotional problems of young ODD children also may interact with their ER; that is, both callous–unemotional features *and* low emotional arousal as assessed by the ERC lability/negativity scale predicted poor emotion recognition (O'Kearney, Chng, & Salmon, 2021).

Regarding ER specifically, another recent study has shown that lower levels of ER (as measured by the Emotional Control scale of the Brief Rating Inventory of Executive Function) and *higher* levels of lability/negativity as measured by the ERC, along with a

[1] Few girls evidenced high levels of callous–unemotional traits.

higher level of callous–unemotional traits, predicted comorbid diagnoses of ODD and ADHD (Garcia, Dick, & Graziano, 2020). When there are difficulties in both areas of emotional competence (emotion knowledge and ER), this disturbing way of viewing and interacting with others was more evident. In sum, callous–unemotional traits and ER problems, along with nonsupportive socialization, together augur particular emotion knowledge difficulties for boys already dealing with the hurdles that their ODD often poses.

## SUMMARY: Early Disruptive Behavior Diagnoses and Emotional Competence

Disruptive behavior diagnoses during the preschool period are marked by emotional competence deficits, and the emergence of these disorders hampers further emotional competence development. Detrimental emotional expressiveness patterns are evident, although perhaps they are different for boys and girls. Emotion knowledge is compromised, particularly in combination with callous–unemotional traits, and ER also is distorted. Continued examination of the bidirectional relationship between emotional competence and diagnosable behavior disorders is warranted, along with programming that specifically targets emotional competence.

## Adverse Childhood Experiences

Biological, environmental, and the mixed contribution of diagnosed behavior disorder are not the only factors related to difficulties with young children's emotional competence. The myriad converging circumstances of ACEs can contribute to this risk (Morris et al., 2014). Such circumstances can include (1) low income; (2) low maternal education (i.e., not graduating from high school); (3) young maternal age at the birth of the first child; (4) single parenthood; (5) lack of employment; (6) receiving public assistance; (7) physical, emotional, or sexual maltreatment; (8) neglect; (9) parental discord and domestic violence; (10) caregiver mental health difficulties, antisocial activity, cognitive impairment, and/or (11) substance use; (12) parent–child separation; and (13) unsafe neighborhood. These conditions involve both (1) deprivation, or atypical learning experiences, inadequate scaffolding and parent–child interactions and (2) a threat, or any situation that instills fear. The circumstances on this staggering list have cumulative effects on the brain (especially the neural circuits related to fear learning and physiological reactivity to negative emotional stimuli, including the hypothalamic pituitary adrenal axis). Given these biological effects, there are subsequent impairments in learning, in behavior, and in both short- and long-term physical and mental well-being (Shonkoff et al., 2012). Not surprisingly, any combination of these situations also can render acquiring emotional competence very difficult for preschool-age children.

Lack of emotion knowledge is particularly troublesome for these children; understanding emotions consciously is necessary to solve problems that occur with peers (Burton & Denham, 1999; see also Cicchetti, Toth, & Bush, 1988). Emotion knowledge, however, could be an important buffer of the effects of ACEs, particularly in its role supporting ER. In fact, because sadness can be so prominent for young children experiencing ACEs, understanding the intensity of sadness can help them avoid depression; specifically, when children had a poor or moderate identification of sadness, each additional ACE added one more depression symptom (Sudit, Luby, & Gilbert, 2021). The postulated link between being able to consider one's own emotions so that regulation can be undertaken seems clear—perhaps one must know what one is feeling to regulate it. This linkage is one more reason to help young children acquire emotion knowledge.

Children experiencing ACEs and lacking in emotion knowledge also have few means of regulating emotions, again in part because they lack experience in attaching labels to internal feelings and they subsequently are unable to bring their own or others' feelings to consciousness. Qualitative analyses of year-long observations suggest that preschoolers who experience ACEs often express felt emotions impulsively (Burton & Denham, 1999).

Thus children with emotion knowledge and ER deficits are at a distinct disadvantage because these competencies are so vital to social relationships. If these children do not recognize feelings in themselves, they certainly cannot empathize with the feelings seen in others. They may take a toy out of the hands of another child without any consideration for the other person or push another child away simply because he or she is in the way of a desired goal. When provoked by another child, they often respond with unregulated anger and physical aggression. Angry and without ER strategies, they hit back without thinking. In short, children who are at risk owing to ACEs have difficulties gleaning the social advantages of emotional competence.

Attention is being paid recently to how accumulated risk status via multiple ACEs contributes to preschoolers' difficulty with ER. Along with the threat/deprivation dichotomy, a distinction also has been made between two types of ACEs derived from (1) negative neighborhood conditions, such as a poor physical environment, lack of safety, and lack of facilities and (2) negative family conditions, including a change of intimate partner, substance abuse, or involvement in the justice system.

Cumulative indices of both types of adversity were related to low-income preschoolers' negative emotion dysregulation (Brown & Ackerman, 2011; see also Brophy-Herb, Martoccio, et al., 2013; Ellis et al., 2014). However, it should be noted that low income by itself may not portend ill effects on ER; in one study, low-income preschoolers used ER strategies with peers that were similar to those of higher-income children—that is, constructive strategies for sadness and more nonconstructive ones for anger experienced during peer interactions (Garner & Spears, 2000).

Emotion socialization patterns associated with family adversity are predictive of negative emotion dysregulation for low-income preschoolers. Importantly, family adversity was not only directly, but also indirectly via its relation with maternal emotional negativity, related to negative emotion dysregulation for low-income preschoolers; effects for neighborhood adversity were *only* indirect (Brown & Ackerman, 2011). Further, mothers' relative inability to sensitively converse about emotions with children can mediate the effect of family adversity on their preschoolers' dysregulation (Ellis et al., 2014), similar to the finding I reported for maltreating mothers. Family adversity disrupts relationships and routines, as well as the overall emotional environment, and such perturbations are conducive to dysregulating children's emotions, especially when mothers also express high negativity—a model of dysregulation—or do not scaffold children's emotional learning.

At times the attributes of the children themselves moderate the contribution of ACEs to their emotion dysregulation. For example, a combination of neighborhood and family adversity was related to preschoolers' observed ER while waiting for a cookie *if* the children had been rated in toddlerhood as high in temperamental negativity (Chang et al., 2012). The highly negative toddlers were more deeply affected by adversity. Their expressiveness patterns may have been affected early in life by the adversity they experienced, as well as being rooted in biological differences associated with experiencing adversity prenatally; these early difficulties in emotional competence multiplied as developmental expectations became greater.

Even preschoolers can participate in reporting on conditions of threat and deprivation. When preschoolers added their own thoughts on adversity to its evaluation, threat-related ACEs were again related to their emotion dysregulation, both as reported by mothers and observed in physiological reactions within a fear-extinction paradigm (Milojevich et al., 2020). This relationship was mediated by maternal emotion dysregulation, again implicating the entire family system experiencing ACEs in their import for young children's ER.

The picture painted so far of the contributions of ACEs to preschoolers' emotional competence problems seems dismal, and implicates parents, children—indeed the whole family system—in the dire trajectory. Although it is important to examine ACEs via cumulative risk factors, however, several factors can be profitably examined separately. I have already discussed two of them, maltreatment and maternal depression, at some length. In addition, poverty can be seen as a proxy for a variable set of ACEs, extending beyond the fact of low income. For example, poverty's stressors prominently include parents' struggle to pay bills and "make ends meet." Among other deleterious effects, these stressors may elicit overwhelming negative emotions within the family, with concomitant negative emotionality, diminished positive emotionality, and gaps in ER during preschoolers' peer interactions (Denham, Bassett, Mincic, et al., 2012; Denham, Bassett, & Wyatt, 2014). These stressors also render children's acquisition of emotion knowledge more difficult (Denham, Bassett, Mincic, et al., 2012; Denham, Bassett, Way, et al., 2012; Denham, Bassett, Zinsser, et al., 2014; National Scientific Council on the Developing Child, 2005/2014; Raver et al., 2015). More broadly, children's ability to detect and appraise emotional stimuli is greater in the absence of environmental adversities such as poverty, household chaos, and interparental aggression (Raver et al., 2015; see also Erhart, Dmitrieva, Blair, & Kim, 2019).

As already suggested, socioeconomic risk also is related to differences in emotion socialization in the family, via the emotional climate that poverty can induce. For example, the stress of living in poverty and/or lacking education understandably can dampen maternal positive expressiveness, even controlling for depression (Davis, Suveg, & Shaffer, 2015a; Dereli, 2016). At the same time, such stress may exacerbate mothers' hostile, punitive, or dismissing reactions to children's emotions (Martini, Root, & Jenkins, 2004; Shaffer, Suveg, Thomassin, & Bradbury, 2012). Considering this potential effect of poverty on emotion socialization in conjunction with its detrimental effect on the development of emotional competence, promoting emotional competence is especially important for low-income children (Nix et al., 2016)—and in fact for all children experiencing ACEs—so that they can understand and manage their emotions well (Denham & Burton, 2003; Greenberg, 2006).

### SUMMARY: ACEs and Young Children's Emotional Competence

ACEs represent the accumulation of pernicious contributors to the optimal development of emotional competence in preschoolers. Growing up in such conditions seems to me to be a "perfect storm." We need more careful research examining the contributions of varying combinations and types of adversity to components of emotional competence, similar to Raver et al. (2015). And, of course, preventive and indicated programming for these children, as advocated in Chapter 13, is necessary and only fair.

## CONCLUSION

Disruptions within the child, the environment, or both are often associated with patterns of deficits in emotional competence. Nonetheless, many gaps in our knowledge of both the emotional strengths and weaknesses of children who experience these disruptions remain to be filled. Given the importance of emotional competence to success in the peer world and beyond, it is especially important for the parents, teachers, and caregivers of children with varying problems to do what they can to identify children with special needs in the area of emotional competence and to foster its growth. To this end, I next describe ways to assess strengths and weaknesses in emotional competence within the preschool period. I then discuss existing intervention programs that directly address milestones of emotional competence.

# 13

# Educating for Emotional Competence

## INTRODUCTION

In this chapter, assessment and instructional programming for emotional competence are considered. As already amply illustrated in this book and elsewhere, young children's emotional competence is important because of its conceptual and empirical linkages with children's (1) successful social relationships, (2) lack of behavior problems, (3) personal well-being and mental health, (4) ultimate workplace performance, and (5) general adaptive resilience in the face of stressful circumstances (e.g., Brackett, Rivers, & Salovey, 2011; Denham, 2006; Greenberg et al., 2003; Jones et al., 2015; Raver & Knitzer, 2002).

As Zins and colleagues (2007, p. 191) have noted, "schools are social places, and learning is a social process." Students learn alongside and in collaboration with teachers and peers and must be able to utilize their emotions, emotion knowledge, and ER to facilitate learning. More specifically, children with emotional competencies participate more in the classroom, have more positive attitudes about and involvement with school, and are more accepted by classmates and given more instruction and positive feedback by teachers. Without emotional competencies, young children are more likely to dislike school and perform poorly on academic tasks and to later experience grade retention and drop out.

Knowing how crucial children's emotional competence is and the contributions made by adults' socialization, it is vital to examine how these matters are dealt with in early childhood education. Therefore, both programming and assessment must be discussed. First, though, I note some boundaries for what I discuss in this chapter. Much excellent work has been done in the last 20 years regarding social–emotional learning (SEL), which includes self-awareness, self-management, social awareness, relationship skills, and responsible decision making (see Figure 13.1). This model supports both assessment and intervention and is used worldwide to describe central abilities within each domain (Mahoney et al., 2021). Obviously, each of these domains can include aspects of emotional competence, but given the focus of this book and to narrow an increasingly large and complex literature, I discuss *only* the assessment tools and programming specific to the emotional competence of 3- to 6-year-olds, following this similar framework of emotional competence (see Figure 13.2). Although much assessment and programming appropriately refer to the prevention of behavior problems, unless this prevention is connected to the building of emotional competence strengths, is not discussed here. To be of assistance, however, I briefly note assessment tools that are broader in nature but still include only preschoolers and kindergartners, the age range discussed in this book.

## AN EDUCATIONAL SYSTEM FOR PROMOTING EMOTIONAL COMPETENCE

Given these parameters, it is helpful to frame assessment and programming for emotional competence in a system of early childhood educational practice. For our purposes here, I adapt a previously developed system (Denham, 2015; Figure 13.3).

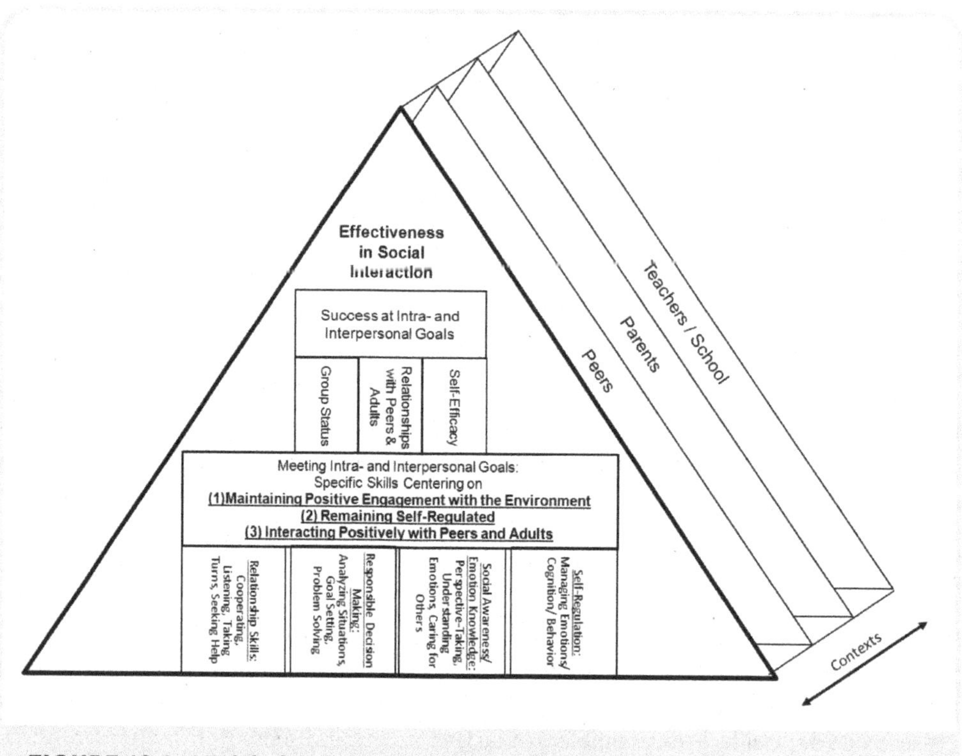


**FIGURE 13.1.** Model of social–emotional learning.

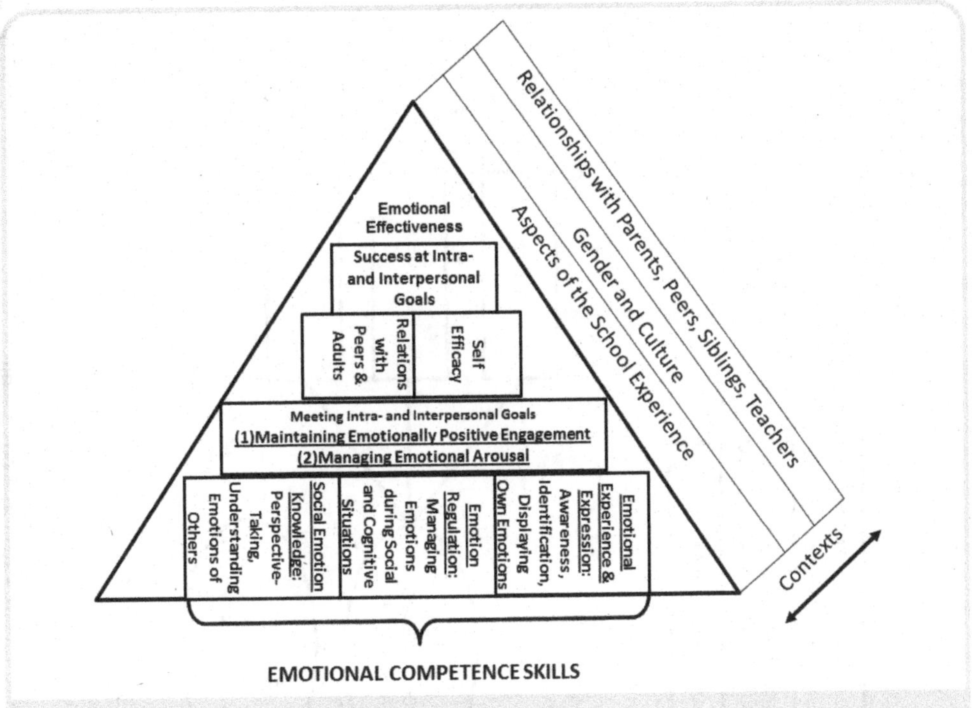


**FIGURE 13.2.** Modified model: emotional competence embedded within developmental tasks, intra- and interpersonal goals, and contexts.

Age-appropriate developmental tasks are the substrate upon which specific emotional competence skills are demonstrated and developed. Clear educational standards must be created emanating from these important competencies as road maps of what skills to look for, expect, and teach (National Association for the Education of Young Children & National Association of Early Childhood Specialists in State Departments of Education, 2003). Educational standards inform the choice of assessment tools, and the use of assessment tools can inform iterations of standards. Both educational standards and assessment are useful in that they lead to instruction and teaching practices related to emotional competence. These efforts by teachers often can lead to the need for additional regular assessment and revised standards, and can be supported by both professional development for teachers as emotion socializers as well as evidence-based curricula or less structured programming (see Humphrey, 2013). Ultimately, of course, we strive for growth in young children's emotional competence. The rubric presented in Figure 13.3 can inform how we situate preschoolers' emotional competence within early childhood education. I now go into more detail about its elements.

I have already defined the developmental tasks and components of emotional competence for this age period, but they are noted again in Figure 13.3. I enumerate them as (1) maintaining positive emotional engagement with the physical and social world; (2) making and maintaining relationships with other children and adults; and (3) managing emotional arousal in the context of social interaction and new cognitive

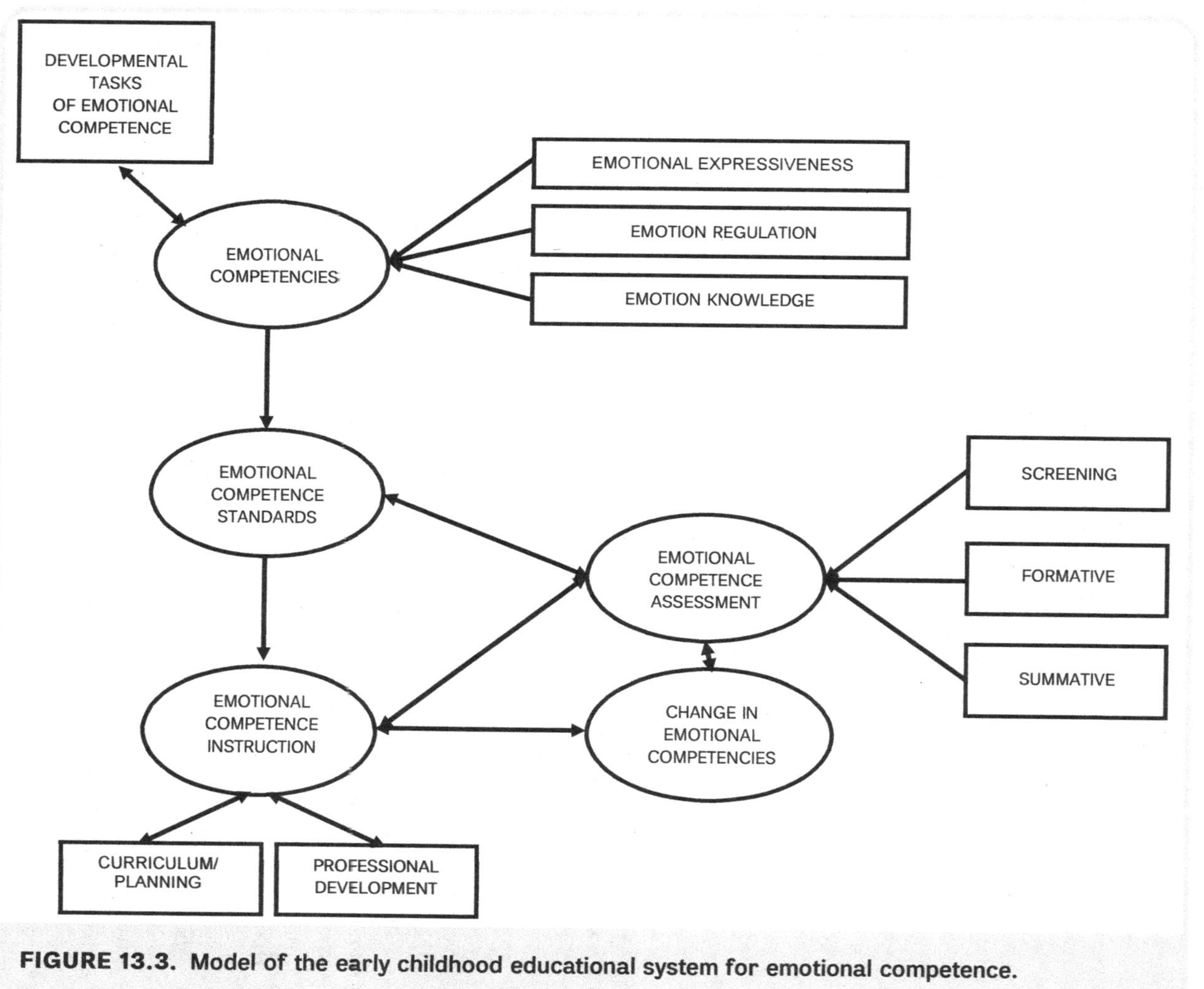


**FIGURE 13.3.** Model of the early childhood educational system for emotional competence.

demands (Parker & Gottman, 1989). These developmental tasks can be difficult to navigate.

Standards are statements about "what students should know and be able to do as a result of educational instruction" (Dusenbury et al., 2011, p. 3; see also Dusenbury et al., 2015) and reflect key stakeholders' decisions about optimal development. They can be useful as reference points for planning, teaching, and learning activities; supporting positive learning environments; and even for assessing children's progress. Standards are thus the foundation by which states, other local education agencies, and early childhood education governing bodies enunciate educational goals, select evidence-based methods, support teachers' high-quality instruction, and monitor student progress. These functions are implied in the pivotal placement of standards in Figure 13.3.

To unite emotional competence standards with assessment and instruction, as shown in Figure 13.3, one must search out exemplars of emotional competence standards that as clearly as possible cover all aspects of emotional competence. As already noted in Chapter 11, most states now have such early childhood SEL standards (Dusenbury et al., 2015; Zinsser, Weissberg, et al., 2013), and often they include an explicit reference to emotional competence skills. When emotional competence standards are in place, it becomes more necessary to develop and/or adopt emotional competence assessment tools. First, I describe the functions that such assessment could (and should) take in the classroom. Then, I detail the evaluation criteria for such assessments to be used for information gathering and decision-making within schools.

## ASSESSMENT OF EMOTIONAL COMPETENCE

Before (and while) implementing programming for emotional competence, teachers will want to know where students stand on their knowledge of emotional competence skills. "What's measured gets treasured"—if emotional competence is assessed well, better decisions about how to facilitate children's emotional competence can be made (Denham, 2006). Emotional competence assessment can serve multiple purposes, including (1) highlighting the specific needs and progress of individual children; (2) guiding instruction and programming; (3) tracking the success of such programming across classrooms, schools, and school systems, so that program-related decisions can be made; (4) showing the overall effects of programming for accountability to governing bodies, such as Head Start and public prekindergartens; and (5) making recommendations for policy changes (Darling-Churchill & Lippman, 2016; Denham, Ji, & Hamre, 2010; Denham, Wyatt, Bassett, Echeverria, & Knox, 2009; Olson, 2021). In what follows, I make suggestions in line with these purposes, although as Darling-Churchill and Lippman (2016) asserted, alignment of these purposes with specific assessment tools is still lagging.

### Functions of SEL Assessment

Screening and formative assessment tools can serve most of these purposes in early childhood educational settings. Brief screening tools allow for the implementation of a three-tiered model of instruction—from universally providing SEL instruction to all children, to targeted interventions for those at risk, to individualized work for those presenting persistent challenges (Halle & Darling-Churchill, 2016; Hemmeter, Ostrosky, & Fox, 2006). That is, screening cutoffs can demarcate targeted and at-risk children whose educational needs may differ from those not at risk. Quick identification of problems or risks, confirmation of suspected problems, or evaluation of readiness to enter formal schooling can be accomplished via screening tools. However, because of their brevity, my opinion is that screening tools do not completely describe a child's emotional competence abilities (see also Halle & Darling-Churchill, 2016). Naglieri, LeBuffe, and Shapiro (2011) though have argued that screeners can be sensitive enough to use for formative progress monitoring, so their extended use is up for some debate. Finally, although they are not a focus of this volume, other assessment measures can assist in the diagnosis of behavior problems in addition to screener evidence.

Next, formative assessment can be seen as minute-by-minute "assessment *for* learning," and integrated into instruction, with the primary purpose of monitoring students' progress and planning instruction (Darling-Churchill & Lippman, 2016; National Research Council, 2012; Perie, Marion, & Gong, 2009). Classroom teachers use such assessment to identify gaps in children's skills, so that they can adjust their approach to improving a particular student's emotional competence. Meta-analytic findings on the use of formative assessment in nonemotional competence content areas show that its use is associated with positive student outcomes, especially when teachers are given professional development in its use, and when it is delivered via computer-based systems (Kingston & Nash, 2011).

Formative assessment can be a criterion-referenced endeavor (i.e., with results interpretable in terms of a defined set of learning tasks, e.g., standards) or a norm-referenced one (i.e., with results interpretable in terms of an individual's relative standing in some known group).

That is, there could be various uses for and means of approaching such assessment (Shavelson et al., 2008; Van der Kleij, Vermeulen, Schildkamp, & Eggen 2015). First, as already suggested, formative assessment can be used for assessment for learning; this use could be criterion-referenced, largely based on observing and interacting with children. Thus for this sort of formative assessment, teachers could use standards as their starting point in gathering information. Or tasks presented in formative assessment can be modified from one student to another, depending on a student's current emotional competencies. Second, formative assessment can also take the form of diagnostic testing, which would ideally be norm referenced. In this chapter, I discuss norm-referenced measures that include useful information for formative assessment.

The major take-home message, then, is that formative assessment is used by teachers to learn about specific children and their classroom as a whole so that instruction can be fine-tuned. At times formative assessment also may supplement screeners for diagnostic workups. Further, formative assessment data, especially norm-referenced data, can be aggregated by classroom, school, and/or district to monitor progress toward various goals and carefully used to assist with policy decisions (National Association for the Education of Young Children & National Association of Early Childhood Specialists in State Departments of Education, 2003). More specifically, such aggregated data can be used to evaluate programs' effectiveness: are programs actually working as intended and helping children become more emotionally competent? This information can assist local and state decision makers in determining whether to strengthen programs or to continue them, as well as in comparing a program's impacts on other programs or deciding whether to have a program at all (Halle & Darling-Churchill, 2016). Additionally, policy decisions can utilize such data; numerous recent U. S. initiatives refer to the promotion of young children's emotional competence (O'Connor et al., 2017), and having hard evidence of the need for and feasibility of such programming can be gathered from these aggregated assessments.

To use formative assessment for these additional functions, users need to decide whether a given assessment can be used for classroom, school, district, and/or policy decision making, while simultaneously and microanalytically contributing to teachers' understanding of what to do day by day with a classroom or particular child. This may be no mean task; in fact, Darling-Churchill and Lippman (2016) assert that separate assessment tools should serve the two sorts of purposes. However, to begin to promote unification of these assessment purposes, recent reports have indicated that some states are working to align such assessments with both standards and curricula (Caron, Kendall, Wilson, & Hash, 2017; Olson, 2021); this is a very promising possibility. Nonetheless, some of these uses have not yet been evaluated sufficiently specifically with respect to emotional competence assessment. Evaluating assessment tools requires clear criteria, to which I now turn.

## Criteria for Quality Assessment

Given these functions of emotional competence assessment, attention must be paid to their quality—both in terms of the measure's integrity and its applications. I now describe the criteria by which we should choose high-quality emotional competence assessments for potential usability for each function. The criteria for choosing "best-bet" measures are first outlined, followed by a description of assessment tools and further commentary on how to plan effective SEL assessment in schools.

Most broadly, a number of criteria need to be met for any assessment tool to adequately measure emotional competence in early childhood. First and of paramount importance, there needs to be a good reason *why* children are assessed (i.e., one of the functions already noted here), the measures must be developmentally appropriate for specific skills, and there needs to be a system in place to *use* the resultant information, especially as connected to instruction (Jones, Zaslow, Darling-Churchill, & Halle, 2016). Thus early childhood emotional competence assessment should be integrated with curricula, beneficial to all parties, based often on ongoing teacher observation, and primarily reliant on the child's everyday activities.

To choose an assessment tool, one must be able to judge its content as germane before one is able to consider more technical and pragmatic concerns. Hence, emotional competence assessment tools should have a manual that contains a description of the measure, the constructs assessed, and assignment of items to scales (with sufficient items per construct if using as formative assessment). Furthermore, the presence of a screening tool parallel to the assessment tool can be very useful.

The manual also should make it clear whether, and if so how, the measure is useful for multiple purposes (e.g., for screening or formative assessment or aggregated for classroom, school, district, or policy uses). Assessment tools are increasingly making these possible uses clear, but this area of concern is far from systematized and still requires much planning from users. It is helpful, furthermore, if a detailed behavioral definition is given for each item; very few emotional competence assessments include such rubrics. Almost no such assessments add even hints extending their results to instruction. These problems are endemic to the assessment of social–emotional competence in general.

Several more detailed criteria are paramount. First, the qualities of the actual assessment tool, or its psychometric properties, must be considered. Assessment tools should have at least adequate reliability and validity (of various types), and as far as possible should be fair, unbiased, and generalizable across ages and demographic groups. All measures I cite here meet these psychometric requirements, but information on generalizability is sometimes less complete. For example, norms and psychometric data for assessments are needed for diverse samples, including dual language learners, children from different cultures, and children with disabilities where possible (Darling-Churchill & Lippman, 2016; Halle & Darling-Churchill, 2016; Jones et al., 2016). Native language and dialect must be considered when selecting and using self- or parent-reports. However, *most* assessment tools of any kind fall short of adequately meeting at least some of these diversity needs.

Second, we must think about utility; it is helpful for assessments to have benchmarks or external anchors, such as norms and/or a connection with standards, to assist in meaningful interpretations of scores and their change over time and to be useful in tracking the results of instruction and programming. Also in terms of utility, such tools should be administrable within a reasonable time frame (e.g., 10–20 minutes). The acceptability of administration time in part depends on whether all children in a school or classroom, or only select children (i.e., for purposes other than student progress and tailored instruction, such as classroom, school, and/or district aggregation) are assessed.

Training and certification of assessors, where necessary, must be standardized and potentially repeated at intervals to maintain quality control (as already implied, I would argue that not only observers, but also raters, must be trained to understand the constructs and methodology involved, for any assessment to be valid).

This issue puts a spotlight on another problem. Even carefully created rating systems, which have rubrics for scoring items and explanations of the construct, can be difficult for users who are not sufficiently trained. Moreover, there is evidence that teachers can have trouble using them accurately (Olson, 2021). The time needed to administer and analyze comprehensive ratings, such as Teaching Strategies GOLD (Lambert, Kim, & Burta, 2014), is substantial (Olson, 2021). Other methods, including direct assessment and observation, also have training and reliability and/or certification issues, in terms of time, expense, and accuracy. In fact, the criteria already mentioned regarding utility are reflected in cost: costs of assessment tools in terms of completion time; the skills, training, and equipment required; and the test forms and/or scoring must be reasonable. This need is especially pronounced given that domains other than emotional competence also need assessment.

Electronic administration and scoring of ratings, observations, and direct assessments also can be desirable because they are faster and less expensive than paper-based administration and hand scoring. Additionally, in the age of mini-laptops, smartphones, and apps, two new possibilities have turned up. For example, computerized batteries of direct assessments for all aspects of emotional competence have been created (Denham, Bassett, Zinsser, et al., 2020; In-Albon et al., 2021). Further, there are beginning to be applications on smart phones that are proving advantageous for early childhood teacher use (Olson, 2021), and other researchers are working on the capability to perform emotional competence assessment virtually (Bogat et al., 2021). Any such technological tool can have several helpful characteristics for tracking children's progress, such as (1) assisting in observation and/or ratings; (2) uploading of such data, as well as notes, videos, and images about children's behaviors and interactions; (3) allowing for scoring; (4) suggesting activities to promote student progress; and (5) even including aspects of direct assessment (Denham, Bassett, Zinsser, et al., 2020; Olson, 2021).

Finally, where possible, multiple informants of the same dimension's measurement are recommended, given that behavior is often rater and context specific and is subject to bias. In the case of school-based emotional competence assessment, aggregating information from multiple sources (e.g., teachers, mental health professionals, and parents) could be especially powerful, although probably is rarely done because of constraints on time and effort.

### SUMMARY: Choosing Assessment Tools

In sum, the criteria of importance that I consider when evaluating assessment tools are as follows: (1) a manual that describes the construct and offers content validity, as well as rubrics to follow in scoring; (2) psychometric quality; (3) generalizability across diverse groups; (4) reference to norms or standards; (5) connections to instruction; (6) time constraints, including training; and (7) scoring considerations. No measure is likely to meet all these criteria, but I continue to search is for those that best capture emotional expressiveness, emotion knowledge, and ER.

## Emotional Competence Assessments for Early Childhood

A number of assessment tools have been developed and evaluated as useful for determining the ways in which more broadly defined social–emotional competencies, such as those depicted in Figure 13.1, promote positive outcomes from infancy through late childhood. Many of these instruments have been included in compendia and reviews (e.g., Crowe, Beauchamp, Catroppa, & Anderson, 2011; Denham, 2015; Denham, Ji, et al., 2010; Denham, Wyatt, et al., 2009; Humphrey et al., 2011; Ringwalt, 2008; Sosna & Mastergeorge, 2005). In general, the compendia are targeted at either mainly research (e.g., Denham et al., 2009, 2010) or applied usage (Ringwalt, 2008; Sosna & Mastergeorge, 2005). The authors of these compendia have searched for more general social–emotional measures, across a broad range of criteria similar to those I have enumerated here. These materials form an important adjunct to this chapter, supplementing the assessments referring specifically to emotional competence that I review here (see, for example, the Devereux Early Childhood Assessment, LeBuffe & Naglieri, 1991; LeBuffe, Shapiro, Naglieri, 2009; the SSiS SEL Brief Scales—Preschool Forms, Anthony, Elliott, DiPerna, & Lei, 2020).

What is obvious from these compendia and reviews is that although specific emotional competencies of expressiveness, regulation, and knowledge have been measured via a wide variety of mechanisms, including informant ratings, direct assessment, and observation (Denham, Ji, et al., 2010), these specific abilities are not represented as often as broader aspects of social–emotional development in extant assessment tools. This scarcity makes the search more difficult, but not impossible.

Mention should be made of the various ways that data are gathered via the assessment tools that I have selected. As already noted, in many cases the time required for direct assessments and observations and for training and observer/coder reliability render such tools more difficult to use in educational or other applied settings. In contrast, rating systems, when carefully crafted to meet as many of the above-referenced criteria as possible, may be used more efficiently in terms of time, and as Duckworth and Yager (2015) note, they can be "cheap, quick, reliable, and in many cases, remarkably predictive" (p. 239; see also Anthony et al., 2020). Other advantages of rating systems include that their time-saving features can allow teachers to rate whole groups of children efficiently, and multiple informants can easily rate children to average out emotional competence over time and context, relative to a standardized reference group (LeBuffe, Shapiro, Robitaille, 2018).

Actually, however, as I have already hinted, neither type of measurement is free of problems nor lacking in strengths. Although it is important to acknowledge the difficulties in using direct assessment and observation (Denham, Bassett, Zinsser, et al., 2014; McKown, 2015, 2017), at the same time such measurement methods arguably may be especially useful for better understanding the emotional competencies for children who are a risk or already showing difficulties. Direct assessment may be needed as well to access children's internalized *understanding* of concepts, such as emotions, which cannot be directly observed (McKown, 2015, 2017). And solely using rating measures may subject data to monorater bias, as well as raising the concern that training in the rubrics for rating measures is very rarely given. Further, the frequent turnover of early childhood personnel begs the question of whether knowledge of children across many contexts, a criterion for the sound use of rating scales, can be attained (Olson, 2021). I have already mentioned that assessors very rarely get any training on rating scales, and that rubrics are almost nonexistent.

Thus, although I never preclude the use of rating scales, I have some preference for direct assessment and observation wherever possible. I see the above issues regarding direct assessment and observation as hurdles to be overcome, perhaps with the use of computerization to standardize and simplify administration. What's more, I argue that actually observing or eliciting indices of emotional competence allows for invaluable knowledge about children.

Given these considerations, I now describe several assessment measures, including rating scales, direct assessment, and observational tools, which directly refer to emotional competence, and attempt to evaluate them given the criteria I have enumerated for quality assessment. I reiterate that I include *only* measures or scales within measures that address preschoolers' emotional competence, including emotional expressiveness (including empathy), emotion knowledge, and ER. Note also that I do not include measures useful in toddlerhood (i.e., prior to 36 months); the measures reviewed here are intended for use with 3- to 6-year-olds. Measures that include only children in kindergarten or the elementary grades are not reviewed, despite their usefulness for other aspects of social–emotional development (e.g., the Devereux Student Strengths Assessment, LeBuffe, et al., 2009; the Social–Emotional Assets and Resilience Scale, Merrell, Cohn, & Tom, 2011; Merrell, Felver-Gant, & Tom, 2011). Table 13.1 illustrates the chosen measures and their qualities according to criteria I have enunciated (see also Campbell et al., 2016, for a critical review of social–emotional measures for early childhood).

## *Measures of Emotional Expressiveness*

Four rating scales and an observational tool are recommended for general use to assess emotional expressiveness. Specifically, Rothbart's Children's Behavior Questionnaire (CBQ; Rothbart, Ahadi, Hershey, & Fisher, 2001), the Social Competence and Behavior Evaluation—30-item scale (SCBE-30; LaFreniere & Dumas, 1996), and part of the Social Skills Improvement System (SSiS; Frey, Elliott, & Kaiser, 2014) appear promising as rating scales. The Positive and Negative Affect Schedule (PANAS; Watson, Clark, & Tellegen, 1988) could also be utilized. For an observational tool, the Minnesota Preschool Affect Checklist, Revised/Shortened (MPAC-R/S; Denham, Bassett, Thayer, et al., 2012) is recommended.

### RATING SCALES: TEMPERAMENT MEASURES

Rothbart's CBQ and its Very Short Form (CBQ-VSF) are useful in describing a preschooler's typical patterns of emotional expressiveness, across many everyday contexts (Putnam & Rothbart, 2006; Rothbart et al., 2001). It is important to note that these measures include both *negative* and *positive* emotionality. The questionnaires are generally parent reported, although some modifications for teacher-reported versions have been undertaken (Teglasi et al., 2015).

In general, the CBQ includes two higher-order temperament factors pertinent to the assessment of emotional expressiveness: (1) negative affectivity, and (2) surgency. Negative affectivity items involve discomfort experienced in overstimulating situations, and in frustration, anger, an inability to soothe oneself, fearfulness, and sadness. It is easy to see how this potent combination could make interacting with both peers and adults problematic.

Surgency is an aspect of temperament measured with items on approach to novel stimuli, smiling, high activity level, and high-level pleasure. Hence, a child high on this dimension of temperament might be a lot of fun to be around—eagerly initiating contact with others, finding interesting things to do, and sharing positive affect. On the other hand, these attractive qualities of surgent children can become too intense, so that they are seen as overly active and boisterous, risky, and impulsive (Degnan et al., 2011; Tarullo et al., 2011).

**TABLE 13.1. Summary Information on Final Preschool Emotional Competence Assessment Battery**

| Assessment tool | Age level | Informant | Emotional expressiveness | Emotion regulation | Emotion knowledge | Adequacy of manual | Reliabilities | Validity | Cost[a] | Time required (in minutes) | Electronic administration/ Scoring | Screener | Formative | Notes |
|---|---|---|---|---|---|---|---|---|---|---|---|---|---|---|
| *Recommended for battery usage* | | | | | | | | | | | | | | |
| AKT-S | PK | C | | | ✓ | ✓ | Good IC, T/RT | ✓ | N/A | 10 | ~ | | ✓ | Norms<br>Translated in Spanish and adapted in many countries<br>Standardized training<br>Used with diverse populations |
| ERC | PK–3 | T, P | | ✓ | | ? | Excellent IC | ✓ | N/A | 10 | ? | ✓ | ✓ | Large research base |
| MPAC-R/S | PK | O | ✓ | ✓ | | ✓ | Adequate IC,T/ RT, IRR | ✓ | N/A | 10–20 | ~ | | ✓ | Norms<br>Standardized training<br>Used with diverse populations |
| Rothbart CBQ | PK | T, P | ✓ | ✓- | | ✓ | Good IC, IRR [b] | ~ | ~[c] | 10 VSF<br>60 CBQ | ? | ✓ | ✓ | Large research base |
| SCBE-30 | PK–1 | T, P | ✓ | ✓ | | ✓ | Good–excellent T/RT, IC, IRR | ✓ | ~[d] | 10 | ? | ✓ | ✓ | Norms |

| *Other potentially useful assessment tools* | | | | | | | | | | | | | | |
|---|---|---|---|---|---|---|---|---|---|---|---|---|---|---|
| BRIEF-P | PK | T, P | | ✓ | | ✓ | Good to excellent T/RT, IC<br>Adequate IRR | ✓ | $260 | 10–15 whole inventory | ✓ | ✓ | ✓ | Norms<br>Translated into Spanish |
| SSiS-RS Empathy Scale | PK–12 | T, P | ✓ | | | ✓ | Good to excellent IC, T/RT, IRR[b] | ✓ | $261–$342 | 10–25 whole inventory | Scoring only | | ✓ | Norms for total scale<br>Large research base |
| Emotion Matching Test | PK | C | | | ✓ | ? | Excellent IC | ✓ | — | 15 | | | ✓ | Promising |
| PANAS | PK–adult | T, P | ✓ | | | — | Excellent IC | ✓ | — | 15 split half | | ✓ | ✓ | |

*Note.* AKT-S = Affect Knowledge Test—Short Version; ERC = Emotion Regulation Checklist; MPAC-R/S = Minnesota Preschool Affect Checklist—Revised/Shortened; CBQ = Children's Behavior Questionnaire; SCBE-30 = Social Competence and Behavior Evaluation Scale—30 Item; SSiS-RS = Social Skills Improvement System Rating Scales; PK= prekindergarten; T = teacher; P = parent; O = observer; ✓ = quality present; — = quality partially present based on available information; ? = unknown as of this writing; T/RT = test–retest reliability; IRR = interrater reliability; IC, internal consistency (coefficient alpha).

[a]Costs depend on whether multiple informant versions are purchased, for example; publishers should be contacted.

[b]Reported reliabilities are for the teacher version of the measure, Very Short Form.

[c]Dr. Rothbart's laboratory allows the use of the temperament questionnaires as long as researchers share with her lab the study's results; use by educational agencies would likely be given permission as well.

[d]The SCBE-30 is published by Western Psychological Services, and they request the option to "approve" use of short form.

For greater specificity regarding emotional expressiveness, along with a shorter length, separate CBQ scales targeting emotional expressiveness could be chosen. The use of emotional expressiveness subscales (e.g., Sadness, Anger, Soothability, High-Intensity Pleasure) could allow a focus on emotional expressiveness across both positive and negative valences. These scales are long enough to be comfortable to use them in a stand-alone fashion. The CBQ-VSF could be used as a screener. Both forms have adequate-to-excellent psychometric qualities (e.g., Putnam & Rothbart, 2006; see Table 13.1).

### RATING SCALES: SCBE-30

For the SCBE-30 (LaFreniere & Dumas, 1996), teachers or parents rate children on 10-item scales, including Angry/Aggressive (e.g., "easily frustrated"), Sensitive/Cooperative (e.g., "comforts or assists children in difficulty"), and Anxious/Withdrawn (e.g., "avoids new situations"). The measure's reliability in terms of internal consistency, stability over time, and across raters is excellent. The validity of the SCBE has been shown with normative, clinical, and cross-cultural samples (Denham, Blair, et al., 2003; LaFreniere & Dumas, 1996; LaFreniere et al., 2002). The SCBE-30 is extensively normed with stratified samples of French Canadian and American preschoolers and shows cross-cultural value. The measure also has been translated into Spanish (Dumas, Martinez, & LaFreniere, 1998; Dumas, Martinez, LaFreniere, & Dolz, 1998). The item content allows evaluations to be completed by anyone who knows the child well. The responses of experienced teachers tend to be distributed differently from inexperienced teachers, which is an issue to take into account generally when using data from teacher reports.

### RATING SCALES: PANAS

The PANAS (Watson et al., 1988) has been modified for older children's self-report and parent report for preschoolers (Ebesutani et al., 2012; Laurent et al., 1999). It assesses how the child "feels on average" for 12 negative emotions (e.g., sad, angry) and 3 positive emotions (e.g., excited, enthusiastic). In fact, Ebesutani and colleagues (2012) used item-response theory to boil down the scales to five items each: negative (miserable, mad, afraid, scared, and sad) and positive (joyful, cheerful, happy, lively, and proud). Thus, it is brief and has excellent psychometric properties. I believe it could be used profitably with preschoolers.

### RATINGS OF EMPATHIC CONCERN

A few assessment tools include scales for examining young children's empathic concern. One is the SSiS, which has both parent and teacher forms (Frey et al., 2014). Thus, six items are included referring to empathy, including identification with or understanding of another's situation, feelings, thoughts, attitudes, or motives and the ability to imagine how another person is feeling and to understand his or her mood. In general I eschew extracting items from an existing assessment measure, but these items have been evaluated as a separate scale and have excellent reliability, as well as negative associations with problem-behavior ratings (Frey et al., 2014).

Recently a parent measure was created for clinical use (Kimonis, Jain, Neo, Fleming, & Briggs, 2021); its 35 items include five factors: Attention to Others' Emotions, Personal Distress (i.e., Emotional Contagion/Affective Empathy), Personal Distress—Fictional Characters, Prosocial Behavior, and Sympathy. Total and subscale scores are internally consistent. More validity data are necessary for this measure to be of use, and it is a bit lengthy, but it holds promise.

#### OBSERVATIONAL MEASURES: MPAC-R/S

The MPAC-R/S (Denham, Bassett, Thayer, et al., 2012) includes 18 items. Regarding emotional expressiveness and regulation, these are scales for positive and negative emotion (e.g., "The child displays positive/negative emotion in any manner (i.e., facial, vocal, or bodily) as well as reactions to frustration (ER, e.g., "The child promptly verbally expresses feelings arising from a problem situation, then moves on to the same or a new activity"). Other scales include productive/unproductive involvement (e.g., "The child is engrossed . . . emotionally invested in [an] activity that has a positive emotional function), peer skills (e.g., "The child smoothly approaches an already ongoing activity and gets actively involved"), and prosocial behaviors (e.g., taking turns, sharing) that could be useful to address social competence in components, below. Each child is observed for four 5-minute epochs across the data collection period of approximately 8 weeks. The scores for items equal the sum of occurrences across all four epochs.

Structure of the MPAC-R/S shows emotionally negative/aggressive, emotionally regulated/prosocial, and emotionally positive/productive components (Denham, Bassett, Thayer, et al., 2012). As such, both emotional expressiveness and ER are captured by this observational assessment. In terms of psychometrics, its internal consistency, test–retest reliability, and construct stability are good. Age, gender, and risk differences have been found, as well as other aspects of emotional competence (i.e., children's emotion knowledge contributed to later emotionally regulated/prosocial behavior) and achievement (i.e., preschool emotionally negative and aggressive behaviors contributed to concurrent and kindergarten school success; Herndon et al., 2013). The measure is now computerized and is being adapted more specifically for teacher use. Further, the computerized version is accompanied by activity suggestions and includes the capability for individualized as well as classwide profiles and data preservation.

The MPAC-R/S is a good example of an observational measure that can be used to glean information on emotional competence and was considered promising in a recent special issue on early childhood emotional competence assessment (Halle & Darling-Churchill, 2016). In many cases, important information about children is acquired by watching them, and given that the MPAC-R/S requires just 20 minutes, it could provide information relatively economically. Moreover, the adaptation of the measure for use by teachers is ongoing.

### *Direct Assessment of Emotional Expressiveness*

No direct assessment of children's emotional expressiveness is available. My research group has performed some initial work (Fettig, Howarth, Watanabe, Denham, &

Bassett, n.d.). Further, in In-Albon et al.'s (2021) computerized assessment, the MeKKI, there is a task in which children are asked to express happiness, sadness, fear, and anger. However, neither the In-Albon et al. nor Fettig et al. measures require much work to be usable at scale. The Preschool Laboratory Temperament Assessment Battery (PS Lab-TAB; Goldsmith, Reilly, Lemery, Longley, & Prescott, 1993) has facility at gathering information on expressiveness and already-reported robust psychometric qualities compared to either other measure but it too is unlikely to be usable at scale because of its complexity in administration and coding.

### **SUMMARY:** Recommended Measures of Emotional Expressiveness

Considering the criteria established here, several suggestions should be made. To meet the need for brevity, the selected scales of the Rothbart measures or the CBQ-VSF would need to be used, and there is evidence that the MPAC-R/S could capture emotional expressiveness with brief (e.g., two 5-minute) epochs. Some elements of necessary documentation, as in a rubric explanation of measure items to improve raters' comprehension of each item, could be improved for the CBQ and SCBE-30 (for MPAC-R/S documentation, see Denham, Bassett, Thayer, et al., 2012). To examine the important quality of empathy, the SSiS could be useful. Norms exist for all these measures, including for diverse populations (although extracting one scale from the SSiS, for example, could be considered problematic). More research on cultural fairness would be useful. Most of these measures can be used for formative and screening purposes (see Table 13.1).

## *Measures of Emotion Knowledge*

Although there are currently only direct assessments of preschoolers' emotion knowledge, actually it remains unclear whether parent and teacher reports could ever garner a level of detail on this aspect of emotional competence, due to the amount of inference required. Research supporting the development of other means of assessing preschool emotion knowledge would be valuable.

### DIRECT ASSESSMENT: AFFECT KNOWLEDGE TEST, SHORT VERSION

The Affect Knowledge Test, Short Version (AKT-S; Denham, Bassett, Brown, et al., 2015; see also Chapter 4), utilizes puppets to measure preschoolers' developmentally appropriate understanding of emotional expressions and situations; it has recently been computerized utilizing videos matching the race and gender of the child. These recent changes (e.g., shorter length and parallel versions) render the test more useful for educational purposes (see Denham, Ji, et al., 2010, for evidence on the earlier version). The AKT-S shows good psychometric properties, with appropriate documentation, as well as parallel versions that could be used for multiple assessment points. However, its norms should be published, and cultural fairness explored further (Darling-Churchill & Lippman, 2016; Humphrey et al., 2011). Bassett et al. (2012) did find measurement equivalence across gender and race and partial equivalence across age and socioeconomic status.

Children's understanding of emotion is assessed using puppets with detachable faces that depict happy, sad, angry, and afraid expressions. First, children are asked to both verbally name the emotions depicted on these faces, and then to nonverbally identify them by pointing. This procedure taps their ability to recognize expressions of emotion. Then, in two subtests of emotion situation knowledge, the puppeteer makes standard facial and vocal expressions of emotions while enacting emotion-laden stories, such as fear during a nightmare or happiness at getting some ice cream. Children place on the puppet the face that depicts the puppet's feeling in each situation. In the first subtest, the puppet feels emotions that would be common to most people, such as those just mentioned. In the second subtest, children are asked to make inferences about emotions in equivocal situations. This individualized subtest measures how well children identify others' feelings in situations in which the "other" feels differently from the child, and that could easily elicit one of two different emotions in different people, as in feeling happy or afraid to get into a swimming pool.

The AKT-S and its computerized version (Denham, Bassett, Zinsser, et al., 2020) require about 10 minutes to administer and have been studied with three diverse samples totaling over 900 children. Reliability and validity are good to excellent (Denham, Bassett, Brown, et al., 2015). The longer version from which the AKT-S was adapted shows similar good-to-excellent reliability (internal consistency and stability), with validity from a wide variety of sources, both in terms of early school success and social competence (see also Denham, Ji, et al., 2010).

### DIRECT ASSESSMENT: EMOTION MATCHING TASK

Another emotion knowledge direct assessment that could be useful is the Emotion Matching Task (EMT; Izard, Haskins, Schultz, Trentacosta, & King, 2003). Considering the emotions happiness, sadness, anger, and fear/surprise, the EMT assesses (1) emotion expression matching, (2) emotion situation knowledge, (3) expressive EK (emotion labeling), and (4) receptive EK. It was specifically developed with multiethnic and well-standardized emotion expression photographs for use with diverse groups. The EMT gives an overall score and a score for each dimension, which enables an in-depth analysis of the development and acquisition of the different components of EK. It has been adapted to non-U.S. cultures (e.g., Alonso-Alberca et al., 2012; DiMaggio, Zappulla, Page, & Izard, 2013), showing adequate psychometric properties in each version. Convergent and criterion validity have also been established (Morgan et al., 2010). At 48 items, it is rather long, but two halves have been created to get around this problem (Finlon et al., 2015), and internal consistency of these halves is excellent.

### DIRECT ASSESSMENT: MEKKI

The MeKKI was developed as a computer-based measure assessing several components of emotional competence in children between 4 and 10 years of age (In-Albon et al.,

2021). It includes emotion vocabulary, emotion identification, and emotion situation vignette subtests, which show good internal consistency. Children completed the test in a one-on-one setting with an assessor. The measure, which also includes emotional expression and regulation subtests, takes about 30 minutes in total, which is rather lengthy (but perhaps it could be performed in two sessions). This intriguing measure requires much further study. However, it could be, along with Denham, Bassett, Zinsser, et al. (2020), ushering in direct, computerized assessment that would ease teachers' assessment burden in terms of time and training for administration. Denham. Bassett, Zinsser, et al.'s (2020) computerized AKT, in fact, does not even require the teacher to do anything other than set up the device and earphones for the child, who takes it from there.

## **SUMMARY:** Recommended Measures of Emotion Knowledge

It is unclear whether parent and teacher reports could ever garner a level of detail on this aspect of emotional competence because of the amount of inference required; thus, direct assessment is seen as more appropriate. The AKT-S shows good properties, with appropriate documentation, and the ability to be used for formative assessment, especially given that it includes two parallel versions that could be used for multiple assessment points. The EMT also is promising, and the MeKKI may become more frequently used with time. Research supporting the development of other means of assessing preschool emotion knowledge would be valuable.

### *Measures of ER*

Overall, there is one almost universally used rating measure of ER, which has been often mentioned in this book, the Emotion Regulation Checklist (ERC). Additionally, the MPAC-R/S, which I have already described, is considered a promising observational tool.

#### RATINGS OF ER: ERC

The ERC (Shields & Cicchetti, 1997; Shields et al., 2001) is a 24-item teacher report including items on lability, intensity, valence, flexibility, and appropriateness of expressed emotions. The measure consists of two subscales, "Lability/Negativity" (e.g., "Is prone to negative outbursts") and "Emotion Regulation" (e.g., "Is empathetic to others"). Specifically, prevalent emotional expressiveness and regulation, including lability, intensity, valence, flexibility, and contextual appropriateness are assessed. The measure demonstrates high internal consistency for each subscale as well as concurrent and predictive validity (Shields & Cicchetti, 1997; Shields et al., 2001). More specifically, the ERC distinguishes regulated from dysregulated children. Further, ER scores predict later school adjustment, whereas emotional lability/negativity predicts poorer outcomes.

Despite these strengths, it should be noted that the measure does conflate regulation with expressiveness within its subscales. The ERC also unfortunately largely assesses the outcomes of regulation (e.g., emotional state, empathy) rather than regulatory skills per se, and it may be contaminated with measures of maladjustment (Weems & Pina, 2010). However, if an overall summary of these two aspects of emotional competence, focusing on negative expressiveness and its control, is warranted, this is a good choice for a teacher or parent report.

#### RATINGS OF ER: BEHAVIOR RATING INVENTORY OF EXECUTIVE FUNCTION

Two other scales could be promising in the assessment of ER. First, the Behavior Rating Inventory of Executive Function, Preschool (BRIEF-P; both teacher and parent forms) includes an "Emotional Control" scale that reflects emotional reactivity and intensity in emotional reactions. In a recent report (Skogan et al., 2016), seven items constituted an internally consistent Emotion Dysregulation factor (e.g., "Has outbursts for little reason"; "Overreacts to small problems"; "Angry or tearful outbursts are intense but end suddenly"), indicating construct validity. Further, Duku and Vaillancourt (2014) found adequate parent–teacher agreement and both construct and convergent validity. This scale (which also may combine in a factor with Inhibitory Control Problems) may be prone, to a lesser degree however, to the same issues as the ERC (e.g., conflating emotional expressiveness with ER).

### *Assessing ER: Promising Developments*

There also are two emerging possibilities for rating children's use of ER strategies (Mirabile, 2014; In-Albon et al., 2021). For example, Mirabile's (2014) new scales measure children's tendencies to use self-directed speech, instrumental coping, information gathering, social distraction, object distraction, self-soothing, comfort seeking, and support seeking. The maladaptive ER scale consists of children's focus on the distressing object, venting, aggression, avoidance, and suppression. The MeKKI computerized measure of ER consists of vignettes that children respond to by choosing ER strategies (In-Albon et al., 2021). Given further validation and usage, these scales could be interesting additions to this group of measures. It also should be noted that I did not include the CBQ's Effortful Control scale because it gets at, to my mind, self-regulation abilities that are more "cool" than ER. It does what it does excellently, but is not truly a measure of ER.

### **SUMMARY: Recommended Measures of Emotion Regulation**

The ERC is the only ER measure that appears "ready to go." It has moderate-to-adequate reported psychometrics and is brief. Documentation is sparse and more evaluation of fair usage with diverse samples are still needed, but the research base (as noted in earlier chapters here!) is truly formidable, and thus formative assessment and potentially screening could be accomplished using this measure. I recommend it as long as users realize its conflation of expressiveness and regulation, along with the items examining a few other areas like empathy. The BRIEF-P also holds promise. Clearly there are gaps that necessitate research on both parent- and teacher-report ratings systems, as well as any sort of brief but ecologically valid observation, for assessing early childhood ER.

## Battery Usage

Because of the significance of emotional competence to positive outcomes, and the multiplicity of skills within its components, we suggest using a battery of measures targeting all components. Given the measures previously described, parents and teachers do have several assessment tools with which to try to capture children's emotional competence. Assessors should aim for the most practical, which is often also the most efficient, method for data collection, using measures that are, cumulatively, the least taxing. Thus, a battery consisting of the MPAC-R/S, the CBQ (and the CBQ-VSF), the SCBE-30, the ERC, and the AKT-S, when fully administered together, would allow professionals to collect data on emotional expression, emotion knowledge, and ER, the three cornerstones of emotional competence. Full-battery administration also provides a multimethod approach to assessment, allowing for a more comprehensive profile of the child's social–emotional competencies, as each tool offers a unique perspective.

Of course, the burdens of time and training are important issues. Further, certain situations may call for only a single facet of emotional competence to be addressed. Depending on the goals for assessment, whole classrooms or only selected students in each classroom may be assessed. In such cases, a careful review of the tools comprising my proposed battery should provide practitioners a guide as to what would best meet their needs. Although a few of the measures proposed (e.g., MPAC-R/S, AKT-S), require training for administration in their current state, the arrival of specifically targeted teacher- and parent-friendly computerized assessments (currently under development) should reduce prerequisite training to a minimum without overburdening assessors cognitively or financially.

It should be clear by now that emotional competence assessment is a complex matter that needs to be addressed from a number of simultaneous directions and by a number of constituents, and that to some extent it lags behind current assessment methods in other domains. Along with Kendziora, Weissberg, and Dusenbury (2011), I can make several recommendations to hopefully identify clear action steps for educators' emotional competence measurement. First and foremost, it is imperative that schools, school systems, and states evaluate the system depicted in Figure 13.3 from the standpoint of emotional competence, and determine the specific, defined needs for and the functions of *their usage* of emotional competence assessment (hopefully after creating freestanding standards).

Presumably, the main goal of emotional competence assessment is to elucidate children's strengths and weaknesses in the area and assist in making data-informed decisions that help to facilitate their development, thereby fostering broad, long-term positive outcomes. The means by which these outcomes can be realized is via planning assessment-based classroom instruction and broader emotional competence programming. These goals, as illustrated in Figure 13.3, are the main reasons to undertake the process of emotional competence assessment, which requires personal and economic resources from everyone concerned—from students, to teachers, to administrators (Kendziora et al., 2011). However, there are other important uses of such a battery of measures: as already mentioned, emotional competence assessment can also be used for tracking the success of programming, making fiscal decisions, and demonstrating evidence for policy changes. It is encouraging that states are beginning to make alignments among these purposes and assessment (Caron et al., 2017; Olson, 2021).

In theory, any technology that enables educators at the classroom, school, district, and/or state levels to store data and generate multiple reports for multiple audiences allows them to not only gather data from students but to analyze it in ways that serve these different purposes. Thus, future developers and users of emotional competence assessments should work together to ascertain the uses for specific tools and the ability of any one assessment to perform multiple assessment functions. Clearly the field needs to come to a resolution of these issues—even if some solutions are somewhat parochial—concerning how any emotional competence assessment is best used.

After such functional decisions are made, the strengths and limitations of individual assessment tools must be recognized and choices must be made by states, school systems, and schools as to which ones to use. In this battery, I included what I consider to be useful emotional competence assessment tools for educational settings, but each set of stakeholders must evaluate what tools to use given their own specific needs. And, of course, the broader social–emotional measures already mentioned, including those for emotional competence, could be utilized when systems need to examine more comprehensive outcomes.

How can this rather daunting task be accomplished? One method is by returning to the criteria enumerated earlier following Denham, Wyatt, et al. (2009) and Kendziora et al. (2011), and creating a system to check in detail that these criteria are met as best as possible. In Table 13.1, I attempted to depict each assessment measure for both the suggested battery and possible other uses, according to as many criteria for which I could find information.

### SUMMARY: Battery Usage and Emotional Competence Assessment

Even given my suggestions for such an emotional competence battery, much work needs to be done—from the very acknowledgment of the importance of emotional competence, to the creation of standards, to their connections with assessment and instruction, and to the implementation of professional development for teachers in both SEL instruction and assessment. Although these endeavors are likely to be effortful, the rewards promise to be well worth it. I now address what I consider to be useful programming that could be enriched by the assessment tools already described.

## EFFECTIVE EMOTIONAL COMPETENCE PROGRAMMING

All children deserve to develop emotional competence, and caring adults want to assist in this developmental endeavor. Universal emotional competence programming needs to be part of all early childhood education and figures prominently in the educational system I propose in Figure 13.3. Further, when some aspect of the development of emotional expressiveness, such as the understanding of emotion or ER, is hindered during the preschool years—whether because of contributions from the child or the environment or some mixture of the two, as noted in Chapter 12—targeted interventions are necessary.

If potential problems have been flagged because of these conditions, and appropriate assessment of emotional competence has been conducted, then targeted instructional programming is even more necessary. For example, a child with autistic tendencies may have a particular difficulty attending to and understanding emotional cues in his or her environment. Another child, with a history of physical abuse, may have episodes of freezing when peers express anger, alternating with her or his own unbridled expressions of rage. A third child, who is at risk owing to living in a chaotic, low-income environment and having adverse childhood experiences, may understandably experience real ER difficulties. Fine-grained interventions targeted at milestones of emotional competence are clearly called for in these cases.

Despite the importance of targeted programming, however, a good way to start is to investigate the proliferating universal programming available for preschool children, which often supports children with targeted needs as well. First, several meta-analyses have noted the efficacy of programming for kindergartners' and older children's SEL (which includes the components of emotional competence; e.g., Durlak et al., 2011; Sklad, Diekstra, Ritter, Ben, & Gravesteijn, 2012; Taylor, Oberle, Durlak, & Weissberg, 2017). In Durlak et al. (2011) the reviewed programs showed improvement compared to control groups in social–emotional skills, behavior problems, and academic performance (see also Sklad et al., 2012). The benefits of programming held true from kindergarten through high school in urban, suburban, and rural schools. The benefits were as equally great in both teacher-led and researcher-led programming, but documentation of appropriate, accurate implementation of any program surfaced as a key issue. No program can be truly successful if it is improperly undertaken.

Taylor et al. (2017) provided evidence that the programs' benefit for social–emotional skills, behavior problems, and academic performance was significant at follow-up periods from 6 months to 18 years, and that such benefits did not vary by students' race, SES, or geographical location. Moreover, there were significant positive effect sizes for outcomes, such as school attendance, dropout rates, safe sexual behavior, and juvenile justice involvement. Thus, social–emotional programming works (although this statement is not without some controversy; Humphrey, 2013). These were obviously groundbreaking studies that confirmed a key tenet of this book, the importance of social–emotional development.

There are several criteria for quality programming identified in these earlier meta-analyses that are pertinent for promoting young children's emotional competence. Durlak et al. (2011) summarize these criteria by the acronym SAFE: (1) Sequenced—lessons are connected and coordinated, consistent in providing clear objectives and activities, clear in their contribution to the overall program goals; (2) Active—active rather than passive modes of learning are used; (3) Focused—any useful program involves at least one of the components of emotional competence considered important here; and (4) Explicit—lessons are explicit in terms of the component emotional competence skill that is the goal. Individual lesson plans or activities need to be consistent in providing clear objectives and activities as well as a clear rationale for their contribution to the overall program goals. There is nothing surer to hamper the momentum of programming than a lesson or series of lessons that "don't make sense" to the teacher or parent.

In addition, for the most positive, long-lasting results the following actions are crucial: (1) infusing emotional competence throughout all teaching, (2) individualizing emotional competence program goals as much as possible, (3) creating opportunities for emotional competence skills application throughout the day, and (4) rewarding students for using their emotional competence in daily interactions. It's also crucial that all the adults and all the environments in a child's life, both proximal and distal (e.g., parents, teachers, and all school personnel), should be involved in emotional competence programming. Thus, for the best possible outcomes, this goal requires schoolwide coordination and, ultimately, school–family and school–community partnerships (Payton et al., 2000; see Denham & Bassett, 2018, for more details).

The quality of program implementation also must be assessed as it relates to emotional competence outcomes. Implementation assistance must exist in the form of formal, in-depth training and technical support, and performance feedback to teachers, as well as in guidelines, procedures, and instruments for planning and monitoring program implementation. Users need to be able to see whether programming is proceeding as expected, and if not, why—so that they may modify and improve our programming.

Given these criteria for quality programming, I now shift to examining preschool emotional competence programming more explicitly. In what follows I focus, except where indicated, on universal programming in preschool (both public and private) and childcare facilities. Several recent meta-analyses confirm the efficacy of such programs (e.g., Blewitt, Fuller-Tyszkiewicz, et al., 2018). First, Blewitt, Fuller-Tyszkiewicz, and colleagues' (2018) analysis of universal, center-based implementation of social–emotional programs indicated medium effect sizes for emotional competence outcomes (i.e., emotion knowledge and ER). These authors suggested that social–emotional programs delivered at a relatively low intensity, despite some differences in theory of change, breadth of domains, and the specific skills addressed, may promote positive outcomes in 2- to 6-year-olds. Second, Luo, Reichow, Snyder, Harrington, and Polignano (2022) used 30 studies involving over 10,000 children and found small effect sizes for emotional competence outcomes of programming. In these studies effects did not differ by various moderating factors.

Third, Murano, Sawyer, and Lipnevich (2020) also undertook a meta-analysis of 48 studies with over 15,000 preschool students, specifically those whose classes participated in randomized control trials or rigorous quasi-experimental studies. They too found a small overall effect for emotional competence. Importantly, these authors found larger overall effect sizes for at-risk children, showing that emotional competence programming may benefit children differentially. They also noted, even though the data were sparse, that lower fidelity and more randomization were associated with smaller overall effect sizes. The direct assessment of children was associated with larger effect sizes.

Fourth, Yang, Datu, Lin, Lau, and Li (2019) examined 29 studies, and found a small effect size for emotion knowledge, a medium effect size for lessening negative emotions, and a large effect size for increasing positive feelings; however, these outcomes were included in relatively few studies. This meta-analysis contrasted SEL-focused and non-SEL-focused programming, and, unsurprisingly, the effects on positive and negative social–emotional outcomes were larger for SEL-focused programs; they were also larger for programs with a greater fidelity of implementation.

Fifth, one meta-analysis that I discovered examined a single aspect of emotional competence. Sprung, Münch, Harris, Ebesutani, and Hofmann (2015) examined whether emotion knowledge training was effective for improving the emotion knowledge constructs in Pons et al.'s (2004) theory. They found robust medium-to-large effect sizes for early childhood emotion knowledge training, unrelated to the length of training and other moderators.

Finally, the federally funded Head Start CARES project was a large evaluation of social–emotional programming for preschoolers. The project was a large-scale endeavor including a total of 307 classrooms and over 3,600 children (Mattera, Lloyd, Fishman, & Bangser, 2013). In contrast to an overall examination of emotional competence programming exemplified in the meta-analyses, its goal was to put in place a large-scale demonstration of preschool programming for social–emotional competence that was different from small studies that have tight controls and extensive resources. Specifically, even though the project did include ongoing teacher training and coaching, technical assistance, and continuous monitoring that extended beyond "typical" implementation of such programming, Head Start CARES can be considered an effectiveness study. That is, investigators sought to understand whether fully developed interventions that already have been shown efficacious under ideal or limited conditions can be well implemented under more typical conditions. The demonstration evaluation indicated that teacher practice did change according to specific program goals, and social–emotional child outcomes that were key or even more ancillary to each program were affected (Hsueh, Lowenstein, Morris, Mattera, & Bangser, 2014; Mattera et al., 2013; Morris et al., 2014). I remark upon the findings from this project in evaluating two of the programs included within it.

Taken as a whole, these results are very encouraging, but it is necessary to remember that many evaluation studies included in meta-analyses do have limitations, in areas such as variability in delivery, the type and adequacy of assessment, the outcomes measured, the use of control groups, random assignment, and follow-up procedures (Mondi, Giovanelli, & Reynolds, 2021). Much improvement can be made.

Nonetheless, given these very positive meta-analytic findings, I introduce five comprehensive programs that specifically address emotional competence skills and have been evaluated: Preschool PATHS, Incredible Years, Al's Pals, Emotion Based Prevention, and Preschool RULER programs. The first two programs were studied recently by the Head Start CARES project (Hsueh et al., 2014; Morris et al., 2014) (see also Camras & Halberstadt, 2017, and Denham & Bassett, 2018, for other descriptions of exemplary programs), and the other three are included because they centrally refer to emotional competence. All five programs have been evaluated for use with low-income preschoolers.

A theory of change can be put forward regarding emotional competence programming (Morris et al., 2014). First, plans for programming include support for implementation, such as training, coaching, resources, understanding contextual factors affecting children (e.g., poverty, cultural factors), and resultant teacher delivery. Given the support for implementation, teachers' practices in the classroom must change, to allow for improvements in classroom support for emotional competence and positive behavior management, and, ultimately, children developing emotional competence skills.

The following important aspects of programming flesh out this theory of change (White, Moore, Fleer, & Anderson, 2017): (1) a strong rationale for the program, which affects stakeholders' (i.e., all school personnel and parents) buy-in; (2) specific programmatic content that facilitates student engagement, such as use of puppets and scripted lessons; (3) intensity of programming (frequency and duration); (4) family involvement; and (5) racial/ethnic/linguistic and other inclusive diversity factors. Further, Humphries and Keenan (2006) assert the need to consider the following when evaluating programs: (1) theoretical orientation, to guide the creation of programs and production of supportive research; (2) developmental appropriateness; (3) cultural relevance; and (4) symptom reduction versus behavior promotion. I consider the five key programs, keeping this theory of change and these important elements in mind (see also Bierman & Motamedi, 2015).

## Preschool PATHS

The Preschool PATHS curriculum, a newer extension of an effective elementary school program, Promoting Alternative Thinking Strategies (PATHS; Greenberg, Kusché, & Mihalic, 1998), has been evaluated as effective both by CASEL (2012) and the Head Start CARES project (Morris et al., 2014). Preschool PATHS' goals are to maximize the environmental conditions that nurture and reward the development and application of the skills of SEL (not only emotional competence, but also social problem solving and social behaviors).

The preschool version of PATHS delivers 33 brief "circle-time" lessons to promote social–emotional competences, including (1) giving compliments; (2) friendship skills and prosocial behaviors; (3) understanding basic and advanced feelings via enriched linguistic experiences, concentrated on mediating the understanding of emotions in self and other; (4) social problem solving (i.e., integrating emotional understanding with cognitive and linguistic skills to analyze and solve problems; children learn that feelings are signals that communicate useful social information); and (5) the "Turtle Technique" as a tool to promote ER. Lessons are performed once or twice a week and use many supportive materials, such as stories, role plays, pictures, and puppets.

A fuller description of the Turtle Technique is warranted here. Children are taught this clever method to control negative feelings (Kusché & Greenberg, 1995a, 1995b; Robin, Schneider, & Dolnick, 1976; Schneider & Robin, 1978). They are encouraged to retreat into their "turtle shell" when they feel hurt or angry, crossing their arms in front of their body to comfort themselves and make disruptive behavior more difficult, and taking deep breaths. This practice can give them time to reflect on their feelings and decide how to react to the cause of these feelings when they come out of their shell.

Teachers also talk through the emotions being felt and help children express and channel these feelings effectively.

Thus regarding emotional competence, Preschool PATHS aims to develop children's awareness of their own and others' emotions and to teach ER. Crucial to the success of the PATHS curriculum is the training and ongoing support that teachers receive to use extension activities and integrate PATHS concepts throughout the preschool day whenever children experience an emotional reaction or a challenging situation. Using language to support ER also is a particular goal that is maximized by such scaffolding. Teachers are trained to use emotion language and to help children use their own and to dialogue with children to manage frustration and conflicts.

In terms of evaluation, in one randomized trial Preschool PATHS increased children's emotion knowledge, social skills, social competence, and social independence, and decreased social withdrawal, when compared to the control group (Domitrovich, Cortes, & Greenberg, 2007). A second study included Preschool PATHS as part of the Head Start REDI program, which also included a literacy intervention. In this study too children demonstrated increased emotion knowledge (Bierman, Domitrovich, et al., 2008; Bierman, Nix, Greenberg, Blair, & Domitrovich, 2008). In a third study, which included a web-based professional development program (Hamre, Pianta, Mashburn, & Downer, 2012), children's frustration tolerance increased.

Two studies examined the program under more "normal" conditions. In the Head Start CARES evaluation, Preschool PATHS showed small-to-moderate improvements in children's emotion knowledge, as well as in their social problem-solving skills and social behaviors (Morris et al., 2014). The demonstration evaluation found that teachers became better at teaching about emotions, supporting children's emotional expression and ER, and facilitating the understanding of peers' emotions, with good implementation. In another study of a scaled-up version of Preschool PATHS, Moore et al. (2015) evaluated a comprehensive public prekindergarten program that combined Preschool PATHS with the more overarching High Scope curriculum. The findings included increases in emotion knowledge in kindergarten, and that 2-year rather than 1-year attendance in the program resulted in greater kindergarten scores on the Head Start Social Competence Scale, which heavily incorporates emotion knowledge and ER. It is encouraging to see Preschool PATHS adopted as part of successful public prekindergarten programming, but unfortunately the effects of the Preschool PATHS and High Scope curriculum could not be disentangled.

Echoing and integrating these studies, a systematic review of five studies showed mild-to-moderate impact of the program on emotion knowledge and ER (Stanley, 2019; see also Fishbein et al., 2016; Powell & Dunlap, 2009). Of note, Fishbein et al. (2016) point out that the training and support teachers receive from a PATHS coordinator is essential to excellent implementation, and that their evidence of children's increased ER was especially notable given the children's baseline level of problems and lack of social–emotional competence as well as the relative brevity of programming. Further, cross-cultural evaluations of Preschool PATHS have been performed in Croatia, Hong Kong, and Turkey (Gershon & Pelliterri, 2018). In countries other than the United States, these evaluations indicated improvements in emotion knowledge, ER, and increased positive expressiveness.

Over and above these specific improvements in emotional competence, Powell and Dunlap (2009) also note that Preschool PATHS is efficacious in terms of treatment fidelity and generalization, and in terms of use with ethnically and racially diverse groups of children. It is clear that Durlak et al.'s (2011) SAFE criteria are met by Preschool PATHS, and the CASEL evaluation highlights the program's attention to both schoolwide and family contexts, as well as the existence of tools not only to monitor children's progress but also the implementation of the program. As already noted, and to continue examining the evaluation criteria I have put forward, Preschool PATHS trains teachers to integrate the program throughout daily interactions with students and to acknowledge children's emotional competence accomplishments. Taken together, these findings are very impressive.

## The Incredible Years

The Incredible Years curriculum for preschoolers aims to reduce challenging behaviors in children by reinforcing programmatic themes both in school and at home. The multicomponent program includes: (1) teacher training on classroom management techniques and promoting children's prosocial behavior; (2) parent workshops focusing on behavior management; and (3) a child curriculum called Dinosaur School, with targeted outcomes including more than emotional competence (e.g., social problem solving, social behavior). In Dinosaur School, children also receive training emphasizing empathy, emotional literacy, and self-control (see also *www.incredibleyears.com*).

More specifically, the curriculum includes 30 lessons per year, implemented at least twice per week, with 15- to 20-minute large-group circle times followed by 20 minutes of small-group skill practice activities, with the following seven units: (1) learning school rules; (2) how to be successful in school; (3) emotional literacy, empathy, and perspective taking; (4) interpersonal problem solving; (5) anger management; (6) social skills; and (7) communication skills. The program includes the use of life-size puppets, Dinosaur homework activities, picture cue cards, and games to stimulate group discussion, cooperation, and skill building. In the classroom, teachers were encouraged to promote the skills taught in circle time lessons throughout the day during less-structured settings, such as during choice time, in the lunchroom, or on the playground (Webster-Stratton, Reid, & Stoolmiller, 2008).

Posttests immediately following the conclusion of programming including some elements of Dinosaur School (Brotman et al., 2005; Webster-Stratton, Reid, & Hammond, 2004) have shown program-specific improvements in child conduct problems at home and at school, and improvements in social competence with peers. Focusing specifically on outcomes of the full Dinosaur School program (implemented along with the teacher module), Webster-Stratton, Reid, and Stoolmiller (2008) found increases in children's ER and identification of positive emotions, along with teachers' positive classroom management strategies.

Still, perhaps because of the broad focus of The Incredible Years, its outcomes in emotional competence as defined here were not highlighted well until the Head Start CARES evaluation, which found improvements in children's emotion knowledge, as well as social problem-solving skills and social behaviors, and in teachers' positive behavior management (Morris et al., 2014). In this evaluation, The Incredible Years did not produce the expected impacts on children's problem behavior and self-regulation, except for the highest-risk children.

Similar to Preschool PATHS, Powell and Dunlap (2009) assert in their technical report that the Incredible Years program overall is efficacious in terms of treatment fidelity, replication across settings, and use with ethnically and racially diverse children. The program also follows Durlak et al.'s (2011) SAFE criteria. The CASEL evaluation highlights its attention to family but not schoolwide contexts, as well as the existence of tools to monitor the implementation of the program, but not program-specific child measures. In examining the evaluation criteria I have put forward, individualization and infusion are not emphasized. In short, The Incredible Years has much to offer, but from my viewpoint its focus is not quite as attuned to emotional competence as Preschool PATHS. It does what it does very well, but this is not its emphasis.

### *Significance of Preschool PATHS and Incredible Years Programming*

Improving children's understanding of emotions and ER (along with their social problem-solving skills and associated prosocial behaviors) may be accomplished either by supporting teachers' positive classroom management practices (as was done in The Incredible Years' teacher module) or their explicit teaching of emotional understanding and social skills through a more lessons-based approach and teacher scaffolding (as was done in Preschool PATHS and The Incredible Year's Dinosaur School). Head Start and other programs may therefore have some options in selecting models that best meet the needs of their teachers and centers, with likely benefits for the children they are serving. The Head Start CARES evaluation, which found positive results for both these approaches, was especially important because it shows that scaled-up, evidence-based models can have nearly the same results as those from smaller, controlled studies—when the programming is supported by more comprehensive professional development (see also Bierman & Motamedi, 2015).

## Al's Pals

Al's Pals is an early childhood prevention program and comprehensive social–emotional curriculum for children ages 3 to 8. It was included in CASEL's evaluation of programming, but not the Head Start CARES evaluation. Specifically for our purposes here, among numerous other goals, Al's Pals curriculum teaches young children to regulate their feelings and behaviors. A variety of materials are utilized during lessons, including puppets, books, and original music. Lessons consist of two 15- to 20-minute interventions per week for 23 weeks in total.

Al's Pals social–emotional curriculum has been implemented in 700 early childhood centers, preschools, childcare centers, and Head Start programs in 34 states in the United States, as of an early report (Lynch, Geller, & Schmidt, 2004). In the multiyear, multistate evaluation, findings indicated that Al's Pals strengthened children's social–emotional competence and positive coping skills, but the only emotional-competence outcome parallel to what I am covering here was a lessening of emotional distress. Moreover, a limitation of the study is that child outcome data were based primarily on teacher ratings; as noted earlier, such reliance could be subject to bias.

Even given the limitation of few emotional-competence outcomes, Powell and Dunlap (2009) classified Al's Pals as efficacious in terms of treatment fidelity, replication across investigators and locations, and use with ethnically and racially diverse groups. The CASEL Guide to Effective Social and Emotional Learning Programs deemed Al's Pals effective in increasing social behavior, reducing conduct problems, and reducing emotional distress based on a quasi-experimental design with both African American and White American students. It is weaker than Preschool PATHS and The Incredible Years regarding schoolwide and family contexts, and I am unsure of its focus on expanding the curricular contact to the day-to-day interaction between teachers and children or individualization with specific children. It does have program-specific measures of implementation and child outcomes. There have been no cross-cultural studies conducted with the Al's Pals program. So, like The Incredible Years program, Al's Pals has advantages, but given the lack of emotional-competence outcomes and recent research, as well as difficulties noted here, I am less enthusiastic about it.

## Emotion-Based Prevention for Head Start Children

This program was not evaluated by Head Start CARES or by CASEL. Nonetheless, I consider it potentially very important because of its complete dedication to emotional competence. The Emotion-Based Prevention (EBP) program for Head Start Children (Izard, King, et al., 2008; Izard, Trentacosta, King, & Mostow, 2004) uses differential emotions theory (see Chapter 1) to teach preschool-age children how to understand, regulate, and utilize emotions appropriately (i.e., effective and constructive use of emotion motivation, such as when modulated, vicarious sadness promotes sympathy). EBP uses puppets, vignettes, storybooks, interactive reading, and teacher–child dialoguing during difficult emotional experiences, to help structure children's learning. Each weekly lesson begins with a puppet show and ends with a storybook.

Teachers actively eliciting children's participation to label or demonstrate emotions, talk about feeling different intensities of emotions and what causes. Parents also receive weekly messages summarizing current lessons, with suggestions to extend the learning. Unique to this program is the substantial focus on the four "basic" emotions: happiness, sadness, anger, and fear, as well as its reliance on the intrinsic rewards associated with greater emotional competence (Izard, King, et al., 2008). Teachers are trained to react appropriately to children's emotions, and to provide emotion-specific support during their dialoguing with distressed children.

This program was first tested by Izard and colleagues in rural Head Start centers (Izard, Trentacosta, et al., 2004). A second study (Finlon et al., 2015) reevaluated the program in inner city Head Start classrooms after adaptations were made based on previous results. Both studies used randomized controlled trials of the EBP program, and the second study added the comparison of EBP to the established treatment program, I Can Problem Solve (Shure, 1993). Results of the two studies were drawn from teacher reports, direct child assessments, and independent observations, showing that

EBP showed increases in participating children's emotion knowledge and regulation (i.e., decreased negative emotion expression) when compared to the control groups. Additionally, EBP had beneficial impacts on positive social behaviors and on maladaptive and aggressive behaviors. In the second study, the findings showed that children experiencing stressful family circumstances or less-supportive classroom environments particularly benefited from EBP programming, more than from I Can Problem Solve.

Overall, I appreciate this program's clear emotional competence goals and find results on its use encouraging. In particular, its use with racially diverse groups and its explicit emphasis on infusion and individualization, as well as on family involvement are important. Scarce evaluation data and lack of information on attention to implementation somewhat limit my full recommendation for its use, but I definitely encourage further research.

## Preschool RULER

Finally, I would like to describe one more emotion-focused program that has not yet been as fully evaluated as the others reviewed here. Regarding emotional competence, Preschool RULER, based on emotional intelligence theory, emphasizes the explicit teaching of social and emotional skills with opportunities for real-life practice and exposure to strong teacher and parent modeling of these skills (Hoffman, Brackett, Bailey, & Willner, 2020; Rivers et al., 2013a, 2013b). Five key emotional skills are highlighted: recognizing, understanding, labeling, expressing, and regulating emotions.

Preschool RULER is an approach embedded throughout the preschool day rather than an approach that involves discrete weekly lessons. A feelings vocabulary is a central focus of the program, especially to aid with ER, and strategies for expressing emotions are role-played. The emotions of characters are highlighted when reading storybooks, and personal stories are shared with students to highlight teachers' experiences with emotion. Emotion-focused discussions take place throughout the school day (Rivers et al., 2013a, 2013b). The program employs several key tools to help young children with emotional self-regulation, including the mood meter, the blueprint, and the meta-moment (Rivers et al., 2013a, 2013b). The mood meter is used to help children learn how to identify their emotions throughout the classroom day, whereas the meta-moment is a several-step technique to help children stop and figure out a strategy to regulate their emotions. The blueprint is a process to help children identify feelings, their causes, and ways to handle them.

A pilot study of Preschool RULER was performed with ethnically diverse 3- to 5-year-olds, using the mood meter and tests of emotional labeling and recognition. Specifically, children's mood meter scores were associated significantly with social and emotional skills. In addition, during a second year of Preschool RULER implementation, children exhibited significantly higher scores on both emotional labeling and recognition than children at a control site (Bailey et al., 2019; Rivers et al., 2013a). Further emerging findings suggest that Preschool RULER may also have an impact on preliteracy skills. These results should be considered preliminary, despite a clear focus on emotional competence, because evaluation lacked randomization and follow-up. In any case, Preschool RULER bears watching.

## SUMMARY: Potential Emotional Competence Programming for Preschoolers

Preschool PATHS, the EBP program, and, given more evaluation, Preschool RULER, focus the most on specific emotional competencies of the programs I have presented here. More information on implementation quality (and the ease of implementation by early childhood personnel) and necessary treatment dosage is needed, and the ability to deliver programming across the diversity of early childhood settings should be considered when choosing emotional competence programming.

## Other Comprehensive Programs of Interest Around the World

Emotional competence programming also has been initiated outside the United States. I describe examples for which the focused measures of emotional competence were outcomes. Some of these programs are limited in scope (e.g., number of child participants, as in Wu, Zhang, Lin, Wu, & Li, 2021), but I include them here to give a sense of the current international scope and impetus behind emotional competence programming for young children.

For example, Ștefan and Miclea (2012; see also Ștefan, 2008; Ștefan & Miclea, 2010) evaluated a hybrid universal and indicated program they created in Romania. Components of the program addressed emotion knowledge, expression of empathy, and ER. Teachers were trained in behavior management, sharing the program with parents, and effective implementation. Children at risk for emotional competence problems improved on emotion knowledge, with sustained medium-to-large treatment effects. A later study (Ștefan & Miclea, 2013) found smaller effects for emotion expressive knowledge, whereas the findings from an earlier version (Ștefan, 2008) included not only increased emotion knowledge, but also greater observed positive emotion and empathy. Although these problem are not uncommon, Mondi and colleagues (2021) note that in these programs teachers both implemented and most often evaluated the programs, and program facets were not separately evaluated, limiting generalizability.

Emotional competence programming for preschoolers also is being carried out in Asia. For example, Wu and colleagues (2021) created a universal program for Chinese 5- to 6-year-olds, replete with ingenious lessons and activities about the causes and features of emotion, as well as hands-on practice and consideration of ER. Results showed that children's emotion knowledge increased, and parents reported that children increased their use of cognitive and problem-solving ER strategies, along with less-frequent venting. Lam and Wong (2017) created a program in Hong Kong that included teachers' work on their own emotional competence, as well as the implementation of a specially designed curriculum; the results included children's improvement in anger and anxiety.

## SUMMARY: International Emotional Competence Programs

It is clear that early childhood emotional competence is of major interest outside the United States, and many promising results have been found. More efforts need to be made, and, equally important, results of these programs need to be shared internationally. Moving forward to consider a "scaling up" of such programs needs to be monitored as well.

## Component-Specific Programs

### *Emotion Knowledge*

A program created in Italy shows that even toddlers, as well as preschoolers, can benefit from simple programming aimed at teaching them about emotion terms (Grazzani & Ornaghi, 2011; Grazzani, Ornaghi, Agliati, et al., 2016; Grazzani, Ornaghi, & Brockmeier, 2016; Ornaghi, Brazzelli, et al., 2017; Ornaghi, Brockmeier, & Gavazzi, 2011; Ornaghi et al., 2014, 2015; see also Fernández-Sánchez et al., 2015). The interventions were only 1 to 2 months in duration. Almost all involved 2- and 3-year-olds, with some findings accruing most strongly to the 3-year-olds. After teachers read specially prepared books including an enriched emotional and/or mental state lexicon, children then conversed about the books' content with teachers in structured, often game-like, ways.

Children who experienced this intervention showed growth in emotion knowledge, and where measured, emotion talk and prosocial orientation (mediated by emotion knowledge), independent of gains in verbal ability. Prosocial orientation was assessed via stories such as "Lucy is going to school with Francie. Francie is crying because she tripped on a stone and fell down and hurt herself. How do you think the story will end?" In another study (Ornaghi et al., 2015) with 4- and 5-year-old children, their poststory conversations also included a discussion of ER; the 6 weeks of training prompted increases in emotion knowledge and prosocial orientation.

The simplicity of this programming, its short duration, and the young age of many participants benefiting from it, are of interest. The stories read by the teachers are very engaging, and teachers are trained to also augment their postreading conversations with emotion and mental state language, and to direct the conversation in a game-like fashion, involving all the children, to help them grasp the link between feelings and behavior. The training is notable in enhancing the emotion knowledge of young preschoolers at a time when it is rapidly developing.

In Spain, a program focusing on improving emotion knowledge and social competence with 4- and 5-year-olds used dialoguing and Socratic questioning to involve children deeply in issues within their everyday lives (Giménez-Dasí, Quintanilla, & Daniel, 2013). Both target behaviors showed improvement for the older children, but only social competence improved for the 4-year-olds. Perhaps the deep questioning was more useful to the older group. Finally, German teachers were taught language support strategies that they then applied during emotion talk accompanying picture book reading, emotion reminiscing, and everyday conversations with preschoolers. This intervention resulted in children's increased emotion knowledge (Voltmer & von Salisch, 2022). Language thus plays a large role in teachers' promotion of preschoolers' emotion knowledge, and successful programming emanates from its successful use.

### *Emotion Regulation*

Another program focused on emotion knowledge and ER, as well as on social competence (Giménez-Dasí, Fernández-Sánchez, & Quintanilla, 2015). For 6 months, 2-year-olds experienced activities on emotion identification (e.g., finding pictures of specific emotions around the room); emotion labeling/expression (e.g., naming or expressing an emotion on a die after rolling it); the cause of emotions (e.g., puppets enact an emotion, children name it and say why it happened); and ER strategies (e.g., "What can the puppet do to feel better?"). The results of the program indicated that children improved in emotion knowledge and slightly on ER as measured by the ERC.

One program focused even more specifically on ER. Romero-López, Pichardo, Justicia-Arráez, and Bembibre-Serrano (2021) taught children to use the Turtle Technique and progressive relaxation as supports for ER when they were upset. Further, they used many other games and activities, such as social dilemmas in which one protagonist had strong negative feelings that needed to be resolved—the ensuing discussion also included children's reflections on similar situations and how they felt and dealt with their feelings. There were also many other activities, such as the "emotion dice"—a dice with different emotions on each side. After rolling the dice, children could reflect on how to control or deal with emotions and draw situations in which they felt the same way as the emotion depicted on the dice. At the end of the program, children who had experienced it had fewer ER difficulties as assessed by the BRIEF-P.

### **SUMMARY:** Component-Specific Programming

There may be situations that call for focus on one or another component of emotional competence, or systems that wish to exercise control over choosing different programming across these components. These programs seem to have been largely developed in Europe, so that exporting them to other areas would require testing in new settings. Nonetheless, their focus on specific aspects of emotional competence is very comprehensive and should be studied further.

## Multicomponent "Overall" Programs

So far, I have discussed programming that deals specifically with emotional competence (or more broadly on social–emotional competence), as delivered by teachers, parents, and the media. It also is important to consider the impact of preschool programming in general—can quality preschool and childcare, both curricular and otherwise, impact children's emotional competence. It may. For example, the Child–Parent Center Early Educational Intervention program in Chicago serves many low-income, racially, and ethnically diverse prekindergartens. Founded in the 1960s, it is embedded in public school settings and emphasizes (1) collaborative leadership, (2) effective learning experiences, (3) alignment between evidence-based curricula and instructional practices, (4) parent involvement and engagement, (5) professional development for educators, and (6) continuity and stability from prekindergarten through third grade

(Reynolds & Mondi, 2016). The program focuses on enhancing children's overall development and school readiness.

Children who participated in this program showed slightly higher social–emotional skills at the beginning of kindergarten and greater growth over the kindergarten year (Mondi & Reynolds, 2021; see also Reynolds, Richardson, Hayakawa, Englund, & Ou, 2016). The assessment tool in this study was broader than emotional competence, however; teachers completed the social–emotional domain of the Gold assessment—this assessment includes nine items, of which one refers specifically to ER, and one to emotion knowledge. To bolster this argument, however there are several other evaluations of emotional competence within programs not necessarily focusing on this outcome, but with salutary effects (Mondi et al., 2021; Reynolds & Mondi, 2016).

### SUMMARY: Comprehensive Programming

Given the push for quality improvement in early childhood education (Olson, 2021), it makes sense to query whether comprehensive prekindergarten programming also can promote children's emotional competence. The results of Reynolds's work especially suggest paying further attention to the potential usefulness of excellent, comprehensive early childhood programs promoting emotional competence even without zeroing in on more specific programming, such as Preschool PATHS. Perhaps the most efficacious method of all would be to implement both excellent comprehensive programming and emotion-specific curriculum elements.

## "Kernels" of Practice: Teacher Behaviors That Work for Emotional Competence

At the same time, an even more molecular view of teaching may be useful.

In Chapter 9, teachers' contributions as emotion socializers were discussed. In this discussion, their actual socialization *behaviors* were highlighted. The findings reported suggest that many interactions that preschoolers have with their teachers are important for the growth of emotional competence, irrespective of specific curricula, interventions, or training programs. To reiterate, showing authentic, often positive emotions, responding with support but also promoting growth in children's emotions, and teaching about emotions are behaviors that I endorsed. And recall the notion that there are moment-to-moment "kernels" of instruction that promote emotional competence. Thus I remind the reader of the importance of such emotion-rich interactions with children, as well as teachers' own emotional competence.

Aside from the lessons, activities, and materials that teachers provide, a consideration of the ways in which teachers learn to interact with children while implementing the programs mentioned here also could be useful. Several specifics have been uncovered. These include, for example, incidental teaching, scaffolding, and coaching of emotion knowledge and ER, along with individualizing learning for specific children, giving them feedback and opportunities for rehearsal (Moore et al., 2015). Further, it is worth stressing here the large literature on the salutary effects of a warm teacher–child relationship (Blewitt, Morris, et al., 2018).

### SUMMARY: "Kernels" of Everyday Teaching Interactions

Thus there is much that teachers can do and *be* that promotes emotional competence in young children. Zinsser et al. (2018) call this "social–emotional teaching," and as noted in Chapter 9, reiterate the importance of preschool teachers' own emotional competence. More emphasis is needed on how teachers, in doing what they normally do in the classroom and in just being themselves, promote emotional competence for the children under their care. Also, as discussed in Chapter 9, support for teachers' classroom practices and their own emotional competence is needed to fully realize the value of "kernels" of everyday teaching.

## Parent- and Media-Based Programming for Emotional Competence

Parents can also learn to be more effective emotion socializers. There are several efficacious programs for parents as socializers of emotion. England-Mason and Gonzalez (2020) have reviewed evaluations of such programming. One program, Tuning into Kids (TIK; Havighurst & Harley, 2007; Havighurst, Wilson, Harley, & Prior, 2009) teaches parents to be more positive emotion socializers to ultimately foster children's emotional competence. The main goals are to becoming less dismissing of children's emotions and more able to help them understand and regulate emotions. The participants are trained in the following steps: (1) awareness of children's emotions, (2) viewing children's emotions as a time for support and teaching, (3) helping children labeling emotions, (4) validating children's emotions, and (5) helping children problem-solve in upsetting situations. In one randomized trial evaluation of the program and another more recent evaluation on extending the study to Norway, parents participating in the intervention reported significant improvements in their own emotion awareness and regulation, increases in emotion coaching, decreases in emotionally dismissive beliefs and behaviors, and increases in emotion talk and encouragement for children to talk about emotions (Bjørk, Bølstad, Pons, & Havighurst, 2022; Havighurst, Wilson, Harley, Prior, & Kehoe, 2010). They were more likely to view their children's anger and sadness as times for closeness rather than avoidance. Obviously, all these aspects of socialization of emotion have been shown to be very important, as discussed in Chapters 7 through 9. Consequently, in studies in which the authors assessed young children's emotional competence, improvements were evident. For example, in Havighurst et al. (2010), children evidence less lability/negativity on the ERC, as well as greater teacher-rated emotion skills; in two other studies, preschoolers' child emotional knowledge improved (Bjørk et al., 2022; Havighurst et al., 2013). Subsequent programming has been extended to parents of toddlers (Lauw, Havighurst, Wilson, Harley, & Northam, 2014) and to fathers (Havighurst, Wilson, Harley, & Kehoe, 2019).

TIK also has been introduced in Asia. In one trial (Chan, Qui, & Shum, 2021; Qiu & Shum, 2021), mothers of preschoolers were randomly assigned to either participate in the intervention or be placed on a waiting list. Mothers in the training group demonstrated increases in positive emotion socialization, including more expressive encouragement and emotion-focused reactions to children's emotion expressions, and lower levels of punitive and emotional-dismissing reactions. These improvements persisted and were accompanied by other, delayed improvements as well as decreases in children's negativity/lability (Chan et al., 2021). Collectively, these findings are the first evidence in a non-Western sample to support the effectiveness of the TIK program. However, even more child outcomes would be useful.

Parents (usually mothers) also have participated in even more focused training, such as learning to reminisce productively about emotional experiences so as to facilitate their young children's development of emotion knowledge. Mothers' emotion-rich, elaborative reminiscing about emotions, which I have discussed in Chapters 8 and 12 (e.g., Van Bergen, Salmon, Dadds, & Allen, 2009), increased with training and facilitated children's emotion knowledge (Valentino et al., 2019). Even more specifically, maltreated preschoolers' emotion knowledge approximated that of nonmaltreated youngsters, even controlling for baseline levels and verbal ability, after their mothers participated in training that included live reminiscence practice focusing on emotion identification and causal thinking, along with learning the Turtle Technique (although child ER was not measured, this technique could allow maltreated children a way to feel safe in emotional situations and to allow them to learn about emotions more readily).

Even media programming can be useful in promoting preschoolers' emotional competence, although not much has been done in this area. However, there is emotion-focused content in some children's TV and apps. The use of the PBS *Daniel Tiger* app and watching the *Daniel Tiger's Neighborhood* show were associated with preschoolers' learning to use the ER strategies taught in these media: (1) counting to four and taking a deep breath to calm down when angry, (2) finding ways to pass the time until feeling better when feeling sad, and (3) looking for some good in a situation when disappointed. Further, for 3- and 4-year-olds (the younger group in this study) who used the *Daniel Tiger* app, emotion knowledge was greater 1 month after the intervention. These media also facilitated parents' participation, although such participation did not mediate program effects on emotional competence in this brief intervention (Rasmussen et al., 2019).

Educational media also have the potential to augment emotional competence programming in preschool classrooms. One such program is Sesame Workshop's toolkit, Little Children, Big Challenges: General Resilience, to foster social–emotional skills (LCBC; Sesame Workshop, 2013; Oades-Sese, Cahill, Allen, Rubic, & Mahmood, 2021). The toolkit provides teachers with resources and video clips that enable them to take an interactive, multisensory, integrated pedagogical approach to help children cope with and understand challenging situations in the classroom and at home. To date, there has been no research on the effectiveness of this toolkit on improving social–emotional competence of preschool children, however.

## SUMMARY: Parent- and Media-Based Programming

Despite being somewhat ancillary to classroom-based programming, given my focus on early childhood education, the parenting and media programs mentioned here deserve close scrutiny. The TIK suite holds promise to engage parents; means of embedding it in early childhood education. Media programming like *Daniel Tiger* could be introduced profitably to parents as well, although methods of embedding it in early childhood education have not, to my knowledge been undertaken. In contrast, Sesame Workshop's program could be used, perhaps extracting emotional competence-pertinent aspects. The conclusion I reach here is one of enthusiasm for these programs, but caution as well in determining how to utilize them to their full benefit while integrating them with other suggestions I've already made here.

## SUMMARY: Programming

Thus there are programs that offer useful evidence on their capacity to enhance preschoolers' emotional competence. However, continued evaluation research would of course be welcome. Even though I have tried to present excellent research here, we must continue to push for *quality* research—we need to move beyond single, nonblind informants and lack of appropriate control groups. We need to *require* information on implementation fidelity, figure out how to evaluate different parts of programs, such as the components of The Incredible Years, and more often offer longitudinal follow-up.

I humbly offer a program that I developed with my colleague Rosemary Burton to show what went right and what went wrong, to bolster these arguments. Even before the creation of Preschool PATHS, we created a social–emotional intervention for at-risk 4-year-olds (Denham & Burton, 1996). Teachers were trained in behavior management and in performing activities associated with relationship building, emotional understanding, and social problem solving over a 32-week period. The children's social–emotional status was assessed via observation and teacher questionnaire at the beginning and end of the period and compared to a group who did not experience the intervention. Children who had the intervention, compared to children who did not experience it, were observed showing decreases in negative emotion and increases in positive expressiveness, greater involvement, and more initiative in positive peer activity, and were seen as improving socially by their teachers. Children who had the lowest pretest scores benefited the most. So, although I was not yet in a position—theoretically or practically—to focus solely on emotional competence outcomes, these promising results did occur.

These were good outcomes, and there also were more qualitative ones. Some stories related by the children and teachers tell volumes.

> One little boy, who initially had trouble controlling his anger, had a protracted, heated argument in which he and another child negotiated their difficulty over ownership of a toy. He proudly announced, "See, I used my words, not my hands!"
>
> Another boy was frightened at a doctor's appointment and happened to see his teacher; he asked her to please read him the "Turtle Story" because he needed it "right now!" (to help him gain control of scary feelings). She did read it to him, and it helped!

Giving these boys tools of emotional competence assisted them during difficult moments. Moreover, qualitative analyses also show that teachers' efforts to make their whole curriculum emotion centered were vital contributors to individual growth (Burton & Denham, 1999).

But we made mistakes, many due to lack of support. We could not randomize our treatment and control groups, and teachers obviously were not uninformed as to treatment (see also Mondi et al., 2021; Reynolds & Mondi, 2016). Our implementation checks were very elementary.

Further, and importantly, even though the teachers were very enthusiastic, and it felt like a team had been created, we nonetheless were somewhat unclear in some of our cultural assumptions (e.g., how our techniques suited the largely African American culture of the teachers and children—ideas that I put forward in the discussion of culture and ethnicity issues in Chapter 9). It is *imperative* to consider matters of culture when enacting emotional competence programming (Humphries & Keenan, 2006; Humphries et al., 2018). Although we made an effort to take culture into account, the matter may go even deeper: as emphasized by Humphries et al. (2018), as a field we need to *listen to teachers*; they are not fond of scripted curricula, especially those that do not include the voices and faces familiar to the children in their care. Teachers know they have a responsibility to teach emotional competence but require contextual relevance and support from administrators and parents.

Additionally, although we did implement individualization and infusion, we were not clear enough on how we did that to be useful to future researchers and users (Humphries & Keenan, 2006). We had great difficulties involving parents despite what we felt were heroic efforts. These parents were under stresses severe enough to likely engender ACEs in their children, and no amount of support could allow them the freedom to attend nighttime meetings, for example.

Finally, follow-up was lacking. After progressing into kindergarten, one girl told her former teacher, whom she sought out during extended childcare, "I know you taught me to talk instead of hit, but in kindergarten everyone hits. What do I do? Hit back?" Clearly, she had absorbed the basic message of this program and was straining to retain it in the new culture of primary school. It would have been best practice to follow her (and others') progress and even to transition to continued programming.

In short, we were very glad when Preschool PATHS was developed. Thus despite the clear needs that our intervention attempted to satisfy, subsequent developments have been encouraging, and teachers can utilize with confidence the programming put forward here.

To select from among the programs I have outlined to follow the general plan in Figure 13.3, several points should be made. Obviously, the cost and ease of implementation must be considered, and decisions about whether to implement it universally or as a prevention after screening are required. An examination of extant research to determine any program's scale-up potential also is necessary. Given the issues brought up in Chapter 9 about the lack of training, professional development and *ongoing* support is a must (Bierman & Motamedi, 2015). Allowance for the "kernels of teaching" ingredient is important, as is the connection of any competence programming with existing curricula.

Involving parents also is crucial, because parents are still their children's first socializers, with whom they spend many hours. But engaging parents can be difficult, and as we learned in our project, many efforts to engage parents as partners in emotional competence programming show disappointing rates of enrollment and attendance (Bierman & Motamedi, 2015). Consideration of cultural meaning is paramount.

## CONCLUSION

It should be obvious both how much work has been done on developing both emotional-competence assessment tools and programming for early childhood educational systems. I have presented criteria for how emotional competence training fits within early childhood education, discussed important considerations for assessment and programming, and introduced both assessment tools and many varied programs.

I agree wholeheartedly with Jones, Barnes, Bailey, and Doolittle (2017) about aligning assessment and programming. As I've illustrated by limiting my discussion of assessment tools to only those addressing emotional competence, we must use excellent, developmentally appropriate, narrow but deeper, emotional competence measures, matched to the skills that programs seek to impart. Similarly, I agree with these authors, as I've suggested in Chapter 9, that we must focus on changes in teachers' own emotional competence and the classroom emotional environment. At the same time, I heed Humphries and colleagues' (2018) calls for needed attention to culturally embedded program design, training, and implementation. Clearly *much* work remains to be done, but we stand in a good position to carry on this effort.

# 14

# Concluding Remarks

What is needed now, given the relative explosion of research into preschoolers' emotional competence, within the last 15 years? There is still much for researchers to do; they should not think that all has been solved! First, there are theoretical issues to consider. Conceptualization of ER and emotional experience still raises questions. The role of culture in the demonstration and socialization of emotional competence should be given even more attention because society is now global.

There also are empirical and applied issues for researchers to evaluate. Much more consideration of teachers' own emotional competence and their means of socializing young children's emotional competence is sorely needed at this point, along with integrating this knowledge with current approaches to professional development programming and assessment. Ways to help parents promote their children's emotional competence, and more research on the role of their own emotional competence that capitalizes on newer findings on their emotion regulation, are also required. These are challenges for the field that cannot be overlooked.

## ADVICE FOR PARENTS AND EARLY CHILDHOOD EDUCATORS

It is true that much research work awaits. But there is still a lot that is known. So what is the "takeaway message" here? What practical points can be gleaned from the information covered in this book? In order to answer this question, I point out what adults need to be aware of in terms of preschoolers' emotional competence and what they can do to foster it.

## What Adults Need to Be Aware of: Emotional Competence in General

Adults who play important roles in young children's lives need to know how children differ in terms of emotional competence, to be able to live harmoniously with them day by day and to help them develop into healthy, productive people. Specifically, caregivers and parents must recognize that there are important developmental and individual differences in preschoolers' emotional competence. If we are to interact with and nurture young children successfully, we need to be prepared for the differences in the emotional makeup between children at any one age level, as well as between children who differ in age.

Further, caregivers need to recognize that despite preschoolers' formidable abilities in emotional competence, limiting factors do exist. For example, before expecting certain levels of emotion knowledge, or particular expressive patterns, or specific means of ER, it would be wise to consider each individual child's age as well as his or her intellectual level. Other specific aspects of emotional competence must also be considered.

## What Adults Need to Be Aware of: Expressiveness

It is vital to keep up with preschoolers' increased emotional sophistication. The increasing subtlety and complexity of preschoolers' emotionality also need to be acknowledged, so that adults in their lives can support their development. For instance, the mother of a 4-year-old girl needs to be aware when her daughter shows a mixture of sadness and anger when arguing about getting ready for school; this blend has a different meaning than unalloyed defiance does. Assuming that the child is "fine" at school just because she does not appear overtly afraid is also a mistake. Too often adults "barrel ahead" without considering the growing emotional competence of their charges. So adults' accuracy in receiving their young charges' emotional signals and the subsequent appropriateness of their own emotional signals are especially important.

The manifestations and implications of toddlers' and preschoolers' new social and self-conscious emotions deserve careful attention. Parents, caregivers, and educators are motivated to promote the experience of sympathy, because of its association with concern and prosocial behavior. Emphasizing the importance of empathy and distinguishing between the subcomponents of sympathy and personal distress are the first steps. Then, if we can focus in on important parameters of the development of sympathy (e.g., similarity of experience), we can help facilitate children's healthy and rewarding interpersonal relationships.

The important adults in young children's lives will also want to be able to recognize guilt and shame when the children express them and to act in a supportive manner. They will want to cheer along when the children experience pride. No doubt they will also want to carefully assess their own role in engendering the experience of these complicated emotions.

With respect to embarrassment, caregivers, parents, and early childhood educators can help young children modify their perception that an audience is making fun of them, because of the potential debilitating effects of this belief. In everyday settings, children may think they are being made fun of when they are not. If a preschool boy freezes in fear and embarrassment when asked to sing a song with his classmates, he can be reassured that no one will laugh at him so that the discomfort of embarrassment can be avoided.

## What Adults Need to Be Aware of: Emotion Knowledge

Adult caregivers can make use of their preschoolers' emotion knowledge. For example, they can tailor their help in ER to those strategies that young children best understand. Consider a 5-year-old boy's feelings of great sadness when his pet dies. It may be a good idea for his father to suggest a visit to the amusement park together—after all, sadness *can* turn into happiness. He can also suggest that his son think about his upcoming fun at day camp. But telling him any variation on the theme of "time heals all wounds" will not be worthwhile!

The limits of young children's emotion knowledge need to be kept in mind as well. Recall that preschoolers do not really discern either guilt or shame as separate emotions; they just feel "sad" about transgression and failures. Parents, teachers, and caregivers need to know that this apparent lag in emotion knowledge is perfectly normal, and not an indication of budding sociopathy. Young children are very unlikely to say "I'm guilty" about a transgression, no matter how significant it is.

As important as it is to realize what young children do *not* understand about emotions, it is also necessary to think about what they *may* understand. In situations where they can be expected to experience ambivalent emotions, for example, young children may understand their caregivers' appropriate reference to such feelings even if they themselves do not spontaneously comment on them. Imagine a mother acting as if it were the most natural thing in the world for her 5-year-old daughter to feel happy and sad about the end of the school year. She mentions both those feelings in introducing the topic to the child as they drive home from the last day of kindergarten. The girl joins in this discussion freely, in relief; her mother has "hit the nail on the head," opening up talk about emotions that the child could not begin by herself.

## What Adults Need to Be Aware of: ER

Adults also need to consider how much support preschoolers in general need in order to accomplish ER. Often children under 6 need the comfort of a lap to soothe the physiological arousal of sadness or fear, a quiet conversation with a parent to give a name to their disquietude, and a big person's ideas about what to do about an emotional experience. As noted earlier (Chapter 5), preschoolers are taking their first small steps toward handling ER processes on their own.

In addition, particular preschoolers may have more or less ease in either supported or independent ER. Highly reactive children (who are easy to recognize!) need more support in their ER, and may need their supporters to be especially skillful in picking

ER strategies tailored to their needs. A little girl whose latency to express fear around animals is extremely short, accompanied by high-intensity arousal and a long recovery time, may be best served by an adult companion who plans ahead to avoid such situations and has a few tried-and-true means to help her feel better. A boy who is very *un*reactive may need an equally skillful adult to help him discern the mild arousal he does experience as emotion.

In short, ER is an area where adult partners are often vital across contexts and emotions. It is also important for adults to be attuned to ER and to know that their children can manage alone. An intrusive adult could have disrupted the fruitful ER "practice" of a girl who was quite capable of soothing her own ankle. As in any partnership, balance is the key.

## WHAT ADULTS CAN DO: SOCIALIZATION PRACTICES SPECIFIC TO EMOTIONAL COMPETENCE

Let me reiterate the gist of the model put forward in Figure 1.2. Parents and all other adults with whom young children interact—through their own emotions, the ways they react to the children's emotions, and they ways they teach about emotions—affect vital emotional competence that is developing during the preschool years. Furthermore, children who understand emotions better, show more positive emotions, and regulate the "tougher" emotions are seen by preschool teachers as more socially able, are better liked by their peers, and can respond more appropriately to their friends' feelings. So adults are vitally important in this area.

Overall, caregivers' emotions, reactions to their kids' emotions, and teaching about emotions wield a potent "double whammy": They affect both emotional and social competence. And what a child practices in terms of emotional competence with adults translates to the realm of peers. So these conclusions reached from the current state of research should give caregivers and parents pause. For preschoolers' benefit, important adults can make adjustments in their own expressiveness and in their reactions to children's emotions. Parents and caregivers can also benefit from a more careful consideration of, and from open (though not overwhelming) discussions of, their own feelings. Here is more detail on what has been learned so far. For economy's sake, I use the word *parents*, but I really mean any important adults with whom children have a relationship.

### Parents' Expressiveness

- Children whose parents are more emotionally positive tend to be more positive themselves around their peers, whereas children whose parents are more negative appear less socially competent in preschool.
- Parents who report that they can remain emotionally positive during challenging circumstances have children who are more adept at understanding emotions. These findings include fathers as well as mothers.

- Young girls' ability to regulate negative emotions is especially vulnerable to the detrimental effects of parents' negative emotions and parents' "mean" reactions to their emotions, as well as to the positive effects of parents' own positive emotions. Little girls are exquisite barometers of parents' emotions. This may be both a blessing and a curse!

### Parents' Reactions to Children's Emotions

- Parental reactions to children's own emotional displays are important, because children generalize them to their own expressiveness and use them in building emotion knowledge. For example, discouraging a child's emotion (e.g., by saying, "Stop that crying!") is a powerful deterrent of self-reflection regarding emotions, and hence a barrier to emotion knowledge.
- Paying attention to and positively reinforcing children's emotions by accepting them, acknowledging them, and responding to meet the children's pragmatic needs may pave the way for children to learn more about their own and others' emotions, as reflected in their social competence.

### Parents' Teaching about Emotions

- Parents who are better teachers about emotions have children who understand emotions better and are more socially competent in preschool. Talking about feelings is vital. (Not surprisingly, though, some of this depends on whether the child is younger or older during the preschool years, and whether the child is male or female.)
- However, parents' use of guiding and socializing emotion language is a negative predictor of both emotional and social competence. Parents use guiding language (e.g., "You really made me sad that time; I wish you wouldn't scream like that") and socializing language (e.g., "Big kids don't cry so much") with children who most actively need this kind of teaching, such as those who are more prone to exhibit sadness and fear, to react immaturely to others' emotions, or to experience more difficult social relations. Preschoolers may also be "wise" to being bullied or preached at via emotion language, so not all emotion talk is created equal!

As I have noted, many of these points pertain to preschool teachers' emotion socialization as well, but not always owing to the nature of the preschool classroom and important ethnic, racial, and cultural differences.

## CONCLUSION

The ways we pay attention to, understand, and promote emotional competence in the early years will reap incalculable rewards. It is my fervent hope that we begin now to act upon this knowledge.

# References


Abraham, K. G., Kuehl, R. O., & Christopherson, V. A. (1983). Age-specific influence of parental behaviors on the development of empathy in preschool children. *Child Study Journal, 13*, 175–185.

Abramovitch, R., & Daly, E. M. (1979). Inferring attributes of a situation from the facial expressions of peers. *Child Development, 50*(2), 586–589.

Ackerman, B. P., Abe, J. A. A., & Izard, C. E. (1998). Differential emotions theory and emotional development. In M. F. Mascolo & S. Griffin (Eds.), *What develops in emotional development?* (pp. 85–106). Springer.

Acland, E. L., Jambon, M., & Malti, T. (2021). Children's emotion recognition and aggression: A multicohort longitudinal study. *Aggressive Behavior, 47*(6), 646–658.

Adams, S., Kuebli, J., Boyle, P. A., & Fivush, R. (1995). Gender differences in parent–child conversations about past emotions: A longitudinal investigation. *Sex Roles, 33*, 309–323.

Ahn, H. J. (2005a). Child care teachers' beliefs and practices regarding socialization of emotion in young children. *Journal of Early Childhood Teacher Education, 26*(3), 283–295.

Ahn, H. J. (2005b). Teachers' discussions of emotion in child care centers. *Early Childhood Education Journal, 32*, 237–242.

Ahn, H. J., & Stifter, C. (2006). Child care teachers' response to children's emotional expression. *Early Education and Development, 17*, 253–270.

Akbag, M., & Imamoglu, S. E. (2010). The prediction of gender and attachment styles on shame, guilt, and loneliness. *Educational Sciences: Theory and Practice, 10*(2), 669–682.

Alessandri, S. M., & Lewis, M. (1993). Parental evaluation and its relation to shame and pride in young children. *Sex Roles, 29*, 335–343.

Alessandri, S. M., & Lewis, M. (1996). Differences in pride and shame in maltreated and normal preschoolers. *Child Development, 67*, 1857–1870.

Alonso-Alberca, N., Vergara, A. I., Fernández-Berrocal, P., Johnson, S. R., & Izard, C. E. (2012). The adaptation and validation of the Emotion Matching Task for preschool children in Spain. *International Journal of Behavioral Development, 36*(6), 489–494.

Alvarenga, P., Zucker, T. A., Tambyraja, S., & Justice, L. (2020). Contingency in teacher–child emotional state talk during shared book reading in early childhood classrooms. *Early Education and Development, 31*(8), 1187–1205.

Alwaely, S. A., Yousif, N. B. A., & Mikhaylov, A. (2020). Emotional development in preschoolers and socialization. *Early Child Development and Care, (16)*, 2484–2493.

Anthony, C. J., Elliott, S. N., DiPerna, J. C., & Lei, P.-W. (2020). Multi-rater assessment of young children's social and emotional learning via the SSIS SEL Brief Scales—Preschool Forms. *Early Childhood Research Quarterly, 53*, 625–637.

Arbeau, K. A., Coplan, R. J., & Weeks, M. (2010). Shyness, teacher-child relationships, and socioemotional adjustment in grade 1. *International Journal of Behavioral Development, 34*(3), 259–269.

Are, F., & Shaffer, A. (2016). Family emotion expressiveness mediates the relations between maternal emotion regulation and child emotion regulation. *Child Psychiatry and Human Development, 47*, 708–715.

Armer, M. (2004). *A longitudinal investigation of the stabil-*

*ity and outcomes of shyness from preschool to early elementary school.* Doctoral dissertation, Carleton University, Ottawa.

Arsenio, W. (2006). Happy victimization: Emotion dysregulation in the context of children's instrumental proactive aggression. In D. Snyder, J. Simpson, & J. Hughes (Eds.), *Emotion regulation in families: Pathways to dysfunction and health* (pp. 101–121). American Psychological Association.

Arsenio, W., Gold, J., & Adams, E. (2006). Children's conceptions and displays of moral emotions. In M. Killen & J. Smetana (Eds.), *Handbook of moral development* (pp. 581–608). Erlbaum.

Arsenio, W. F., Cooperman, S., & Lover, A. (2000). Affective predictors of preschoolers' aggression and peer acceptance: Direct and indirect effects. *Developmental Psychology, 36*(4), 438–448.

Arsenio, W. F., & Kramer, R. (1992). Victimizers and their victims: Children's conceptions of the mixed emotional consequences of moral transgression. *Child Development, 63*, 915–927.

Arsenio, W. F., & Lover, A. (1995). Children's conceptions of sociomoral affect: Happy victimizers, mixed emotions, and other expressions. In M. Killen & D. Hart (Eds.), *Morality in everyday life: Developmental perspectives* (pp. 87–128). Cambridge University Press.

Arsenio, W. F., & Lover, A. (1997). Emotions, conflicts, and aggression during preschoolers' freeplay. *British Journal of Developmental Psychology, 15*, 531–542.

Arsenio, W. F., Lover, A., Cooperman, J., Fein, A., Gordy, A., & Preiser, L. (1997). Emotions, conflicts, and preschoolers' peer acceptance. In J. Hubbard (Chair), *The role of emotions in children's peer relationships.* Symposium conducted at the biennial meeting of the Society for Research in Child Development, Washington, DC.

Arslan, E., Durmuşoğlu-Saltali, N., & Yilmaz, H. (2011). Social skills and emotional and behavioral traits of preschool children. *Social Behavior and Personality, 39*(9), 1281–1287.

Asendorpf, J. B. (1990). Beyond social withdrawal: Shyness, unsociability, and peer avoidance. *Human Development, 33*(4–5), 250–259.

Auerbach-Major, S. T., Kochanoff, A. T., & Queenan, P. (1997, April). *The interactive contributions of child temperament and parent disciplinary style on preschoolers' social competence.* Poster presented at the biennial meeting of the Society for Research in Child Development, Washington, DC.

August, E. G., Stack, D. M., Martin-Storey, A., Serbin, L. A., Ledingham, J., & Schwartzman, A. E. (2017). Emotion regulation in at-risk preschoolers: Longitudinal associations and influences of maternal histories of risk. *Infant and Child Development, 26*(1), e1954.

Aznar, A., & Tenenbaum, H. R. (2013). Spanish parents' emotion talk and their children's understanding of emotion. *Frontiers in Psychology, 4*, 670.

Aznar, A., & Tenenbaum, H. R. (2020). Gender comparisons in mother-child emotion talk: A meta-analysis. *Sex Roles, 82*(3), 155–162.

Bafunno, D., & Camodeca, M. (2013). Shame and guilt development in preschoolers: The role of context, audience and individual characteristics. *European Journal of Developmental Psychology, 10*(2), 128–143.

Bailey, C. S., Denham, S. A., & Curby, T. W. (2013). Questioning as a component of scaffolding in predicting emotion knowledge in preschoolers. *Early Child Development and Care, 183*(2), 265–279.

Bailey, C. S., Denham, S. A., Curby, T. W., & Bassett, H. H. (2016). Emotional and organizational supports for preschoolers' emotion regulation: Relations with school adjustment. *Emotion, 16*(2), 263–279.

Bailey, C. S., Rivers, S. E., Tominey, S. L., O'Bryon, E. C., Olsen, S. G., Sneeden, C. K., . . . Brackett, M. A. (2019). Promoting early childhood social and emotional learning with Preschool RULER. Manuscript submitted for publication.

Bailey Bisson, J. (2019). It's written all over their faces: Preschoolers' emotion understanding. *Social Development, 28*(1), 74–89.

Band, E. B., & Weisz, J. R. (1988). How to feel better when it feels bad: Children's perspectives on coping with everyday stress. *Developmental Psychology, 24*, 247–253.

Banerjee, M. (1997a). Hidden emotions: Preschoolers' knowledge of appearance–reality and emotion display rules. *Social Cognition, 15*, 107–132.

Banerjee, M. (1997b). Peeling the onion: A multi-layered view of children's emotional development. In S. Hala (Ed.), *The development of social cognition* (pp. 241–272). Psychology Press.

Banerjee, M., & Eggleston, R. (1993, April). *Preschoolers' and parents' understanding of emotion regulation.* Poster presented at the biennial meeting of the Society for Research in Child Development, New Orleans, LA.

Barden, R. C., Zelko, F. A., Duncan, S. W., & Masters, J. C. (1980). Children's consensual knowledge about the experiential determinants of emotion. *Journal of Personality and Social Psychology, 39*, 968–976.

Barisnikov, K., Theurel, A., & Lejeune, F. (2022). Emotion knowledge in neurotypical children and in those with down syndrome. *Applied Neuropsychology: Child*, 1–15.

Barisnikov, K., Thomasson, M., Stutzmann, J., & Lejeune, F. (2020). Relation between processing facial identity and emotional expression in typically developing school-age children and those with Down syndrome. *Applied Neuropsychology: Child, 9*(2), 179–192.

Barnett, L. A. (1984). Research note: Young children's resolution of distress through play. *Journal of Child Psychology and Psychiatry, 25*, 477–483.

Barnett, M. A. (1984). Similarity of experience and empathy in preschoolers. *Journal of Genetic Psychology, 145*, 241–250.

Barnett, M. A., Howard, J. A., & Melton, E. M. (1982). Effect of inducing sadness about self or other on behavior in high- and low-empathic children. *Child Development, 53*, 920–923.

Barnett, M. A., King, L. M., Howard, J. A., & Dino, G. A. (1980). Empathy in young children: Relation to parents' empathy, affection, and emphasis on feelings of others. *Developmental Psychology, 16*, 243–244.

Barnett, W. S., Epstein, D. J., Friedman, A. H., Sansanelli, R. A., & Hustedt, J. T. (2009). *The state of preschool 2009: State preschool yearbook*. National Institute for Early Education Research, Rutgers University.

Baron-Cohen, S. (1991). Do people with autism understand what causes emotion? *Child Development, 62*, 385–395.

Barrett, K. (2005). The origins of social emotions and self-regulation in toddlerhood: New evidence. *Cognition and Emotion, 19*(7), 953–979.

Barrett, K. C. (2020). Emotional development is complicated. *Developmental Psychology, 56*(4), 833–836.

Barrett, K. C., & Campos, J. J. (1987). Perspectives on emotional development: II. A functionalist approach to emotions. In J. D. Osofsky (Ed.), *Handbook of infant development* (pp. 555–578). Wiley.

Barrett, K. C., & Campos, J. J. (1991). A diacritical function approach to emotions and coping. In E. M. Cummings, A. L. Greene, & K. H. Karraker (Eds.), *Lifespan developmental psychology: Perspectives on stress and coping* (pp. 21–41). Erlbaum.

Barrett, K. C., Zahn-Waxler, C., & Cole, P. M. (1993). Avoiders versus amenders—Implications for the investigation of guilt and shame during toddlerhood? *Cognition and Emotion, 7*, 481–505.

Barry, R. A., & Kochanska, G. (2010). A longitudinal investigation of the affective environment in families with young children: From infancy to early school age. *Emotion, 10(2)*, 237–249.

Barth, J. M., & Bastiani, A. (1997). A longitudinal study of emotional recognition and preschool children's social behavior. *Merrill–Palmer Quarterly, 43*, 107–128.

Bassett, H. H., Denham, S. A., Fettig, N. B., Curby, T. W., Mohtasham, M., & Austin, N. (2017). Temperament in the classroom: Children low in surgency are more sensitive to teachers' reactions to emotions. *International Journal of Behavioral Development, 41*, 4–14.

Bassett, H. H., Denham, S. A., Mincic, M. M., & Graling, K. (2012). The structure of preschoolers' emotion knowledge: Model equivalence and validity using a structural equation modeling approach. *Early Education and Development, 23*, 259–279.

Bassett, H. H., Denham, S. A., Mohtasham, M., & Austin, N. (2020). Psychometric properties of the Book Readings for an Affective Classroom Education (BRACE) coding system. *Reading Psychology, 41*(4), 322–346.

Bassok, D., Markowitz, A. J., Bellows, L., & Sadowski, K. (2021). New evidence on teacher turnover in early childhood. *Educational Evaluation and Policy Analysis, 43*(1), 172–180.

Batson, C. D. (1991). *The altruism question: Toward a social psychological answer*. Erlbaum.

Baumgartner, J. J., Carson, R. L., Apavaloaie, L., & Tsouloupas, C. (2009). Uncovering common stressful factors and coping strategies among childcare providers. *Child and Youth Care Forum, 38*, 239–251.

Beaudoin, M. J., Poirier, N., & Nader-Grosbois, N. (2021). Relationships between mother–child conversations about emotion and socioemotional development of children with autism spectrum disorder. *Journal of Autism and Developmental Disorders*, 1–13.

Beck, L., Kumschick, I. R., Eid, M., & Klann-Delius, G. (2012). Relationship between language competence and emotional competence in middle childhood. *Emotion, 12*(3), 503–514.

Becker, E. S., Keller, M. M., Goetz, T., Frenzel, A. C., & Taxer, J. L. (2015). Antecedents of teachers' emotions in the classroom: an intraindividual approach. *Frontiers in Psychology, 6*, 635.

Bedford, R., Wagner, N. J., Rehder, P. D., Propper, C., Willoughby, M. T., & Mills-Koonce, R. W. (2017). The role of infants' mother-directed gaze, maternal sensitivity, and emotion recognition in childhood callous unemotional behaviours. *European Child and Adolescent Psychiatry, 26(8)*, 947–956.

Beeghly, M., & Cicchetti, D. (1994). Child maltreatment, attachment, and the self-system: Emergence of an internal state lexicon in toddlers at high social risk. *Development and Psychopathology, 6*, 5–30.

Begeer, S., Koot, H. M., Rieffe, C., Terwogt, M. M., & Stegge, H. (2008). Emotional competence in children with autism: Diagnostic criteria and empirical evidence. *Developmental Review, 28*(3), 342–369.

Behrendt, H. F., Wade, M., Bayet, L., Nelson, C. A., & Enlow, M. B. (2020). Pathways to social-emotional functioning in the preschool period: The role of child temperament and maternal anxiety in boys and girls. *Development and Psychopathology, 32*(3), 961–974.

Belacchi, C., & Farina, E. (2010). Prosocial/hostile roles and emotion comprehension in preschoolers. *Aggressive Behavior, 36*(6), 371–389.

Belacchi, C., & Farina, E. (2012). Feeling and thinking of others: Affective and cognitive empathy and emotion comprehension in prosocial/hostile preschoolers. *Aggressive Behavior, 38*(2), 150–165.

Bellas, V. M. (2009). *Emotion in the classroom: A theory-based exploration of teachers' emotion socialization beliefs and behaviors* [Dissertation]. Clark University.

Bennett, D. S., Bendersky, M., & Lewis, M. (2005). Antecedents of emotion knowledge: Predictors of individual differences in young children. *Cognition and Emotion, 19*(3), 375–396.

Bennett, D. S., Sullivan, M. W., & Lewis, M. (2005). Young children's adjustment as a function of maltreatment, shame, and anger. *Child Maltreatment, 10*(4), 311–323.

Bennett, M. (1989). Children's self-attributions of embarrassment. *British Journal of Developmental Psychology, 7*, 207–217.

Bennett, M., & Gillingham, K. (1991). The role of self-focused attention in children's attributions of social emotions to the self. *Journal of Genetic Psychology, 152*, 303–309.

Bergen, P. V., Salmon, K., Dadds, M. R., & Allen, J. (2009). The effects of mother training in emotion-rich, elaborative reminiscing on children's shared recall and emotion knowledge. *Journal of Cognition and Development, 10*(3), 162–187.

Bergman Deitcher, D., Aram, D., Khalaily-Shahadi, M., & Dwairy, M. (2020). Promoting preschoolers' mental-emotional conceptualization and social understanding: A shared book-reading study. *Early Education eand Development, 32*(4), 501–515.

Berkovits, L., Eisenhower, A., & Blacher, J. (2017). Emotion regulation in young children with autism spectrum disorders. *Journal of Autism and Developmental Disorders, 47*(1), 68–79.

Berlin, L. J., & Cassidy, J. (2003). Mothers' self-reported control of their preschool children's emotional expressiveness: A longitudinal study of associations with infant–mother attachment and children's emotion regulation. *Social Development, 12*, 478–495.

Bernier, A., Marquis-Brideau, C., Dusablon, C., Lemelin, J. P., & Sirois, M. S. (2021). From negative emotionality to aggressive behavior: Maternal and paternal parenting stress as intervening factors. *Research on Child and Adolescent Psychopathology, 50*(4), 477–487.

Berti, A. E., Garattoni, C., & Venturini, B. A. (2000). The understanding of sadness, guilt, and shame in 5-, 7-, and 9-year-old children. *Genetic, Social, and General Psychology Monographs, 126*, 293–318.

Bierman, K. L., Domitrovich, C. E., Nix, R. L., Gest, S. D., Welsh, J. A., Greenberg, M. T., . . . Gill, S. (2008). Promoting academic and social-emotional school readiness: The Head Start REDI program. *Child Development, 79*(6), 1802–1817.

Bierman, K. L., & Motamedi, M. (2015). Social and emotional learning programs for preschool children. In J. A. Durlak, C. E. Domitrovich, R. P. Weissberg, & T. P. Gullotta (Eds.), *Handbook of social and emotional learning: Research and practice* (pp. 135–151). Guilford Press.

Bierman, K. L., Nix, R. L., Greenberg, M. T., Blair, C., & Domitrovich, C. E. (2008). Executive functions and school readiness intervention: Impact, moderation, and mediation in the Head Start REDI program. *Development and Psychopathology, 20*(3), 821–843.

Bierman, K. L., Nix, R. L., Heinrichs, B. S., Domitrovich, C. E., Gest, S. D., Welsh, J. A., & Gill, S. (2014). Effects of Head Start REDI on children's outcomes 1 year later in different kindergarten contexts. *Child Development, 85*(1), 140–159.

Bischof-Kohler, D. (1988). On the connection between empathy and the ability to recognize oneself in the mirror. *Schweizerische Zeitschrift für Psychologie, 47*, 147–159.

Bisharat, R., Mattar, M., & Jehan, W. (2020). *Emotional regulation and its relation to school readiness among first grade students in private schools in Amman. Jordanian Educational Journal, 6*(4), 1–27.

Bjørk, R. F., Bølstad, E., Pons, F., & Havighurst, S. S. (2022). Testing TIK (Tuning in to Kids) with TEC (Test of Emotion Comprehension): Does enhanced emotion socialization improve child emotion understanding? *Journal of Applied Developmental Psychology, 78*, 101368.

Blair, B. L., Perry, N. B., O'Brien, M., Calkins, S. D., Keane, S. P., & Shanahan, L. (2015). Identifying developmental cascades among differentiated dimensions of social competence and emotion regulation. *Developmental Psychology, 51*(8), 1062–1073.

Blair, K. A., Denham, S. A., Kochanoff, A., & Whipple, B. (2004). Playing it cool: Temperament, emotion regulation, and social behavior in preschoolers. *Journal of School Psychology, 42*(6), 419–443.

Blandon, A. Y., Calkins, S. D., Grimm, K. J., Keane, S. P., & O'Brien, M. (2010). Testing a developmental cascade model of emotional and social competence and early peer acceptance. *Development and Psychopathology, 22*(4), 737–748.

Blankson, A. N., O'Brien, M., Leerkes, E. M., Marcovitch, S., Calkins, S. D., & Weaver, J. M. (2013). Developmental dynamics of emotion and cognition processes in preschoolers. *Child Development, 84*(1), 346–360.

Blankson, A. N., Weaver, J. M., Leerkes, E. M., O'Brien, M., Calkins, S. D., & Marcovitch, S. (2017). Cognitive and emotional processes as predictors of a successful transition into school. *Early Education and Development, 28*(1), 1–20.

Blewitt, C., Fuller-Tyszkiewicz, M., Nolan, A., Bergmeier, H., Vicary, D., Huang, T., . . . Skouteris, H. (2018). Social and emotional learning associated with universal curriculum-based interventions in early childhood education and care centers: A systematic review and meta-analysis. *JAMA Network Open, 1*(8), e185727.

Blewitt, C., Morris, H., Nolan, A., Jackson, K., Barrett, H., & Skouteris, H. (2018). Strengthening the quality of educator-child interactions in early childhood education and care settings: A conceptual model to improve mental health outcomes for preschoolers. *Early Child Development and Care, 190*(7), 991–1004.

Blurton-Jones, N. (2017). An ethological study of some aspects of social behaviour of children in nursery school. In D. Morris (Ed.), *Primate ethology* (pp. 347–368). Weidenfeld and Nicolson.

Bogat, G. A., Wong, K., Muzik, M., Lonstein, J. S., Nuttall, A. K., Levendosky, A. A., . . . Stein, S. F. (2021). Conducting virtual assessments in developmental research: COVID-19 restrictions as a case example. *Applied Developmental Science*, 1–17.

Boiger, M., & Mesquita, B. (2012). The construction of emotion in interactions, relationships, and cultures. *Emotion Review, 4*(3), 221–229.

Bondy, E., & Ross, D. D. (2008). The teacher as warm demander. *Educational Leadership, 66*(1), 54–58.

Borke, H. (1971). Interpersonal perception of young children: Egocentrism or empathy? *Developmental Psychology, 5*, 263–269.

Bornstein, M. H., Hahn, C. S., Putnick, D. L., & Pearson, R. (2019). Stability of child temperament: Multiple moderation by child and mother characteristics. *British Journal of Developmental Psychology, 37*(1), 51–67.

Bosacki, S. L., & Moore, C. (2004). Preschoolers' understanding of simple and complex emotions: Links with gender and language. *Sex Roles, 50*(9), 659–675.

Boyatzis, C. J., & Satyaprasad, C. (1994). Children's facial and gestural decoding and encoding: Relations between skills and with popularity. *Journal of Nonverbal Behavior, 18*(1), 37–55.

Boyum, L. A., & Parke, R. D. (1995). The role of family emotional expressiveness in the development of children's social competence. *Journal of Marriage and the Family, 57*, 593–608.

Bowling, B., & Jones, D. C. (1993). Family expressiveness and display rule knowledge. In D. C. Jones (Chair), *Emotions and the family*. Symposium conducted at the biennial meeting of the Society for Research in Child Development, New Orleans, LA.

Brackett, M. A., & Katulak, N. A. (2006). Emotional intelligence in the classroom: Skill-based training for teachers and students. In J. Ciarrochi & J. D. Mayer (Eds.), *Applying emotional intelligence: A practitioner's guide* (pp. 1–27). Psychology Press.

Brackett, M. A., Rivers, S. E., & Salovey, P. (2011). Emotional intelligence: Implications for personal, social, academic, and workplace success. *Social and Personality Psychology Compass, 5*, 88–103.

Brajsa-Zganec, A. (2014). Emotional life of the family: Parental meta-emotions, children's temperament and internalising and externalising problems. *Drustvena Istrazivanja, 23(1)*, 25–45.

Braza, F., Azurmendi, A., Muñoz, J. M., Carreras, M. R., Braza, P., García, A., . . . Sánchez-Martín, J. R. (2009). Social cognitive predictors of peer acceptance at age 5 and the moderating effects of gender. *British Journal of Developmental Psychology, 27*(3), 703–716.

Bretherton, I., & Beeghly, M. (1982). Talking about internal states: The acquisition of an explicit theory of mind. *Developmental Psychology, 18*, 906–921.

Bretherton, I., Fritz, J., Zahn-Waxler, C., & Ridgeway, D. (1986). Learning to talk about emotions: A functionalist perspective. *Child Development, 57*, 529–548.

Bridgeland, J., Bruce, M., & Hariharan, A. (2013). *The missing piece: A national teacher survey on how social and emotional learning can empower children and transform schools. A Report for CASEL*. Civic Enterprises.

Bridges, L. J., & Grolnick, W. S. (1995). The development of emotional self-regulation in infancy and early childhood. In N. Eisenberg (Ed.), *Review of personality and social psychology: Vol. 15. Social development* (pp. 185–211). SAGE.

Brock, L. L., Kim, H., Gutshall, C. C., & Grissmer, D. W. (2018). The development of theory of mind: Predictors and moderators of improvement in kindergarten. *Early Child Development and Care, 189(12)*, 1914–1924.

Brody, L. R., & Harrison, R. H. (1987). Developmental changes in children's abilities to match and label emotionally laden situations. *Motivation and Emotion, 11*, 347–365.

Brooker, R. J., & Buss, K. A. (2010). Dynamic measures of RSA predict distress and regulation in toddlers. *Developmental Psychobiology, 52*(4), 372–382.

Brophy-Herb, H. E., Martoccio, T. L., Hillaker, B., Stansbury, K. E., Harewood, T., Senehi, N., & Fitzgerald, H. (2013). Profiles of low-income maternal well-being and family climate: Relations to toddler boys' and girls' behaviors. *Family Relations, 62*(2), 326–340.

Brophy-Herb, H. E., Schiffman, R. F., Bocknek, E. L., Dupuis, S. B., Fitzgerald, H. E., Horodynski, M., . . . Hillaker, B. (2011). Toddlers' social-emotional competence in the contexts of maternal emotion socialization and contingent responsiveness in a low-income sample. *Social Development, 20*(1), 73–92.

Brophy-Herb, H. E., Zajicek-Farber, M. L., Bocknek, E. L., McKelvey, L. M., & Stansbury, K. (2013). Longitudinal connections of maternal supportiveness and early emotion regulation to children's school readiness in low-income families. *Journal of the Society for Social Work and Research, 4*(1), 2–19.

Brotman, L. M., Gouley, K. K., Chesir-Teran, D., Dennis, T., Klein, R. G., & Shrout, P. (2005). Prevention for preschoolers at high risk for conduct problems: Immediate outcomes on parenting practices and child social competence. *Journal of Clinical Child and Adolescent Psychology, 34*(4), 724–734.

Brown, E. D., & Ackerman, B. P. (2011). Contextual risk, maternal negative emotionality, and the negative emotion dysregulation of preschool children from economically disadvantaged families. *Early Education and Development, 22*(6), 931–944.

Brown, E. L., Vesely, C. K., Mahatmya, D., & Visconti, K. J. (2018). Emotions matter: The moderating role of emotional labour on preschool teacher and children interactions. *Early Child Development and Care, 188*(12), 1773–1787.

Brown, J. R., Donelan-McCall, N., & Dunn, J. (1996). Why talk about mental states?: The significance of children's conversations with friends, siblings, and mothers. *Child Development, 67*, 836–849.

Brown, J. R., & Dunn, J. (1991). "You can cry, Mum": The social and developmental implications of talk about internal states. *British Journal of Developmental Psychology, 9*, 237–256.

Brown, J. R., & Dunn, J. (1992). Talk with your mother or your sibling?: Developmental changes in early family conversations about feelings. *Child Development, 63*, 336–349.

Brown, J. R., & Dunn, J. (1996). Continuities in emotion understanding from three to six years. *Child Development, 67*, 789–802.

Brown, K., Covell, K., & Abramovitch, R. (1991). Time course and control of emotion: Age differences in understanding and recognition. *Merrill–Palmer Quarterly, 37*, 273–287.

Brownell, C. A., Svetlova, M., Anderson, R., Nichols, S. R., & Drummond, J. (2013). Socialization of early prosocial behavior: Parents' talk about emotions is associated with sharing and helping in toddlers. *Infancy, 18*(1), 91–119.

Buettner, C. K., Hur, E. H., Jeon, L., & Andrews, D. W. (2016). What are we teaching the teachers?: Child development curricula in US higher education. *Child and Youth Care Forum, 45*, 155–175.

Buettner, C. K., Jeon, L., Hur, E., & Garcia, R. E. (2016). Teachers' social–emotional capacity: Factors associated with teachers' responsiveness and professional commitment. *Early Education and Development, 27*, 1–22.

Bullock, M., & Russell, J. (1984). Preschool children's interpretations of facial expressions of emotion. *International Journal of Behavioral Development, 7*, 193–214.

Bullock, M., & Russell, J. (1985). Further evidence on preschoolers' interpretation of facial expressions. *International Journal of Behavioral Development, 8*, 15–38.

Bullock, M., & Russell, J. (1986). Conceptual emotions

in developmental psychology. In C. E. Izard & P. Read (Eds.), *Measurement of emotions in children* (Vol. 2, pp. 203–237). Cambridge University Press.

Bullough, R. V., Hall-Kenyon, K. M., & MacKay, K. L. (2012). Head Start teacher well-being: Implications for policy and practice. *Early Childhood Education Journal, 40*(6), 323–331.

Burley, D. T., Hobson, C. W., Adegboye, D., Shelton, K. H., & Van Goozen, S. H. M. (2021). Negative parental emotional environment increases the association between childhood behavioral problems and impaired recognition of negative facial expressions. *Development and Psychopathology, 34*(3), 936–945.

Burton, R., & Denham, S. A. (1999). "Are you my friend?": A qualitative analysis of a social-emotional intervention for at-risk four-year-olds. *Journal of Research in Childhood Education, 12*, 210–224.

Buss, A. H. (1986). A theory of shyness. In W. H. Jones, J. M. Cheek, & S. R. Briggs (Eds.), *Shyness: Perspectives on research and treatment* (pp. 39–46). Plenum Press.

Buss, K. A., Cho, S., Morales, S., McDoniel, M., Webb, A. F., Schwartz, A., . . . Teti, D. M. (2021). Toddler dysregulated fear predicts continued risk for social anxiety symptoms in early adolescence. *Development and Psychopathology, 33*(1), 252–263.

Buss, K. A., Cole, P. M., & Zhou, A. M. (2019). Theories of emotional development: Where have we been and where are we now? In V. LoBue, K. Pérez-Edgar, & K. A. Buss (Eds.), *Handbook of emotional development* (pp. 7–25). Springer.

Buss, K. A., Davis, E. L., Kiel, E. J., Brooker, R. J., Beekman, C., & Early, M. C. (2013). Dysregulated fear predicts social wariness and social anxiety symptoms during kindergarten. *Journal of Clinical Child and Adolescent Psychology, 42*, 1–14.

Butkovsky, L. L. (1991, April). *Emotional expressiveness in the family: Connection to children's peer relations.* Poster presented at the biennial meeting of the Society for Research in Child Development, Seattle, WA.

Caiozzo, C. N., Yule, K., & Grych, J. (2018). Caregiver behaviors associated with emotion regulation in high-risk preschoolers. *Journal of Family Psychology, 32*(5), 565–574.

Calkins, S. D., & Dedmon, S. A. (2000). Physiological and behavioral regulation in two-year-old children with aggressive/destructive behavior problems. *Journal of Abnormal Child Psychology, 28*(2), 103–118.

Calkins, S. D., Dollar, J. M., & Wideman, L. (2019). Temperamental vulnerability to emotion dysregulation and risk for mental and physical health challenges. *Development and Psychopathology, 31*(3), 957–970.

Calkins, S. D., & Mackler, J. S. (2011). Temperament, emotion regulation, and social development. In M. K. Underwood & L. H. Rosen (Eds.), *Social development: Relationships in infancy, childhood, and adolescence* (pp. 44–70). Guilford Press.

Calkins, S. D., & Marcovitch, S. (2010). Emotion regulation and executive functioning in early development: Integrated mechanisms of control supporting adaptive functioning. In S. D. Calkins & M. A. Bell (Eds.), *Child development at the intersection of emotion and cognition* (pp. 37–57). American Psychological Association.

Camodeca, M., & Coppola, G. (2016). Bullying, empathic concern, and internalization of rules among preschool children: The role of emotion understanding. *International Journal of Behavioral Development, 40*, 459–465.

Camodeca, M., & Coppola, G. (2019). Participant roles in preschool bullying: The impact of emotion regulation, social preference, and quality of the teacher–child relationship. *Social Development, 28*(1), 3–21.

Campbell, S. B., Denham, S. A., Howarth, G. Z., Jones, S. M., Whittaker, J. V., Williford, A. P., . . . Darling-Churchill, K. (2016). Commentary on the review of measures of early childhood social and emotional development: Conceptualization, critique, and recommendations. *Journal of Applied Developmental Psychology, 45*, 19–41.

Campbell, S., & Ewing, L. J. (1990). Follow-up of hard-to-manage preschoolers: Adjustment at age 9 and predictors of continuing symptoms. *Journal of Child Psychology and Psychiatry, 31*, 871–889.

Campos, J. J., & Barrett, K. C. (1984). Toward a new understanding of emotions and their development. In C. E. Izard, J. Kagan, & R. B. Zajonc (Eds.), *Emotions, cognition, and behavior* (pp. 229–263). Cambridge University Press.

Campos, J. J., Campos, R. G., & Barrett, K. C. (1989). Emergent themes in the study of emotional development and emotion regulation. *Developmental Psychology, 25*, 394–402.

Campos, J. J., Mumme, D. L., Kermoian, R., & Campos, R. G. (1994). A functionalist perspective on the nature of emotion. In N. A. Fox (Ed.), The development of emotion regulation: Biological and behavioral considerations. *Monographs of the Society for Research in Child Development, 59*(2–3, Serial No. 240), 284–303.

Camras, L. A., & Allison, K. (1985). Children's understanding of emotional facial expressions and verbal labels. *Journal of Nonverbal Behavior, 9*, 84–94.

Camras, L. A., & Fatani, S. S. (2010). The facial development of expressions. In M. Lewis, J. Haviland-Jones, & L. F. Barrett (Eds.) *Handbook of emotions* (3rd ed., pp. 291–303). Guilford Press.

Camras, L. A., & Halberstadt, A. G. (2017). Emotional development through the lens of affective social competence. *Current Opinion in Psychology, 17*, 113–117.

Camras, L. A., Oster, H., Campos, J., Campos, R., Ujiie, T., Miyake, K., . . . Meng, Z. (1998). Production of emotional facial expressions in European American, Japanese, and Chinese infants. *Developmental Psychology, 34*(4), 616–628.

Camras, L., Ribordy, S., & Hill, J. (1988). Recognition and posing of emotional expressions by abused children and their mothers. *Developmental Psychology, 24*, 776–781.

Camras, L., Ribordy, S., Hill, J., Martino, S., Sachs, V., Spaccarelli, S., & Ştefani, R. (1990). Maternal facial behavior and the recognition and production of emotional expression by maltreated and nonmaltreated children. *Developmental Psychology, 26*, 304–312.

Camras, L. A., Sachs-Alter, E., & Ribordy, S. C. (1996). Emotion understanding in maltreated children: Recognition of facial expressions and integration with other emotion cues. In M. Lewis & M. W. Sullivan (Eds.), *Emotional development in atypical children* (pp. 203–225). Erlbaum.

Camras, L. A., & Witherington, D. C. (2005). Dynamical systems approaches to emotional development. *Developmental Review, 25*, 328–350.

Carlson, C. R., Felleman, E. S., & Masters, J. C. (1983). Influence of children's emotional states on the recognition of emotion in peers and social motives to change another's emotional state. *Motivation and Emotion, 7*, 61–79.

Carlson, S. M., & Wang, T. S. (2007). Inhibitory control and emotion regulation in preschool children. *Cognitive Development, 22*(4), 489–510.

Caron, B., Kendall, R., Wilson, G., & Hash. M. (2017). *Taking on the challenge: Building a strong foundation for early learning.* Early Learning Challenge Summary Report. AEM Corp.

Carrera, P., Jiménez-Morago, J. M., Román, M., & León, E. (2020). Differential associations of threat and deprivation with emotion understanding in maltreated children in foster care. *Child and Family Social Work, 25*(4), 973–982.

Carreras, M. R., Braza, P., Muñoz, J. M., Braza, F., Azurmendi, A., Pascual-Sagastizabal, E., . . . Sánchez-Martín, J. R. (2014). Aggression and prosocial behaviors in social conflicts mediating the influence of cold social intelligence and affective empathy on children's social preference. *Scandinavian Journal of Psychology, 55*(4), 371–379.

Carson, J., & Parke, R. D. (1996). Reciprocal negative affect in parent–child interactions and children's peer competency. *Child Development, 67*, 2217–2226.

Carson, R. L., Baumgartner, J. J., Matthews, R. A., & Tsouloupas, C. N. (2010). Emotional exhaustion, absenteeism, and turnover intentions in childcare teachers: Examining the impact of physical activity behaviors. *Journal of Health Psychology, 15*, 905–914.

Casey, R. J., & Fuller, L. (1994). Maternal regulation of children's emotions. *Journal of Nonverbal Behavior, 18*, 57–89.

Casey, R. J., Fuller, L., & Johll, T. (1993). Parental regulation of children's emotional responses: Will wishing make it so? In D. C. Jones (Chair), *Emotions and the family.* Symposium conducted at the biennial meeting of the Society for Research in Child Development, New Orleans, LA.

Cassidy, D. J., King, E. K., Wang, Y. C., Lower, J. K., & Kintner-Duffy, V. L. (2017). Teacher work environments are toddler learning environments: Teacher professional well-being, classroom emotional support, and toddlers' emotional expressions and behaviours. *Early Child Development and Care, 187*, 1666–1678.

Cassidy, J., Parke, R. D., Butkovsky, L., & Braungart, J. M. (1992). Family–peer connections: The roles of emotional expressiveness within the family and children's understanding of emotions. *Child Development, 63*, 603–618.

Castro, V. L., Cooke, A. N., Halberstadt, A. G., & Garrett-Peters, P. (2018). Bidirectional linkages between emotion recognition and problem behaviors in elementary school children. *Journal of Nonverbal Behavior, 42*(2), 155–178.

Cavadini, T., Richard, S., Dalla-Libera, N., & Gentaz, E. (2021). Emotion knowledge, social behaviour and locomotor activity predict the mathematic performance in 706 preschool children. *Scientific Reports, 11*(1), 1–13.

Cebula, K. R., Wishart, J. G., Willis, D. S., & Pitcairn, T. K. (2017). Emotion recognition in children with down syndrome: Influence of emotion label and expression intensity. *American Journal on Intellectual and Developmental Disabilities, 122*(2), 138–155.

Cefai, C., Bartolo P. A., Cavioni. V, & Downes, P. (2018). *Strengthening social and emotional education as a core curricular area across the EU: A review of the international evidence* (NESET II report). Publications Office of the European Union.

Cervantes, C. A., & Callanan, M. A. (1998). Labels and explanations in mother–child emotion talk: Age and gender differentiation. *Developmental Psychology, 34*(1), 88–98.

Chan, M. H., Feng, X., Inboden, K., Hooper, E., & Gerhardt, M. (2021). Dynamic, bidirectional influences of children's emotions and maternal regulatory strategies. *Emotion.*

Chan, R. F. Y., Qiu, C., & Shum, K. K. M. (2021). Tuning in to kids: A randomized controlled trial of an emotion coaching parenting program for Chinese parents in Hong Kong. *Developmental Psychology, 57*(11), 1796–1809.

Chang, L., Schwartz, D., Dodge, K. A., & McBride-Chang, C. (2003). Harsh parenting in relation to child emotion regulation and aggression. *Journal of Family Psychology, 17*(4), 598.

Chang, H., Shelleby, E. C., Cheong, J., & Shaw, D. S. (2012). Cumulative risk, negative emotionality, and emotion regulation as predictors of social competence in transition to school: A mediated moderation model. *Social Development, 21*(4), 780–800.

Channell, M. M., Conners, F. A., & Barth, J. M. (2014). Emotion knowledge in children and adolescents with Down syndrome: A new methodological approach. *American Journal on Intellectual and Developmental Disabilities, 119*(5), 405–421.

Chaplin, T. M., & Aldao, A. (2013). Gender differences in emotion expression in children: A meta-analytic review. *Psychological Bulletin, 139*(4), 735–765.

Chaplin, T. M., Cole, P. M., & Zahn-Waxler, C. (2005). Parental socialization of emotion expression: Gender differences and relations to child adjustment. *Emotion, 5*(1), 80–88.

Chaplin, T. M., Klein, M. R., Cole, P. M., & Turpyn, C. C. (2017). Developmental change in emotion expression in frustrating situations: The roles of context and gender. *Infant and Child Development, 26*(6), e2028.

Chapman, M., Zahn-Waxler, C., Cooperman, G., & Iannotti, R. (1987). Empathy and responsibility in the motivation of children's helping. *Developmental Psychology, 23*, 140–145.

Chen, D., Sullivan, M., & Lewis, M. (1995, March-April). *Shame and pride, sadness and joy expressions in 4- and 5-year-old children.* Poster presented at the biennial meeting of the Society for Research in Child Development, Indianapolis, IN.

Chen, X., Fu, R., Li, D., Chen, H., Wang, Z., & Wang, L. (2020). Behavioral inhibition in early childhood and adjustment in late adolescence in China. *Child Development, 92(3),* 994–1010.

Chen, X., Rubin, K. H., & Li, Z. Y. (1995). Social functioning and adjustment in Chinese children: A longitudinal study. *Developmental Psychology, 31*(4), 531–539.

Chen, X., Wu, X., & Wang, Y. (2018). Mothers' emotional expression and discipline and preschoolers' emotional regulation strategies: Gender differences. *Journal of Child and Family Studies, 27*(11), 3709–3716.

Cheng, F., Wang, Y., Zhao, J., & Wu, X. (2018). Mothers' negative emotional expression and preschoolers' negative emotional regulation strategies in Beijing, China: The moderating effect of maternal educational attainment. *Child Abuse and Neglect, 84,* 74–81.

Cheyne, J. A. (1976). Development of forms and functions of smiling in preschoolers. *Child Development, 47,* 820–823.

Cho, H. J., & Lee, D.-G. (2015). The mediating effect of mothers' emotional expressiveness in the relationship between their beliefs about children's emotion and the children's emotional regulation as it is perceived by their mothers. *Korean Journal of Child Studies, 36(3),* 1–18.

Chobhthaigh, S. N., & Wilson, C. (2015). Children's understanding of embarrassment: Integrating mental time travel and mental state information. *British Journal of Developmental Psychology,* 33(3), 324–339.

Chronaki, G., Garner, M., Hadwin, J. A., Thompson, M. J., Chin, C. Y., & Sonuga-Barke, E. J. (2015). Emotion-recognition abilities and behavior problem dimensions in preschoolers: Evidence for a specific role for childhood hyperactivity. *Child Neuropsychology, 21(1),* 25–40.

Chung, K. S., & Kim, M. (2020). How parenting anxiety, number of children, and employment status affect the parental anger of mothers with young children in Korea. 아동학회지, *Korean Journal of Child Studies, 11*(5), 1–12.

Cibralic, S., Kohlhoff, J., Wallace, N., McMahon, C., & Eapen, V. (2019). A systematic review of emotion regulation in children with Autism Spectrum Disorder. *Research in Autism Spectrum Disorders,* 68, 101422.

Cicchetti, D., Toth, S., & Bush, M. (1988). Developmental psychopathology and incompetence in childhood: Suggestions for intervention. In B. Lahey & A. Kazdin (Eds.), *Advances in clinical child psychology* (pp. 1–72). Plenum Press.

Cohen, J. S. & Mendez, J. L. (2009). Emotion regulation, language ability, and the stability of preschool children's peer play behavior. *Early Education and Development,* 20(6), 1016–1037.

Colasante, T., Zuffianò, A., Bae, N. Y., & Malti, T. (2014). Inhibitory control and moral emotions: Relations to reparation in early and middle childhood. *Journal of Genetic Psychology, 175(5–6),* 511–527.

Cole, P. M. (1985). Display rules and the socialization of affective displays. In G. Zivin (Ed.), *The development of expressive behavior* (pp. 269–290). Academic Press.

Cole, P. M. (1986). Children's spontaneous control of facial expressions. *Child Development 57,* 1309–1321.

Cole, P. M., Armstrong, L. M., & Pemberton, C. K. (2010). The role of language in the development of emotion regulation. In S. D. Calkins & M. A. Bell (Eds.), *Child development at the intersection of emotion and cognition* (pp. 59–77). American Psychological Association.

Cole, P. M., Barrett, K. C., & Zahn-Waxler, C. (1992). Emotion displays in two-year-olds during mishaps. *Child Development, 63,* 314–324.

Cole, P. M., Bendezú, J. J., Ram, N., & Chow, S. M. (2017). Dynamical systems modeling of early childhood self-regulation. *Emotion, 17*(4), 684–699.

Cole, P. M., Dennis, T. A., Smith-Simon, K. E., & Cohen, L. H. (2009). Preschoolers' emotion regulation strategy understanding: Relations with emotion socialization and child self-regulation. *Social Development, 18*(2), 324–352.

Cole, P. M., & Jacobs, A. E. (2018). From children's expressive control to emotion regulation: Looking back, looking ahead. *European Journal of Developmental Psychology, 15*(6), 658–677.

Cole, P. M., LeDonne, E. N., & Tan, P. Z. (2013). A longitudinal examination of maternal emotions in relation to young children's developing self-regulation. *Parenting, 13,* 113–132.

Cole, P. M., Lougheed, J. P., Chow, S. M., & Ram, N. (2020). Development of emotion regulation dynamics across early childhood: A multiple time-scale approach. *Affective Science, 1*(1), 28–41.

Cole, P. M., Lougheed, J. P., & Ram, N. (2018). The development of emotion regulation in early childhood. In P. M. Cole & T. Hollerstein (Eds.), *Emotion regulation: A matter of time* (pp. 52–69). Routledge.

Cole, P. M., Martin, S. E., & Dennis, T. A. (2004). Emotion regulation as a scientific construct: Methodological challenges and directions for child development research. *Child Development, 75*(2), 317–333.

Cole, P. M., Michel, M. K., & Teti, L. O. (1994). The development of emotion regulation and dysregulation: A clinical perspective. In N. A. Fox (Ed.), The development of emotion regulation: Biological and behavioral considerations. *Monographs of the Society for Research in Child Development, 59*(2–3, Serial No. 240), 73–102.

Cole, P. M., Tamang, B. L., & Shrestha, S. (2006). Cultural variations in the socialization of young children's anger and shame. *Child Development, 77*(5), 1237–1251.

Cole, P. M., & Tan, P. Z. (2007). Emotion socialization from a cultural perspective. In J. E. Grusec & P. D. Hastings (Eds.), *Handbook of socialization: Theory and research* (pp. 516–542). Guilford Press.

Cole, P. M., Tan, P. Z., Hall, S. E., Zhang, Y., Crnic, K. A., Blair, C. B., & Li, R. (2011). Developmental changes in anger expression and attention focus: Learning to wait. *Developmental Psychology, 47(4),* 1078–1089.

Cole, P. M., & Zahn-Waxler, C. (1988). *Prediction of conduct problems during the transition from preschool to school age* (Protocol No. 88-M-0217). National Institute of Mental Health.

Cole, P. M., Zahn-Waxler, C., Fox, N. A., Usher, B. A., & Welsh, J. D. (1996). Individual differences in emotion regulation and behavior problems in preschool children. *Journal of Abnormal Psychology, 103,* 518–529.

Cole, P. M., Zahn-Waxler, C., & Smith, K. D. (1994). Expressive control during a disappointment: Variations related to preschoolers' behavior problems. *Developmental Psychology, 30*, 833–846.

Collaborative for Academic, Social, and Emotional Learning (CASEL). (2012). *2013 CASEL guide: Effective social and emotional learning programs—Preschool and elementary school edition*. Collaborative for Academic, Social, and Emotional Learning.

Collaborative for Academic and Social-Emotional Learning (2018). *Federal policy*. Collaborative for Academic, Social, and Emotional Learning. Retrieved from *www.casel.org/federal-policy-and-legislation*.

Colonnesi, C., Nikolić, M., de Vente, W., & Bögels, S. M. (2017). Social anxiety symptoms in young children: Investigating the interplay of theory of mind and expressions of shyness. *Journal of Abnormal Child Psychology, 45*(5), 997–1011.

Conte, E., Grazzani, I., & Pepe, A. (2018). Social cognition, language, and prosocial behaviors: A multitrait mixed-methods study in early childhood. *Early Education and Development, 29*(6), 814–830.

Conte, E., Ornaghi, V., Grazzani, I., Pepe, A., & Cavioni, V. (2019). Emotion knowledge, theory of mind, and language in young children: Testing a comprehensive conceptual model. *Frontiers in Psychology, 10*, 2144.

Contreras, J. M., Kerns, K. A., Weimer, B. L., Gentzler, A. L., & Tomich, P. L. (2000). Emotion regulation as a mediator of associations between mother-child attachment and peer relationships in middle childhood. *Journal of Family Psychology, 14*, 111–124.

Conway, A., Mcdonough, S. C., Mackenzie, M., Miller, A., Dayton, C., Rosenblum, K., . . . & Sameroff, A. (2014). Maternal sensitivity and latency to positive emotion following challenge: Pathways through effortful control. *Infant Mental Health Journal, 35*(3), 274–284.

Cooper, S., Hobson, C. W., & van Goozen, S. H. (2020). Facial emotion recognition in children with externalising behaviours: A systematic review. *Clinical Child Psychology and Psychiatry, 25*(4), 1068–1085.

Cooper, A. M., Pradera, L., Sorensen, K., & Reschke, P. J. (2021, April). *Emotion learning through questions: How parental questions differentiate in reference to self-conscious emotions*. Poster presented at the biennial meeting of the Society for Research in Child Development, Virtual.

Coplan, R. J., & Armer, M. (2005). Talking yourself out of being shy: Shyness, expressive vocabulary, and socioemotional adjustment in preschool. *Merrill–Palmer Quarterly 51*(1), 20–41.

Coplan, R. J., & Evans, M. A. (2009). At a loss for words? Introduction to the special issue on shyness and language in childhood. *Infant and Child Development, 18*, 211–215.

Coplan, R. J., Prakash, K., O'Neil, K., & Armer, M. (2004). Do you "want" to play?: Distinguishing between conflicted shyness and social disinterest in early childhood. *Developmental Psychology, 40*(2), 244–258.

Çorapçı, F., Friedlmeier, W., Benga, O., Strauss, C., Pitica, I., & Susa, G. (2018). Cultural socialization of toddlers in emotionally charged situations. *Social Development, 27*(2), 262–278.

Cortez, V. L., & Bugental, D. B. (1994). Children's visual avoidance of threat: A strategy associated with low social control. *Merrill–Palmer Quarterly, 40*, 82–97.

Costin, S. E., & Jones, D. C. (1992). Friendship as a facilitator of emotional responsiveness and prosocial interventions among young children. *Developmental Psychology, 28*, 941–947.

Covell, K., & Abramovitch, R. (1987). Understanding of emotion in the family: Children's and parents' attributions of happiness, sadness, and anger. *Child Development, 58*, 985–991.

Covell, K., & Abramovitch, R. (1988). Children's understanding of maternal anger: Age and source of anger differences. *Merrill–Palmer Quarterly, 34*, 353–368.

Covell, K., & Miles, B. (1992). Children's beliefs about strategies to reduce parental anger. *Child Development, 63*, 381–390.

Crespo, L. M., Trentacosta, C. J., Aikins, D., & Wargo-Aikins, J. (2017). Maternal emotion regulation and children's behavior problems: The mediating role of child emotion regulation. *Journal of Child and Family Studies, 26*(10), 2797–2809.

Crockenberg, S. B. (1985). Toddlers' reactions to maternal anger. *Merrill–Palmer Quarterly, 31*, 361–373.

Crowe, L. M., Beauchamp, M. H., Catroppa, C., & Anderson, V. (2011). Social function assessment tools for children and adolescents: A systematic review from 1988 to 2010. *Clinical Psychology Review, 31*, 767–785.

Crozier, W. R., & Hostettler, K. (2003). The influence of shyness on children's test performance. *British Journal of Educational Psychology, 73*(3), 317–328.

Cummings, E. M. (1995a). Security, emotionality, and parental depression: A commentary. *Developmental Psychology, 31*, 425–427.

Cummings, E. M. (1995b). Usefulness of experiments for the study of the family. *Journal of Family Psychology, 9*, 175–185.

Cummings, E. M., & Cummings, J. L. (1988). A process-oriented approach to children's coping with adult's angry behavior. *Developmental Review, 8*, 296–321.

Cummings, E. M., Iannotti, R. J., & Zahn-Waxler, C. (1985). Influence of conflict between adults on the emotions and aggression of young children. *Developmental Psychology, 21*, 495–507.

Cummings, E. M., Simpson, K. S., & Wilson, A. (1993). Children's responses to interadult anger as a function of information about resolution. *Developmental Psychology, 29*, 978–985.

Cummings, E. M., Zahn-Waxler, C., & Radke-Yarrow, M. (1981). Young children's responses to expressions of anger and affection by others in the family. *Child Development, 52*, 1274–1282.

Cummings, E. M., Zahn-Waxler, C., & Radke-Yarrow, M. (1984). Developmental changes in children's reactions to anger in the home. *Journal of Child Psychology and Psychiatry, 25*(1), 63–74.

Cunningham, J. G., & Odom, R. D. (1986). Differential salience of facial features in children's perception of affective expression. *Child Development, 57*, 136–142.

Curby, T. W., Brock, L. L., & Hamre, B. K. (2013). Teachers' emotional support consistency predicts children's achievement gains and social skills. *Early Education and Development, 24,* 292–309.

Curby, T. W., Brown, C. A., Bassett, H. H., & Denham, S. A. (2015). Associations between preschoolers' social–emotional competence and preliteracy skills. *Infant and Child Development, 24*(5), 549–570.

Curby, T. W., Downer, J. T., & Booren, L. (2014). Behavioral exchanges between teachers and children over the course of a typical preschool day: Testing bidirectional associations. *Early Childhood Research Quarterly, 29,* 193–204.

Curenton, S. M., & Wilson, M. N. (2003). "I'm happy with my mommy": Low-income preschoolers' causal attributions for emotions. *Early Education and Development, 14*(2), 199–214.

Cutting, A. L., & Dunn, J. (1999). Theory of mind, emotion understanding, language, and family background: Individual differences and interrelations. *Child Development, 70*(4), 853–865.

Dadds, M. R., Sanders, M. R., Morrison, M., & Rebetz, M. (1992). Childhood depression and conduct disorder: II. An analysis of family interaction patterns in the home. *Journal of Abnormal Psychology, 101,* 505–513.

Darling-Churchill, K. E., & Lippman, L. (2016). Early childhood social and emotional development: Advancing the field of measurement. *Journal of Applied Developmental Psychology, 45,* 1–7.

da Silva, B. M., Ketelaar, L., Veiga, G., Tsou, Y. T., & Rieffe, C. (2022). Moral emotions in early childhood: Validation of the Moral Emotions Questionnaire (MEQ). *International Journal of Behavioral Development, 46*(2), 157–168.

Davidov, M., Paz, Y., Roth-Hanania, R., Uzefovsky, F., Orlitsky, T., Mankuta, D., & Zahn-Waxler, C. (2020). Caring babies: Concern for others in distress during infancy. *Developmental Science, 24*(2), e13016.

Davidov, M., Zahn-Waxler, C., Roth-Hanania, R., & Knafo, A. (2013). Concern for others in the first year of life: Theory, evidence, and avenues for research. *Child Development Perspectives, 7*(2), 126–131.

Davies, P. T., & Cummings, E. M. (1995). Children's emotions as organizers of their reactions to interadult anger: A functionalist perspective. *Developmental Psychology, 31,* 677–684.

Davis, E. L., Levine, L. J., Lench, H. C., & Quas, J. A. (2010). Metacognitive emotion regulation: children's awareness that changing thoughts and goals can alleviate negative emotions. *Emotion, 10*(4), 498–510.

Davis, M., Suveg, C., & Shaffer, A. (2015a). Maternal positive affect mediates the link between family risk and preschoolers' positive affect. *Child Psychiatry and Human Development, 46,* 167–175

Davis, M., Suveg, C., & Shaffer, A. (2015b). The value of a smile: Child positive affect moderates relations between maternal emotion dysregulation and child adjustment problems. *Journal of Child and Family Studies, 24,* 2441–2452.

Dawson, G., Hill, D., Spencer, A., Galpert, L., & Watson, L. (1990). Affective exchanges between young autistic children and their mothers. *Journal of Abnormal Child Psychology, 18,* 335–345.

Day, C., & Hong, J. (2016). Influences on the capacities for emotional resilience of teachers in schools serving disadvantaged urban communities: Challenges of living on the edge. *Teaching and Teacher Education, 59,* 115–125.

De Castro, B. O., Veerman, J. W., Koops, W., Bosch, J. D., & Monshouwer, H. J. (2002). Hostile attribution of intent and aggressive behavior: A meta-analysis. *Child Development, 73*(3), 916–934.

De Leersnyder, J., Boiger, M., & Mesquita, B. (2015). Emerging trends: Cultural differences in emotions. *Emerging Trends in the Social Sciences,* 1–22.

De Rosnay, M., Fink, E., Begeer, S., Slaughter, V., & Peterson, C. (2014). Talking theory of mind talk: Young school-aged children's everyday conversation and understanding of mind and emotion. *Journal of Child Language, 41*(5), 1179–1193.

De Rosnay, M. D., & Harris, P. L. (2002). Individual differences in children's understanding of emotion: The roles of attachment and language. *Attachment and Human Development, 4*(1), 39–54.

de Santana, C. C., Souza, W. C. D., & Feitosa, M. A. G. (2014). Recognition of facial emotional expressions and its correlation with cognitive abilities in children with Down syndrome. *Psychology and Neuroscience, 7,* 73–81.

De Stasio, S., Fiorilli, C., & Di Chiacchio, C. (2014). Effects of verbal ability and fluid intelligence on children's emotion understanding. *International Journal of Psychology, 49*(5), 409–414.

Decety, J., & Jackson, P. L. (2006). A social-neuroscience perspective on empathy. *Current Directions in Psychological Science, 15*(2), 54–58.

Decety, J., & Svetlova, M. (2012). Putting together phylogenetic and ontogenetic perspectives on empathy. *Developmental Cognitive Neuroscience, 2*(1), 1–24.

Degnan, K. A., Hane, A. A., Henderson, H. A., Moas, O. L., Reeb-Sutherland, B. C., & Fox, N. A. (2011). Longitudinal stability of temperamental exuberance and social–emotional outcomes in early childhood. *Developmental Psychology, 47*(3), 765–780.

Deichmann, F., & Ahnert, L. (2021). The terrible twos: How children cope with frustration and tantrums and the effect of maternal and paternal behaviors. *Infancy, 26*(3), 469–493.

DeMorat, M. G. (1998). *Emotion socialization in the classroom context: A functionalist analysis.* University of California, Santa Barbara. Retrieved from *http://media.proquest.com.*

Deneault, J., & Ricard, M. (2013). Are emotion and mind understanding differently linked to young children's social adjustment?: Relationships between behavioral consequences of emotions, false belief, and SCBE. *Journal of Genetic Psychology, 174*(1), 88–116.

Denham, S. A. (1986). Social cognition, social behavior, and emotion in preschoolers: Contextual validation. *Child Development, 57,* 194–201.

Denham, S. A. (1989). Maternal affect and toddlers' social-emotional competence. *American Journal of Orthopsychiatry, 59,* 368–376.

Denham, S. A. (1993). Maternal emotional responsiveness and toddlers' social-emotional functioning. *Journal of Child Psychology and Psychiatry, 34,* 725–728.

Denham, S. A. (1996a). *Preschoolers' understanding of parents' emotions: Implications for emotional competence.* Unpublished manuscript.

Denham, S. A. (1996b). *Maternal child-rearing practices: Contributions to preschoolers' understanding of emotion.* Unpublished manuscript.

Denham, S. A. (1997). "When I have a bad dream, Mommy holds me": Preschoolers' consequential thinking about emotions and social competence. *International Journal of Behavioral Development, 20,* 301–319.

Denham, S. A. (1998). *Emotional development in young children.* Guilford Press.

Denham, S. A. (2006). Social-emotional competence as support for school readiness: What is it and how do we assess it? *Early Education and Development, 17,* 57–89.

Denham, S. A. (2015). Assessment of SEL in educational contexts. In J. A. Durlak, C. E. Domitrovich, R. P. Weissberg, & T. P. Gullotta (Eds), *Handbook of social and emotional learning: Research and practice* (pp. 285–300). Guilford Press.

Denham, S. A. (2019). Emotional competence during childhood and adolescence. In V. LoBue, K. Perez-Edgar, & K. Buss (Eds.), *Handbook of emotional development* (pp. 493–542). Springer.

Denham, S. A., & Auerbach, S. (1995). Mother–child dialogue about emotions. *Genetic, Social, and General Psychology Monographs, 121,* 311–338.

Denham, S. A., & Bassett, H. H. (2018). Implications of preschoolers' emotional competence in the classroom. In K. Keefer, J. Parker, & D. Saklofske (Eds.), *Emotional intelligence in education* (pp. 135–171). Springer.

Denham, S. A., & Bassett, H. H. (2019). Early childhood teachers' socialization of children's emotional competence. *Journal of Research in Innovative Teaching and Learning, 12(2),* 133–150.

Denham, S. A., Bassett, H. H., Brown, C., Way, E., & Steed, J. (2015). "I know how you feel": Preschoolers' emotion knowledge contributes to early school success. *Journal of Early Childhood Research, 13*(3), 252–262.

Denham, S. A., Bassett, H. H., & Miller, S. (2017). Early childhood teachers' socialization of emotion: Contextual and individual contributors. *Child and Youth Care Forum, 46,* 805–824.

Denham, S. A. Bassett, H. H., Mincic, M. M., Kalb, S. C., Way, E., Wyatt, T., & Segal, Y. (2012). Social-emotional learning profiles of preschoolers' early school success: A person-centered approach. *Learning and Individual Differences, 22*(2), 178–189.

Denham, S. A., Bassett, H. H., Sirotkin, Y., & Zinsser, K. (2013). Head Start preschoolers' emotional positivity and emotion regulation predict their social-emotion behavior, classroom adjustment, and early school success. *National Head Start Association Dialog, 16(2).*

Denham, S. A., Bassett, H. H., Thayer, S. K., Mincic, M., Sirotkin, Y. S., & Zinsser, K. (2012). Observing preschoolers' social-emotional behavior: Structure, foundations, and prediction of early school success. *Journal of Genetic Psychology, 173,* 246–278.

Denham, S. A., Bassett, H. H., Way, E., Mincic, M., Zinsser, K., & Graling, K. (2012). Preschoolers' emotion knowledge: Self-regulatory foundations, and predictions of early school success. *Cognition and Emotion,* 26, 667–679.

Denham, S. A., Bassett, H. H., & Wyatt, T. M. (2010). Gender differences in the socialization of preschoolers' emotional competence. *New Directions for Child and Adolescent Development,* 128, 29–49.

Denham, S. A., Bassett, H. H., & Wyatt, T. (2014). The socialization of emotional competence. In J. Grusec & P. Hastings (Eds.), *Handbook of socialization* (2nd ed., pp. 590–613). Guilford Press.

Denham, S. A., Bassett, H. H., & Zinsser, K. (2012). Early childhood teachers as socializers of young children's emotional competence. *Early Childhood Education Journal,* 40, 137–143.

Denham, S. A., Bassett, H. H., Zinsser, K. M., Bradburn, I. S., Bailey, C. S., Shewark, E. A., . . . Kianpour, S. (2020). Computerized social-emotional assessment measures for early childhood settings. *Early Childhood Research Quarterly, 51,* 55–66.

Denham, S. A., Bassett, H. H., Zinsser, K., & Wyatt, T. M. (2014). How preschoolers' social–emotional learning predicts their early school success: Developing theory-promoting, competency-based assessments. *Infant and Child Development, 23,* 426–454.

Denham, S. A., Blair, K. A., DeMulder, E., Levitas, J., Sawyer, K. S., Auerbach-Major, S. T., & Queenan, P. (2003). Preschoolers' emotional competence: Pathway to social competence? *Child Development, 74,* 238–256.

Denham, S. A., Blair, K., Schmidt, M., & DeMulder, E. (2002). Compromised emotional competence: Seeds of violence sown early? *American Journal of Orthopsychiatry, 72,* 70–82.

Denham, S. A., Brown, C. A., & Domitrovich, C. E. (2010). "Plays nice with others": Social-emotional learning and academic success. *Early Education and Development, 21,* 652–680.

Denham, S. A., & Burger, C. (1991). Observational validation of teacher rating scales. *Child Study Journal, 21,* 185–202.

Denham, S. A., & Burton, R. (1996). A social-emotional intervention program for at risk four-year-olds. *Journal of School Psychology, 34,* 225–245.

Denham, S. A., & Burton, R. (2003). *Social and emotional prevention and intervention programming for preschoolers.* Kluwer Academic/Plenum.

Denham, S. A., Caal, S., Bassett, H. H., Benga, O., & Geangu, E. (2004). Listening to parents: Cultural variations in the meaning of emotions and emotion socialization. *Cognitie Creier Comportament, 8,* 321–350.

Denham, S. A., Caverly, S., Schmidt, M., Blair, K., DeMulder, E., Caal, S, . . . Mason, T. (2002). Preschool understanding of emotions: Contributions to classroom anger and aggression. *Journal of Child Psychology and Psychiatry,* 43, 901–916.

Denham, S. A., Cook, M. C., & Zoller, D. (1992). "Baby looks *very* sad": Discussions about emotions between mother and preschooler. *British Journal of Developmental Psychology, 10*, 301–315.

Denham, S. A., & Couchoud, E. A. (1990a). Young preschoolers' ability to identify emotions in equivocal emotion situations. *Child Study Journal, 20*, 153–170.

Denham, S. A., & Couchoud, E. A. (1990b). Young preschoolers' understanding of emotion. *Child Study Journal, 20*, 171–192.

Denham, S. A., & Couchoud, E. A. (1991). Social-emotional contributors to preschoolers' responses to an adult's negative emotions. *Journal of Child Psychology and Psychiatry, 32*, 595–608.

Denham, S. A., Ferrier, D. E., & Bassett, H. H. (2020). Preschool teachers' socialization of emotion knowledge: Considering socioeconomic risk. *Journal of Applied Developmental Psychology, 69*, 101160.

Denham, S. A., Grant, S., & Hamada, H. (2002, June). *"I have two first teachers about emotions: Contributions of mothers and teachers in promoting preschoolers' self-regulation and social competence.* Poster presented at the National Head Start Research Conference, Washington, DC.

Denham, S. A., & Grout, L. (1992). Mothers' emotional expressiveness and coping: Topography and relations with preschoolers' social-emotional competence. *Genetic, Social, and General Psychology Monographs, 118*, 75–101.

Denham, S. A., & Grout, L. (1993). Socialization of emotion: Pathway to preschoolers' affect regulation. *Journal of Nonverbal Behavior, 17*, 205–227.

Denham, S. A., & Holt, R. (1993). Preschoolers' peer status: A cause or consequence of behavior? *Developmental Psychology, 29*, 271–275.

Denham, S., Ji, P., & Hamre, B. K. (2010). *Compendium of social-emotional learning and associated assessment measures.* Collaborative for Academic, Social, and Emotional Learning.

Denham, S., & Kochanoff, A. T. (2002). Parental contributions to preschoolers' understanding of emotion. *Marriage and Family Review, 34*(3–4), 311–343.

Denham, S. A., Lehman, E. B., Moser, M. H., & Reeves, S. (1995). Continuity and change in emotional components of temperament. *Child Study Journal, 25*, 289–304.

Denham, S. A., Mason, T., & Couchoud, E. A. (1995). Situational contributors to preschoolers' responses to adults' sadness, anger, and pain. *International Journal of Behavioral Development, 18*, 489–504

Denham, S. A., Mason, T., Caverly, S., Schmidt, M., Hackney, R., Caswell, C., & DeMulder, E. (2001). Preschoolers at play: Co-socializers of emotional and social competence. *International Journal of Behavioral Development, 25*, 290–301.

Denham, S. A., & McKinley, M. (1993). Sociometric nominations of preschoolers: A psychometric analysis. *Early Education and Development, 4*, 109–122.

Denham, S. A., McKinley, M., Couchoud, E. A., & Holt, R. (1990). Emotional and behavioral predictors of peer status in young preschoolers. *Child Development, 61*, 1145–1152.

Denham, S. A., Mitchell-Copeland, J., Strandberg, K., Auerbach, S., & Blair, K. (1997). Parental contributions to preschoolers' emotional competence: Direct and indirect effects. *Motivation and Emotion, 27*, 65–86.

Denham, S. A., Mortari, L., & Silva, R. (2022). Preschool teachers' emotion socialization and child social-emotional behavior in two countries. *Early Education and Development, 33*(5), 806–831.

Denham, S. A., Renwick, S., & Holt, R. (1991). Working and playing together: Prediction of preschool social-emotional competence from mother–child interaction. *Child Development, 62*, 242–249.

Denham, S. A., Renwick-DeBardi, S., & Hewes, S. (1994). Affective communication between mothers and preschoolers: Relations with social-emotional competence. *Merrill–Palmer Quarterly, 40*, 488–508.

Denham, S. A., Way, E., Kalb, S. C., Warren-Khot, H. K., & Bassett, H. H. (2013). Preschoolers' social information processing and early school success: The Challenging Situations Task. *British Journal of Developmental Psychology, 31*, 180–197.

Denham, S. A., & Weissberg, R. P. (2004). Social-emotional learning in early childhood: What we know and and where to go from here? In E. Chesebrough, P. King, T. P. Gullotta, & M. Bloom (Eds.), *A blueprint for the promotion of prosocial behavior in early childhood* (pp. 13–50). Kluwer/Academic.

Denham, S. A., Workman, E., Cole, P., Weissbrod, C., Kendziora, K., & Zahn-Waxler, C. (2000). Parental contributions to externalizing and internalizing patterns in young children at risk for conduct disorder. *Development and Psychopathology, 12*, 23–45.

Denham, S. A., Wyatt, T. M., Bassett, H. H., Echeverria, D., & Knox, S. S. (2009). Assessing social-emotional development in children from a longitudinal perspective. *Journal of Epidemiology and Community Health, 63*(Suppl. 1), 137–152.

Denham, S. A., Zahn-Waxler, C., Cummings, E. M., & Iannotti, R. J. (1991). Social competence in young children's peer relationships: Patterns of development and change. *Child Psychiatry and Human Development, 22*, 29–43.

Denham, S. A., & Zoller, D. (1990, March). *"When Mommy's angry, I feel sad": Preschoolers' understanding of emotion and its socialization.* Poster presented at the biennial Conference on Human Development, Richmond, VA.

Denham, S. A., & Zoller, D. (1991). "When my hamster died, I cried": Preschoolers' attributions of the causes of emotions. *Journal of Genetic Psychology, 152*, 371–373.

Denham, S. A., Zoller, D., & Couchoud, E. A. (1994). Socialization of preschoolers' understanding of emotion. *Developmental Psychology, 30*, 928–936.

Dennis, T. A., & Kelemen, D. A. (2009). Preschool children's views on emotion regulation: Functional associations and implications for social-emotional adjustment. *International Journal of Behavioral Development, 33*, 243–252.

Dereli, E. (2016). Prediction of emotional understanding and emotion regulation skills of 4–5 age group children with parent-child relations. *Journal of Education and Practice, 7*(21), 42–54.

Desmarais, E. E., French, B. F., Ahmetoglu, E., Acar, I., Gonzalez-Salinas, C., Kozlova, E., . . . Gartstein, M. A. (2021). Cultural contributors to negative emotionality: A multilevel analysis from the Joint Effort Toddler Temperament Consortium. *International Journal of Behavioral Development, 45*(6), 545–552.

Di Maggio, R., Zappulla, C., & Pace, U. (2016). The relationship between emotion knowledge, emotion regulation and adjustment in preschoolers: A mediation model. *Journal of Child and Family Studies, 25*, 2626–2635.

Di Maggio, R., Zappulla, C., Pace, U., & Izard, C. E. (2013). La conoscenza delle emozioni in età prescolare: un contributo alla validazione italiana dell'Emotion Matching Task (EMT) [Knowledge of emotions in preschool age: a contribution to the Italian validation of the Emotion Matching Task (EMT)]. *Psicologia clinica dello sviluppo* [*Clinical Developmental Psychology*], *17*(3), 521–532.

Diamond, A., Stuss, D. T., & Knight, R. T. (2002). Normal development of prefrontal cortex from birth to young adulthood: Cognitive functions, anatomy, and biochemistry. In D. Stuss & R. Knight (Eds.), *Principles of frontal lobe function* (pp. 466–503). Oxford University Press.

Diaz, A., Eisenberg, N., Valiente, C., VanSchyndel, S., Spinrad, T. L., Berger, R., . . . Southworth, J. (2017). Relations of positive and negative expressivity and effortful control to kindergarteners' student–teacher relationship, academic engagement, and externalizing problems at school. *Journal of Research in Personality, 67*, 3–14.

Diener, M. L., & Kim, D. Y. (2004). Maternal and child predictors of preschool children's social competence. *Journal of Applied Developmental Psychology, 25*(1), 3–24.

Dissanayake, C., Sigman, M., & Kasari, C. (1996). Long-term stability of individual differences in the emotional responsiveness of children with autism. *Journal of Child Psychology and Psychiatry, 37*, 461–467.

Dix, T. (1991). The affective organization of parenting: Adaptive and maladaptive processes. *Psychological Bulletin, 110*, 3–25.

Doan, S. N., Lee, H. Y., & Wang, Q. (2019). Maternal mental state language is associated with trajectories of Chinese immigrant children's emotion situation knowledge. *International Journal of Behavioral Development, 43*(1), 43–52.

Doan, S. N., & Wang, Q. (2010). Maternal discussions of mental states and behaviors: Relations to emotion situation knowledge in European American and immigrant Chinese children. *Child Development, 81*(5), 1490–1503.

Doan, S. N., & Wang, Q. (2018). Children's emotion knowledge and internalizing problems: The moderating role of culture. *Transcultural Psychiatry, 55*(5), 689–709.

Dodge, K. A. (2006). Translational science in action: Hostile attributional style and the development of aggressive behavior problems. *Development and Psychopathology, 18*, 791–814.

Dodge, K. A., & Frame, C. L. (1982). Social cognitive biases and deficits in aggressive boys. *Child Development, 53*, 620–635.

Doey, L., Coplan, R. J., & Kingsbury, M. (2014). Bashful boys and coy girls: A review of gender differences in childhood shyness. *Sex Roles, 70*(7–8), 255–266.

Dollar, J. M., Perry, N. B., Calkins, S. D., Shanahan, L., Keane, S. P., Shriver, L., & Wideman, L. (2022). Longitudinal associations between specific types of emotional reactivity and psychological, physical health, and school adjustment. *Development and Psychopathology*, 1–15. [Epub ahead of print]

Dollar, J. M., & Stifter, C. A. (2012). Temperamental surgency and emotion regulation as predictors of childhood social competence. *Journal of Experimental Child Psychology, 112*(2), 178–194.

Domitrovich, C. E., Cortes, R. C., & Greenberg, M. T. (2007). Improving young children's social and emotional competence: A randomized trial of the preschool "PATHS" curriculum. *Journal of Primary Prevention, 28*(2), 67–91.

Donaldson, S. K., & Westerman, M. A. (1986). Development of children's understanding of ambivalence and causal theories of emotions. *Developmental Psychology, 22*, 655–662.

Downs, A., Strand, P., & Cerna, S. (2007). Emotion understanding in English- and Spanish-speaking preschoolers enrolled in Head Start. *Social Development, 16(3)*, 410–439.

Drummond, J. D., Hammond, S. I., Satlof-Bedrick, E., Waugh, W. E., & Brownell, C. A. (2017). Helping the one you hurt: Toddlers' rudimentary guilt, shame, and prosocial behavior after harming another. *Child Development, 88*(4), 1382–1397.

Drummond, J., Paul, E. F., Waugh, W. E., Hammond, S. I., & Brownell, C. A. (2014). Here, there and everywhere: Emotion and mental state talk in different social contexts predicts empathic helping in toddlers. *Frontiers in Psychology, 5*, 361.

Duckworth, A. L., & Yeager, D. S. (2015). Measurement matters: Assessing personal qualities other than cognitive ability for educational purposes. *Educational Researcher, 44*(4), 237–251.

Duku, E., & Vaillancourt, T. (2014). Validation of the BRIEF-P in a sample of Canadian preschool children. *Child Neuropsychology, 20*(3), 358–371.

Dumas, J. E., Martinez, A., & LaFreniere, P. J. (1998). The Spanish version of the Social Competence and Behavior Evaluation (SCBE)—Preschool edition: Translation and field testing. *Hispanic Journal of Behavioral Sciences*. 20, 255–269.

Dumas, J. E., Martinez, A., LaFreniere, P. J., & Dolz, L. (1998). Spanish version of the Social Competence and Behavior Evaluation—Preschool Edition (SCBE): Adaptation and validation. *Psicologica. 19*, 107–121.

Dunbar, A. S., Leerkes, E. M., Coard, S. I., Supple, A. J., & Calkins, S. (2017). An integrative conceptual model of parental racial/ethnic and emotion socialization and links to children's social-emotional development among African American families. *Child Development Perspectives, 11*(1), 16–22.

Dunn, J. (1988). *The beginnings of social understanding.* Harvard University Press.

Dunn, J. (1994). Understanding others and the social world: Current issues in developmental research and their relation to preschool experiences and practice. *Journal of Applied Developmental Psychology, 15*(4), 571–583.

Dunn, J. (1995). Children as psychologists: The later correlates of individual differences in understanding of emotions and other minds. *Cognition and Emotion, 9*, 187–201.

Dunn, J., Bretherton, I., & Munn, P. (1987). Conversations about feeling states between mothers and their young children. *Developmental Psychology, 23*, 132–139.

Dunn, J., & Brown, J. R. (1994). Affect expression in the family: Children's understanding of emotions and their interactions with others. *Merrill–Palmer Quarterly, 40*, 120–137.

Dunn, J., Brown, J. R., & Beardsall, L. (1991). Family talk about feeling states and children's later understanding of others' emotions. *Developmental Psychology, 27*, 448–455.

Dunn, J., Brown, J. R., & Maguire, M. (1995). The development of children's moral sensibility: Individual differences and emotion understanding. *Developmental Psychology, 31*, 649–659.

Dunn, J., Brown, J. R., Slomkowski, C., Tesla, C., & Youngblade, L. (1991). Young children's understanding of other people's feelings and beliefs: Individual differences and their antecedents. *Child Development, 62*, 1352–1366.

Dunn, J., & Hughes, C. (1998). Young children's understanding of emotions within close relationships. *Cognition and Emotion, 12*, 171–190.

Dunn, J., & Munn, P. (1985). Becoming a family member: Family conflict and the development of social understanding in the second year. *Child Development, 56*, 480–492.

Dunn, J., Slomkowski, C., Donelan, N., & Herrera, C. (1995). Conflict, understanding, and relationships: Developments and differences in the preschool years. *Early Education and Development, 6*(4), 303–316.

Dunsmore, J. C., Her, P., Halberstadt, A. G., & Perez-Rivera, M. B. (2009). Parents' beliefs about emotions and children's recognition of parents' emotions. *Journal of Nonverbal Behavior, 33*(2), 121–140.

Dunsmore, J. C., & Karn, M. A. (2004). The influence of peer relationships and maternal socialization on kindergartners' developing emotion knowledge. *Early Education and Development, 15*, 39–56.

Dunsmore, J. C., Noguchi, R. J., Garner, P. W., Casey, E. C., & Bhullar, N. (2008). Gender-specific linkages of affective social competence with peer relations in preschool children. *Early Education and Development, 19*(2), 211–237.

During, S. M., & McMahon, R. J. (1991). Recognition of emotional facial expressions by abusive mothers and their children. *Journal of Clinical Child Psychology, 20*, 132–139.

Durlak, J. A., Weissberg, R. P., Dymnicki, A. B., Taylor, R. D., & Schellinger, K. B. (2011). The impact of enhancing students' social and emotional learning: A meta-analysis of school-based universal interventions. *Child Development, 82*, 405–432.

Dusenbury, L., Newman, J. A., Weissberg, R. P., Goren, P., Domitrovich, C. E., Mart, A. K., & Cascarino, J. (2015). Developing a blueprint for preschool through high school education in social and emotional learning: The case for state learning standards. In J. A. Durlak, C. E. Domitrovich, R. P. Weissberg, & T. P. Gullotta (Eds.), *Handbook of social and emotional learning: Research and practice* (pp. 532–548). Guilford Press.

Dusenbury, L., Zadrazil, J., Mart, A., & Weissberg, R. (2011). *State learning standards to advance social and emotional learning.* Collaborative for Academic, Social, and Emotional Learning.

Ebesutani, C., Regan, J., Smith, A., Reise, S., Higa-McMillan, C., & Chorpita, B. F. (2012). The 10-item positive and negative affect schedule for children, child and parent shortened versions: Application of item response theory for more efficient assessment. *Journal of Psychopathology and Behavioral Assessment, 34*(2), 191–203.

Edwards, A., Eisenberg, N., Spinrad, T. L., Reiser, M., Eggum-Wilkens, N. D., & Liew, J. (2015). Predicting sympathy and prosocial behavior from young children's dispositional sadness. *Social Development* 24(1), 76–94.

Egeland, B., Kalkoske, M., Gottesman, N., & Erickson, M. F. (1990). Preschool behavior problems: Stability and factors accounting for change. *Journal of Child Psychology and Psychiatry, 31*, 891–909.

Eggum, N. D., Eisenberg, N., Kao, K., Spinrad, T. L., Bolnick, R., Hofer, C., . . . Fabricius, W. V. (2011). Emotion understanding, theory of mind, and prosocial orientation: Relations over time in early childhood. *Journal of Positive Psychology, 6*(1), 4–16.

Eggum, N. D., Eisenberg, N., Spinrad, T. L., Reiser, M., Gaertner, B. M., Sallquist, J., & Smith, C. L. (2009). Development of shyness: Relations with children's fearfulness, sex, and maternal behavior. *Infancy, 14*(3), 325–345.

Eggum-Wilkens, N. D., Lemery-Chalfant, K., Aksan, N., & Goldsmith, H. H. (2015). Self-conscious shyness: Growth during toddlerhood, strong role of genetics, and no prediction from fearful shyness. *Infancy, 20*(2), 160–188.

Eisenberg, N. (1986). *Altruism, emotion, cognition, and behavior.* Erlbaum.

Eisenberg, N. (2020). Findings, issues, and new directions for research on emotion socialization. *Developmental Psychology, 56*(3), 664–670.

Eisenberg, N., Bernzweig, J., & Fabes, R. A. (1991). Coping and vicarious emotional responding. In T. M. Field, P. M. McCabe, & N. Schneiderman (Eds.), *Stress and coping in infancy and childhood* (pp. 101–117). Erlbaum.

Eisenberg, N., Cumberland, A., & Spinrad, T. L. (1998). Parental socialization of emotion. *Psychological Inquiry, 9*(4), 241–273.

Eisenberg, N., & Eggum, N. D. (2009). Empathic responding: Sympathy and personal distress. *Social Neuroscience of Empathy, 6*, 71–830.

Eisenberg, N., & Fabes, R. A. (1992). Emotion, regulation, and the development of social competence. In

M. S. Clark (Ed.), *Review of personality and social psychology: Vol. 14. Emotion and social behavior* (pp. 119–150). SAGE.

Eisenberg, N., & Fabes, R. A. (1994). Mothers' reactions to children's negative emotions: Relations to children's temperament and anger behavior. *Merrill–Palmer Quarterly, 40*, 138–156.

Eisenberg, N., Fabes, R. A., Bernzweig, J., Karbon, M., Poulin, R., & Hanish, L. (1993). The relations of emotionality and regulation to preschoolers' social skills and sociometric status. *Child Development, 64*, 1418–1438.

Eisenberg, N., Fabes, R. A., Carlo, G., & Karbon, M. (1992). Emotional responsivity to others: Behavioral correlates and socialization antecedents. In N. Eisenberg & R. A. Fabes (Eds.), *New Directions for Child Development: No. 55. Emotion and its regulation in early development* (pp. 57–73). Jossey-Bass.

Eisenberg, N., Fabes, R. A., Murphy, B., Karbon, M., Smith, M., & Maszk, P. (1996). The relations of children's dispositional empathy-related responding to their emotionality, regulation, and social functioning. *Developmental Psychology, 32*, 195–209.

Eisenberg, N., Fabes, R. A., Murphy, B., Maszk, P., Smith, M., & Karbon, M. (1995). The role of emotionality and regulation in children's social functioning: A longitudinal study. *Child Development, 66*, 1360–1384.

Eisenberg, N., Fabes, R. A., Nyman, M., Bernzweig, J., & Pinuelas, A. (1994). The relation of emotionality and regulation to preschoolers' anger-related reactions. *Child Development, 65*, 1352–1366.

Eisenberg, N., Fabes, R. A., Schaller, M., Carlo, G., & Miller, P. (1991). The relations of parental characteristics and practices to children's vicarious emotional responding. *Child Development, 62*, 1393–1408.

Eisenberg, N., Fabes, R. A., Shepard, S. A., Murphy, B. C., Guthrie, I. K., Jones, S., . . . Maszk, P. (1997). Contemporaneous and longitudinal prediction of children's social functioning from regulation and emotionality. *Child Development, 68*(4), 642–664.

Eisenberg, N., Ma, Y., Chang, L., Zhou, Q., West, S. G., & Aiken, L. (2007). Relations of effortful control, reactive undercontrol, and anger to Chinese children's adjustment. *Development and Psychopathology, 19*(2), 385–409.

Eisenberg, N., McCreath, H., & Ahn, R. (1988). Vicarious emotional responsiveness and prosocial behavior: Their interrelations in young children. *Personality and Social Psychology Bulletin, 14*, 298–311.

Eisenberg, N., Pasternack, J. F., Cameron, E., & Tryon, K. (1984). The relations of quantity and mode of prosocial behavior to moral cognitions and social style. *Child Development, 55*, 1479–1485.

Eisenberg, N., Sadovsky, A., & Spinrad, T. L. (2005). Associations of emotion-related regulation with language skills, emotion knowledge, and academic outcomes. *New Directions for Child and Adolescent Development, 2005*(109), 109–118.

Eisenberg, N., Sadovsky, A., Spinrad, T. L., Fabes, R. A., Losoya, S. H., Valiente, C., . . . Shepard, S. A. (2005). The relations of problem behavior status to children's negative emotionality, effortful control, and impulsivity: concurrent relations and prediction of change. *Developmental Psychology, 41*(1), 193–211.

Eisenberg, N., Schaller, M., Fabes, R. A., Bustamante, D., Mathy, R., Shell, R., & Rhodes, K. (1988). Differentiation of personal distress and sympathy in children and adults. *Developmental Psychology, 24*, 766–775.

Eisenberg, N., Shepard, S. A., Fabes, R. A., Murphy, B. C., & Guthrie, I. K. (1998). Shyness and children's emotionality, regulation, and coping: Contemporaneous, longitudinal, and across-context relations. *Child Development, 69*(3), 767–790.

Eisenberg, N., Spinrad, T. L., & Morris, A. (2014). Empathy-related responding in children In M. Killen & J. Smetana (Eds.), *Handbook of moral development* (pp. 184–207). Psychology Press.

Ekerim-Akbulut, M., Şen, H. H., Beşiroğlu, B., & Selçuk, B. (2020). The role of theory of mind, emotion knowledge and empathy in preschoolers' disruptive behavior. *Journal of Child and Family Studies, 29*(1), 128–143.

Ekman, P., & Friesen, W. V. (1975). *Unmasking the face*. Prentice-Hall.

Ellis, B. H., Alisic, E., Reiss, A., Dishion, T., & Fisher, P. A. (2014). Emotion regulation among preschoolers on a continuum of risk: The role of maternal emotion coaching. *Journal of Child and Family Studies, 23*(6), 965–974.

Else-Quest, N. M., Hyde, J. S., Goldsmith, H. H., & Van Hulle, C. A. (2006). Gender differences in temperament: A meta-analysis. *Psychological Bulletin, 132*(1), 33–72.

El-Sheikh, M., Cummings, E. M., & Reiter, S. (1996). Preschoolers' responses to ongoing interadult conflict: The role of prior exposure to resolved versus unresolved arguments. *Journal of Abnormal Child Psychology, 24*, 665–679.

Emde, R. N. (2009). Facilitating reflective supervision in an early child development center. *Infant Mental Health Journal: Official Publication of the World Association for Infant Mental Health, 30*(6), 664–672.

Engel, S. (1995). *The stories children tell: Making sense of the narratives of childhood*. W. H. Freeman.

England-Mason, G., & Gonzalez, A. (2020). Intervening to shape children's emotion regulation: A review of emotion socialization parenting programs for young children. *Emotion, 20*(1), 98–104.

Ensor, R., Spencer, D., & Hughes, C. (2011). 'You feel sad?' Emotion understanding mediates effects of verbal ability and mother–child mutuality on prosocial behaviors: Findings from 2 years to 4 years. *Social Development, 20*(1), 93–110.

Erhart, A., Dmitrieva, J., Blair, R. J., & Kim, P. (2019). Intensity, not emotion: The role of poverty in emotion labeling ability in middle childhood. *Journal of Experimental Child Psychology, 180*, 131–140.

Erickson, M. F., Egeland, B., & Pianta, R. (1989). The effects of maltreatment on the development of young children. In D. Cicchetti & V. Carlson (Eds.), *Child maltreatment: Theory and research on the courses and consequences of child abuse and neglect* (pp. 647–684). Cambridge University Press.

Ersan, C. (2020). Physical aggression, relational aggression and anger in preschool children: The mediating role of emotion regulation. *Journal of General Psychology, 147*(1), 18–42.

Ersan, C., & Tok, Ş. (2020). The study of the aggression levels of preschool children in terms of emotion expression and emotion regulation. *Education & Science/Egitim ve Bilim, 45*(201), 359–391.

Ersay, E. (2007). *Preschool teachers' emotional experience traits, awareness of their own emotions and their emotional socialization practices.* Retrieved from ProQuest Dissertations and Theses.

Ersay, E. (2015). Preschool teachers' emotional awareness levels and their responses to children's negative emotions. *Procedia-Social and Behavioral Sciences, 191,* 1833–1837.

Fabes, R. A., & Eisenberg, N. (1992). Young children's coping with interpersonal anger. *Child Development, 63,* 116–128.

Fabes, R. A., Eisenberg, N., & Bernzweig, J. (1990). *The Coping with Children's Negative Emotions Scale: Description and scoring.* Unpublished manuscript, Department of Family and Human Development, Arizona State University.

Fabes, R. A., Eisenberg, N., Hanish, L. D., & Spinrad, T. L. (2001). Preschoolers' spontaneous emotion vocabulary: Relations to likability. *Early Education and Development, 12*(1), 11–27.

Fabes, R. A., Eisenberg, N., Karbon, M., Bernzweig, J., Speer, A. L., & Carlo, G. (1994). Socialization of children's vicarious emotional responding and prosocial behavior: Relations with mothers' perceptions of children's emotional reactivity. *Developmental Psychology, 30,* 44–55.

Fabes, R. A., Eisenberg, N., McCormick, S. E., & Wilson, M. S. (1988). Preschoolers' attributions of the situational determinants of others' naturally occurring emotions. *Developmental Psychology, 24,* 376–385.

Fabes, R. A., Eisenberg, N., & Miller, P. A. (1990). Maternal correlates of children's vicarious emotional responsiveness. *Developmental Psychology, 26,* 639–648.

Fabes, R. A., Eisenberg, N., Nyman, M., & Michealieu, Q. (1991). Young children's appraisal of others' spontaneous emotional reactions. *Developmental Psychology, 27,* 858–866.

Fabes, R. A., Leonard, S. A., Kupanoff, K., & Martin, C. L. (2001). Parental coping with children's negative emotions: Relations with children's emotional and social responding. *Child Development, 72*(3), 907–920.

Fabes, R. A., Poulin, R. E., Eisenberg, N., & Madden-Derdich, D. A. (2002). The Coping with Children's Negative Emotions Scale (CCNES): Psychometric properties and relations with children's emotional competence. *Marriage and Family Review, 34,* 285–310.

Farina, E., & Belacchi, C. (2014). The relationship between emotional competence and hostile/prosocial behavior in Albanian preschoolers: An exploratory study. *School Psychology International, 35*(5), 475–484.

Farrant, B. M., Devine, T. A., Maybery, M. T., & Fletcher, J. (2012). Empathy, perspective taking and prosocial behaviour: The importance of parenting practices. *Infant and Child Development, 21*(2), 175–188.

Farrell, C. B., & Gilpin, A. T. (2021). Longitudinal bidirectionality of emotion knowledge and inhibitory control in low-income children using cross-lagged panels. *Social Development, 30*(4), 1106–1022.

Farver, J. M., & Branstetter, W. H. (1994). Preschoolers' prosocial responses to their peers' distress. *Developmental Psychology, 30,* 334–341.

Feito, J. A. (1997). *Children's belief about the social consequences of emotional expression.* Universal.

Feldman, R., Dollberg, D., & Nadam, R. (2011). The expression and regulation of anger in toddlers: Relations to maternal behavior and mental representations. *Infant Behavior and Development, 34*(2), 310–320.

Felleman, E. S., Barden, R. C. Carlson, C. R., Rosenberg, L., & Masters, J. C. (1983). Children's and adults' recognition of spontaneous and posed emotional expressions in young children. *Developmental Psychology, 19,* 405–413.

Feng, X., Shaw, D. S., Kovacs, M., Lane, T., O'Rourke, F. E., & Alarcon, J. H. (2008). Emotion regulation in preschoolers: The roles of behavioral inhibition, maternal affective behavior, and maternal depression. *Journal of Child Psychology and Psychiatry, 49*(2), 132–141.

Feng, X., Shaw, D. S., & Moilanen, K. L. (2011). Parental negative control moderates the shyness–emotion regulation pathway to school-age internalizing symptoms. *Journal of Abnormal Child Psychology, 39*(3), 425–436.

Feng, X., Shaw, D. S., Skuban, E. M., & Lane, T. (2007). Emotional exchange in mother-child dyads: Stability, mutual influence, and associations with maternal depression and child problem behavior. *Journal of Family Psychology, 21*(4), 714–725.

Fenning, R. M., Baker, J. K., & Moffitt, J. (2018). Intrinsic and extrinsic predictors of emotion regulation in children with autism spectrum disorder. *Journal of Autism and Developmental Disorders, 48*(11), 3858–3870.

Ferguson, T., & Stegge, H. (1995). Emotional states and traits in children: The case of guilt and shame. In J. P. Tangney & K. W. Fischer (Eds.), *Self-conscious emotions: The psychology of shame, guilt, embarrassment, and pride* (pp. 174–197). Guilford Press.

Ferguson, T. J., Stegge, H., Miller, E. R., & Olsen, M. E. (1999). Guilt, shame, and symptoms in children. *Developmental Psychology, 35*(2), 347–357.

Fergusson, A. S., Hopkins, S. W., Stark, A. M., Tousignant, O. H., & Fireman, G. D. (2020). Children expressing mixed emotion in a nonsocial context. *Journal of Genetic Psychology, 181*(5), 348–364.

Fernandes, C., Fernandes, M. S., Santos, A. J., Antunes, M., Monteiro, L., Vaughn, B. E., & Verissimo, M. (2021). Early attachment to mothers and fathers: Contributions to preschoolers' emotional regulation. *Frontiers in Psychology, 12,* 2395.

Fernandes, C., Veríssimo, M., Fernandes, M., Antunes, M., Santos, A. J., & Vaughn, B. E. (2019). Links between use of the secure base script and preschool children's knowledge about emotions. *Análise Psicológica, 37*(1), 71–80.

Fernández-Sánchez, M., Quintanilla, L., & Giménez-Dasí, M. (2015). Thinking emotions with two-year-old children: An educational programme to improve emotional knowledge in young preschoolers. *Cultura y Educación, 27*(4), 802–838.

Ferreira, M., Reis-Jorge, J., & Batalha, S. (2021). Social and emotional learning in preschool education: A qualitative study with preschool teachers. *International Journal of Emotional Education, 13(1)*, 51–66.

Ferrier, D., Karalus, S. P., Denham, S. A., & Bassett, H. H. (2018). Indirect effects of cognitive self-regulation on the relation between emotion knowledge and emotionality. *Early Child Development and Care, 188(7)*, 966–979.

Fettig, N., Howarth, G., Watanabe, N., Denham, S. A., & Bassett, H. H. (nd). *The Emotion Elicitation and Regulation Assessment (EERA)*. George Mason University.

Field, T. M., & Walden, T. A. (1982). Production and discrimination of facial expressions by preschool children. *Child Development, 53*, 1299–1311.

Fields-Olivieri, M. A., Cole, P. M., & Maggi, M. C. (2017). Toddler emotional states, temperamental traits, and their interaction: Associations with mothers' and fathers' parenting. *Journal of Research in Personality, 67*, 106–119.

Findlay, L. C., Girardi, A., & Coplan, R. J. (2006). Links between empathy, social behavior, and social understanding in early childhood. *Early Childhood Research Quarterly, 21*(3), 347–359.

Fine, S. E., Izard, C. E., Mostow, A. J., Trentacosta, C. J., & Ackerman, B. P. (2003). First grade emotion knowledge as a predictor of fifth grade self-reported internalizing behaviors in children from economically disadvantaged families. *Development and Psychopathology, 15*(2), 331–342.

Finlon, K. J., Izard, C. E., Seidenfeld, A., Johnson, S. R., Cavadel, E. W., Ewing, E. S. K., & Morgan, J. K. (2015). Emotion-based preventive intervention: Effectively promoting emotion knowledge and adaptive behavior among at-risk preschoolers. *Development and Psychopathology, 27*(4pt1), 1353–1365.

Fiorilli, C., De Stasio, S., Di Chicchio, C., & Chan, S. M. (2015). Emotion socialization practices in Italian and Hong Kong-Chinese mothers. *SpringerPlus, 4*(1), 1–9.

Fischer, K. W., Shaver, P. R., & Carnochan, P. (1989). A skill approach to emotional development: From basic- to superordinate-category emotions. In W. Damon (Ed.), *Child development today and tomorrow* (pp. 107–136). Jossey-Bass.

Fishbein, D. H., Domitrovich, C., Williams, J., Gitukui, S., Guthrie, C., Shapiro, D., & Greenberg, M. (2016). Short-term intervention effects of the PATHS curriculum in young low-income children: Capitalizing on plasticity. *Journal of Primary Prevention, 37*(6), 493–511.

Fivush, R. (1989). Exploring sex differences in the emotional content of mother–child conversations about the past. *Sex Roles, 20*, 675–691.

Fivush, R. (2021). The development of an emotional self-concept through narrative reminiscing. *Emotion Researcher*, 30–36.

Flores-Kanter, P. E., & Medrano, L. A. (2020). Commentary: Putting 'emotional intelligences' in their place: Introducing the integrated model of affect-related individual differences. *Frontiers in Psychology, 11*, 574.

Fogel, A., & Reimers, M. (1989). On the psychobiology of emotions and their development. *Monographs of the Society for Research in Child Development, 54*(1–2, Serial No. 219) 105–113.

Fox, N. A., & Calkins, S. D. (2003). The development of self-control of emotion: Intrinsic and extrinsic influences. *Motivation and Emotion, 27*(1), 7–26.

Fox, N. A., Schmidt, L. A., Calkins, S. D., Rubin, K. H., & Coplan, R. J. (1996). The role of frontal activation in the regulation and dysregulation of social behavior during the preschool years. *Development and Psychopathology, 8*(1), 89–102.

Frenzel, A. C., Goetz, T., Ludtke, O., Pekrun, R., & Sutton, R. E. (2009). Emotional transmission in the classroom: Exploring the relationship between teacher and student enjoyment. *Journal of Educational Psychology, 101*, 705–716.

Frey, J. R., Elliott, S. N., & Kaiser, A. P. (2014). Social skills intervention planning for preschoolers: Using the SSiS-Rating Scales to identify target behaviors valued by parents and teachers. *Assessment for Effective Intervention, 39*(3), 182–192.

Fridenson-Hayo, S., Berggren, S., Lassalle, A., Tal, S., Pigat, D., Bölte, S., . . . Golan, O. (2016). Basic and complex emotion recognition in children with autism: Cross-cultural findings. *Molecular Autism, 7*(1), 1–11.

Friedlmeier, W., Çorapçı, F., & Benga, O. (2015). Early emotional development in cultural perspective. In L. A. Jensen (Ed.), *The Oxford handbook of human development and culture: An interdisciplinary perspective* (pp. 127–148). Oxford University Press.

Friedlmeier, W., Çorapçı, F., & Cole, P. M. (2011). Emotion socialization in cross-cultural perspective. *Social and Personality Psychology Compass, 5*, 410–427.

Frydenberg, E., Martin, A. J., & Collie, R. J. (2017). *Social and emotional learning in Australia and the Asia-Pacific: Social and emotional learning in the Australasian context*. Springer Social Sciences.

Fu, C. S., Lin, S. T., Syu, S. H., & Guo, C. Y. (2010). What's the matter in class?: Preschool teachers' emotions expression. *Procedia-Social and Behavioral Sciences, 2*(2), 4887–4891.

Fuchs, D., & Thelen, M. H. (1988). Children's expected interpersonal consequences of communicating their affective state and reported likelihood of expression. *Child Development, 59*, 1314–1322.

Gaertner, B. M., Spinrad, T. L., & Eisenberg, N. (2008). Focused attention in toddlers: Measurement, stability, and relations to negative emotion and parenting. *Infant and Child Development, 17*(4), 339–363.

Gagne, J. R., Spann, C. A., & Prater, J. C. (2013). Parent depression symptoms and child temperament outcomes: A family study approach. *Journal of Applied Biobehavioral Research, 18*(4), 175–197.

Gagnon, M., Gosselin, P., Hudon-ven Der Buhs, I., Larocque, K., & Milliard, K. (2010). Children's recognition and discrimination of fear and disgust facial expressions. *Journal of Nonverbal Behavior, 34*(1), 27–42.

Galarneau, E., Colasante, T., Speidel, R., & Malti, T. (2022). Correlates of children's sympathy: Recognition and regulation of sadness and anger. *Social Development, 31*(3), 829–845.

Gal-Szabo, D. E., Spinrad, T. L., Eisenberg, N., & Sulik, M. J. (2019). The relations of children's emotion knowledge to their observed social play and reticent/uninvolved behavior in preschool: Moderation by effortful control. *Social Development, 28*(1), 57–73.

Gao, M., & Han, Z. R. (2016). Family expressiveness mediates the relation between cumulative family risks and children's emotion regulation in a Chinese sample. *Journal of Child and Family Studies, 25*(5), 1570–1580.

Garcia, A., Dick, A., & Graziano, P. A. (2020). A multimodal assessment of emotion dysregulation in young children with and without ADHD. Preprint.

Gardner, F. E. M. (1989). Inconsistent parenting: Is there evidence for a link with children's conduct problems? *Journal of Abnormal Child Psychology, 17*, 223–233.

Garner, P. W. (1995). Toddlers' emotion regulation behaviors: The role of social context and family expressiveness. *Journal of Genetic Psychology, 156*, 417–430.

Garner, P. W. (2006). Prediction of prosocial and emotional competence from maternal behavior in African American preschoolers. *Cultural Diversity and Ethnic Minority Psychology, 12*(2), 179–198

Garner, P. W. (2010). Emotional competence and its influences on teaching and learning. *Educational Psychology Review, 22*(3), 297–321.

Garner, P. W., Bolt, E., & Roth, A. N. (2019). Emotion-focused curricula models and expressions of and talk about emotions between teachers and young children. *Journal of Research in Childhood Education, 33*(2), 180–193

Garner, P. W., Dunsmore, J. C., & Southam-Gerrow, M. (2008). Mother–child conversations about emotions: Linkages to child aggression and prosocial behavior. *Social Development, 17*(2), 259–277.

Garner, P. W., & Estep, K. M. (2001). Emotional competence, emotion socialization, and young children's peer-related social competence. *Early Education and Development, 12*, 29–48.

Garner, P. W., Jones, D. C., Gaddy, G., & Rennie, K. (1997). Low income mothers' conversations about emotions and their children's emotional competence. *Social Development, 6*, 37–52.

Garner, P. W., Jones, D. C., & Miner, J. L. (1994). Social competence among low-income preschoolers: Emotion socialization practices and social cognitive correlates. *Child Development, 65*, 622–637.

Garner, P. W., Jones, D. C., & Palmer, D. J. (1994). Social cognitive correlates of preschool children's sibling caregiving behavior. *Developmental Psychology, 30*, 905–911.

Garner, P. W., & Lemerise, E. A. (2007). The roles of behavioral adjustment and conceptions of peers and emotions in preschool children's peer victimization. *Development and Psychopathology, 19*(1), 57–71.

Garner, P. W., & Parker, T. S. (2018). Young children's picture-books as a forum for the socialization of emotion. *Journal of Early Childhood Research, 16*(3), 291–304.

Garner, P. W., Parker, T. S., & Prigmore, S. B. (2019). Caregivers' emotional competence and behavioral responsiveness as correlates of early childcare workers' relationships with children in their care. *Infant Mental Health Journal, 40*(4), 496–512.

Garner, P. W., & Power, T. G. (1996). Preschoolers' emotional control in the disappointment paradigm and its relation to temperament, emotion knowledge, and family expressiveness. *Child Development, 67*, 1406–1419.

Garner, P. W., Robertson, S., & Smith, G. (1997). Preschool children's emotional expressions with peers: The roles of gender and emotion socialization. *Sex Roles, 36*, 675–691.

Garner, P. W., & Spears, F. M. (2000). Emotion regulation in low-income preschoolers. *Social Development, 9*(2), 246–264.

Garner, P. W., & Toney, T. D. (2020). Financial strain, maternal attributions, emotion knowledge and children's behavioral readiness for school. *Journal of Applied Developmental Psychology, 67*, 101122.

Garner, P. W., & Waajid, B. (2008). The associations of emotion knowledge and teacher-child relationships to preschool children's school-related developmental competence. *Journal of Applied Developmental Psychology, 29*, 89–100.

Garner, P. W., & Waajid, B. (2012). Emotion knowledge and self-regulation as predictors of preschoolers' cognitive ability, classroom behavior, and social competence. *Journal of Psychoeducational Assessment, 30*, 330–343.

Gartstein, M. A., Putnam, S. P., & Kliewer, R. (2016). Do infant temperament characteristics predict core academic abilities in preschool-aged children? *Learning and Individual Differences, 45*, 299–306.

George, C., & Main, M. (1979). Social interactions of young abused children: Approach, avoidance, and aggression. *Child Development, 50*, 306–318.

Gergen, K. J. (1985). The social constructionist movement in modern psychology. *American Psychologist, 40*, 266–275.

Gerhardt, M., Feng, X., Wu, Q., Hooper, E. G., Ku, S., & Chan, M. H. (2020). A naturalistic study of parental emotion socialization: Unique contributions of fathers. *Journal of Family Psychology, 34*(2), 204–214.

Gershon, P., & Pellitteri, J. (2018). Promoting emotional intelligence in preschool education: A review of programs. *International Journal of Emotional Education, 10*(2), 26–41.

Gev, T., Avital, H., Rosenan, R., Aronson, L. O., & Golan, O. (2021). Socio emotional competence in young children with ASD during interaction with their typically developing peers. *Research in Autism Spectrum Disorders, 86*, 101818.

Ghassabian, A., Székely, E., Herba, C. M., Jaddoe, V.

W., Hofman, A., Oldehinkel, A. J., . . . Tiemeier, H. (2014). From positive emotionality to internalizing problems: The role of executive functioning in preschoolers. *European Child and Adolescent Psychiatry, 23*(9), 729–741.

Gibb, B. E., Pollak, S. D., Hajcak, G., & Owens, M. (2016). Attentional biases in children of depressed mothers: An event-related potential (ERP) study. *Journal of Abnormal Psychology, 125*(8), 1166–1178.

Giesbrecht, G. F., Miller, M. R., & Müller, U. (2010). The anger–distress model of temper tantrums: Associations with emotional reactivity and emotional competence. *Infant and Child Development, 19*, 478–497.

Gilkerson, L. (2004). Reflective supervision in infant–family programs: Adding clinical process to nonclinical settings. *Infant Mental Health Journal, 25*, 424–439.

Giménez-Dasí, M., Fernández-Sánchez, M., & Quintanilla, L. (2015) Improving social competence through emotion knowledge in 2-year-old children: A pilot study. *Early Education and Development, 26* (8), 1128–1144.

Giménez-Dasí, M., Fernández-Sánchez, M., Quintanilla, L., & Daniel, M. F. (2013). Improving emotion comprehension and social skills in early childhood through philosophy for children. *Childhood & Philosophy*, 9(17), 63–89.

Giménez-Dasí, M., Quintanilla, L., & Lucas-Molina, B. (2018). Scripts or components?: A comparative study of basic emotion knowledge in Roma and non-Roma children. *Early Education and Development, 29*(2), 178–191.

Gnepp, J. (1983). Children social sensitivity: Inferring emotions from conflicting cues. *Developmental Psychology, 19*, 805–814.

Gnepp, J. (1989a). Children's use of personal information to understand other people's feelings. In P. Harris & C. Saarni (Eds.), *Children's understanding of emotion* (pp. 151–177). Cambridge University Press.

Gnepp, J. (1989b). Personalized inferences of emotions and appraisals: Component processes and correlates. *Developmental Psychology, 25*, 277–288.

Gnepp, J., & Chilamkurti, C. (1988). Children's use of personality attributions to predict other people's emotional and behavioral reactions. *Child Development, 59*, 743–754.

Gnepp, J., & Gould, M. E. (1985). The development of personalized inferences: Understanding other people's emotional reactions in light of their prior experiences. *Child Development, 56*, 1455–1464.

Gnepp, J., & Hess, D. L. R. (1986). Children's understanding of verbal and facial display rules. *Developmental Psychology, 22*, 103–108.

Gnepp, J., Klayman, J., & Trabasso, T. (1982). A hierarchy of information sources for inferring emotional reactions. *Journal of Experimental Child Psychology, 33*, 111–123.

Gnepp, J., McKee, E., & Domanic, J. A. (1987). Children's use of situational information to infer emotion: Understanding emotionally equivocal situations. *Developmental Psychology, 23*, 114–123.

Goagoses, N., Bolz, T., Eilts, J., Schipper, N., Schütz, J., Rademacher, A., . . . & Koglin, U. (2022). Parenting dimensions/styles and emotion dysregulation in childhood and adolescence: A systematic review and Meta-analysis. *Current Psychology, 1*–25.

Goldman, J. A., Corsini, D. A., & de Urioste, R. (1980). Implications of positive and negative sociometric status for assessing social competence of young children. *Journal of Applied Developmental Psychology, 1*, 209–220.

Goldsmith, H. H., Buss, K. A., & Lemery, K. S. (1997). Toddler and childhood temperament: Expanded content, stronger genetic evidence, new evidence for the importance of environment. *Developmental Psychology, 33*, 891–905.

Goldsmith, H. H., Reilly, J., Lemery, K. S., Longley, S., & Prescott, A. (1993). *Preschool Laboratory Temperament Assessment Battery (PS Lab-TAB; Version 1.0)*. University of Wisconsin–Madison, Department of Psychology.

Goleman, D. (1995). *Emotional intelligence*. Bantam Books.

Goodvin, R., Carlo, G., & Torquati, J. (2006). The role of child emotional responsiveness and maternal negative emotion expression in children's coping strategy use. *Social Development, 15*(4), 591–611.

Gordis, F., Rosen, A. B., & Grand, S. (1989, April). *Young children's understanding of simultaneous conflicting emotions*. Poster presented at the biennial meeting of the Society for Research in Child Development, Kansas City, MO.

Gosselin, P., & Simard, J. (1999). Children's knowledge of facial expressions of emotions: Distinguishing fear and surprise. *Journal of Genetic Psychology, 160*(2), 181–193.

Gottman, J. M., Katz, L. F., & Hooven, C. (1996a). *Meta-emotion: How families communicate emotionally, links to child peer relations, and other developmental outcomes*. Erlbaum.

Gottman, J. M., Katz, L. F., & Hooven, C. (1996b). Parental meta-emotion philosophy and the emotional life of families: Theoretical model and preliminary data. *Journal of Family Psychology, 10*, 249–268.

Gould, M. E. (1984). *Children's recognition and resolution of ambiguity in making affective judgements*. Paper presented at the annual meeting of the Midwestern Psychological Association, Chicago.

Gove, F., & Keating, D. P. (1979). Empathic role-taking precursors. *Developmental Psychology, 15*, 594–600.

Grady, J. S. (2018). Parents' reactions to toddlers' emotions: Relations with toddler shyness and gender. *Early Child Development and Care, 190(12)*, 1855–1862.

Grant, A. A., Jeon, L., & Buettner, C. K. (2019). Relating early childhood teachers' working conditions and well-being to their turnover intentions. *Educational Psychology, 39*(3), 294–312.

Graziano, P., & Derefinko, K. (2013). Cardiac vagal control and children's adaptive functioning: A meta-analysis. *Biological Psychology, 94*(1), 22–37.

Graziano, P. A., Reavis, R. D., Keane, S. P., & Calkins, S. D. (2007). The role of emotion regulation in children's early academic success. *Journal of School Psychology, 45*, 3–19.

Grazzani, I., & Ornaghi, V. (2011). Emotional state talk and emotion understanding: A training study with preschool children. *Journal of Child Language, 38*(5), 1124–1139.

Grazzani, I., Ornaghi, V., Agliati, A., & Brazzelli, E. (2016). How to foster toddlers' mental-state talk, emotion understanding, and prosocial behavior: A conversation-based intervention at nursery school. *Infancy, 21*, 199–227.

Grazzani, I., Ornaghi, V., & Brockmeier, J. (2016) Conversation on mental states at nursery: Promoting social cognition in early childhood, *European Journal of Developmental Psychology, 13 (5)*, 563–581.

Greenberg, M. T. (2006). Promoting resilience in children and youth: Preventive interventions and their interface with neuroscience. *Annals of the New York Academy of Sciences, 1094*(1), 139–150.

Greenberg, M. T., Kusche, C. A., & Mihalic, S. F. (1998). *Blueprints for violence prevention, book ten: Promoting alternative thinking strategies*. Center for the Study and Prevention of Violence.

Greenberg, M. T., Weissberg, R. P., O'Brien, M. U., Zins, J. E., Fredericks, L., Resnik, H., & Elias, M. J. (2003). Enhancing school-based prevention and youth development through coordinated social, emotional, and academic learning. *American Psychologist, 58*(6–7), 466–474.

Greif, E. B., Alvarez, M., & Tone, M. (1984, April). *Parents' teaching of emotions to preschool children*. Paper presented at the annual meeting of the Eastern Psychological Association, Baltimore.

Grolnick, W. S, Bridges, L. J., & Connell, J. P. (1996). Emotion regulation in two-year-olds: Strategies and emotional expression in four contexts. *Child Development, 67*, 928–941.

Grolnick, W. S., Kurowski, C. O., McMenamy, J. M., Rivkin, I., & Bridges, L. J. (1998). Mothers' strategies for regulating their toddlers' distress. *Infant Behavior and Development, 21*(3), 437–450.

Gross, D. (1993, March). *Young children's understanding of misleading emotional displays*. Poster presented at the biennial meetings of the Society for Research in Child Development, New Orleans, LA.

Gross, D., & Harris, P. (1988). Understanding false beliefs about emotion. *International Journal of Behavioral Development, 11*, 475–488.

Gross, J. J. (2013). Emotion regulation: Taking stock and moving forward. *Emotion, 13*(3), 359–365.

Gross, J. J. (2015). Emotion regulation: Current status and future prospects. *Psychological Inquiry, 26*(1), 1–26.

Grosse, G., Streubel, B., Gunzenhauser, C., & Saalbach, H. (2021). Let's talk about emotions: The development of children's emotion vocabulary from 4 to 11 years of age. *Affective Science, 2*(2), 150–162.

Grusec, J. E., & Goodnow, J. J. (1994). Impact of parental discipline methods on the child's internalization of values: A reconceptualization of current points of view. *Developmental Psychology, 30*, 4–19.

Gulsrud, A. C., Jahromi, L. B., & Kasari, C. (2010). The co-regulation of emotions between mothers and their children with autism. *Journal of Autism and Developmental Disorders, 40*(2), 227–237.

Gündüz, G., Yagmurlu, B., & Harma, M. (2015). Self-regulation mediates the link between family context and socioemotional competence in Turkish preschoolers. *Early Education and Development, 26*(5–6), 729–748.

Gunzenhauser, C., Fäsche, A., Friedlmeier, W., & von Suchodoletz, A. (2014). Face it or hide it: Parental socialization of reappraisal and response suppression. *Frontiers in Psychology, 4*, 992.

Gust, N., Koglin, U., & Petermann, F. (2014). An understanding of emotion regulation strategies in preschool age. *Zeitschrift Fur Entwicklungspsychologie Und Padagogische Psychologie* [German Journal of Developmental and Educational Psychology], *46*, 191–200.

Hadwin, J., Baron-Cohen, S., Howlin, P., & Hill, K. (1996). Can we teach children with autism to understand emotions, belief, or pretence? *Development and Psychopathology, 8*, 345–365.

Hadwin, J., & Perner, J. (1991). Pleased and surprised: Children's cognitive theory of emotion. *British Journal of Developmental Psychology, 9*, 215–234.

Halberstadt, A. G. (1991). Socialization of expressiveness: Family influences in particular and a model in general. In R. S. Feldman & S. Rimé (Eds.), *Fundamentals of emotional expressiveness* (pp. 106–162). Cambridge University Press.

Halberstadt, A. G., Denham, S. A., & Dunsmore, J. C. (2001). Affective social competence. *Social Development, 10*(1), 79–119.

Halberstadt, A. G., Dunsmore, J. C., Bryant, A. Jr., Parker, A. E., Beale, K. S., & Thompson, J. A. (2013). Development and validation of the Parents' Beliefs About Children's Emotions Questionnaire. *Psychological Assessment, 25*, 1195–1210.

Halberstadt, A. G., & Fox, N. A. (1990, April). *Mothers' and their children's expressiveness and emotionality*. Poster presented at the biennial Conference on Human Development, Richmond, VA.

Halberstadt, A. G., & Lozada, F. T. (2011). Emotional development in infancy through the lens of culture. *Emotion Review 3*, 158–168.

Halberstadt, A. G., Thompson, J. A., Parker, A. E., & Dunsmore, J. C. (2008). Parents' emotion-related beliefs and behaviours in relation to children's coping with the 11 September 2001 terrorist attacks. *Infant and Child Development, 17*, 557–580.

Hale-Jinks, C., Knopf, H., & Kemple, K. (2006). Tackling teacher turnover in child care: Understanding causes and consequences, identifying solutions. *Childhood Education, 82*(4), 219–226.

Halle, T. G., & Darling-Churchill, K. E. (2016). Review of measures of social and emotional development. *Journal of Applied Developmental Psychology, 45*, 8–18.

Halligan, S. L., Cooper, P. J., Fearon, P., Wheeler, S.,L., Crosby, M., & Murray, L. (2013). The longitudinal development of emotion regulation capacities in children at risk for externalizing disorders. *Development and Psychopathology, 25*(2), 391–406.

Hamaidi, D. A., Mattar, J. W., & Arouri, Y. M. (2021). Emotion regulation and its relationship to social competence among kindergarten children in Jordan. *European Journal of Contemporary Education, 10(1)*, 66–76.

Hamre, B. K., Pianta, R. C., Mashburn, A. J., & Downer, J. T. (2012). Promoting young children's social competence through the preschool PATHS curriculum and MyTeachingPartner professional development resources. *Early Education and Development, 23*(6), 809–832.

Han, P. G., Wu, Y. P., Yu, T., Xia, X. M., & Gao, F. Q. (2016). The relationship between shyness and externalizing problem in Chinese preschoolers: The moderating effect of teacher-child relationship. *Journal of Education and Training Studies, 4*(3), 167–173.

Harden, B. J., Morrison, C., & Clyman, R. B. (2014). Emotion labeling among young children in foster care. *Early Education and Development, 25*(8), 1180–1197

Harris, P. L. (1983). Children's understanding of the link between situation and emotion. *Journal of Experimental Child Psychology, 36*, 490–509.

Harris, P. L. (1989). *Children and emotion: The development of psychological understanding.* Blackwell.

Harris, P. L. (1993). Understanding of emotions. In M. Lewis & J. Haviland (Eds.), *Handbook of emotions* (pp. 237–246). Guilford Press.

Harris, P. L. (2008). Children's understanding of emotion. In M. Lewis, J. M. Haviland, & L. F. Barrett (Eds.), *Handbook of emotions* (3rd ed., pp. 320–331). Guilford Press.

Harris, P. L., & Cheng, L. (2022). Evidence for similar conceptual progress across diverse cultures in children's understanding of emotion. *International Journal of Behavioral Development, 46*(3), 238–250.

Harris, P. L., & Gross, D. (1988). Children's understanding of real and apparent emotion. In J. W. Astington, P. L. Harris & D. R. Olson (Eds.), *Developing theories of mind* (pp. 295–314). Cambridge University Press.

Harris, P. L., Johnson, C. N., Hutton, D., Andrews, G. M., & Cooke, T. (1989). Young children's theory of mind and emotion. *Cognition and Emotion, 3*, 379–400.

Harter, S., & Buddin, B. J. (1987). Children's understanding of the simultaneity of two emotions: A five-stage developmental acquisition sequence. *Developmental Psychology, 23*, 388–399.

Harter, S., & Whitesell, N. R. (1989). Developmental changes in children's understanding of single, multiple, and blended emotion concepts. In P. Harris & C. Saarni (Eds.), *Children's understanding of emotion* (pp. 81–116). Cambridge University Press.

Hasegawa, M. (2021). Preschoolers' and third graders' understanding of the causal relations of emotions and behaviors in moral situations. *Japanese Psychological Research, 64*(3), 333–342.

Havighurst, S., & Harley, A. (2007). *Tuning in to kids: Emotionally intelligent parenting: Program manual.* University of Melbourne.

Havighurst, S. S., Wilson, K. R., Harley, A. E., Kehoe, C., Efron, D., & Prior, M. R. (2013). "Tuning into Kids": Reducing young children's behavior problems using an emotion coaching parenting program. *Child Psychiatry and Human Development, 44*(2), 247–264.

Havighurst, S. S., Wilson, K. R., Harley, A. E., & Kehoe, C. E. (2019). Dads tuning in to kids: A randomized controlled trial of an emotion socialization parenting program for fathers. *Social Development, 28*(4), 979–997.

Havighurst, S. S., Wilson, K. R., Harley, A. E., & Prior, M. R. (2009). Tuning in to Kids: An emotion-focused parenting program—initial findings from a community trial. *Journal of Community Psychology, 37*(8), 1008–1023.

Havighurst, S. S., Wilson, K. R., Harley, A. E., Prior, M. R., & Kehoe, C. (2010). Tuning in to Kids: Improving emotion socialization practices in parents of preschool children–findings from a community trial. *Journal of Child Psychology and Psychiatry, 51*(12), 1342–1350.

Heinze, J. E., Miller, A. L., Seifer, R., Dickstein, S., & Locke, R. L. (2015). Emotion knowledge, loneliness, negative social experiences, and internalizing symptoms among low-income preschoolers. *Social Development, 24*, 240–265.

Helmsen, J., Koglin, U., & Petermann, F. (2012). Emotion regulation and aggressive behavior in preschoolers: The mediating role of social information processing. *Child Psychiatry and Human Development, 43*(1), 87–101.

Hemmeter, M. L., Ostrosky, M., & Fox, L. (2006). Social and emotional foundations for early learning: A conceptual model for intervention. *School Psychology Review, 35*(4), 583–601.

Hernández, M. M., Eisenberg, N., Valiente, C., Diaz, A., VanSchyndel, S. K., Berger, R. H., . . . Southworth, J. (2017a). Concurrent and longitudinal associations of peers' acceptance with emotion and effortful control in kindergarten. *International Journal of Behavioral Development, 41*, 30–40.

Hernández, M. M., Eisenberg, N., Valiente, C., Spinrad, T. L., Johns, S. K., Berger, R. H., . . . Southworth, J. (2022). Effortful control and extensive observations of negative emotion as joint predictors of teacher–student conflict in childhood. *Early Education and Development, 33*, 1–16.

Hernández, M. M., Eisenberg, N., Valiente, C., Spinrad, T. L., VanSchyndel, S. K., Diaz, A., . . . Piña, A. A. (2015). Observed emotion frequency versus intensity as predictors of socioemotional maladjustment. *Emotion, 15*(6), 699–704.

Hernández, M. M., Eisenberg, N., Valiente, C., Spinrad, T. L., VanSchyndel, S. K., Diaz, A., . . . Southworth, J. (2017b). Observed emotions as predictors of quality of kindergartners' social relationships. *Social Development, 26*, 21–39.

Hernández, M. M., Eisenberg, N., Valiente, C., VanSchyndel, S. K., Spinrad, T. L., Silva, K. M., . . . Southworth, J. (2016). Emotional expression in school context, social relationships, and academic adjustment in kindergarten. *Emotion, 16*(4), 553–566.

Herndon, K. J., Bailey, C. S., Shewark, E. A., Denham, S. A., & Bassett, H. H. (2013). Preschoolers' emotion expression and regulation: Relations with school adjustment. *Journal of Genetic Psychology, 174*(6), 642–663.

Hipson, W. E., Coplan, R. J., & Séguin, D. G. (2019). Active emotion regulation mediates links between shyness and social adjustment in preschool. *Social Development, 28*(4), 893–907.

Hirschler-Guttenberg, Y., Golan, O., Ostfeld-Etzion, S., & Feldman, R. (2015). Mothering, fathering, and the regulation of negative and positive emotions in high-functioning preschoolers with autism spectrum disorder. *Journal of Child Psychology and Psychiatry, 56*(5), 530–539.

Hochschild, A. R. (1979). Emotion work, feeling rules, and social structure. *American Journal of Sociology, 85*, 551–575.

Hoemann, K., Devlin, M., & Barrett, L. F. (2020). Comment: emotions are abstract, conceptual categories that are learned by a predicting brain. *Emotion Review, 12*(4), 253–255.

Hoemann, K., Xu, F., & Barrett, L. F. (2019). Emotion words, emotion concepts, and emotional development in children: A constructionist hypothesis. *Developmental Psychology, 55*(9), 1830–1849.

Hoffman, M. L. (1975). Altruistic behavior and the parent–child relationship. *Journal of Personality and Social Psychology, 31*, 937–943.

Hoffman, M. L. (1984). Interaction of affect and cognition in empathy. In C. E. Izard, J. Kagan, & R. B. Zajonc (Eds.), *Emotions, cognition, and behavior* (pp. 103–131). Cambridge University Press.

Hoffman, M. L., & Saltzstein, H. D. (1967). Parent discipline and the child's moral development. *Journal of Personality and Social Psychology, 5*, 45–57.

Hoffmann, J. D., Brackett, M. A., Bailey, C. S., & Willner, C. J. (2020). Teaching emotion regulation in schools: Translating research into practice with the RULER approach to social and emotional learning. *Emotion, 20*(1), 105–109.

Hoffner, C., & Badzinski, D. M. (1989). Children's integration of facial and situations cues to emotion. *Child Development, 60*, 415–422.

Holodynski, M., & Seeger, D. (2019). Expressions as signs and their significance for emotional development. *Developmental Psychology, 55*, 1812–1829.

Hooper, E. G., Wu, Q., Ku, S., Gerhardt, M., & Feng, X. (2018). Maternal emotion socialization and child outcomes among African Americans and European Americans. *Journal of Child and Family Studies, 27*(6), 1870–1880.

Hooven, C., Katz, L., & Gottman, J. M. (1994). The family as a meta-emotion culture. *Cognition and Emotion, 9*, 229–264.

Howe, N. (1991). Sibling-directed internal state language, perspective-taking, and affective behavior. *Child Development, 62*, 1503–1512.

Howes, C., & Eldredge, R. (1985). Responses of abused, neglected, and non-maltreated children to the behaviors of their peers. *Journal of Applied Developmental Psychology, 6*, 261–270.

Howse, R. B., Calkins, S. D., Anastopoulos, A. D., Keane, S. P., & Shelton, T. L. (2003). Regulatory contributors to children's kindergarten achievement. *Early Education and Development, 14*(1), 101–120.

Hsueh, J., Lowenstein, A. E. Morris, P., Mattera, S. K., & Bangser, M. (2014). *Impacts of social-emotional curricula on three-year-olds: Exploratory findings from the Head Start CARES Demonstration*. OPRE Report 2014–78. Office of Planning, Research and Evaluation.

Hudson, A., & Jacques, S. (2014). Put on a happy face! Inhibitory control and socioemotional knowledge predict emotion regulation in 5- to 7-year-olds. *Journal of Experimental Child Psychology, 123*, 36–52.

Hughes, C., & Dunn, J. (1998). Understanding mind and emotion: Longitudinal associations with mental-state talk between young friends. *Developmental Psychology, 34*(5), 1026–1037.

Hughes, C., White, A., Sharpen, J., & Dunn, J. (2000). Antisocial, angry, and unsympathetic: "Hard-to-manage" preschoolers' peer problems and possible cognitive influences. *Journal of Child Psychology and Psychiatry and Allied Disciplines, 41*(2), 169–179.

Hughes, K., & Coplan, R. J. (2010). Exploring processes linking shyness and academic achievement in childhood. *School Psychology Quarterly, 25*(4), 213–222.

Hughes, M., & Kasari, C. (2000). Caregiver-child interaction and the expression of pride in children with down syndrome. *Education and Training in Mental Retardation and Developmental Disabilities*, 35(1), 67–77.

Humphrey, N. (2013) *Social and emotional learning: A critical appraisal*. SAGE.

Humphrey, N., Kalambouka, A., Wigelsworth, M., Lendrum, A., Deighton, J., & Wolpert, M. (2011). Measures of social and emotional skills for children and young people: A systematic review. *Educational and Psychological Measurement, 71*(4), 617–637.

Humphries, M. L., & Keenan, K. E. (2006). Theoretical, developmental and cultural orientations of school-based prevention programs for preschoolers. *Clinical Child and Family Psychology Review, 9*(2), 135–148.

Humphries, M. L., Williams, B. V., & May, T. (2018). Early childhood teachers' perspectives on social-emotional competence and learning in urban classrooms. *Journal of Applied School Psychology, 34*(2), 157–179.

Hyson, M. C. (1994). *The emotional development of young children: Building an emotion-centered curriculum*. Teachers College Press.

Hyson, M. (2002). Emotional development and school readiness: Professional development. *Young Children, 57*(6), 76–78.

Hyson, M. C., & Lee, K.-M. (1996). Assessing early childhood teachers' beliefs about emotions: Content, contexts, and implications for practice. *Early Education and Development, 7*, 59–78.

In-Albon, T., Shafiei, M., Christiansen, H., Könen, T., Gutzweiler, R., & Schmitz, J. (2021). Development and psychometric properties of a computer-based standardized emotional competence inventory (MeKKi) for preschoolers and school-aged children. *Child Psychiatry and Human Development*, 1–14.

Ince, S., & Ersay, E. (2022). Okul Öncesi Dönem çocuğuna sahip anne ve babaların duygu sosyalleştirme davranışlarnın incelenmesi [Investigation of Emotional Socialization Behaviors of Parents with Preschool Children]. *Gelişim ve Psikoloji Dergisi* [Journal of Development and Psychology], 3(5), 1–17.

Ip, K. I., Jester, J. M., Sameroff, A., & Olson, S. L. (2019). Linking Research Domain Criteria (RDoC) constructs to developmental psychopathology: The role of self-regulation and emotion knowledge in the development of internalizing and externalizing growth trajectories from ages 3 to 10. *Development and Psychopathology, 31*(4), 1557–1574.

Ip, K. I., Miller, A. L., Karasawa, M., Hirabayashi, H., Kazama, M., Wang, L., . . . Tardif, T. (2021). Emotion expression and regulation in three cultures: Chinese, Japanese, and American preschoolers' reactions to disappointment. *Journal of Experimental Child Psychology, 201*, 104972.

Isley, S. L., O'Neil, R., Clatfelter, D., & Parke, R. D. (1999). Parent and child expressed affect and children's social competence: Modeling direct and indirect pathways. *Developmental Psychology, 35*, 547–560.

Izard, C. E. (1991). *The psychology of emotions*. Plenum Press.

Izard, C. E. (1993a). Four systems for emotion activation: Cognitive and noncognitive processes. *Psychological Review, 100*, 68–90.

Izard, C. E. (1993b). Organizational and motivational functions of discrete emotions. In M. Lewis & J. Haviland (Eds.), *Handbook of emotions* (pp. 631–642). Guilford Press.

Izard, C. E. (2002). Emotion knowledge and emotion utilization facilitate school readiness. *Social Policy Report, 16*(3), 7.

Izard, C. E. (2007). Basic emotions, natural kinds, emotion schemas, and a new paradigm. *Perspectives on Psychological Science, 2*(3), 260–280.

Izard, C. E. (2010). The many meanings/aspects of emotion: Definitions, functions, activation, and regulation. *Emotion Review, 2*(4), 363–370.

Izard, C. E., Dougherty, L., & Hembree, E. A. (1980). *System for identifying affect expressions by holistic judgment (AFFEX)*. University of Delaware, Instructional Resources Center.

Izard, C., Fine, S., Schultz, D., Mostow, A., Ackerman, B., & Youngstrom, E. (2001). Emotion knowledge as a predictor of social behavior and academic competence in children at risk. *Psychological Science, 12*, 18–23.

Izard, C. E., Haskins, F. W., Schultz, D., Trentacosta, C. J., & King, K. A.(2003). *Emotion Matching Test*. Unpublished manuscript, University of Delaware, Newark, Department of Psychology.

Izard, C. E., King, K. A., Trentacosta, C. J., Laurenceau, J. P., Morgan, J. K., Krauthamer-Ewing, E. S., & Finlon, K. J. (2008). Accelerating the development of emotion competence in Head Start children. *Development and Psychopathology, 20*, 369–397.

Izard, C., Stark, K., Trentacosta, C., & Schultz, D. (2008). Beyond emotion regulation: Emotion utilization and adaptive functioning. *Child Development Perspectives, 2*(3), 156–163.

Izard, C. E., Trentacosta, C. J., King, K. A., & Mostow, A. J. (2004). An emotion-based prevention program for Head Start children. *Early Education and Development, 15*, 407–422.

Izard, C. E., Woodburn, E. M., Finlon, K. J., Krauthamer-Ewing, E. S., Grossman, S. R., & Seidenfeld, A. (2011). Emotion knowledge, emotion utilization, and emotion regulation. *Emotion Review, 3*(1), 44–52.

Jahromi, L. B., Bryce, C. I., & Swanson, J. (2013). The importance of self-regulation for the school and peer engagement of children with high-functioning autism. *Research in Autism Spectrum Disorders, 7*(2), 235–246.

Jahromi, L. B., Gulsrud, A., & Kasari, C. (2008). Emotional competence in children with Down syndrome: Negativity and regulation. *American Journal on Mental Retardation, 113*(1), 32–43.

Jahromi, L. B., Kirkman, K. S., Friedman, M. A., & Nunnally, A. D. (2021). Associations between emotional competence and prosocial behaviors with peers among children with autism spectrum disorder. *American Journal on Intellectual and Developmental Disabilities, 126*(2), 79–96.

Jahromi, L. B., Meek, S. E., & Ober-Reynolds, S. (2012). Emotion regulation in the context of frustration in children with high functioning autism and their typical peers. *Journal of Child Psychology and Psychiatry, 53*(12), 1250–1258.

Jambon, M., Colasante, T., Peplak, J., & Malti, T. (2019). Anger, sympathy, and children's reactive and proactive aggression: Testing a differential correlate hypothesis. *Journal of Abnormal Child Psychology, 47(6)*, 1013–1024.

Jennings, P. A. (2015). Early childhood teachers' well-being, mindfulness, and self-compassion in relation to classroom quality and attitudes towards challenging students. *Mindfulness, 6*, 732–743.

Jennings, J. L., & DiPrete, T. A. (2010). Teacher effects on social and behavioral skills in early elementary school. *Sociology of Education, 83*, 135–159.

Jennings, P. A. (2015). Early childhood teachers' well-being, mindfulness, and self-compassion in relation to classroom quality and attitudes towards challenging students. *Mindfulness, 6*, 732–743.

Jennings, P. A., & Greenberg, M. T. (2009). The prosocial classroom: Teacher social and emotional competence in relation to student and classroom outcomes. *Review of Educational Research, 79*, 491–525.

Jeon, L., Buettner, C. K., Grant, A. A., & Lang, S. N. (2019). Early childhood teachers' stress and children's social, emotional, and behavioral functioning. *Journal of Applied Developmental Psychology, 61*, 21–32.

Jeon, L., Buettner, C. K., & Hur, E. (2016). Preschool teachers' professional background, process quality, and job attitudes: A person-centered approach. *Early Education and Development, 27*, 551–571.

Jeon, L., Hur, E., & Buettner, C. K. (2016). Child-care chaos and teachers' responsiveness: The indirect associations through teachers' emotion regulation and coping. *Journal of School Psychology, 59*, 83–96.

Jessee, A. (2020). Associations between maternal reflective functioning, parenting beliefs, nurturing, and preschoolers' emotion understanding. *Journal of Child and Family Studies, 29*(11), 3020–3028.

Jin, Z., Zhang, X., & Han, Z. R. (2017). Parental emotion socialization and child psychological adjustment among Chinese urban families: Mediation through child emotion regulation and moderation through dyadic collaboration. *Frontiers in Psychology, 8*, 2198.

Jones, D. C., Abbey, B. B., & Cumberland, A. (1998). The development of display rule knowledge: Linkages with family expressiveness and social competence. *Child Development, 69*(4), 1209–1222.

Jones, D. E., Greenberg, M., & Crowley, M. (2015). Early social-emotional functioning and public health: The relationship between kindergarten social competence and future wellness. *American Journal of Public Health, 105*(11), 2283–2290.

Jones, S. M., Barnes, S. P., Bailey, R., & Doolittle, E. J. (2017). Promoting social and emotional competencies in elementary school. *The Future of Children, 27*(1), 49–72.

Jones, S. M., & Bouffard, S. M. (2012). Social and emotional learning in schools: From programs to strategies and commentaries. *Social Policy Report, 26*(4), 1–33.

Jones, S. M., Zaslow, M., Darling-Churchill, K. E., & Halle, T. G. (2016). Assessing early childhood social and emotional development: Key conceptual and measurement issues. *Journal of Applied Developmental Psychology, 45*, 42–48.

Josephs, I. (1994). Display rule behavior and understanding in preschool children. *Journal of Nonverbal Behavior, 18*, 301–326.

Joshi, M. S., & MacLean, M. (1994). Indian and English children's understanding of the distinction between real and apparent emotion. *Child Development, 65*(5), 1372–1384.

Junge, C., Valkenburg, P. M., Deković, M., & Branje, S. (2020). The building blocks of social competence: contributions of the Consortium of Individual Development. *Developmental Cognitive Neuroscience, 45*, 100861.

Kahle, S., Miller, J. G., Troxel, N. R., & Hastings, P. D. (2021). The development of frustration regulation over early childhood: Links between attention diversion and parasympathetic activity. *Emotion, 21*(6), 1252–1267.

Kam, C. M., Greenberg, M. T., Bierman, K. L., Coie, J. D., Dodge, K. A., Foster, M. E., . . . Pinderhughes, E. E. (2011). Maternal depressive symptoms and child social preference during the early school years: Mediation by maternal warmth and child emotion regulation. *Journal of Abnormal Child Psychology, 39*(3), 365–377.

Kao, K., Tuladhar, C. T., & Tarullo, A. R. (2020). Parental and family-level sociocontextual correlates of emergent emotion regulation: Implications for early social competence. *Journal of Child and Family Studies, 29*, 1630–1641.

Karalus, S. P., Herndon, K., Bassett, H. H., & Denham, S. A. (2016). *Childcare teachers' socialization practices and beliefs on children's social emotional competence and the moderating contribution of classroom age.* Unpublished manuscript. Fairfax, VA: George Mason University.

Karevold, E., Ystrom, E., Coplan, R. J., Sanson, A. V., & Mathiesen, K. S. (2012). A prospective longitudinal study of shyness from infancy to adolescence: Stability, age-related changes, and prediction of socio-emotional functioning. *Journal of Abnormal Child Psychology, 40*(7), 1167–1177.

Kårstad, S. B., Wichstrøm, L., Reinfjell, T., Belsky, J., & Berg-Nielsen, T. S. (2015). What enhances the development of emotion understanding in young children?: A longitudinal study of interpersonal predictors. *British Journal of Developmental Psychology, 33(3)*, 340–354.

Kasari, C., Freeman, S. F., & Bass, W. (2003). Empathy and response to distress in children with Down syndrome. *Journal of Child Psychology and Psychiatry, 44*(3), 424–431.

Kasari, C., Freeman, S. F., & Hughes, M. A. (2001). Emotion recognition by children with Down syndrome. *American Journal on Mental Retardation, 106*(1), 59–72.

Kasari, C., Mundy, P., Yirmiya, N., & Sigman, M. (1990). Affect and attention in children with Down syndrome. *American Journal on Mental Retardation, 95*, 55–67.

Kasari, C., & Sigman, M. (1996). Expression and understanding of emotion in atypical development: Autism and Down syndrome. In M. Lewis & M. E. Sullivan (Eds.), *Emotional development in atypical children* (pp. 109–130). Erlbaum.

Kasari, C., Sigman, M., Baumgartner, P., & Stipek, D. (1993). Pride and mastery in children with autism. *Journal of Child Psychology and Psychiatry, 34*, 353–362.

Keating, C. T., & Cook, J. L. (2020). Facial expression production and recognition in autism spectrum disorders: A shifting landscape. *Child and Adolescent Psychiatric Clinics, 29*(3), 557–571.

Kemeny, M. E., Foltz, C., Cavanagh, J. F., Cullen, M., Giese-Davis, J., Jennings, P., . . . Ekman, P. (2012). Contemplative/emotion training reduces negative emotional behavior and promotes prosocial responses. *Emotion, 12*, 338–350.

Kendziora, K., Weissberg, R. P., & Dusenbury, L. (2011). *Strategies for social and emotional learning: Preschool and elementary grade student learning standards and assessment.* National Center for Mental Health Promotion and Youth Violence Prevention, Education Development Center.

Kerr, M. L., Rasmussen, H. F., Buttitta, K. V., Smiley, P. A., & Borelli, J. L. (2021). Exploring the complexity of mothers' real-time emotions while caregiving. *Emotion, 21*(3), 545–556.

Kestenbaum, R., Farber, E. A., & Sroufe, L. A. (1989). Individual differences in empathy among preschoolers: Relation to attachment history. In N. Eisenberg & R. A. Fabes (Eds.), *New Directions for Child Development: No. 44. Emotion and its regulation in early development* (pp. 51–64). Jossey-Bass.

Kestenbaum, R., & Gelman, S. (1995). Preschool children's identification and understanding of mixed emotions. *Cognitive Development, 10*, 443–458.

Kieras, J. E., Tobin, R. M., Graziano, W. G., & Rothbart, M. K. (2005). You can't always get what you want: Effortful control and children's responses to undesirable gifts. *Psychological Science, 16*(5), 391–396.

Kiliç, S. (2015a). Emotional competence and emotion socialization in preschoolers: The viewpoint of preschool teachers. *Educational Sciences: Theory and Practice, 15*(4), 1007–1020.

Kiliç, S. (2015b). Preschool teachers' emotional socialization responses to 4–6-year-old Turkish preschoolers' emotional expressions. *European Journal of Research on Education, 3*(1), 53–63.

Kim, J., Carlson, G. A., Meyer, S. E., Bufferd, S. J., Dougherty, L. R., Dyson, M. W., . . . Klein, D. N.

(2012). Correlates of the CBCL-dysregulation profile in preschool-aged children. *Journal of Child Psychology and Psychiatry, 53*(9), 918–926.

Kim, S., & Kochanska, G. (2017). Relational antecedents and social implications of the emotion of empathy: Evidence from three studies. *Emotion, 17*(6), 981–992.

Kim, S., & Kochanska, G. (2021, August). Family sociodemographic resources moderate the path from toddlers' hard-to-manage temperament to parental control to disruptive behavior in middle childhood. *Development and Psychopathology, 33*(1), 160–172.

Kimonis, E. R., Jain, N., Neo, B., Fleming, G. E., & Briggs, N. (2021). Development of an empathy rating scale for young children. *Assessment*. [Epub ahead of print]

King, E. K. (2020). Fostering toddlers' social emotional competence: considerations of teachers' emotion language by child gender. *Early Child Development and Care, 191*(16), 2494–2507.

King, E. K., Johnson, A. V., Cassidy, D. J., Wang, Y. C., Lower, J. K., & Kintner-Duffy, V. L. (2015). Preschool teachers' financial well-being and work time supports: Associations with children's emotional expressions and behaviors in classrooms. *Early Childhood Education Journal, 44*, 545–553.

King, E. K., & La Paro, K. M. (2018). Teachers' emotion minimizing language and toddlers' social emotional competence. *Early Education and Development, 29*(8), 989–1003.

Kingston, N., & Nash, B. (2011). Formative assessment: A meta-analysis and a call for research. *Educational Measurement: Issues and Practice, 30*, 28–37.

Kiselica, M. S., & Levin, G. R. (1987, April). *Young children's responses to a crying peer*. Paper presented at the biennial meeting of the Society for Research in Child Development, Baltimore.

Kitzmann. K. M., Gaylord. N. K., Holt, A. R., & Kenny, E. D. (2003). Child witnesses to domestic violence: A meta-analytic review. *Journal of Consulting & Clinical Psychology, 71(2)*, 339–352.

Klein, M. R., Moran, L., Cortes, R., Zalewski, M., Ruberry, E. J., & Lengua, L. J. (2018). Temperament, mothers' reactions to children's emotional experiences, and emotion understanding predicting adjustment in preschool children. *Social Development, 27*(2), 351–365.

Klimes-Dougan, B., & Kistner, J. (1990). Physically abused preschoolers' responses to peers' distress. *Developmental Psychology, 26*, 599–602.

Knafo, A., Zahn-Waxler, C., Davidov, M., Van Hulle, C., Robinson, J. L., & Rhee, S. H. (2009). Empathy in early childhood: Genetic, environmental, and affective contributions. *Annals of the New York Academy of Sciences, 1167*(1), 103–114.

Knafo, A., Zahn-Waxler, C., Van Hulle, C., Robinson, J. L., & Rhee, S. H. (2008). The developmental origins of a disposition toward empathy: Genetic and environmental contributions. *Emotion 8*, 737–752.

Knitzer, J. (1993). Children's mental health policy: Challenging the future. *Journal of Emotional and Behavioral Disorders, 1*, 8–16.

Knothe, J. M., & Walle, E. A. (2018). Parental communication about emotional contexts: Differences across discrete categories of emotion. *Social Development, 27*(2), 247–261.

Kochanska, G. (1987, April). *Socialization of young children's anger by well and depressed mothers*. Paper presented at the biennial meeting of the Society for Research in Child Development, Baltimore.

Kochanska, G., & Aksan, N. (2004). Conscience in childhood: Past, present, and future. *Merrill–Palmer Quarterly, 50*(3), 299–310.

Kochanska, G., Casey, R. J., & Fukumoto, A. (1995). Toddlers' sensitivity to standard violations. *Child Development, 66*, 643–656.

Kochanska, G., Gross, J. N., Lin, M. H., & Nichols, K. E. (2002). Guilt in young children: Development, determinants, and relations with a broader system of standards. *Child Development, 73*(2), 461–482.

Kolak, A. M., & Volling, B. L. (2022). Amenders and avoiders: An examination of guilt and shame for toddlers and their older siblings. *Cognition and Emotion*, 1–16.

Kolmodin, K. E. (2007). *Exploring links between children's understanding of emotion, parent-child reminiscing about emotional events, and the kindergarten classroom affective environment*. Dissertation, ProQuest Information & Learning.

Koludrović, M., & Mrsić, A. (2021): The attitudes of initial teacher education students towards teacher socioemotional competence, *Ekonomska Istraživanja* [Economic Research], *35*(1), 4113–4127.

Komsi, N., Räikkönen, K., Pesonen, A. K., Heinonen, K., Keskivaara, P., Järvenpää, A. L., & Strandberg, T. E. (2006). Continuity of temperament from infancy to middle childhood. *Infant Behavior and Development, 29*(4), 494–508.

Kopp, C. B. (1989). Regulation of distress and negative emotions: A developmental view. *Developmental Psychology, 25*, 343–354.

Kornilaki, E. N., & Chloverakis, G. (2004). The situational antecedents of pride and happiness: Developmental and domain differences. *British Journal of Developmental Psychology, 22*, 605–619.

Kremenitzer, J. P., & Miller, R. (2008). Are you a highly qualified, emotionally intelligent early childhood educator? *Young Children, 63*(4), 106–112.

Krettenauer, T., Malti, T., & Sokol, B. W. (2008). The development of moral emotion expectancies and the happy victimizer phenomenon: A critical review of theory and application. *International Journal of Developmental Science, 2*(3), 221–235.

Kuebli, J., Butler, S., & Fivush, R. (1995). Mother–child talk about past emotions: Relations of maternal language and child gender over time. *Cognition and Emotion, 9*, 265–283.

Kuebli, J., & Fivush, R. (1992). Gender differences in parent–child conversations about past emotions. *Sex Roles, 27*, 683–698.

Kuebli, J., & Fivush, R. (1996). Making everyday events emotional: The construal of emotion in parent–child conversations about the past. In N. L. Stein, P. A. Ornstein, B. Tversky, & C. J. Brainerd (Eds.), *Memory for everyday and emotional events* (pp. 15–48). Erlbaum.

Kuhnert, R. L., Begeer, S., Fink, E., & de Rosnay, M. (2017). Gender-differentiated effects of theory of mind, emotion understanding, and social preference on prosocial behavior development: A longitudinal study. *Journal of Experimental Child Psychology, 154*, 13–27.

Kujawa, A., Dougherty, L. E. A., Durbin, C. E., Laptook, R., Torpey, D., & Klein, D. N. (2014). Emotion recognition in preschool children: Associations with maternal depression and early parenting. *Development and Psychopathology, 26*(1), 159–170.

Kujawa, A. J., Torpey, D., Kim, J., Hajcak, G., Rose, S., Gotlib, I. H., & Klein, D. N. (2011). Attentional biases for emotional faces in young children of mothers with chronic or recurrent depression. *Journal of Abnormal Child Psychology, 39(1)*, 125–135.

Kurki, K., Järvenoja, H., Järvelä, S., & Mykkänen, A. (2016). How teachers co-regulate children's emotions and behaviour in socio-emotionally challenging situations in day-care settings. *International Journal of Educational Research, 76*, 76–88.

Kusché, C. A., & Greenberg, M. T. (1995a). *Promoting social and emotional development in deaf children: The PATHS project*. University of Washington Press.

Kusché, C. A., & Greenberg, M. K. (1995b). *The PATHS curriculum*. Developmental Research and Programs.

Kwon, K., & Min, H. (2021). The Influence of preschoolers' emotionality and social competence on play behavior. *Journal of Korean Child Care and Education, 17*(4), 73–91.

Kwon, K-A., Ford, T. G., Salvatore, A. L., Randall, K., Jeon, L., Malek-Lasater, A., . . . Han, M. (2022). Neglected elements of a high-quality early childhood workforce: Whole teacher well-being and working conditions. *Early Childhood Education Journal, 50*, 157–168.

Labella, M. H. (2018). The sociocultural context of emotion socialization in African American families. *Clinical Psychology Review, 59*, 1–15.

Labella, M. H., Lind, T., Sellers, T., Roben, C. K., & Dozier, M. (2020). Emotion regulation among children in foster care versus birth parent care: Differential effects of an early home-visiting intervention. *Journal of Abnormal Child Psychology, 48*(8), 995–1006.

LaBounty, J., Wellman, H. M., Olson, S., Lagattuta, K., & Liu, D. (2008). Mothers' and fathers' use of internal state talk with their young children. *Social Development, 17*(4), 757–775.

LaFreniere, P. J., & Dumas, J. (1996). Social Competence and Behavior Evaluation in children aged three to six: The Short Form (SCBE-30). *Psychological Assessment, 8*, 369–377.

LaFreniere, P, Masataka, N., Butovskaya, M., Chen, Q., Dessen, M. A., Atwanger, K., . . . Frigerio, A., (2002). Cross-cultural analysis of social competence and behavior problems in preschoolers. *Early Education and Development, 13*, 201–219.

LaFreniere, P. J., & Sroufe, L. A. (1985). Profiles of peer competence in the preschool: Interrelations between measures, influence of social ecology, and relation to attachment history. *Developmental Psychology, 21*(1), 56–69.

Lagattuta, K. H. (2005). When you shouldn't do what you want to do: Young children's understanding of desires, rules, and emotions. *Child development, 76*(3), 713–733.

Lagattuta, K. (2007). Thinking about the future because of the past: Young children's knowledge about the causes of worry and preventative decisions. *Child Development, 78*(5), 1492–1509.

Lagattuta, K. H. (2014). Linking past, present, and future: Children's ability to connect mental states and emotions across time. *Child Development Perspectives, 8*(2), 90–95.

Lagattuta, K. H., & Thompson, R. A. (2007). The development of self-conscious emotions: Cognitive processes and social influences. In J. L. Tracy, R. W. Robins, & J. P. Tangney (Eds), *The self-conscious emotions: Theory and research* (pp. 91–113). Guilford Press.

Lagattuta, K. H., & Wellman, H. M. (2001). Thinking about the past: Early knowledge about links between prior experience, thinking, and emotion. *Child Development, 72*(1), 82–102.

Lagattuta, K. H., & Wellman, H. M. (2002). Differences in early parent–child conversations about negative versus positive emotions: implications for the development of psychological understanding. *Developmental Psychology, 38*(4), 564–580.

Lagattuta, K. H., Wellman, H. M., & Flavell, J. H. (1997). Preschoolers' understanding of the link between thinking and feeling: Cognitive cueing and emotional change. *Child Development, 68*, 1081–1104.

Laible, D. (2004). Mother-child discourse in two contexts: Links with child temperament, attachment security, and socioemotional competence. *Developmental Psychology, 40*(6), 979–992.

Laible, D. (2011). Does it matter if preschool children and mothers discuss positive vs. negative events during reminiscing?: Links with mother-reported attachment, family emotional climate, and socioemotional development. *Social Development, 20*(2), 394–411.

Laible, D., Carlo, G., Murphy, T., Augustine, M., & Roesch, S. (2014). Predicting children's prosocial and co-operative behavior from their temperamental profiles: A person-centered approach. *Social Development, 23*(4), 734–752.

Laible, D. J., Kumru, A., Carlo, G., Streit, C., Selcuk, B., & Sayil, M. (2017). The longitudinal associations among temperament, parenting, and Turkish children's prosocial behaviors. *Child Development, 88*(4), 1057–1062.

Laible, D., Panfile, T., & Makariev, D. (2008). The quality and frequency of mother–toddler conflict: Links with attachment and temperament. *Child Development, 79*(2), 426–443.

Laible, D., Panfile Murphy, T., & Augustine, M. (2013). Constructing emotional and relational understanding: The role of mother–child reminiscing about negatively valenced events. *Social Development, 22*(2), 300–318.

Lam, L. T., & Wong, E. M. (2017). Enhancing social-emotional well-being in young children through improving teachers' social-emotional competence and curriculum design in Hong Kong. *International Journal of Child Care and Education Policy, 11*(1), 1–14.

Lambert, R. G., Kim, D. H., & Burts, D. C. (2014). Using teacher ratings to track the growth and development of young children using the Teaching Strategies GOLD® assessment system. *Journal of Psychoeducational Assessment, 32*(1), 27–39.

Lang, S. N., Jeon, L., Sproat, E. B., Brothers, B. E., & Buettner, C. K. (2020). Social emotional learning for teachers (SELF-T): A short-term, online intervention to increase early childhood educators' resilience. *Early Education and Development, 31*(7), 1112–1132.

Larson, J., Yen, M., & Fireman, G. (2007). Children's understanding and experience of mixed emotions. *Psychological Science*, 18(2), 186–191.

Laurent, J., Catanzaro, S. J., Joiner, T. E. Jr., Rudolph, K. D., Potter, K. I., Lambert, S., . . . Gathright, T. (1999). A measure of positive and negative affect for children: Scale development and preliminary validation. *Psychological Assessment, 11*(3), 326–338.

Lauw, M. S., Havighurst, S. S., Wilson, K. R., Harley, A. E., & Northam, E. A. (2014). Improving parenting of toddlers' emotions using an emotion coaching parenting program: A pilot study of Tuning in to Toddlers. *Journal of Community Psychology, 42*(2), 169–175.

Lavi, I., Katz, L. F., Ozer, E. J., & Gross, J. J. (2019). Emotion reactivity and regulation in maltreated children: A meta-analysis. *Child Development, 90(5)*, 1503–1524.

Lazarus, R. S. (1991). Cognition and motivation in emotion. *American Psychologist, 46*, 352–367.

LeBuffe, P. A., & Naglieri, J. A. (1999). The Devereux Early Childhood Assessment (DECA): A measure of within-child protective factors in preschool children. *NHSA Dialog, 3*(1), 75–80.

LeBuffe, P. A., Shapiro, V. B., & Naglieri, J. A. (2009). *The Devereux Student Strengths Assessment (DESSA)*. Kaplan.

LeBuffe, P. A., Shapiro, V. B., & Robitaille, J. L. (2018). The Devereux Student Strengths Assessment (DESSA) comprehensive system: Screening, assessing, planning, and monitoring. *Journal of Applied Developmental Psychology, 55*, 62–70.

LeDoux, J. E. (1996). *The emotional brain*. Simon & Schuster.

Lee, H. N., & Sung, M. (2021). Mother's emotional expressiveness and children's interpersonal problem solving skills according to children's negative emotionality. *Journal of the Korea Contents Association, 21*(6), 380–391.

Lee, J. H., Eoh, Y., Jeong, A., & Park, S. H. (2017). Preschoolers' emotional understanding and psychosocial adjustment in Korea: The moderating effect of maternal attitude towards emotional expressiveness. *Journal of Child and Family Studies, 26*(7), 1854–1864.

Lee, S., Chang, H., Ip, K. I., & Olson, S. L. (2019). Early socialization of hostile attribution bias: The roles of parental attributions, parental discipline, and child attributes. *Social Development, 28*(3), 549–563.

Leerkes, E. M., Paradise, M. J., O'Brien, M., Calkins, S. D., & Lange, G. (2008). Emotion and cognition processes in preschool children. *Merrill–Palmer Quarterly, 54*, 102–124.

Lemerise, E. A., & Arsenio, W. F. (2000). An integrated model of emotion processes and cognition in social information processing. *Child Development, 71*(1), 107–118.

Lemerise, E. A., & Dodge, K. A. (2008). The development of anger and hostile interactions. In M. Lewis, J. M. Haviland, & L. F. Barrett (Eds.), *Handbook of emotions* (3rd ed., pp. 730–741). Guilford Press.

Lennon, R., & Eisenberg, N. (1987a). Emotional displays associated with preschoolers' prosocial behavior. *Child Development, 58*, 992–1000.

Lennon, R., & Eisenberg, N. (1987b). Gender and age differences in empathy and sympathy. In N. Eisenberg & J. Strayer (Eds.), *Empathy and its development* (pp. 195–217). Cambridge University Press.

Lennon, R., Eisenberg, N., & Carroll, J. (1986). The relation between nonverbal indices of empathy and preschoolers' prosocial behavior. *Journal of Applied Developmental Psychology, 7*, 219–224.

Leyva, D., Catalán Molina, D., Suárez, C., Tamis-Lemonda, C. S., & Yoshikawa, H. (2021). Mother–child reminiscing and first-graders emotion competence in a low-income and ethnically diverse sample. *Journal of Cognition and Development, 22*(4), 501–522.

Lewis, M. (1992). *Shame: The exposed self.* Plenum Press.

Lewis, M. (1993a). Basic psychological processes in emotion. In M. Lewis & J. M. Haviland (Eds.), *Handbook of emotions* (pp. 223–236). Guilford Press.

Lewis, M. (1993b). The development of deception. In M. Lewis & C. Saarni (Eds.), *Lying and deception in everyday life* (pp. 90–105). Guilford Press.

Lewis, M. (2010). The emergence of human emotions. In M. Lewis, J. M. Haviland-Jones, & L. F. Barrett (Eds.), *Handbook of emotions* (3rd ed., pp. 304–319). Guilford Press.

Lewis, M., Alessandri, S. M., & Sullivan, M. (1992). Differences in shame and pride as a function of children's gender and task difficulty. *Child Development, 63*, 630–638.

Lewis, M., & Michalson, L. (1983). *Children's emotions and moods: Developmental theory and measurement*. Plenum Press.

Lewis, M., & Minar, N. J. (2022). Self-recognition and emotional knowledge. *European Journal of Developmental Psychology, 19*(3), 319–342.

Lewis, M., & Ramsay, D. (2002). Cortisol response to embarrassment and shame. *Child Development, 73*(4), 1034–1045.

Lewis, M., Stanger, C., & Sullivan, M. (1989). Deception in three-year-olds. *Developmental Psychology, 25*, 439–443.

Lewis, M., Stanger, C., Sullivan, M., & Barone, P. (1991). Changes in embarrassment as a function of age, sex, and situation. *British Journal of Developmental Psychology, 9*, 485–492.

Lewis, M., Sullivan, M., Stanger, C., & Weiss, M. (1989). Self development and self-conscious emotions. *Child Development, 60*, 146–156.

Lewis, M., Sullivan, M., & Vasen, A. (1987). Making faces: Age and emotion differences in the posing of emotional expressions. *Developmental Psychology, 23*, 690–697.

Lewis, M., Takai-Kawakami, K., Kawakami, K., & Sullivan, M. W. (2010). Cultural differences in emotional responses to success and failure. *International Journal of Behavioral Development, 34*(1), 53–61.

Li, Q., Liu, P., Yan, N., & Feng, T. (2020). Executive function training improves emotional competence for preschool children: The roles of inhibition control and working memory. *Frontiers in Psychology, 11*, 347.

Liang, Z. B., Zhang, G. Z., Chen, H. C., & Zhang, P. (2012). Relations among parental meta-emotion philosophy, parental emotion expressivity, and children's social competence. *Acta Psychologica Sinica, 44*(2), 199–210.

Liao, Z., Li, Y., & Su, Y. (2014). Emotion understanding and reconciliation in overt and relational conflict scenarios among preschoolers. *International Journal of Behavioral Development, 38*, 111–117.

Licardo, M., & Purgaj, M. (2019). Differences in practices for social-emotional learning among preschool teachers who work in age groups 3 to 6 years. In M. Licardo & I. Simões Dias (Eds.), *Contemporary themes in early childhood education and international educational modules* (pp. 43–57). University of Maribor Press.

Liddle, M. J. E., Bradley, B. S., & Mcgrath, A. (2015). Baby empathy: Infant distress and peer prosocial responses. *Infant Mental Health Journal, 36*(4), 446–458.

Lieberman, A. (1993). *The emotional life of the toddler.* Macmillan.

Liebermann, D., Giesbrecht, G. F., & Müller, U. (2007). Cognitive and emotional aspects of self-regulation in preschoolers. *Cognitive Development, 22*(4), 511–529.

Lin, H. L., Lawrence, F. R., & Gorrell, J. (2003). Kindergarten teachers' views of children's readiness for school. *Early Childhood Research Quarterly, 18*, 225–237.

Lind, T., Bernard, K., Ross, E., & Dozier, M. (2014). Intervention effects on negative affect of CPS-referred children: Results of a randomized clinical trial. *Child Abuse and Neglect, 38*(9), 1459–1467.

Lindsey, E. W. (2017). Mutual positive emotion with peers, emotion knowledge, and preschoolers' peer acceptance. *Social Development, 26*, 349–366.

Lindsey, E. W. (2019a). Emotions expressed with friends and acquaintances and preschool children's social competence with peers. *Early Childhood Research Quarterly, 47*, 373–384.

Lindsey, E. W. (2019b). Frequency and intensity of emotional expressiveness and preschool children's peer competence. *Journal of Genetic Psychology, 180*(1), 45–61.

Lipscomb, S. T., Leve, L. D., Shaw, D. S., Neiderhiser, J. M., Scaramella, L. V., Ge, X., . . . Reiss, D. (2012). Negative emotionality and externalizing problems in toddlerhood: Overreactive parenting as a moderator of genetic influences. *Development and Psychopathology, 24*(1), 167–179.

Liu, C., Moore, G. A., Beekman, C., Pérez-Edgar, K. E., Leve, L. D., Shaw, D. S., . . . Neiderhiser, J. M. (2018). Developmental patterns of anger from infancy to middle childhood predict problem behaviors at age 8. *Developmental Psychology, 54*(11), 2090–2100.

Liu, J. L., Harkness, S., & Super, C. M. (2020). Chinese mothers' cultural models of children's shyness: Ethnotheories and socialization strategies in the context of social change. *New Directions for Child and Adolescent Development, 170*, 69–92.

Liu, R., Calkins, S. D., & Bell, M. A. (2018). Fearful inhibition, inhibitory control, and maternal negative behaviors during toddlerhood predict internalizing problems at age 6. *Journal of Abnormal Child Psychology, 46*(8), 1665–1675.

Liu, R., Calkins, S. D., & Bell, M. A. (2021). Frontal EEG asymmetry moderates the associations between negative temperament and behavioral problems during childhood. *Development and Psychopathology, 33*(3), 1016–1025.

LoBue, V., Pérez-Edgar, K., & Buss, K. A. (2019). Introduction: Emotional development, past, and present. In V. LoBue, K. Pérez-Edgar, & K. A. Buss (Eds.), *The handbook of emotional development.* (pp. 7–26). Springer.

Locke, R. L., Davidson, R. J., Kalin, N. H., & Goldsmith, H. H. (2009). Children's context inappropriate anger and salivary cortisol. *Developmental Psychology, 45*, 1284–1297.

Locke, R. L., Miller, A. L., Seifer, R., & Heinze, J. E. (2015). Context-inappropriate anger, emotion knowledge deficits, and negative social experiences in preschool. *Developmental Psychology, 51*(10), 1450.

Loinaz, E. S. (2019). Teachers' perceptions and practice of social and emotional education in Greece, Spain, Sweden and the United Kingdom. *International Journal of Emotional Education, 11*(1), 31–48.

Lopez, F. G., Gover, M. R., Leskela, J., Sauer, E. M., Schirmer, L., & Wyssmann, J. (1997). Attachment styles, shame, guilt, and collaborative problem-solving orientations. *Personal Relationships, 4*, 187–199.

López-Pérez, B., Gummerum, M., Wilson, E., & Dellaria, G. (2017). Studying children's intrapersonal emotion regulation strategies from the process model of emotion regulation. *Journal of Genetic Psychology, 178*(2), 73–88.

López-Pérez, B., Wilson, E. L., Dellaria, G., & Gummerum, M. (2016). Developmental differences in children's interpersonal emotion regulation. *Motivation and Emotion, 40*(5), 767–780.

Lord, C., & Magill-Evans, J. (1995). Peer interactions of autistic children and adolescents. *Development and Psychopathology, 7*, 611–626.

Losoya, S., Eisenberg, N., & Fabes, R. A. (1998). Developmental issues in the study of coping. *International Journal of Behavioral Development, 22*(2), 287–313.

Louie, J. Y., Oh, B. J., & Lau, A. S. (2013). Cultural differences in the links between parental control and children's emotional expressivity. *Cultural Diversity and Ethnic Minority Psychology, 19*(4), 424–434.

Louie, J. Y., Wang, S. W., Fung, J., & Lau, A. (2015). Children's emotional expressivity and teacher perceptions of social competence: A cross-cultural comparison. *International Journal of Behavioral Development, 39*, 497–507.

Luby, J., Belden, A., Sullivan, J., Hayen, R., McCadney, A., & Spitznagel, E. (2009). Shame and guilt in preschool depression: Evidence for elevations in self-conscious emotions in depression as early as age 3. *Journal of Child Psychology and Psychiatry, 50*(9), 1156–1166.

Lucas-Molina, B., Quintanilla, L., Sarmento-Henrique, R., Martín Babarro, J., & Giménez-Dasí, M. (2020). The relationship between emotion regulation and emotion knowledge in preschoolers: A longitudinal study. *International Journal of Environmental Research and Public Health, 17*(16), 5726.

Luebbe, A. M., Kiel, E. J., & Buss, K. A. (2011). Toddlers' context-varying emotions, maternal responses to emotions, and internalizing behaviors. *Emotion, 11*, 697–703.

Lugo-Candelas, C., Flegenheimer, C., McDermott, J. M., & Harvey, E. (2017). Emotional understanding, reactivity, and regulation in young children with ADHD symptoms. *Journal of Abnormal Child Psychology, 45*, 1297–1310.

Lugo-Candelas, C. I., Harvey, E. A., & Breaux, R. P. (2015). Emotion socialization practices in Latina and European-American mothers of preschoolers with behavior problems. *Journal of Family Studies, 21*(2), 144–162.

Luke, N., & Banerjee, R. (2013). Differentiated associations between childhood maltreatment experiences and social understanding: A meta-analysis and systematic review. *Developmental Review, 33*(1), 1–28.

Lunkenheimer, E. S., Olson, S. L., Hollenstein, T., Sameroff, A. J., & Winter, C. (2011). Dyadic flexibility and positive affect in parent–child coregulation and the development of child behavior problems. *Development and Psychopathology, 23*(2011), 577–591.

Luo, L., Reichow, B., Snyder, P., Harrington, J., & Polignano, J. (2022). Systematic review and meta-analysis of classroom-wide social–emotional interventions for preschool children. *Topics in Early Childhood Special Education, 2*(1), 4–19.

Luo, L., Snyder, P., Huggins-Manley, A. C., Conroy, M., & Hong, X. (2021). Chinese preschool teachers' implementation of practices to support young children's social-emotional competence. *Early Education and Development, 32*(8), 1083–1102.

Lynch, K. B., Geller, S. R., & Schmidt, M. G. (2004). Multi-year evaluation of the effectiveness of a resilience-based prevention program for young children. *Journal of Primary Prevention, 24*, 335–353.

Macari, S., DiNicola, L., Kane-Grade, F., Prince, E., Vernetti, A., Powell, K., . . . Chawarska, K. (2018). Emotional expressivity in toddlers with autism spectrum disorder. *Journal of the American Academy of Child & Adolescent Psychiatry, 57*(11), 828–836.

Maccoby, E., & Martin, J. (1983). Socialization in the context of the family: Parent–child interaction. In P. H. Mussen (Series Ed.) & E. M. Hetherington (Vol. Ed.), *Handbook of child psychology: Vol. 4. Socialization, personality, and social development* (4th ed., pp. 1–101). Wiley.

MacGowan, T. L., & Schmidt, L. A. (2021). Helping as prosocial practice: Longitudinal relations among children's shyness, helping behavior, and empathic response. *Journal of Experimental Child Psychology, 209*, 105154.

Mahoney, J. L., Weissberg, R. P., Greenberg, M. T., Dusenbury, L., Jagers, R. J., Niemi, K., . . . Yoder, N. (2021). Systemic social and emotional learning: Promoting educational success for all preschool to high school students. *American Psychologist, 76*(7), 1128–1142.

Main, M., & George, C. (1985). Responses of abused and disadvantaged toddlers to distress in agemates: A study in the day care setting. *Developmental Psychology, 21*, 407–412.

Malatesta, C. Z. (1981). Infant emotion and the vocal affect lexicon. *Motivation and Emotion, 5*, 1–23.

Malatesta, C. Z. (1990). The role of emotions in the development and organization of personality. In R. A. Thompson (Ed.), *Nebraska Symposium on Motivation: Vol. 36. Socioemotional development* (pp. 1–56). University of Nebraska Press.

Malatesta, C. Z., Culver, C., Tesman, J. R., & Shepard, B. (1989). The development of emotional expression during the first two years of life. *Monographs of the Society for Research in Child Development, 54*(1–2, Serial No. 219), i–136.

Malatesta, C. Z., & Haviland, J. M. (1982). Learning display rules: The socialization of emotion expression in infancy. *Child Development, 53*, 991–1003.

Malatesta-Magai, C., Leak, S., Tesman, J., Shepard, B., Culver, C., & Smaggia, B. (1994). Profiles of emotional development: Individual differences in facial and vocal expression of emotion during the second and third years of life. *International Journal of Behavioral Development, 17*, 239–269.

Malti, T., Gummerum, M., Keller, M., & Buchmann, M. (2009). Children's moral motivation, sympathy, and prosocial behavior. *Child Development, 80*(2), 442–460.

Mann, T. D., Hund, A. M., Hesson-McInnis, M. S., & Roman, Z. J. (2017). Pathways to school readiness: Executive functioning predicts academic and social–emotional aspects of school readiness. *Mind, Brain, and Education, 11*(1), 21–31.

Marcus, R. F. (1980). Empathy and popularity. *Child Study Journal, 10*, 133–145.

Marcus, R. F. (1987). The role of affect in children's cooperation. *Child Study Journal, 17*, 153–168.

Mark, I. L. V. D., IJzendoorn, M. H. V., & Bakermans-Kranenburg, M. J. (2002). Development of empathy in girls during the second year of life: Associations with parenting, attachment, and temperament. *Social Development, 11*(4), 451–468.

Marlow, L., & Inman, D. (2002, November). *Pro-social literacy? Are educators being prepared to teach social and emotional competence?* Paper presented at the annual meeting of the National Council of Teachers of English, Atlanta, GA.

Martin, R. M., & Green, J. A. (2005). The use of emotion explanations by mothers: Relation to preschoolers' gender and understanding of emotions. *Social Development, 14*(2), 229–249.

Martin, S. E., Boekamp, J. R., McConville, D. W., & Wheeler, E. E. (2010). Anger and sadness perception in clinically referred preschoolers: Emotion processes and externalizing behavior symptoms. *Child Psychiatry and Human Development, 41*(1), 30–46.

Martin, S. E., Williamson, L. R., Kurtz-Nelson, E. C., & Boekamp, J. R. (2015). Emotion understanding (and misunderstanding) in clinically referred preschoolers: The role of child language and maternal depressive symptoms. *Journal of Child and Family Studies, 24*, 24–37.

Martini, T. S., Root, C. A., & Jenkins, J. M. (2004). Low and middle income mothers' regulation of negative emotion: Effects of children's temperament and situational emotional responses. *Social Development, 13*(4), 515–530.

Martins, E. C., Osório, A., Veríssimo, M., & Martins, C. (2016). Emotion understanding in preschool children: The role of executive functions. *International Journal of Behavioral Development, 40*(1), 1–10.

Mascolo, M. F., & Fischer, K. W. (2007). The co-development of self and socio-moral emotions during the toddler years. In C. A. Brownell & C. B. Kopp (Eds.), *Transitions in early socioemotional development: The toddler years* (pp. 66–99). Guilford Press.

Mashburn, A. J., Hamre, B. K., Downer, J. T., & Pianta, R. C. (2006). Teacher and classroom characteristics associated with teachers' ratings of prekindergartners' relationships and behaviors. *Journal of Psychoeducational Assessment, 24*(4), 367–380.

Mathiesen, K. S., & Tambs, K. (1999). The EAS Temperament Questionnaire—Factor structure, age trends, reliability, and stability in a Norwegian sample. *Journal of Child Psychology and Psychiatry, 40*(3), 431–439.

Mattar, J., Hamaidi, D., Al Anati, J. (2018). Emotion regulation and its relationship to academic difficulties among Jordanian first grade students. *Early Child Development and Care, 190*(8), 1313–1322.

Mattera, S., Lloyd, C. M., Fishman, M., & Bangser, M. (2013). *A first look at the Head Start CARES demonstration: Large-scale implementation of programs to improve children's social-emotional competence*. OPRE Report 2013-47. Office of Planning, Research and Evaluation.

Matthews, C. M., Thierry, S. M., & Mondloch, C. J. (2022). Recognizing, discriminating, and labeling emotional expressions in a free-sorting task: A developmental story. *Emotion, 22*(5), 945–953.

Maughan, A., & Cicchetti, D. (2002). Impact of child maltreatment and interadult violence on children's emotion regulation abilities and socioemotional adjustment. *Child Development, 73*(5), 1525–1542.

Maughan, A., Cicchetti, D., Toth, S. L., & Rogosch, F. A. (2007). Early-occurring maternal depression and maternal negativity in predicting young children's emotion regulation and socioemotional difficulties. *Journal of Abnormal Child Psychology, 35*(5), 685–703.

Mazzone, S., & Nader-Grosbois, N. (2016). How are parental reactions to children's emotions related to their theory of mind abilities? *Psychology, 7*(2), 166–179.

McCord, B. L., & Raval, V. V. (2016). Asian Indian immigrant and white American maternal emotion socialization and child socio-emotional functioning. *Journal of Child and Family Studies, 25*, 464–474.

McCoy, C. L., & Masters, J. C. (1985). The development of children's strategies for the social control of emotion. *Child Development, 56*, 1214–1222.

McDonald, N. M., & Messinger, D. S. (2011). The development of empathy: How, when, and why. *Free Will, Emotions, and Moral Actions: Philosophy and Neuroscience in Dialogue, 23*, 333–359.

McElwain, N. L., Halberstadt, A. G., & Volling, B. L. (2007). Mother- and father-reported reactions to children's negative emotions: Relations to young children's emotional understanding and friendship quality. *Child Development, 78*(5), 1407–1425.

McGee, G. G., Feldman, R. S., & Chernin, L. (1991). A comparison of emotional facial display by children with autism and typical preschoolers. *Journal of Early Intervention, 15*, 237–245.

McKee, L. G., DiMarzio, K., Parent, J., Dale, C., Acosta, J., & O'Leary, J. (2022). Profiles of emotion socialization across development and longitudinal associations with youth psychopathology. *Research on Child and Adolescent Psychopathology, 50*(2), 193–210.

McKown, C. (2015). Challenges and opportunities in the direct assessment of children's social and emotional comprehension. In J. A. Durlak, C. E. Domitrovich, R. P. Weissberg, & T. P. Gullotta (Eds.), *Handbook of social and emotional learning research and practice*. (pp. 320–335). Guilford Press.

McKown, C. (2017). Social-emotional assessment, performance, and standards. *The Future of Children, 27*(1), 157–178.

McMullen, M. B., Lee, M. S., McCormick, K. I., & Choi, J. (2020). Early childhood professional well-being as a predictor of the risk of turnover in child care: A matter of quality. *Journal of Research in Childhood Education, 34*(3), 331–345.

McRae, K., & Gross, J. (2020). Introduction. *Emotion, 20*(1), 1–9.

Melchers, M., Montag, C., Reuter, M., Spinath, F. M., & Hahn, E. (2016). How heritable is empathy?: Differential effects of measurement and subcomponents. *Motivation and Emotion, 40*(5), 720–730.

Melis Yavuz, H., Selcuk, B., Çorapçı, F., & Aksan, N. (2017). Role of temperament, parenting behaviors, and stress on Turkish preschoolers' internalizing symptoms. *Social Development, 26*(1), 109–128.

Melzi, G., & Fernández, C. (2004). Talking about past emotions: Conversations between Peruvian mothers and their preschool children. *Sex Roles, 50*(9), 641–657.

Merrell, K. W., Cohn, B. P., & Tom, K. M. (2011). Development and validation of a teacher report measure for assessing social-emotional strengths of children and adolescents. *School Psychology Review, 40*, 226–241.

Merrell, K. W., Felver-Gant, J. C., & Tom, K. M. (2011). Development and validation of a parent report measure for assessing social-emotional competencies of children and adolescents. *Journal of Child and Family Studies, 20*, 529–540.

Merz, E. C., Zucker, T. A., Landry, S. H., Williams, J. M., Assel, M., Taylor, H. B., . . . School Readiness

Research Consortium. (2015). Parenting predictors of cognitive skills and emotion knowledge in socioeconomically disadvantaged preschoolers. *Journal of Experimental Child Psychology, 132,* 14–31.

Meyer, S., Raikes, H. A., Virmani, E. A., Waters, S., & Thompson, R. A. (2014). Parent emotion representations and the socialization of emotion regulation in the family. *International Journal of Behavioral Development, 38,* 164–173.

Miller, A. L., Fine, S. E., Kiely-Gouley, K., Seifer, R., Dickstein, S., & Shields, A. (2006). Showing and telling about emotions: Interrelations between facets of emotional competence and associations with classroom adjustment in Head Start preschoolers. *Cognition and Emotion, 20*(8), 1170–1192.

Miller, A. L., Gouley, K. K, Seifer, R., Dickstein, S., & Shields, A. (2004). Emotions and behaviors in the Head Start classroom: Associations among observed dysregulation, social competence, and preschool adjustment. *Early Education and Development, 15*(2), 147–166.

Miller, A. L., Gouley, K. K., Seifer, R., Zakriski, A., Eguia, M., & Vergnani, M. (2005). Emotion knowledge skills in low-income elementary school children: Associations with social status and peer experiences. *Social Development, 14,* 637–651.

Miller, A. L., & Olson, S. L. (2000). Emotional expressiveness during peer conflicts: A predictor of social maladjustment among high-risk preschoolers. *Journal of Abnormal Child Psychology, 28*(4), 339–352.

Miller, A. L., Seifer, R., Stroud, L., Sheinkopf, S. J., & Dickstein, S. (2006). Biobehavioral indices of emotion regulation relate to school attitudes, motivation, and behavior problems in a low-income preschool sample. *Annals of the New York Academy of Sciences, 1094*(1), 325–329.

Miller, J. G., Kahle, S., & Hastings, P. D. (2017). Moderate baseline vagal tone predicts greater prosociality in children. *Developmental Psychology, 53*(2), 274–289.

Miller, P. J., & Sperry, L. L. (1987). The socialization of anger and aggression. *Merrill–Palmer Quarterly, 33,* 1–31.

Miller, P. J., & Sperry, L. L. (1988). The socialization and acquisition of emotional meanings, with special reference to language: A reply to Saarni. *Merrill–Palmer Quarterly, 34,* 217–222.

Miller, R. S. (2010). Are embarrassment and social anxiety disorder merely distant cousins, or are they closer kin? In S. G. Hoffmann & P. M. Di Bartolo (Eds.), *Social anxiety* (pp. 93–118). Academic Press.

Mills, R. S. (2005). Taking stock of the developmental literature on shame. *Developmental Review, 25*(1), 26–63.

Mills, R. S., Arbeau, K. A., Lall, D. I., & De Jaeger, A. E. (2010). Parenting and child characteristics in the prediction of shame in early and middle childhood. *Merrill–Palmer Quarterly, 56*(4), 500–528.

Mills, R. S., Imm, G. P., Walling, B. R., & Weiler, H. A. (2008). Cortisol reactivity and regulation associated with shame responding in early childhood. *Developmental Psychology, 44*(5), 1369–1380.

Milojevich, H. M., Machlin, L., & Sheridan, M. A. (2020). Early adversity and children's emotion regulation: Differential roles of parent emotion regulation and adversity exposure. *Development and Psychopathology, 32*(5), 1788–1798.

Mirabile, S. P. (2014). Parents' inconsistent emotion socialization and children's socioemotional adjustment. *Journal of Applied Developmental Psychology, 35*(5), 392–400.

Mirabile, S. P. (2015). Ignoring children's emotions: A novel ignoring subscale for the Coping with Children's Negative Emotions Scale. *European Journal of Developmental Psychology, 12*(4), 459–471.

Mirabile, S. P., Oertwig, D., & Halberstadt, A. G. (2018). Parent emotion socialization and children's socioemotional adjustment: When is supportiveness no longer supportive? *Social Development, 27*(3), 466–481.

Misailidi, P. (2006). Young children's display rule knowledge: Understanding the distinction between apparent and real emotions and the motives underlying the use of display rules. *Social Behavior and Personality: An International Journal, 34*(10), 1285–1296.

Mitchell-Copeland, J., Denham, S. A., & DeMulder, E. K. (1997). Q-sort assessment of child-teacher attachment relationships and social competence in the preschool. *Early Education and Development, 8,* 27–39.

Molina, P., Bulgarelli, D., Henning, A., & Aschersleben, G. (2014). Emotion understanding: A cross-cultural comparison between Italian and German preschoolers. *European Journal of Developmental Psychology, 11*(5), 592–607.

Molina, P., Sala, M. N., Zappulla, C., Bonfigliuoli, C., Cavioni, V., Zanetti, M. A., . . . Cicchetti, D. (2014). The Emotion Regulation Checklist–Italian translation. Validation of parent and teacher versions. *European Journal of Developmental Psychology, 11*(5), 624–634.

Möller, C., Bull, R., & Aschersleben, G. (2022). Culture shapes preschoolers' emotion recognition but not emotion comprehension: A cross-cultural study in Germany and Singapore. *Journal of Cultural Cognitive Science,* 1–17.

Mondi, C. F., Giovanelli, A., & Reynolds, A. J. (2021). Fostering socio-emotional learning through early childhood intervention. *International Journal of Child Care and Education Policy, 15*(1), 1–43.

Mondi, C. F., & Reynolds, A. J. (2021). Socio-emotional learning among low-income prekindergarteners: The roles of individual factors and early intervention. *Early Education and Development, 32*(3), 360–384.

Moore, J. E., Cooper, B. R., Domitrovich, C. E., Morgan, N. R., Cleveland, M. J., Shah, H., . . . Greenberg, M. T. (2015). The effects of exposure to an enhanced preschool program on the social-emotional functioning of at-risk children. *Early Childhood Research Quarterly, 32,* 127–138.

Moran, L. R., Lengua, L. J., & Zalewski, M. (2013). The interaction between negative emotionality and effortful control in early social-emotional development. *Social Development, 22,* 340–362.

Morelen, D., & Thomassin, K. (2013). Emotion socialization and ethnicity: An examination of practices and outcomes in African American, Asian American, and

Latin American families. *The Yale Journal of Biology and Medicine, 86*(2), 168–178.

Morgan, J. K., Izard, C. E., & Hyde, C. (2014). Emotional reactivity and regulation in Head Start children: Links to ecologically valid behaviors and internalizing problems. *Social Development, 23*(2), 250–266.

Morgan, J. K., Izard, C. E., & King, K. A. (2010). Construct validity of the Emotion Matching Task: Preliminary evidence for convergent and criterion validity of a new emotion knowledge measure for young children. *Social Development, 19*(1), 52–70.

Moreira, J. F. G., & Silvers, J. A. (2018). In due time: Neurodevelopmental considerations in the study of emotion regulation. In P. M. Cole & T. Hollenstein (Eds.), *Emotion regulation: A matter of time* (pp. 93–116). Routledge.

Morris, A. S., Silk, J. S., Morris, M. D., Steinberg, L., Aucoin, K. J., & Keyes, A. W. (2011). The influence of mother–child emotion regulation strategies on children's expression of anger and sadness. *Developmental Psychology, 47*(1), 213.

Morris, A. S., Silk, J. S., Steinberg, L., Terranova, A. M., & Kithakye, M. (2010). Concurrent and longitudinal links between children's externalizing behavior in school and observed anger regulation in the mother–child dyad. *Journal of Psychopathology and Behavioral Assessment, 32*(1), 48–56.

Morris, C. A. S., Denham, S. A., Bassett, H. H., & Curby, T. W. (2013). Relations among teachers' emotion socialization beliefs and practices, and preschoolers' emotional competence. *Early Education and Development. 24*(7), 979–999.

Morris, N., Keane, S., Calkins, S., Shanahan, L., & O'Brien, M. (2014). Differential components of reactivity and attentional control predicting externalizing behavior. *Journal of Applied Developmental Psychology, 35*, 121–127.

Morris, P., Mattera, S. K., Castells, N., Bangser, M., Bierman, K., & Raver, C. (2014). *Impact findings from the Head Start CARES demonstration: National evaluation of three approaches to improving preschoolers' social and emotional competence*. OPRE Report 2014-44. Office of Planning, Research and Evaluation.

Mortari, L. (2009). *Ricercare e riflettere: la formazione del docente professionista*. Carocci.

Mortari, L. (2012). Learning thoughtful reflection in teacher education. *Teachers and Teaching, 18*(5), 525–545.

Moskowitz, C. (1997). *Self-evaluation*. Unpublished doctoral dissertation, George Mason University, Fairfax, VA.

Mostow, A. J., Izard, C. E., Fine, S., & Trentacosta, C. J. (2002). Modeling emotional, cognitive, and behavioral predictors of peer acceptance. *Child Development, 73*(6), 1775–1787.

Mullin, B. C., & Hinshaw, S. P. (2007). Emotion regulation and externalizing disorders in children and adolescents. In J. J. Gross (Ed.), *Handbook of emotion regulation* (pp. 523–541). Guilford Press.

Mundy, P., Kasari, C., & Sigman, M. (1992). Nonverbal communication, affective sharing, and intersubjectivity. *Infant Behavior and Development, 15*, 377–381.

Murano, D., Sawyer, J. E., & Lipnevich, A. A. (2020). A meta-analytic review of preschool social and emotional learning interventions. *Review of Educational Research, 90(2)*, 227–263.

Murgatroyd, S. J., & Robinson, E. J. (1993). Children's judgments of emotions following moral transgression. *International Journal of Behavioral Development, 16*, 93–111.

Muris, P., & Meesters, C. (2014). Small or big in the eyes of the other: On the developmental psychopathology of self-conscious emotions as shame, guilt, and pride. *Clinical Child and Family Psychology Review, 17*(1), 19–40.

Murphy, B. C., Eisenberg, N., Fabes, R. A., Shepard, S., & Guthrie, I. K. (1999). Consistency and change in children's emotionality and regulation: A longitudinal study. *Merrill–Palmer Quarterly 45*(3), 413–444.

Murphy, T. P., & Laible, D. J. (2013). The influence of attachment security on preschool children's empathic concern. *International Journal of Behavioral Development, 37*(5), 436–440.

Naglieri, J. A., LeBuffe, P., & Shapiro, V. B. (2011). Universal screening for social–emotional competencies: A study of the reliability and validity of the DESSA-mini. *Psychology in the Schools, 48*, 660–671.

Naito, M., & Seki, Y. (2009). The relationship between second-order false belief and display rules reasoning: the integration of cognitive and affective social understanding. *Developmental Science, 12*(1), 150–164.

Nakamichi, K. (2017). Differences in young children's peer preference by inhibitory control and emotion regulation. *Psychological Reports, 120*(5), 805–823.

Nancarrow, A. F., Gilpin, A. T., Thibodeau, R. B., & Farrell, C. B. (2018). Knowing what others know: Linking deception detection, emotion knowledge, and theory of mind in preschool. *Infant and Child Development, 27*(5), e2097.

National Association for the Education of Young Children & National Association of Early Childhood Specialists in State Departments of Education (2003). *Early childhood curriculum, assessment, and program evaluation: Building an effective, accountable system in programs for children birth through age 8*. Retrieved from *www.naeyc.org/files/naeyc/file/positions/CA3expand.pdf*.

National Research Council. (2012). *Education for life and work: Developing transferable knowledge and skills in the 21st century*. National Academies Press.

National Scientific Council on the Developing Child. (2005/2014). *Excessive stress disrupts the architecture of the developing brain: Working paper 3*. Updated edition.

Nelson, J. A., de Lucca Freitas, L. B., O'Brien, M., Calkins, S. D., Leerkes, E. M., & Marcovitch, S. (2013). Preschool-aged children's understanding of gratitude: Relations with emotion and mental state knowledge. *British Journal of Developmental Psychology, 31*(1), 42–56.

Nelson, J. A., Leerkes, E. M., O'Brien, M., Calkins, S. D., & Marcovitch, S. (2012). African American and European American mothers' beliefs about negative emotions and emotion socialization practices. *Parenting, 12*(1), 22–41.

Nelson, J. A., Leerkes, E. M., Perry, N. B., O'Brien, M., Calkins, S. D., & Marcovitch, S. (2013). European-American and African-American mothers' emotion socialization practices relate differently to their children's academic and social-emotional competence. *Social Development, 22*(3), 485–498.

Nelson, N. L., Hudspeth, K., & Russell, J. A. (2013). A story superiority effect for disgust, fear, embarrassment, and pride. *British Journal of Developmental Psychology, 31*(3), 334–348.

Nelson, N. L., & Russell, J. A. (2012). Children's understanding of nonverbal expressions of pride. *Journal of Experimental Child Psychology, 111*(3), 379–385.

Neppl, T. K., Donnellan, M. B., Scaramella, L. V., Widaman, K. F., Spilman, S. K., Ontai, L. L., & Conger, R. D. (2010). Differential stability of temperament and personality from toddlerhood to middle childhood. *Journal of Research in Personality, 44*(3), 386–396.

Newland, R. P., & Crnic, K. A. (2011). Mother–child affect and emotion socialization processes across the late preschool period: Predictions of emerging behaviour problems. *Infant and Child Development, 20*, 371–388.

Nichols, S. R., Svetlova, M., & Brownell, C. A. (2009). The role of social understanding and empathic disposition in young children's responsiveness to distress in parents and peers. *Cognition, Brain, Behavior, 13*(4), 449–478.

Nix, R. L., Bierman, K. L., Domitrovich, C. E., & Gill, S. (2013). Promoting children's social-emotional skills in preschool can enhance academic and behavioral functioning in kindergarten: Findings from Head Start REDI. *Early Education and Development, 24*, 1000–1019.

Nix, R. L., Bierman, K. L., Heinrichs, B. S., Gest, S. D., Welsh, J. A., & Domitrovich, C. E. (2016). The randomized controlled trial of Head Start REDI: Sustained effects on developmental trajectories of social–emotional functioning. *Journal of Consulting and Clinical Psychology, 84*(4), 310–322.

Nixon, C. L., & Watson, A. C. (2001). Family experiences and early emotion understanding. *Merrill–Palmer Quarterly 47*(2), 300–322.

Nook, E. C., Stavish, C. M., Sasse, S. F., Lambert, H. K., Mair, P., McLaughlin, K. A., & Somerville, L. H. (2020). Charting the development of emotion comprehension and abstraction from childhood to adulthood using observer-rated and linguistic measures. *Emotion, 20*(5), 773–792.

Nunner-Winkler, G., & Sodian, B. (1988). Children's understanding of moral emotions. *Child Development, 59*, 1323–1338.

Nuske, H. J., Hedley, D., Woollacott, A., Thomson, P., Macari, S., & Dissanayake, C. (2017). Developmental delays in emotion regulation strategies in preschoolers with autism. *Autism Research, 10*(11), 1808–1822.

Nwadinobi, O. K., & Gagne, J. R. (2020). Preschool anger, activity level, inhibitory control, and behavior problems: A family study approach. *Merrill–Palmer Quarterly, 66*(4), 339–365.

O'Brien, M., Miner Weaver, J., Nelson, J. A., Calkins, S. D., Leerkes, E. M., & Marcovitch, S. (2011). Longitudinal associations between children's understanding of emotions and theory of mind. *Cognition and Emotion, 25*(6), 1074–1086.

O'Connor, R., DeFeyter, J., Carr, A., Luo, J. L., & Romm, H. (2017). *A review of literature on social and emotional learning for students ages 3–8: Implementation strategies and state and district support policies (part 2 of 4)*. U.S. Department of Education Institute for Education Sciences National Center for Education Evaluation and Regional Assistance: Regional Educational Laboratory (Mid-Atlantic) at ICF International.

O'Kearney, R., Chng, R. Y., & Salmon, K. (2021). Callous-unemotional features are associated with emotion recognition impairments in young odd children with low but not high affective arousal. *Child Psychiatry and Human Development, 52*, 869–879.

O'Kearney, R., Salmon, K., Liwag, M., Fortune, C. A., & Dawel, A. (2017). Emotional abilities in children with oppositional defiant disorder (ODD): Impairments in perspective-taking and understanding mixed emotions are associated with high callous–unemotional traits. *Child Psychiatry and Human Development, 48*(2), 346–357.

O'Neill, D. K., Astington, J. W., & Flavell, J. H. (1992). Young children's understanding of the role that sensory experiences play in knowledge acquisition. *Child Development, 63*, 474–490.

O'Neill, D. K., & Chong, S. (2001). Preschool children's difficulty understanding the types of information obtained through the five senses. *Child Development, 72*(3), 803–815.

Oades-Sese, G. V., Cahill, A., Allen, J. W. P., Rubic, W. L., & Mahmood, N. (2021). Effectiveness of Sesame Workshop's Little Children, Big Challenges: A digital media SEL intervention for preschool classrooms. *Psychology in the Schools, 58*(10), 2041–2067.

Odom, E. C., Garrett-Peters, P., Vernon-Feagans, L., & Family Life Project Investigators. (2016). Racial discrimination as a correlate of African American mothers' emotion talk to young children. *Journal of Family Issues, 37*(7), 970–996.

Ogelman, H. G., & Fetihi, L. (2021). Examination of the relationship between emotional regulation strategies of 5-year-old children and their peer relationships. *Early Child Development and Care, 119*(1), 49–57.

Ogren, M., & Johnson, S. P. (2020). Factors facilitating early emotion understanding development: Contributions to individual differences. *Human Development, 64*, 108–118.

Ogren, M., & Sandhofer, C. M. (2021). Emotion words in early childhood: A language transcript analysis. *Cognitive Development, 60*, 101122.

Olino, T. M., Lopez-Duran, N. L., Kovacs, M., George, C. J., Gentzler, A. L., & Shaw, D. S. (2011). Developmental trajectories of positive and negative affect in children at high and low familial risk for depressive disorder. *Journal of Child Psychology and Psychiatry, 52*(7), 792–799.

Olson, L. (2021). *Tough test: The nations' troubled early learning assessment landscape*. FutureED.

Ongley, S. F., & Malti, T. (2014). The role of moral emotions in the development of children's sharing behavior. *Developmental Psychology, 50*(4), 1148–1159.

Ornaghi, V., Agliati, A., Pepe, A., & Gabola, P. (2020).

Patterns of association between early childhood teachers' emotion socialization styles, emotion beliefs and mind-mindedness. *Early Education and Development, 31*(1), 47–65.

Ornaghi, V., Brazzelli, E., Grazzani, I., Agliati, A., & Lucarelli, M. (2017). Does training toddlers in emotion knowledge lead to changes in their prosocial and aggressive behavior toward peers at nursery? *Early Education and Development, 28*(4), 396–414.

Ornaghi, V., Brockmeier, J., & Gavazzi, I. G. (2011). The role of language games in children's understanding of mental states: A training study. *Journal of Cognition and Development, 12*(2), 239–259.

Ornaghi, V., Brockmeier, J., & Grazzani, I. (2014). Enhancing social cognition by training children in emotion understanding: A primary school study. *Journal of Experimental Child Psychology, 119*, 26–39.

Ornaghi, V., Conte, E., Agliati, A., & Gandellini, S. (2022). Early-childhood teachers' emotion socialization practices: A multi-method study. *Early Child Development and Care, 192*(10), 1608–1625. [Epub ahead of print]

Ornaghi, V., Conte, E., & Grazzani, I. (2020). Empathy in toddlers: The role of emotion regulation, language ability, and maternal emotion socialization style. *Frontiers in Psychology, 11*, 2844.

Ornaghi, V., Grazzani, I., Cherubin, E., Conte, E., & Piralli, F. (2015). 'Let's talk about emotions!' The effect of conversational training on preschoolers' emotion comprehension and prosocial orientation. *Social Development, 24*, 166–183.

Ornaghi, V., Pepe, A., Agliati, A., & Grazzani, I. (2019). The contribution of emotion knowledge, language ability, and maternal emotion socialization style to explaining toddlers' emotion regulation. *Social Development, 28*(3), 581–598.

Orta, I. M., Çorapçı, F., Yagmurlu, B., & Aksan, N. (2013). The mediational role of effortful control and emotional dysregulation in the link between maternal responsiveness and Turkish preschoolers' social competency and externalizing symptoms. *Infant and Child Development, 22*(5), 459–479.

Pala, F. C., & Lewis, C. (2021). Do preschoolers grasp the importance of regulating emotional expression? *European Journal of Developmental Psychology, 18*(4), 494–519.

Panfile, T. M., & Laible, D. J. (2012). Attachment security and child's empathy: The mediating role of emotion regulation. *Merrill–Palmer Quarterly 58*(1), 1–21.

Paquette, D. (2004). Theorizing the father-child relationship: Mechanisms and developmental outcomes. *Human development, 47*(4), 193–219.

Parisette-Sparks, A., Bufferd, S. J., & Klein, D. N. (2017). Parental predictors of children's shame and guilt at age 6 in a multimethod, longitudinal study. *Journal of Clinical Child and Adolescent Psychology, 46*(5), 721–731.

Park, M. H., Tiwari, A., & Neumann, J. W. (2020). Emotional scaffolding in early childhood education. *Educational Studies, 46*(5), 570–589.

Parke, R. D., Cassidy, J., Burks, V. M., Carson, J. L., & Boyum, L. (1992). Familial contribution to peer competence among young children: The role of interactive and affective processes. In R. D. Parke & G. W. Ladd (Eds.), *Family–peer relationships: Modes of linkage* (pp. 107–134). Erlbaum.

Parker, A. E., Halberstadt, A. G., Dunsmore, J. C., Townley, G., Bryant, A. Jr., Thompson, J. A., & Beale, K. S. (2012). Emotions are a window into one's heart: A qualitative analysis of parental beliefs about children's emotions across three ethnic groups. *Monographs of the Society for Research in Child Development, 77*(3), 1–136.

Parker, A. E., Mathis, E. T., & Kupersmidt, J. B. (2013). How is this child feeling?: Preschool-aged children's ability to recognize emotion in faces and body poses. *Early Education and Development, 24*, 188–211.

Parker, J. G., & Gottman, J. M. (1989). Social and emotional development in a relational context: Friendship interaction from early childhood to adolescence. In T. Berndt & G. Ladd (Eds.), *Peer relationships in child development* (pp. 95–131). Wiley.

Parker, J. G., Rubin, K. H., Erath, S. A., Wojslawowicz, J. C., & Buskirk, A. A. (2006). Peer relationships, child development, and adjustment: A developmental psychopathology perspective. In D. Cicchetti & D. J. Cohen (Eds.), *Developmental psychopathology: Theory and method* (pp. 419–493). Wiley.

Pasalich, D. S., Waschbusch, D. A., Dadds, M. R., & Hawes, D. J. (2014). Emotion socialization style in parents of children with callous–unemotional traits. *Child Psychiatry and Human Development, 45*(2), 229–242.

Patterson, G. R. (1980). Mothers: The unacknowledged victims. *Monographs of the Society for Research in Child Development, 45*(5, Serial No. 186), 1–64.

Patterson, G. R., Reid, J. B., & Dishion, T. J. (1992). *Antisocial boys*. Eugene, OR: Castalia.

Pavarini, G., de Hollanda Souza, D., & Hawk, C. K. (2013). Parental practices and theory of mind development. *Journal of Child and Family Studies, 22*(6), 844–853.

Payton, J. W., Wardlaw, D. M., Graczyk, P. A., Bloodworth, M. R., Tompsett, C. J., & Weissberg, R. P. (2000). Social and emotional learning: A framework for promoting mental health and reducing risk behavior in children and youth. *Journal of School Health, 70*, 179–186.

Paz, Y., Davidov, M., Orlitsky, T., Roth-Hanania, R., & Zahn-Waxler, C. (2021). Developmental trajectories of empathic concern in infancy and their links to social competence in early childhood. *Journal of Child Psychology and Psychiatry, 63*(7), 762–770.

Paz, Y., Orlitsky, T., Roth-Hanania, R., Zahn-Waxler, C., & Davidov, M. (2021). Predicting externalizing behavior in toddlerhood from early individual differences in empathy. *Journal of Child Psychology and Psychiatry, 62*(1), 66–74.

Pecora, G., Sette, S., Baumgartner, E., Laghi, F., & Spinrad, T. L. (2016). The moderating role of internalising negative emotionality in the relation of self-regulation to social adjustment in Italian preschool-aged children. *Cognition and Emotion, 30*(8), 1512–1520.

Pekrun, R., & Linnenbrink-Garcia, L. (2012). Academic emotions and student engagement. In S. L. Christenson, A. L. Reschly, and C. Wylie (Eds.), *Handbook of research on student engagement* (pp. 259–-282). Springer.

Penela, E. C., Walker, O. L., Degnan, K. A., Fox, N. A., & Henderson, H. A. (2015). Early behavioral inhibition and emotion regulation: Pathways toward social competence in middle childhood. *Child Development, 86*(4), 1227–1240.

Peng, M., Johnson, C. N., Pollock, J., Glasspool, R., & Harris, P. L. (1992). Training young children to acknowledge mixed emotions. *Cognition and Emotion, 6*, 387–401.

Perie, M., Marion, S., & Gong, B. (2009). Moving toward a comprehensive assessment system: A framework for considering interim assessments. *Educational Measurement: Issues and Practice, 28*(3), 5–13.

Perlman, S. B., Camras, L. A., & Pelphrey, K. A. (2008). Physiology and functioning: Parents' vagal tone, emotion socialization, and children's emotion knowledge. *Journal of Experimental Child Psychology, 100*(4), 308–315.

Perlman, S. B., Kalish, C. W., & Pollak, S. D. (2008). The role of maltreatment experience in children's understanding of the antecedents of emotion. *Cognition and Emotion, 22*(4), 651–670.

Perra, O., Paine, A. L., & Hay, D. F. (2021). Continuity and change in anger and aggressiveness from infancy to childhood: The protective effects of positive parenting. *Development and Psychopathology, 33*(3), 937–956.

Perry, N. B., & Calkins, S. D. (2018). A biopsychosocial perspective on the development of emotion regulation across childhood. In P. M. Cole & T. Hollerstein (Eds.), *Emotion regulation: A matter of time* (pp. 3–30). Routledge.

Perry-Parrish, C., Waasdorp, T. E., & Bradshaw, C. P. (2012). Peer nominations of emotional expressivity among urban children: Social and psychological correlates. *Social Development, 21*(1), 88–108.

Philoppot, P., & Feldman, R. S. (1990). Age and social competence in preschoolers' decoding of facial expression. *British Journal of Social Psychology, 29*, 43–54.

Phillips, W., Baron-Cohen, S., & Rutter, M. (1995). To what extent can children with autism understand desire? *Development and Psychopathology, 7*, 151–169.

Phinney, J. S., Feshbach, N. D., & Farver, J. (1986). Preschool children's response to peer crying. *Early Childhood Research Quarterly, 1*, 207–219.

Piaget, J. (1977/1995). *Sociological studies*. Routledge. (Original work published 1977)

Pintar Breen, A. I., Tamis-LeMonda C. S., & Kahana-Kalman R. (2018). Latina mothers' emotion socialization and their children's emotion knowledge. *Infant and Child Development, 27*(3), e2077.

Piotrkowski, C. S., Botsko, M., & Matthews, E. (2000). Parents' and teachers' beliefs about children's school readiness in a high-need community. *Early Childhood Research Quarterly, 15*, 537–558.

Pitskel, N. B., Bolling, D. Z., Kaiser, M. D., Crowley, M. J., & Pelphrey, K. A. (2011). How grossed out are you?: The neural bases of emotion regulation from childhood to adolescence. *Developmental Cognitive Neuroscience, 1*(3), 324–337.

Pochon, R., & Declercq, C. (2013). Emotion recognition by children with Down syndrome: A longitudinal study. *Journal of Intellectual and Developmental Disability, 38*(4), 332–343.

Pollak, S. D., Cicchetti, D., Hornung, K., & Reed, A. (2000). Recognizing emotion in faces: Developmental effects of child abuse and neglect. *Developmental Psychology, 36*(5), 679–699.

Pollak, S. D., & Sinha, P. (2002). Effects of early experience on children's recognition of facial displays of emotion. *Developmental Psychology, 38*(5), 784–79.

Pollak, S. D., & Tolley-Schell, S. A. (2003). Selective attention to facial emotion in physically abused children. *Journal of Abnormal Psychology, 112*(3), 323–336.

Pons, F., Harris, P. L., & de Rosnay, M. (2004). Emotion comprehension between 3 and 11 years: Developmental periods and hierarchical organization. *European Journal of Developmental Psychology, 1*(2), 127–152.

Pons, F., Lawson, J., Harris, P. L., & De Rosnay, M. (2003). Individual differences in children's emotion understanding: Effects of age and language. *Scandinavian Journal of Psychology, 44*(4), 347–353.

Poon, J., Zeman, J., Miller-Slough, R., Sanders, W., & Crespo, L. (2017). "Good enough" parental responsiveness to children's sadness: Links to psychosocial functioning. *Journal of Applied Developmental Psychology, 48*, 69–78.

Porges, S. W. (2003). The polyvagal theory: Phylogenetic contributions to social behavior. *Physiology and Behavior, 79*, 503–513.

Posner, J., Russell, J. A., & Peterson, B. S. (2005). The circumplex model of affect: An integrative approach to affective neuroscience, cognitive development, and psychopathology. *Development and Psychopathology, 17*(3), 715–734.

Poulou, M. (2005). The prevention of emotional and behavioural difficulties in schools: Teachers' suggestions. *Educational Psychology in Practice*, 21, 37–52.

Poulou, M. S., Garner, P. W., & Bassett, H. H. (2022). Teachers' emotional expressiveness and classroom management practices: Associations with young students' social-emotional and behavioral competence. *Psychology in the Schools, 59*(3), 557–573.

Powell, D., & Dunlap, G. (2009). *Evidence-based social emotional curricula and intervention packages for children 0–5 years and their families: Roadmap to effective intervention practices #2*. Technical Assistance Center on Social Emotional Intervention for Young Children.

Premo, J. E., & Kiel, E. J. (2014). The effect of toddler emotion regulation on maternal emotion socialization: Moderation by toddler gender. *Emotion, 14*, 782–793.

Price, N. N., & Kiel, E. J. (2022). Longitudinal links among mother and child emotion regulation, maternal emotion socialization, and child anxiety. *Research on Child and Adolescent Psychopathology, 50*(2), 241–254.

Profyt, L., & Whissell, C. (1991). Children's understanding of facial expression of emotion: 1. Voluntary creation of emotion-faces. *Perceptual and Motor Skills, 73*, 199–202.

Preston, S. D., & de Waal, F. B. M. (2002). Empathy: Its ultimate and proximate bases. *Behavioral and Brain Sciences, 25*(1), 1–20.

Prosen, S., & Smrtnik Vitulić, H. (2018). Children's emotional expression in the preschool context, *Early Child Development and Care, 188*(12), 1675–1683.

Putnam, S. P., & Rothbart, M. K. (2006). Development of short and very short forms of the Children's Behavior Questionnaire. *Journal of Personality Assessment, 87*(1), 102–112.

Qiu, C., & Shum, K. K. M. (2021). Emotion coaching intervention for Chinese mothers of preschoolers: A randomized controlled trial. *Child Psychiatry and Human Development*, 1–15.

Raikes, H. A., & Thompson, R. A. (2006). Family emotional climate, attachment security and young children's emotion knowledge in a high risk sample. *British Journal of Developmental Psychology, 24*(1), 89–104.

Raikes, H. A., & Thompson, R. A. (2008). Conversations about emotion in high-risk dyads. *Attachment and Human Development, 10*(4), 359–377.

Ramsook, K. A., Benson, L., Ram, N., & Cole, P. M. (2020). Age-related changes in the relation between preschoolers' anger and persistence. *International Journal of Behavioral Development, 44*(3), 216–225.

Rasmussen, E. E., Strouse, G. A., Colwell, M. J., Johnson, C. R., Holiday, S., Brady, K., . . . & Norman, M. S. (2019). Promoting preschoolers' emotional competence through prosocial TV and mobile app use. *Media Psychology, 22(1)*, 1–22.

Ratcliff, K. A., Vazquez, L. C., Lunkenheimer, E. S., & Cole, P. M. (2021). Longitudinal changes in young children's strategy use for emotion regulation. *Developmental Psychology, 57*(9), 1471–1486.

Raval, V. V., Li, X., Deo, N., & Hu, J. (2018). Reports of maternal socialization goals, emotion socialization behaviors, and child functioning in China and India. *Journal of Family Psychology, 32*(1), 81–91.

Raval, V. V., & Walker, B. L. (2019). Unpacking 'culture': Caregiver socialization of emotions and child functioning in diverse families. *Developmental Review, 51*, 146–174.

Raver, C. C., Blair, C., Garrett-Peters, P., & Family Life Project Key Investigators. (2015). Poverty, household chaos, and interparental aggression predict children's ability to recognize and modulate negative emotions. *Development and Psychopathology, 27*(3), 695–708.

Raver, C. C., & Knitzer, J. (2002). *Ready to enter: What research tells policymakers about strategies to promote social and emotional school readiness among three- and four-year-olds*. Harris School of Public Policy Studies, University of Chicago.

Raver, C., & Spagnola, M. (2003). "When my mommy was angry, I was speechless": Children's perceptions of maternal emotional expressiveness within the context of economic hardship. *Marriage and Family Review, 34(1–2)*, 63–88.

Ravindran, N., Genaro, B. G., & Cole, P. M. (2021). Parental structuring in response to toddler negative emotion predicts children's later use of distraction as a self-regulation strategy for waiting. *Child Development, 92*(5), 1969–1983.

Ravindran, N., McElwain, N. L., Berry, D., & Kramer, L. (2018). Mothers' dispositional distress reactivity as a predictor of maternal support following momentary fluctuations in children's aversive behavior. *Developmental Psychology, 54*(2), 209–219.

Rehder, P. D., Mills-Koonce, W. R., Willoughby, M. T., Garrett-Peters, P., & Wagner, N. J. (2017). Emotion recognition deficits among children with conduct problems and callous-unemotional behaviors. *Early Childhood Research Quarterly, 41*, 174–183.

Reimer, K. J. (1997). Emotion socialization and children's emotional expressiveness in the preschool context. *Dissertation Abstracts International Section A: Humanities and Social Sciences, 57*(7), 2848.

Reissland, J., & Harris, P. (1991). Children's use of display rules in pride-eliciting situations. *British Journal of Developmental Psychology, 9*, 431–435.

Ren, Y., Wyver, S., Xu Rattanasone, N., & Demuth, K. (2016). Social competence and language skills in Mandarin–English bilingual preschoolers: The moderation effect of emotion regulation. *Early Education and Development, 27*(3), 303–317.

Reynolds, A. J., & Mondi, C. F. (2016). Child–Parent Centers. In D. Couchenour & J. K. Chrisman (Eds.), *SAGE encyclopedia of contemporary early childhood education*. SAGE.

Reynolds, A. J., Richardson, B. A., Hayakawa, M., Englund, M. M., & Ou, S. (2016). Multi-site expansion of an early childhood intervention and school readiness. *Pediatrics, 138*, e20154587.

Rhee, S. H., Boeldt, D. L., Friedman, N. P., Corley, R. P., Hewitt, J. K., Young, S. E., . . . & Zahn-Waxler, C. (2013). The role of language in concern and disregard for others in the first years of life. *Developmental Psychology, 49*(2), 197–214.

Rhoades, B. L., Warren, H. K., Domitrovich, C. E., & Greenberg, M. T. (2011). Examining the link between preschool social–emotional competence and first grade academic achievement: The role of attention skills. *Early Childhood Research Quarterly, 26*, 182–191.

Richards, D. D., & Siegler, R. S. (1981). Very young children's acquisition of systematic problem-solving strategies. *Child Development, 52*, 1318–1321.

Ridgeway, D., & Kuczaj, S. (1985). Acquisition of emotion-descriptive language: Receptive and productive vocabulary norms for ages 18 months to 6 years. *Developmental Psychology, 21*, 901–908.

Rieffe, C., Meerum Terwogt, M., & Cowan, R. (2005). Children's understanding of mental states as causes of emotions. *Infant and Child Development, 14*(3), 259–272.

Rieffe, C., Meerum Terwogt, M., Koops, W., Stegge, H. & Oomen, A. (2001). Pre-schoolers' appreciation of uncommon desires and subsequent emotions. *British Journal of Developmental Psychology, 19*, 259–274.

Riese, M. L. (1990). Neonatal temperament in monozygotic and dizygotic twin pairs. *Child Development, 61*, 1230–1237.

Rimm-Kaufman, S. E., Pianta, R. C., & Cox, M. J. (2000). Teachers' judgments of problems in the transition to kindergarten. *Early Childhood Research Quarterly, 15*, 147–166.

Ringwalt, S. (2008). *Developmental screening and assessment instruments with an emphasis on social and emotional development for young children ages birth through five*. University of North Carolina, FPG Child Development Institute, National Early Childhood Technical Assistance Center.

Rivers, S. E., Tominey, S. L., Bailey, C. S., O'Bryon, E. C., Olsen, S. G., Sneeden, C. K., . . . Brackett, M. A. *Promoting social and emotional skill development in early childhood with Preschool RULER*. Manuscript submitted for publication.

Rivers, S. E., Tominey, S. L., O' Bryon, E., & Brackett, M. (2013a). Developing emotional skills in early childhood settings using Preschool RULER. *Psychological Education Review, 37*, 20–25.

Rivers, S. E., Tominey, S. L., O'Bryon, E. C., & Brackett, M. A. (2013b). Introduction to the special issue on social and emotional learning in early education. *Early Education and Development, 24*(7), 953–959.

Roben, C. K., Cole, P. M., & Armstrong, L. M. (2013). Longitudinal relations among language skills, anger expression, and regulatory strategies in early childhood. *Child Development, 84*(3), 891–905.

Roberts, W. R., & Strayer, J. (1987). Parents' responses to the emotional distress of their children: Relations with children's competence. *Developmental Psychology, 23*, 415–422.

Roberts, W., Strayer, J., & Denham, S. (2014). Empathy, anger, guilt: Emotions and prosocial behaviour. *Canadian Journal of Behavioural Science, 46*(4), 465–474.

Robin, A. L., Schneider, M., & Dolnick, M. (1976). The Turtle Technique: An extended case study of self-control in the classroom. *Psychology in the Schools, 13*, 449–453.

Robinson, L. R., Morris, A. S., Heller, S. S., Scheeringa, M. S., Boris, N. W., & Smyke, A. T. (2009). Relations between emotion regulation, parenting, and psychopathology in young maltreated children in out of home care. *Journal of Child and Family Studies, 18*(4), 421–434.

Rodrigo-Ruiz, D., Perez-Gonzalez, J. C., & Cejudo, J. (2017). Emotional facial recognition difficulties as primary deficit in children with attention deficit hyperactivity disorder: A systematic review. *Revista de Neurologica, 65*(4), 145–152.

Rogosch, F. A., Cicchetti, D., & Aber, J. L. (1995). The role of child maltreatment in early deviations in cognitive and affective processing abilities and later peer relationship problems. *Development and Psychopathology, 7*, 591–610.

Romano, E., Babchishin, L., Pagani, L. S., & Kohen, D. (2010). School readiness and later achievement: Replication and extension using a nationwide Canadian survey. *Developmental Psychology, 46*, 995–1007.

Romero, N. L. (2017). A pilot study examining a computer-based intervention to improve recognition and understanding of emotions in young children with communication and social deficits. *Research in Developmental Disabilities, 65*, 35–45.

Romero-López, M., Pichardo, M. C., Justicia-Arráez, A., & Bembibre-Serrano, J. (2021). Reducing aggression by developing emotional and inhibitory control. *International Journal of Environmental Research and Public Health, 18*(10), 5263.

Ros-Demarize, R., & Graziano, P. A. (2021). Initial feasibility and efficacy of the Summer Treatment Program (STP-PreK) for preschoolers with autism spectrum disorder and comorbid externalizing behavior problems. *Journal of Early Intervention, 43*(1), 60–79.

Rose, S. L., Rose, S. A., & Feldman, J. F. (1989). Stability of behavior problems in very young children. *Development and Psychopathology, 1*(1), 5–19.

Rose-Krasnor, L., & Denham, S. A. (2008). Social-emotional competence in early childhood. In K., H. Rubin, W. Bukowski, & B. Laursen (Eds.), *Handbook of peer relationships* (pp. 613–637). Guilford Press.

Ross, J. (2017). You and me: Investigating the role of self-evaluative emotion in preschool prosociality. *Journal of Experimental Child Psychology, 155*, 67–83.

Roth-Hanania, R., Davidov, M., & Zahn-Waxler, C. (2011). Empathy development from 8 to 16 months: Early signs of concern for others. *Infant Behavior and Development, 34*(3), 447–458.

Rothbart, M. K., Ahadi, S. A., Hershey, K. L., & Fisher, P. (2001). Investigations of temperament at 3–7 years: The Children's Behavior Questionnaire. *Child Development, 72*, 1394–1408.

Ruba, A. L., Kalia, V., & Wilbourn, M. P. (2022). Happy, sad, or yucky?: Parental emotion talk with infants in a book-sharing task. *Infancy, 27*(2), 277–290.

Rubin, K. D., & Clark, M. L. (1983). Preschool teachers' ratings of behavioral problems: Observational, sociometric, and social-cognitive correlates. *Journal of Abnormal Child Psychology, 11*, 273–286.

Rubin, K. D., & Daniels-Byrness, T. (1983). Concurrent and predictive correlates of sociometric status in kindergarten and grade 1 children. *Merrill–Palmer Quarterly, 29*, 337–352.

Rubin, K. H. (1982). Non-social play in preschoolers: Necessary evil? *Child Development, 53*, 651–657.

Rubin, K. H., Burgess, K. B., Dwyer, K. M., & Hastings, P. D. (2003). Predicting preschoolers' externalizing behaviors from toddler temperament, conflict, and maternal negativity. *Developmental Psychology, 39*(1), 164–178.

Rubin, K. H., Burgess, K. B., & Hastings, P. D. (2002). Stability and social–behavioral consequences of toddlers' inhibited temperament and parenting behaviors. *Child Development, 73*(2), 483–495.

Rubin, K. H., Coplan, R. J., & Bowker, J. C. (2009). Social withdrawal in childhood. *Annual Review of Psychology, 60*, 141–171.

Rubin, K. H., Hemphill, S. A., Chen, X., Hastings, P., Sanson, A., Coco, A. L., . . . Cui, L. (2006). A cross-cultural study of behavioral inhibition in toddlers: East–West–North–South. *International Journal of Behavioral Development, 30*(3), 219–226.

Rudasill, K. M., & Konold, T. R. (2008). Contributions of children's temperament to teachers' judgments of social competence from kindergarten through second grade. *Early Education and Development, 19*(4), 643–666.

Ruffman, T., & Keenan, T. R. (1996). The belief-based emotion of surprise: The case for a lag in understanding relative to false belief. *Developmental Psychology, 32,* 40–49.

Russell, J. A. (1989). Culture, scripts, and children's understanding of emotion. In P. P. Harris & C. Saarni (Eds.), *Children's understanding of emotion* (pp. 293–318). Cambridge University Press.

Russell, J. A. (1990). The preschooler's understanding of the causes and consequences of emotion. *Child Development, 61,* 1872–1881.

Russell, J. A. (1994). Is there universal recognition of emotion from facial expression?: A review of the cross cultural studies. *Psychological Bulletin, 115,* 102–141.

Russell, J. A., & Paris, F. A. (1994). Do children acquire concepts of complex emotions abruptly? *International Journal of Behavioral Development, 17,* 349–365.

Russell, J. A., & Widen, S. C. (2002). A label superiority effect in children's categorization of facial expressions. *Social Development, 11*(1), 30–52.

Rydell, A. M., Berlin, L., & Bohlin, G. (2003). Emotionality, emotion regulation, and adaptation among 5- to 8-year-old children. *Emotion,* 3(1), 30–47.

Saarni, C. (1987). Cultural rules of emotional experience: A commentary on Miller and Sperry's study. *Merrill–Palmer Quarterly, 33,* 535–540.

Saarni, C. (1990). Emotional competence. In R. A. Thompson (Ed.), *Nebraska Symposium on Motivation: Vol. 36. Socioemotional development* (pp. 115–161). University of Nebraska Press.

Saarni, C. (1998). Issues of cultural meaningfulness in emotional development. *Developmental Psychology,* 34(4), 647–652.

Saarni, C. (1999). *The development of emotional competence.* Guilford Press.

Saarni, C. (2001). Cognition, context, and goals: Significant components in social–emotional effectiveness. *Social Development, 10*(1), 125–129.

Saarni, C., Campos, J. J., Camras, L. A., & Witherington, D. (2006). Emotional development: Action, communication, and understanding. In N. Eisenberg, W. Damon, & R. M. Lerner (Eds.), *Handbook of child psychology: Social, emotional, and personality development* (pp. 226–299). Wiley.

Saarni, C., & Crowley, M. (1990). The development of emotion regulation: Effects on emotional state and expression. In E. A. Blechman (Ed.), *Emotions and the family: For better or for worse* (pp. 53–73). Erlbaum.

Saarni, C., & von Salisch, M. (1993). The socialization of emotional dissemblance. In M. Lewis & C. Saarni (Eds.), *Lying and deception in everyday life* (pp. 106–125). Guilford Press.

Sachs-Alter, E. (1989). *The contextual use of facial expressions by maltreating and nonmaltreating mothers.* Unpublished master's thesis, DePaul University, Chicago.

Sachs-Alter, E. (1993). *Maltreated and nonmaltreated children's use of cues in understanding the emotions of others.* Unpublished doctoral dissertation, DePaul University, Chicago.

Sahin Asi, D., Ocak Karabay, S., & Guzeldere Aydin, D. (2019). Emotional correspondence between preschoolers and teachers: What are the effects on child–teacher relationships? *Education 3–13,* 47(8), 969–982.

Sala, M. N., Pons, F., & Molina, P. (2014). Emotion regulation strategies in preschool children. *British Journal of Developmental Psychology, 32,* 440–453.

Sallquist, J., DiDonato, M. D., Hanish, L. D., Martin, C. L., & Fabes, R. A. (2012). The importance of mutual positive expressivity in social adjustment: Understanding the role of peers and gender. *Emotion, 12*(2), 304–313.

Sallquist, J., Eisenberg, N., Spinrad, T. L., Eggum, N. D., & Gaertner, B. M. (2009). Assessment of preschoolers' positive empathy: Concurrent and longitudinal relations with positive emotion, social competence, and sympathy. *Journal of Positive Psychology,* 4(3), 223–233.

Sallquist, J., Eisenberg, N., Spinrad, T. L., Gaertner, B. M., Eggum, N. D., & Zhou, N. (2010). Mothers' and children's positive emotion: Relations and trajectories across four years. *Social Development, 19*(4), 799–821.

Salmon, K., Evans, I. M., Moskowitz, S., Grouden, M., Parkes, F., & Miller, E. (2013). The components of young children's emotion knowledge: Which are enhanced by adult emotion talk? *Social Development, 22*(1), 94–110.

Sanson, A., Pedlow, R., Cann, W., Prior, M., & Oberklaid, F. (1996). Shyness ratings: Stability and correlates in early childhood. *International Journal of Behavioral Development, 19*(4), 705–724.

Santucci, A. K., Silk, J. S., Shaw, D. S., Gentzler, A., Fox, N. A., & Kovacs, M. (2008). Vagal tone and temperament as predictors of emotion regulation strategies in young children. *Developmental Psychobiology, 50,* 205–216.

Sarmento-Henrique, R., Quintanilla, L., Lucas-Molina, B., Recio, P., & Giménez-Dasí, M. (2020). The longitudinal interplay of emotion understanding, theory of mind, and language in the preschool years. *International Journal of Behavioral Development, 14*(3), 236–245.

Sawada, T. (1997). Development of children's understanding of emotional dissemblance in another person. *Japanese Journal of Educational Psychology, 45,* 50–59.

Schapira, R., & Aram, D. (2020). Shared book reading at home and preschoolers' socio-emotional competence. *Early Education and Development, 31*(6), 819–837.

Schmidt, E., & Pyers, J. (2011). Children's understanding of the link between sensory perception and knowledge. *Proceedings of the Annual Meeting of the Cognitive Science Society,* 33(33), 3016–3021.

Schmidt, L. A., & Poole, K. L. (2019). On the bifurcation of temperamental shyness: Development, adaptation, and neoteny. *New Ideas in Psychology, 53,* 13–21.

Schmitz, S., Fulker, D. W., Plomin, R., Zahn-Waxler, C., Emde, R. N., & DeFries, J. C. (1999). Temperament and problem behaviour during early childhood. *International Journal of Behavioral Development, 23*(2), 333–355.

Schneider, M., & Robin, A. L. (1978). *Manual for the Turtle Technique.* Unpublished manual, Department of Psychology, State University of New York at Stony Brook.

Schonert-Reichl, K. A., Kitil, M. J., & Hanson-Peterson, J. (2017). *To reach the students, teach the teachers: A national scan of teacher preparation and social and emotional learning.* A report prepared for the Collaborative for Academic, Social, and Emotional Learning (CASEL). University of British Columbia.

Schoppmann, J., Schneider, S., & Seehagen, S. (2021). Can you teach me not to be angry?: Relations between temperament and the emotion regulation strategy distraction in 2-year-olds. *Child Development.* [Epub ahead of print]

Schuberth, D. A., Zheng, Y., Pasalich, D. S., McMahon, R. J., Kamboukos, D., Dawson-McClure, S., & Brotman, L. M. (2019). The role of emotion understanding in the development of aggression and callous-unemotional features across early childhood. *Journal of Abnormal Child Psychology, 47*(4), 619–631.

Schultz, D., & Izard, C. E. (1998). *Assessment of Children's Emotion Skills (ACES).* University of Delaware.

Schultz, D., Izard, C. E., & Ackerman, B. P. (2000). Children's anger attribution bias: Relations to family environment and social adjustment. *Social Development, 9,* 284–301.

Schultz, D., Izard, C. E., Ackerman, B. P., & Youngstrom, E. A. (2001). Emotion knowledge in economically disadvantaged children: Self-regulatory antecedents and relations to social difficulties and withdrawal. *Development and Psychopathology, 13,* 53–67.

Schultz, D., Izard, C. E., Stapleton, L. M., Buckingham-Howes, S., & Bear, G. A. (2009). Children's social status as a function of emotionality and attention control. *Journal of Applied Developmental Psychology, 30*(2), 169–181.

Schutz, P. A., Aultman, L. P., & Williams-Johnson, M. R. (2009). Educational psychology perspectives on teachers' emotions. In P. A. Schutz, & M. Zembylas (Eds.), *Advances in teacher emotion research: The impact on teachers' lives* (pp. 195- 212). Springer.

Scott-Little, C., Kagan, S. L., & Frelow, V. S. (2006). Conceptualization of readiness and the content of early learning standards: The intersection of policy and research? *Early Childhood Research Quarterly, 21,* 153–173.

Sedgwick, D. A. (2015). *To work together or not?: Examining public-public program collaboration between Head Start and the Virginia Preschool Initiative.* Virginia Polytechnic Institute and State University.

Séguin, D. G., & MacDonald, B. (2018). The role of emotion regulation and temperament in the prediction of the quality of social relationships in early childhood. *Early Child Development and Care, 188*(8), 1147–1163.

Seidenfeld, A. M., Johnson, S. R., Cavadel, E. W., & Izard, C. E. (2014). Theory of mind predicts emotion knowledge development in head start children. *Early Education and Development, 25*(7), 933–948.

Serrat Sellabona, E., Amadó Codony, A., Rostán Sánchez, C., Caparrós Caparrós, B., & Sidera Caballero, F. (2020). Identifying emotional expressions: Children's reasoning about pretend emotions of sadness and anger. *Frontiers in Psychology, 11,* 602385.

Sesame Workshop. (2013). Little children, big challenges educator guide. Retrieved from *www.cfchildren.org/resources/sesame-street-little-children-big-challenges.*

Sette, S., Baldwin, D., Zava, F., Baumgartner, E., & Coplan, R. J. (2019). Shame on me?: Shyness, social experiences at preschool, and young children's self-conscious emotions. *Early Childhood Research Quarterly, 47,* 229–238.

Sette, S., Bassett, H. H., Baumgardner, E., & Denham, S. A. (2015). Structure and validity of affect knowledge test in a sample of Italian preschoolers. *Journal of Genetic Psychology, 176,* 330–347.

Sette, S., Baumgartner, E., Laghi, F., & Coplan, R. J. (2016). The role of emotion knowledge in the links between shyness and children's socio-emotional functioning at preschool. *British Journal of Developmental Psychology, 34,* 471–488.

Sette, S., Baumgartner, E., & Schneider, B. H. (2014). Shyness, child–teacher relationships, and socio-emotional adjustment in a sample of Italian preschool-aged children. *Infant and Child Development, 23*(3), 323–332.

Sette, S., Colasante, T., Zava, F., Baumgartner, E., & Malti, T. (2018). Preschoolers' anticipation of sadness for excluded peers, sympathy, and prosocial behavior. *Journal of Genetic Psychology, 179*(5), 286–296.

Sette, S., Zava, F., Baumgartner, E., Baiocco, R., & Coplan, R. (2017). Shyness, unsociability, and socio-emotional functioning at preschool: The protective role of peer acceptance. *Journal of Child and Family Studies, 26,* 1196–1205.

Shackman, J. E., Shackman, A. J., & Pollak, S. D. (2007). Physical abuse amplifies attention to threat and increases anxiety in children. *Emotion, 7*(4), 838–852.

Shafer, A. E., Wanless, S. B., & Briggs, J. O. (2022). Toddler teachers' responses to tantrums and relations to successful resolutions. *Infant and Child Development,* e2304.

Shaffer, A., Suveg, C., Thomassin, K., & Bradbury, L. L. (2012). Emotion socialization in the context of family risks: Links to child emotion regulation. *Journal of Child and Family Studies, 21*(6), 917–924.

Shala, M. (2013). The impact of preschool social-emotional development on academic success of elementary school students. *Psychology, 4*(11), 787–791.

Shamay-Tsoory, S. G. (2011). The neural bases for empathy. *The Neuroscientist, 17*(1), 18–24.

Shatz, M. (1994). *A toddler's life: Becoming a person.* Oxford University Press.

Shavelson, R. J., Young, D. B., Ayala, C. C., Brandon, P. R., Furtak, E. M., Ruiz-Primo, M. A., . . . Yin, Y. (2008). On the impact of curriculum-embedded formative assessment on learning: A collaboration between curriculum and assessment developers. *Applied Measurement in Education, 21*(4), 295–314.

Shaw, D. S., Schonberg, M., Sherrill, J., Huffman, D., Lukon, J., Obrosky, D., & Kovacs, M. (2006). Responsivity to offspring's expression of emotion among childhood-onset depressed mothers. *Journal of Clinical Child and Adolescent Psychology, 35*(4), 490–503.

Shewark, E. A., & Blandon, A. Y. (2015). Mothers' and fathers' emotion socialization and children's emotion regulation: A within-family model. *Social Development, 24*(2), 266–284.

Shewark, E. A., Zinsser, K. M., & Denham, S. A. (2018). Teachers' perspectives on the consequences of managing classroom climate. *Child and Youth Care Forum, 47*(6), 787–802).

Shields, A., & Cicchetti, D. (1997). Emotion regulation among school-age children: the development and validation of a new criterion Q-sort scale. *Developmental Psychology, 33*(6), 906–916.

Shields, A. M., Cicchetti, D., & Ryan, R. M. (1994). The development of emotional and behavioral self-regulation and social competence among maltreated school age children. *Development and Psychopathology, 6*, 57–75.

Shields, A., Dickstein, S., Seifer, R., Giusti, L., Dodge Magee, K., & Spritz, B. (2001). Emotional competence and early school adjustment: A study of preschoolers at risk. *Early Education and Development, 12*(1), 73–96.

Shin, N., Krzysik, L., & Vaughn, B. E. (2014). Emotion expressiveness and knowledge in preschool-age children: Age-related changes. *Child Studies in Asia-Pacific Contexts, 4*(1), 1–12.

Shin, N., Vaughn, B. E., Akers, V., Kim, M., Stevens, S., Krzysik, L., . . . Korth, B. (2011). Are happy children socially successful?: Testing a central premise of positive psychology in a sample of preschool children. *Journal of Positive Psychology, 6*(5), 355–367.

Shiner, R., & Caspi, A. (2003). Personality differences in childhood and adolescence: Measurement, development, and consequences. *Journal of Child Psychology and Psychiatry, 44*(1), 2–32.

Shipman, K. L., Schneider, R., Fitzgerald, M. M., Sims, C., Swisher, L., & Edwards, A. (2007). Maternal emotion socialization in maltreating and non-maltreating families: Implications for children's emotion regulation. *Social Development, 16*(2), 268–285.

Shonkoff, J. P., Garner, A. S., Siegel, B. S., Dobbins, M. I., Earls, M. F., McGuinn, L., . . . Committee on Early Childhood, Adoption, and Dependent Care. (2012). The lifelong effects of early childhood adversity and toxic stress. *Pediatrics, 129*(1), e232–e246.

Shure, M. B. (1993). I can problem solve (ICPS): Interpersonal cognitive problem-solving for young children. *Early Childhood Development and Care, 96*, 49–64.

Siegler, R. S., & Jenkins, E. (1989). *How children discover new strategies*. Erlbaum.

Sigman, M. D., Kasari, C., Kwon, J. H., & Yirmiya, N. (1992). Responses to the negative emotions of others by autistic, mentally retarded, and normal children. *Child Development, 63*, 796–807.

Silk, J. S., Shaw, D. S., Forbes, E. E., Lane, T. L., & Kovacs, M. (2006). Maternal depression and child internalizing: The moderating role of child emotion regulation. *Journal of Clinical Child and Adolescent Psychology, 35*(1), 116–126.

Silkenbeumer, J. R., Schiller, E. M., & Kärtner, J. (2018). Co-and self-regulation of emotions in the preschool setting. *Early Childhood Research Quarterly, 44*, 72–81.

Silvers, J. A., Insel, C., Powers, A., Franz, P., Helion, C., Martin, R. E., . . . Ochsner, K. N. (2017). vlPFC–vmPFC–amygdala interactions underlie age-related differences in cognitive regulation of emotion. *Cerebral Cortex, 27*(7), 3502–3514.

Singh, A. L., & Waldman, I. D. (2010). The etiology of associations between negative emotionality and childhood externalizing disorders. *Journal of Abnormal Psychology, 119*(2), 376–388.

Sivaratnam, C. S., Newman, L. K., Tonge, B. J., & Rinehart, N. J. (2015). Attachment and emotion processing in children with autism spectrum disorders: Neurobiological, neuroendocrine, and neurocognitive considerations. *Review Journal of Autism and Developmental Disorders, 2*(2), 222–242.

Sklad, M., Diekstra, R., Ritter, M. D., Ben, J., & Gravesteijn, C. (2012). Effectiveness of school-based universal social, emotional, and behavioral programs: Do they enhance students' development in the area of skill, behavior, and adjustment? *Psychology in the Schools, 49*, 892–909.

Skogan, A. H., Egeland, J., Zeiner, P., Øvergaard, K. R., Oerbeck, B., Reichborn-Kjennerud, T., & Aase, H. (2016). Factor structure of the Behavior Rating Inventory of Executive Functions (BRIEF-P) at age three years. *Child Neuropsychology, 22*(4), 472–492.

Smiley, P., & Huttenlocher, J. (1989). Young children's acquisitions of emotion concepts. In P. Harris & C. Saarni (Eds.), *Children's understanding of emotion* (pp. 27–79). Cambridge University Press.

Smith, C. E., Chen, D., & Harris, P. L. (2010). When the happy victimizer says sorry: Children's understanding of apology and emotion. *British Journal of Developmental Psychology, 28*(4), 727–746.

Smith, J. P., Glass, D. J., & Fireman, G. (2015). The understanding and experience of mixed emotions in 3–5-year-old children. *Journal of Genetic Psychology, 176(2)*, 65–81.

Smith, M., & Walden, T. (1998). Developmental trends in emotion understanding among a diverse sample of African-American preschool children. *Journal of Applied Developmental Psychology, 19*(2), 177–197.

Smith, M., & Walden, T. (1999). Understanding feelings and coping with emotional situations: A comparison of maltreated and nonmaltreated preschoolers. *Social Development, 8(1)*, 93–116.

Snow, M. E., Hertzig, M. E., & Shapiro, T. (1987). Expression of emotion in young autistic children. *Journal of the American Academy of Child and Adolescent Psychiatry, 26*, 836–838.

Somerwil, T., Klieve, H., & Exley, B. (2020). Preschool educators' readiness to promote children's emotional competence. *Asia-Pacific Journal of Research in Early Childhood Education, 14*(2), 135–158.

Son, S. H. C., & Chang, Y. E. (2018). Childcare experiences and early school outcomes: The mediating role of executive functions and emotionality. *Infant and Child Development, 27*(4), e2087.

Song, J. H., Colasante, T., & Malti, T. (2018). Helping yourself helps others: Linking children's emotion regulation to prosocial behavior through sympathy and trust. *Emotion, 18*(4), 518–527.

Song, Q., Smiley, P. A., & Doan, S. N. (2022). The moderating effect of facial emotion recognition in maternal emotion socialization and child socioemotional adjustment. *Social Development.*

Sosna, T., & Mastergeorge, A. (2005). *Compendium of screening tools for early childhood social-emotional development.* Sacramento, CA: California Institute for Mental Health.

Speidel, R., Wang, L., Cummings, E. M., & Valentino, K. (2020). Longitudinal pathways of family influence on child self-regulation: The roles of parenting, family expressiveness, and maternal sensitive guidance in the context of child maltreatment. *Developmental Psychology, 56*(3), 608–622.

Spere, K., & Evans, M. A. (2009). Shyness as a continuous dimension and emergent literacy in young children: Is there a relation? *Infant and Child Development, 18*(3), 216–237.

Spinrad, T. L., Losoya, S. H., Eisenberg, N., Fabes, R. A., Shepard, S. A., Cumberland, A., . . . Murphy, B. C. (1999). The relations of parental affect and encouragement to children's moral emotions and behaviour. *Journal of Moral Education, 28*(3), 323–337.

Spinrad, T. L., Stifter, C. A., Donelan-McCall, N., & Turner, L. (2004). Mothers' regulation strategies in response to toddlers' affect: Links to later emotion self-regulation. *Social Development, 13*, 40–55.

Spivak, A. L., & Farran, D. C. (2016). Predicting first graders' social competence from their preschool classroom interpersonal context. *Early Education and Development, 27*, 735–750.

Spritz, B. L., Sandberg, E. H., Maher, E., & Zajdel, R. T. (2010). Models of emotion skills and social competence in the Head Start classroom. *Early Education and Development, 21*(4), 495–516.

Sprung, M., Münch, H. M., Harris, P. L., Ebesutani, C., & Hofmann, S. G. (2015). Children's emotion understanding: A meta-analysis of training studies. *Developmental Review, 37*, 41–65.

Sroufe, L. A. (1996). *Emotional development.* Cambridge University Press.

Sroufe, L. A., & Fleeson, J. (1986). Attachment and the construction of relationships. In W. Hartup & Z. Rubin (Eds.), *Relationships and development* (pp. 51–72). Erlbaum.

Sroufe, L. A., Schork, E., Motti, F., Lawroski, N., & LaFreniere, P. (1984). The role of affect in social competence. In C. E. Izard, J. Kagan, & R. B. Zajonc (Eds.), *Emotions, cognition, and behavior* (pp. 289–319). Cambridge University Press.

Stanley, L. (2019). Is the preschool PATHS curriculum effective?: A review. *Journal of Evidence-Based Social Work, 16*(2), 130–143.

Stansbury, K., & Sigman, M. (1995). *Development of behavioral expressions of emotion regulation in normally developing and at-risk preschool-age children.* Unpublished manuscript.

Stearns, E., Banerjee, N., Mickelson, R., & Moller, S. (2014). Collective pedagogical teacher culture, teacher-student ethno-racial mismatch, and teacher job satisfaction. *Social Science Research, 45*, 56–72.

Steed, E. A., & Roach, A. T. (2017). Childcare providers' use of practices to promote young children's social–emotional competence. *Infants and Young Children, 30*(2), 162–171.

Steele, H., Steele, M., & Croft, C. (2008). Early attachment predicts emotion recognition at 6 and 11 years old. *Attachment and Human Development, 10*(4), 379–393.

Steele, H., Steele, M., Croft, C., & Fonagy, P. (1999). Infant–mother attachment at one year predicts children's understanding of mixed emotions at six years. *Social Development, 8(2)*, 161–178.

Ştefan, C. A. (2008). Short-term efficacy of a primary prevention program for the development of social-emotional competencies in preschool children. *Cognition, Brain, Behavior, 12*(3), 285–307.

Ştefan, C. A., & Avram, J. (2018). The multifaceted role of attachment during preschool: moderator of its indirect effect on empathy through emotion regulation. *Early Child Development and Care, 188*(1), 62–76.

Ştefan, C. A., & Avram, J. (2021). Attachment and externalizing/internalizing problems in preschoolers: Contributions of positive and negative empathic perspective-taking. *Merrill–Palmer Quarterly, 67*(2), 123–148.

Ştefan, C. A., Avram, J., & Miclea, M. (2017). Children's awareness concerning emotion regulation strategies: Effects of attachment status. *Social Development, 26*(4), 694–708.

Ştefan, C. A., & Miclea, M. (2010). A preliminary efficiency study of a multifocused prevention program for children with deficient emotional and social competencies. *Procedia-Social and Behavioral Sciences, 5*, 127–139.

Ştefan, C. A., & Miclea, M. (2012). Classroom effects of a hybrid universal and indicated prevention program for preschool children: A comparative analysis based on social and emotional competence screening. *Early Education and Development, 23*(3), 393–426.

Ştefan, C. A., & Miclea, M. (2013). Effects of a multifocused prevention program on preschool children's competencies and behavior problems. *Psychology in the Schools, 50*(4), 382–402.

Ştefan, C. A., & Negrean, D. (2022). Parent-and teacher-rated emotion regulation strategies in relation to preschoolers' attachment representations: A longitudinal perspective. *Social Development. 31*(1), 180–195.

Stein, N., & Jewett, J. L. (1986). A conceptual analysis of the meaning of negative emotions: Implications for a theory of development. In C. E. Izard & P. Read (Eds.), *Measurement of emotions in children* (Vol. 2, pp. 238–268). Cambridge University Press.

Stein, N., & Levine, L. (1989). The causal organization of emotional knowledge: A developmental study. *Cognition and Emotion, 3*, 343–378.

Stein, N., & Levine, L. (1990). Making sense out of emotion: The representation and use of goal-structured knowledge. In N. Stein, T. Leventhal, & T. Trabasso (Eds.), *Psychological and biological approaches to emotion* (pp. 45–74). Erlbaum.

Stein, N., & Trabasso, T. (1989). Children's understanding of changing emotional states. In P. Harris & C. Saarni (Eds.), *Children's understanding of emotion* (pp. 50–80). Cambridge University Press.

Stein, N., Trabasso, T., & Liwag, M. (1993). The representation and organization of emotional experience: Unfolding the emotion episode. In M. Lewis & J.

Haviland (Eds.), *Handbook of emotions* (pp. 279–300). Guilford Press.

Stern, J. A., & Cassidy, J. (2018). Empathy from infancy to adolescence: An attachment perspective on the development of individual differences. *Developmental Review, 47*, 1–22.

Stifter, C. A., Dollar, J. M., & Cipriano, E. A. (2011). Temperament and emotion regulation: The role of autonomic nervous system reactivity. *Developmental Psychobiology, 53*(3), 266–279.

Stifter, C., & Fox, N. (1987). Preschoolers' ability to identify and label emotions. *Journal of Nonverbal Behavior, 10*, 255–266.

Stipek, D. J., Gralinski, J. H., & Kopp, C. B. (1990). Self-concept development in the toddler years. *Developmental Psychology, 26*(6), 972–977.

Stipek, D., Recchia, S., & McClintic, S. (1992). Self-evaluation in young children. *Monographs of the Society for Research in Child Development, 57*(1, Serial No. 226), 1–84.

Straker, G., & Jacobson, R. S. (1981). Aggression, emotional maladjustment, and empathy in the abused child. *Developmental Psychology, 17*, 762–765.

Strand, P. S., Barbosa-Leiker, C., Arellano Piedra, M., & Downs, A. (2015). Exploring the bidirectionality of emotion understanding and classroom behavior with Spanish- and English-speaking preschoolers attending Head Start. *Social Development, 24*(3), 579–600.

Strand, P. S., Downs, A., & Barbosa-Leiker, C. (2016). Does facial expression recognition provide a toehold for the development of emotion understanding? *Developmental Psychology, 52(8)*, 1182–1191.

Strandberg-Sawyer, K., Denham, S. A., DeMulder, E., Blair, K. A., Auerbach-Major, S. T., & Levitas, J. (2002). The contribution of older siblings' reactions to emotions to preschoolers' emotional and social competence. *Marriage and Family Review, 34*, 183–212.

Strayer, J. (1980). A naturalistic study of empathic behaviors and their relation to affective states and perspective-taking skills in preschool children. *Child Development, 51*, 815–822.

Strayer, J. (1986). Children's attributions regarding the situational determinants of emotion in self and others. *Developmental Psychology, 22*, 649–654.

Strayer, J. (1993). Children's concordant emotions and cognitions in response to observed emotions. *Child Development, 64*, 188–210.

Strayer, J., & Roberts, W. (2004). Empathy and observed anger and aggression in five-year-olds. *Social Development, 13*(1), 1–13.

Strayer, J., & Schroeder, M. (1989). Children's helping strategies: Influences of emotion, empathy, and age. In N. Eisenberg (Ed.), *New Directions for Child Development: No. 44. Empathy and related emotional responses* (pp. 85–105). Jossey-Bass.

Streit, C., Carlo, G., Ispa, J. M., & Palermo, F. (2017). Negative emotionality and discipline as long-term predictors of behavioral outcomes in African American and European American children. *Developmental Psychology, 53*(6), 1013–1026.

Stremmel, A. J., Benson, M. J., & Powell, D. R. (1993). Communication, satisfaction, and emotional exhaustion among child care center staff: Directors, teachers, and assistant teachers. *Early Childhood Research Quarterly, 8*, 221–233.

Streubel, B., Gunzenhauser, C., Grosse, G., & Saalbach, H. (2020). Emotion-specific vocabulary and its contribution to emotion understanding in 4- to 9-year-old children. *Journal of Experimental Child Psychology, 193*, 104790.

Stuewig, J., Tangney, J. P., Kendall, S., Folk, J. B., Meyer, C. R., & Dearing, R. L. (2015). Children's proneness to shame and guilt predict risky and illegal behaviors in young adulthood. *Child Psychiatry and Human Development, 46*(2), 217–227.

Sudit, E., Luby, J., & Gilbert, K. (2021). Sad, sadder, saddest: Recognition of sad and happy emotional intensity, adverse childhood experiences and depressive symptoms in preschoolers. *Child Psychiatry and Human Development*, 1–10.

Suh, B. L., & Kang, M. J. (2020). Maternal reactions to preschoolers' negative emotions and aggression: Gender difference in mediation of emotion regulation. *Journal of Child and Family Studies, 29*(1), 144–154.

Sullivan, M. W., Carmody, D. P., & Lewis, M. (2010). How neglect and punitiveness influence emotion knowledge. *Child Psychiatry and Human Development, 41*(3), 285–298.

Supplee, L. H., Skuban, E. M., Trentacosta, C. J., Shaw, D. S., & Stoltz, E. (2011). Preschool boys' development of emotional self-regulation strategies in a sample at risk for behavior problems. *Journal of Genetic Psychology, 172*(2), 95–120.

Swartz, R. A., & McElwain, N. L. (2012). Preservice teachers' emotion-related regulation and cognition: Associations with teachers' responses to children's emotions in early childhood classrooms. *Early Education and Development, 23*, 202–226.

Székely, E., Tiemeier, H., Arends, L. R., Jaddoe, V. W., Hofman, A., Verhulst, F. C., & Herba, C. M. (2011). Recognition of facial expressions of emotions by 3-years-olds. *Emotion, 11*, 425–435.

Székely, E., Tiemeier, H., Jaddoe, V. W., Hofman, A., Verhulst, F. C., & Herba, C. M. (2014). Associations of internalizing and externalizing problems with facial expression recognition in preschoolers: The generation R study. *Social Development, 23*(3), 611–630.

Takahashi, Y., Kusanagi, E., & Hoshi, N. (1998). Masking of negative emotional expression in 3-year-olds. *Research and Clinical Center for Child Development, 20*, 43–48.

Talley, K., Zhu, D., & Dunsmore, J. (2021, April). *Mothers' and children's coaching and dismissing of positive emotions from early to middle childhood.* Poster presented at the biennial meetings of the Society for Research in Child Development.

Talwar, V., & Crossman, A. (2011). From little white lies to filthy liars: The evolution of honesty and deception in young children. *Advances in Child Development and Behavior, 40*, 139–179.

Talwar, V., & Lee, K. (2002). Development of lying to conceal a transgression: Children's control of expressive behaviour during verbal deception. *International Journal of Behavioral Development, 26*(5), 436–444.

Tan, P. Z., Armstrong, L. M., & Cole, P. M. (2013). Relations between temperament and anger regulation over early childhood. *Social Development, 22*(4), 755–772.

Tan, L., Volling, B. L., Gonzalez, R., LaBounty, J., & Rosenberg, L. (2022). Growth in emotion understanding across early childhood: A cohort-sequential model of firstborn children across the transition to siblinghood. *Child Development, 93*(3), e299–e214.

Tang, Y., Harris, P. L., Pons, F., Zou, H., Zhang, W., & Xu, Q. (2018). The understanding of emotion among young Chinese children. *International Journal of Behavioral Development, 42*(5), 512–517.

Tangney, J. P. (1990). Assessing individual differences in proneness to shame and guilt: Development of the self-conscious affect and attribution inventory. *Journal of Personality and Social Psychology, 59*, 102–111.

Tangney, J. P. (1992). Situational determinants of shame and guilt in young adulthood. *Personality and Social Psychology Bulletin, 18*, 199–206.

Tangney, J. P. (1995). Shame and guilt in interpersonal relationships. In J. P. Tangney & K. W. Fischer (Eds.), *Self-conscious emotions: The psychology of shame, guilt, embarrassment, and pride* (pp. 114–139). Guilford Press.

Tangney, J. P. (1998). How does guilt differ from shame? In J. A. Bybee (Ed.), *Guilt and children* (pp. 1–17). Academic Press.

Tangney, J. P., & Tracy, J. L. (2012). Self-conscious emotions. In M. R. Leary & J. P. Tangney (Eds.), *Handbook of self and identity* (p. 446–478). Guilford Press.

Tarullo, A. R., Mliner, S., & Gunnar, M. R. (2011). Inhibition and exuberance in preschool classrooms: Associations with peer social experiences and changes in cortisol across the preschool year. *Developmental Psychology, 47*(5), 1374–1388.

Taylor, R. D., Oberle, E., Durlak, J. A., & Weissberg, R. P. (2017). Promoting positive youth development through school-based social and emotional learning interventions: A meta-analysis of follow-up effects. *Child Development, 88*, 1156–1171.

Taylor, Z. E., Eisenberg, N., & Spinrad, T. L. (2015). Respiratory sinus arrhythmia, effortful control, and parenting as predictors of children's sympathy across early childhood. *Developmental Psychology, 51*(1), 17–25.

Taylor, Z. E., Eisenberg, N., Spinrad, T. L., Eggum, N. D., & Sulik, M. J. (2013). The relations of ego-resiliency and emotion socialization to the development of empathy and prosocial behavior across early childhood. Emotion, 13(5), 822–831.

Taylor, Z. E., Eisenberg, N., Van Schyndel, S. K., Eggum-Wilkens, N. D., & Spinrad, T. L. (2014). Children's negative emotions and ego-resiliency: Longitudinal relations with social competence. *Emotion, 14(2)*, 397–406.

Teglasi, H., Schussler, L., Gifford, K., Annotti, L. A., Sanders C., & Liu, H. (2015). Child Behavior Questionnaire—Short Form for Teachers: Informant correspondences and divergences. *Assessment, 22(6)*, 730–748.

Tenenbaum, H. R., Visscher, P., Pons, F., & Harris, P. L. (2004). Emotional understanding in Quechua children from an agro-pastoralist village. *International Journal of Behavioral Development, 28*(5), 471–478.

Thompson, R. A. (1990). Emotion and self-regulation. In R. A. Thompson (Ed.), *Nebraska Symposium on Motivation: Vol. 36. Socioemotional development* (pp. 367–468). University of Nebraska Press.

Thompson, R. A. (1993). Socioemotional development: Enduring issues and new challenges. *Developmental Review, 13*, 372–402.

Thompson, R. A. (1994). Emotion regulation: A theme in search of definition. In N. A. Fox (Ed.), The development of emotion regulation: Biological and behavioral considerations. *Monographs of the Society for Research in Child Development, 59*(2–3, Serial No. 240), 25–52.

Thompson, R. A. (2011). Emotion and emotion regulation: Two sides of the developing coin. *Emotion Review*, 3(1), 53–61.

Thompson, R. A. (2014). Socialization of emotion and emotion regulation in the family. In J. J. Gross (Ed.), *Handbook of emotion regulation* (pp. 173–186). Guilford Press.

Thompson, R. A. (2019). Emotion dysregulation: A theme in search of definition. *Development and Psychopathology, 31*(3), 805–815.

Thompson, R. A., & Calkins, S. (1996). The double-edged sword: Emotional regulation for children at risk. *Development and Psychopathology, 8*, 163–182.

Thompson, R. A., Lewis, M. D., & Calkins, S. D. (2008). Reassessing emotion regulation. *Child Development Perspectives, 2*(3), 124–131.

Thompson, S. F., Zalewski, M., Kiff, C. J., Moran, L., Cortes, R., & Lengua, L. J. (2020). An empirical test of the model of socialization of emotion: Maternal and child contributors to preschoolers' emotion knowledge and adjustment. *Developmental Psychology, 56*(3), 418–430.

Thomsen, T., & Lessing, N. (2020). Children's emotion regulation repertoire and problem behavior: A latent cross-lagged panel study. *Journal of Applied Developmental Psychology, 71*, 101198.

Thomson, N. D., Centifanti, L., & Lemerise, E. A. (2017). Emotion regulation and conduct disorder: The role of callous-unemotional traits. In C. A. Essau, S. LeBlanc, & T. H. Ollendick (Eds.), *Emotion regulation and psychopathology in children and adolescents* (pp. 129–153). Oxford University Press.

Tomkins, S. (1962). *Affect, imagery, and consciousness: Vol. 1. The positive affects*. Springer.

Tomkins, S. (1963). *Affect, imagery, and consciousness: Vol. 2. The negative affects*. Springer.

Tomkins, S. (1991). *Affect, imagery, and consciousness: Vol. 3. The negative affects: Anger and fear*. Springer.

Tompkins, V., Benigno, J. P., Kiger Lee, B., & Wright, B. M. (2018). The relation between parents' mental state talk and children's social understanding: A meta-analysis. *Social Development, 27*(2), 223–246.

Tone, E. B., & Tully, E. C. (2014). Empathy as a "risky strength": A multilevel examination of empathy and risk for internalizing disorders. *Development and Psychopathology, 26*(4. Pt. 2), 1547–1565.

Torrente, C., Alimchandani, A., & Aber, J. L. (2015). International perspectives on SEL. In J. A. Durlak, C. E. Domitrovich, R. W. Weissberg, & T. P. Gullotta (Eds.), *Handbook of social and emotional learning* (pp. 566–588). Guilford Press.

Torres, M. M., Domitrovich, C. E., & Bierman, K. L. (2015). Preschool interpersonal relationships predict kindergarten achievement: Mediated by gains in emotion knowledge. *Journal of Applied Developmental Psychology, 39*, 44–52.

Toth, S. L., Manly, J., & Cicchetti, D. (1992). Child maltreatment and vulnerability to depression. *Development and Psychopathology, 4*, 97–112.

Tracy, J. L., Robins, R. W., & Lagattuta, K. H. (2005). Can children recognize pride? *Emotion, 5*(3), 251–257.

Trentacosta, C. J., & Fine, S. E. (2010). Emotion knowledge, social competence, and behavior problems in childhood and adolescence: A meta-analytic review. *Social Development, 19*, 1–29.

Trentacosta, C. J., & Izard, C. E. (2007). Kindergarten children's emotion competence as a predictor of their academic competence in first grade. *Emotion, 7*(1), 77–88.

Trentacosta, C. J., Izard, C. E., Mostow, A. J., & Fine, S. E. (2006). Children's emotional competence and attentional competence in early elementary school. *School Psychology Quarterly, 21*(2), 148–160.

Trommsdorff, G. (2013). *Person-context relations as developmental conditions for empathy and prosocial action: A cross-cultural analysis* (pp. 125–158). Psychology Press.

Trommsdorff, G., & Cole, P. M. (2011). Emotion, self-regulation, and social behavior in cultural context. In X. Chen & K. H. Rubin (Eds.), *Socioemotional development in cultural context* (pp. 131–163). Guilford Press.

Trommsdorff G., & Friedlmeier, W. (2010) Preschool girls distress and mothers' sensitivity in Japan and Germany. *European Journal of Developmental Psychology, 7*, 350–370.

Trommsdorff, G., Friedlmeier, W., & Mayer, B. (2007). Sympathy, distress, and prosocial behavior of preschool children in four cultures. *International Journal of Behavioral Development, 31*(3), 284–293.

Trommsdorff, G., & Heikamp, T. (2013). Socialization of emotions and emotion regulation in cultural context. In S. Barnow & N. Balkir (Eds.), *Cultural variations in psychopathology* (pp. 67– 92). Hogrefe.

Trommsdorff, G., & Rothbaum, F. (2008). *Development of emotion regulation in cultural context.* In M. Vandekerckhove, C. von Scheve, S. Ismer, S. Jung, & S. Kronast (Eds.), *Regulating emotions: Culture, social necessity, and biological inheritance* (pp.85–120). Blackwell.

Tronick, E. (1989). Emotions and emotional communication in infants. *American Psychologist, 44*, 112–119.

Tsujimoto, S. (2008). The prefrontal cortex: Functional neural development during early childhood. *The Neuroscientist, 14*(4), 345–358.

Tully, E. C., & Donohue, M. R. (2017). Empathic responses to mother's emotions predict internalizing problems in children of depressed mothers. *Child Psychiatry and Human Development, 48*(1), 94–106.

Türkmen, S., & Ulutaş, İ. (2018). How do preschool teachers perceive the emotional intelligence? Teaching practices and emotional intelligence in early childhood. *Educational Sciences Research in the Globalizing World, 177*, 170–183.

Ugarte, E., Miller, J. G., Weissman, D. G., & Hastings, P. D. (2021). Vagal flexibility to negative emotions moderates the relations between environmental risk and adjustment problems in childhood. *Development and Psychopathology*, 1–18. [Epub ahead of print]

Ulloa, M., Evans, I. M., & Jones, L. C. (2016). The effects of emotional awareness training on teachers' ability to manage the emotions of preschool children: An experimental study. *Escritos de psicología, 9*(1), 1–14.

Ulrich, F., & Petermann, F. (2017). Parental emotion dysregulation as a risk factor for child development. *Kindheit und Entwicklung, 26*(3), 133–146.

Ursache, A., Dawson-McClure, S., Siegel, J., & Brotman, L. M. (2019). Predicting early emotion knowledge development among children of colour living in historically disinvested neighbourhoods: Consideration of child pre-academic abilities, self-regulation, peer relations and parental education. *Cognition and Emotion, 33*(8), 1562–1576.

Ursache, A., Kiely Gouley, K., Dawson-McClure, S., Barajas-Gonzalez, R. G., Calzada, E. J., Goldfeld, K. S., & Brotman, L. M. (2020). Early emotion knowledge and later academic achievement among children of color in historically disinvested neighborhoods. *Child Development, 91*(6), e1249–e1266.

Vacas, J., Antolí, A., Sánchez-Raya, A., & Pérez-Dueñas, C. (2022). Eye tracking methodology for studying emotional competence in children with autism spectrum disorder (ASD) and specific language impairment (SLI): A comparative research review. *Review Journal of Autism and Developmental Disorders, 9*, 351–365.

Vaish, A. (2018). The prosocial functions of early social emotions: The case of guilt. *Current Opinion in Psychology, 20*, 25–29.

Vaish, A. (2019). Something old, something new: Leveraging what we know to optimize new directions in emotion development research. *Developmental Psychology, 55*(9), 1998–2001.

Vaish, A., Carpenter, M., & Tomasello, M. (2009). Sympathy through affective perspective taking and its relation to prosocial behavior in toddlers. *Developmental Psychology, 45*(2), 534–543.

Vaish, A., Carpenter, M., & Tomasello, M. (2011). Young children's responses to guilt displays. *Developmental Psychology, 47*(5), 1248–1262.

Vaish, A., Carpenter, M., & Tomasello, M. (2016). The early emergence of guilt-motivated prosocial behavior. *Child Development, 87*(6), 1772–1782.

Vaish, A., & Hepach, R. (2020). The development of prosocial emotions. *Emotion Review, 12*(4), 259–273.

Valentino, K., Cummings, E. M., Borkowski, J., Hibel, L. C., Lefever, J., & Lawson, M. (2019). Efficacy of a reminiscing and emotion training intervention on maltreating families with preschool-aged children. *Developmental Psychology, 55(11)*, 2365–2378.

Valentino, K., Hibel, L. C., Speidel, R., Fondren, K., & Ugarte, E. (2020). Longitudinal effects of maltreatment, intimate partner violence, and Reminiscing and Emotion Training on children's diurnal cortisol regulation. *Development and Psychopathology*, 33(3), 868–884.

Valiente, C., Doane, L. D., Clifford, S., Grimm, K. J., & Lemery-Chalfant, K. (2021). School readiness and achievement in early elementary school: Moderation by students' temperament. *Journal of Applied Developmental Psychology*, *74*, 101265.

Valiente, C., Lemery-Chalfant, K., & Swanson, J. (2010). Prediction of kindergartners' academic achievement from their effortful control and emotionality: Evidence for direct and moderated relations. *Journal of Educational Psychology*, *102*, 550–560.

Van Bergen, P., & Salmon, K. (2010). The association between parent–child reminiscing and children's emotion knowledge. *New Zealand Journal of Psychology (Online)*, *39*(1), 51–56.

Van der Kleij, F. M., Vermeulen, J. A., Schildkamp, K., & Eggen, T. J. (2015). Integrating data-based decision making, assessment for learning and diagnostic testing in formative assessment. *Assessment in Education: Principles, Policy and Practice*, *22*(3), 324–343.

van der Pol, L. D., Groeneveld, M. G., van Berkel, S. R., Endendijk, J. J., Hallers-Haalboom, E. T., Bakermans-Kranenburg, M. J., & Mesman, J. (2015). Fathers' and mothers' emotion talk with their girls and boys from toddlerhood to preschool age. *Emotion*, *15*(6), 854–864.

Vaughn, B. E., Contreras, J., & Seifer, R. (1993). Short-term longitudinal study of maternal ratings of temperament in samples of children with Down syndrome and children who are developing normally. *American Journal of Mental Retardation*, *98*, 607–618.

Vernon, H., & Teglasi, H. (2018). Indirect effects of temperament on social competence via emotion understanding. *Early Education and Development*, *29*(5), 655–674.

Vogel, A. C., Jackson, J. J., Barch, D. M., Tillman, R., & Luby, J. L. (2019). Excitability and irritability in preschoolers predicts later psychopathology: The importance of positive and negative emotion dysregulation. *Development and Psychopathology*, *31*(3), 1067–1083.

Volbrecht, M. M., Lemery-Chalfant, K., Aksan, N., Zahn-Waxler, C., & Goldsmith, H. H. (2007). Examining the familial link between positive affect and empathy development in the second year. *Journal of Genetic Psychology*, *168*(2), 105–130.

Voltmer, K., & von Salisch, M. (2017). Three meta-analyses of children's emotion knowledge and their school success. *Learning and Individual Differences*, *59*, 107–118.

Voltmer, K., & von Salisch, M. (2019). Native-born German and immigrant children's development of emotion knowledge: A latent growth curve analysis. *British Journal of Developmental Psychology*, *37*(1), 112–129.

Voltmer, K., & von Salisch, M. (2022). The feeling thinking talking intervention with teachers advances young children's emotion knowledge. *Social Development*, *31*(3), 846–861.

von Salisch, M., Denham, S. A., Benga, O., Chin, J-C., & Geangu, E., & Slough, R. (2022). Emotions and peer relationships. In C. Hart & P. K. Smith (Eds.), *Wiley/Blackwell Handbook of childhood social development* (3rd ed., pp. 631–650). Blackwell.

von Salisch, M., & Denham, S. A., & Koch, T. (2016). Emotion knowledge and attention problems in young children: A cross-lagged panel study on the direction of effects. *Journal of Abnormal Child Psychology*, *45*, 45–56.

von Salisch, M., Häenel, M., & Denham, S. A. (2015). Self-regulation, language skills, and emotion knowledge in young children from Northern Germany. *Early Education and Development*, *26*, 792–806.

von Salisch, M., Häenel, M., & Freund, P. A. (2013). Emotion understanding and cognitive abilities in young children. *Learning and Individual Differences*, *26*, 15–19.

von Salisch, M., & Janke, B. (2010). Development of emotional competence in the preschool age. *Praxis der Kinderpsychologie und Kinderpsychiatrie*, *59*, 509–512.

Waajid, B., Garner, P. W., & Owen, J. E. (2013). Infusing social emotional learning into the teacher education curriculum. *International Journal of Emotional Education*, *5*, 31–48.

Walle, E. A., & Campos, J. J. (2012). Interpersonal responding to discrete emotions: A functionalist approach to the development of affect specificity. *Emotion Review*, *4*(4), 413–422.

Walle, E. A., & Dahl, A. (2020). Definitions matter for studying emotional development. *Developmental Psychology*, *56*(4), 837–840.

Walter, J. L., & LaFreniere, P. J. (2000). A naturalistic study of affective expression, social competence, and sociometric status in preschoolers. *Early Education and Development*, *11*(1), 109–122.

Wang, J., & Barrett, K. C. (2015). Differences between American and Chinese preschoolers in emotional responses to resistance to temptation and mishap contexts. *Motivation and Emotion*, *39*(3), 420–433.

Wang, M., & Saudino, K. J. (2013). Genetic and environmental influences on individual differences in emotion regulation and its relation to working memory in toddlerhood. *Emotion*, *13*(6), 1055–1067.

Wang, Q. (2001). "Did you have fun?": American and Chinese mother–child conversations about shared emotional experiences. *Cognitive Development*, *16*(2), 693–715.

Wang, Q. (2003). Emotion situation knowledge in American and Chinese preschool children and adults. *Cognition and Emotion*, *17*(5), 725–746.

Wang, X., Liu, X., & Feng, T. (2021). The continuous impact of cognitive flexibility on the development of emotion understanding in children aged 4 and 5 years: A longitudinal study. *Journal of Experimental Child Psychology*, *203*, 105018.

Warren, H. K., & Stifter, C. A. (2008). Maternal emotion-related socialization and preschoolers' developing emotion self-awareness. *Social Development*, *17*(2), 239–258.

Waters, E., & Sroufe, L. A. (1983). Social competence as a developmental construct. *Developmental Review*, *3*, 79–97.

Waters, E., Wippman, J., & Sroufe, L. A. (1979). Two studies in construct validation: Attachment, positive affect, and competence in the peer group. *Child Development, 50*, 821–829.

Waters, S. F., & Thompson, R. A. (2014). Children's perceptions of the effectiveness of strategies for regulating anger and sadness. *International Journal of Behavioral Development, 38*(2), 174–181.

Waters, S. F., Virmani, E. A., Thompson, R. A., Meyer, S., Raikes, H. A., & Jochem, R. (2010). Emotion regulation and attachment: Unpacking two constructs and their association. *Journal of Psychopathology and Behavioral Assessment, 32*(1), 37–47.

Watson, D., & Clark, L. A., & Tellegen, A. (1988). Development and validation of brief measures of positive and negative affect: The PANAS Scales. *Journal of Personality and Social Psychology, 54*, 1063–1070.

Webster-Stratton, C., Reid, M. J., & Hammond, M. (2004). Treating children with early-onset conduct problems: Intervention outcomes for parent, child, and teacher training. *Journal of Clinical Child and Adolescent Psychology, 33*(1), 105–124.

Webster-Stratton, C., Reid, J. M., & Stoolmiller, M. (2008). Preventing conduct problems and improving school readiness: Evaluation of The Incredible Years teacher and child training programs in high-risk schools. *Journal of Child Psychology and Psychiatry, 49*(5), 471–488.

Weems, C. F., & Pina, A. A. (2010). The assessment of emotion regulation: Improving construct validity in research on psychopathology in youth—an introduction to the special section. *Journal of Psychopathology and Behavioral Assessment, 32*, 1–7.

Wei, M., Schaffer, P. A., Young, S. K., & Zakalik, R. A. (2005). Adult attachment, shame, depression, and loneliness: The mediation role of basic psychological needs satisfaction. *Journal of Counseling Psychology, 52*, 591–601.

Weimer, A. A., Sallquist, J., & Bolnick, R. R. (2012). Young children's emotion comprehension and theory of mind understanding. *Early Education and Development, 23*(3), 280–301.

Weinberger, N., & Bushnell, E. W. (1994). Young children's knowledge about their senses: Perceptions and misconceptions. *Child Study Journal, 24*, 209–235.

Wellman, H. M., & Banerjee, M. (1991). Mind and emotion: Children's understanding of the emotional consequences of beliefs and desires. *British Journal of Developmental Psychology, 9*, 191–214.

Wellman, H. M., & Woolley, J. D. (1990). From simple desires to ordinary beliefs: The early development of everyday psychology. *Cognition, 35*, 245–275.

Werner, E. E. (1989). High-risk children in young adulthood: A longitudinal study from birth to 32 years. *American Journal of Orthopsychiatry, 59*, 72–81.

Whissell, C. K., & Nicholson, H. (1991). Children's freely produced synonyms for seven key emotions. *Perceptual and Motor Skills, 72*, 1107–1111.

White, A., Moore, D. W., Fleer, M., & Anderson, A. (2017). A thematic and content analysis of instructional and rehearsal procedures of preschool social emotional learning programs. *Australasian Journal of Early Childhood, 42*(3), 82–91.

White, S. F., Briggs-Gowan, M. J., Voss, J. L., Petitclerc, A., McCarthy, K., Blair, R. J. R., & Wakschlag, L. S. (2016). Can the fear recognition deficits associated with callous-unemotional traits be identified in early childhood? *Journal of Clinical and Experimental Neuropsychology, 38(6)*, 672–684.

Whitesell, N. R. (1989, April). *A prototype approach to children's understanding of basic emotions.* Paper presented at the biennial meeting of the Society for Research in Child Development, Kansas City, MO.

Widen, S. C., & Russell, J. A. (2004). The relative power of an emotion's facial expression, label, and behavioral consequence to evoke preschoolers' knowledge of its cause. *Cognitive Development, 19*(1), 111–125.

Widen, S. C., & Russell, J. A. (2008). Children acquire emotion categories gradually. *Cognitive Development, 23*(2), 291–312.

Widen, S. C., & Russell, J. A. (2010a). Children's scripts for social emotions: Causes and consequences are more central than are facial expressions. *British Journal of Developmental Psychology, 28*(3), 565–581.

Widen, S. C., & Russell, J. A. (2010b). Descriptive and prescriptive definitions of emotion. *Emotion Review, 2*(4), 377–378.

Widen, S. C., & Russell, J. A. (2010c). Differentiation in preschooler's categories of emotion. *Emotion, 10*(5), 651–661.

Wiggers, M., & Van Lieshout, C. F. (1985). Development of recognition of emotions: Children's reliance on situational and facial expressive cues. *Developmental Psychology, 21*, 338–349.

Wilson, B. J., & Cantor, J. (1985). Developmental differences in empathy with a television protagonist's fear. *Journal of Experimental Psychology, 39*, 284–299.

Wilson, B. J., Dauterman, H. A., Frey, K. S., Rutter, T. M., Myers, J., Zhou, V., & Bisi, E. (2021). Effortful control moderates the relation between negative emotionality and socially appropriate behavior. *Journal of Experimental Child Psychology, 207*, 105119.

Wilson, S. R., Rack, J. J., Shi, X., & Norris, A. M. (2008). Comparing physically abusive, neglectful, and non-maltreating parents during interactions with their children: A meta-analysis of observational studies. *Child Abuse and Neglect, 32*, 897–911.

Wintre, M., Polivy, J., & Murray, M. A. (1990). Self-predictions of emotional response patterns: Age, sex, and situational determinants. *Child Development, 61*, 1124–1133.

Wintre, M., & Vallance, D. D. (1994). A developmental sequence in the comprehension of emotions: Multiple emotions, intensity and valence. *Developmental Psychology, 30*, 509–514.

Wong, M. S., Chen, X., & McElwain, N. L. (2019). Emotion understanding and maternal sensitivity as protective factors against hostile attribution bias in anger-prone children. *Social Development, 28*(1), 41–56.

Wong, M. S., Diener, M. L., & Isabella, R. A. (2008). Parents' emotion related beliefs and behaviors and child grade: Associations with children's perceptions of peer competence. *Journal of Applied Developmental Psychology, 29*, 175–186.

Wong, M. S., McElwain, N. L., & Halberstadt, A. G.

(2009). Parent, family, and child characteristics: Associations with mother- and father-reported emotion socialization practices. *Journal of Family Psychology, 23*, 452–463.

Wong, Y., & Tsai, J. (2007). Cultural models of shame and guilt. In J. L. Tracy, R. W. Robins, & J. P. Tangney (Eds.), *The self-conscious emotions: Theory and research* (pp. 209–223). Guilford Press.

Woods, S. E., Menna, R., & McAndrew, A. J. (2017). The mediating role of emotional control in the link between parenting and young children's physical aggression. *Early Child Development and Care, 187*, 1157–1169.

Wu, J., Zhang, M., Lin, W., Wu, Y., & Li, H. (2021). School-based training for sustainable emotional development in Chinese preschoolers: A quasi-experiment study. *Sustainability, 13*(11), 6331.

Wu, Q., Feng, X., Hooper, E. G., Gerhardt, M., Ku, S., & Chan, M. H. M. (2019). Mother's emotion coaching and preschooler's emotionality: Moderation by maternal parenting stress. *Journal of Applied Developmental Psychology, 65*, 101066.

Wu, Q., Feng, X., Yan, J., Hooper, E. G., Gerhardt, M., & Ku, S. (2022). Maternal emotion coaching styles in the context of maternal depressive symptoms: Associations with preschoolers' emotion regulation. *Emotion, 22*(6), 1171–1184.

Wu, Q., Hooper, E., Feng, X., Gerhardt, M., & Ku, S. (2019). Mothers' depressive symptoms and responses to preschoolers' emotions: Moderated by child expression. *Journal of Applied Developmental Psychology, 60*, 134–143.

Wu, X., Wang, Y., & Liu, A. (2017). Maternal emotional expressiveness affects preschool children's development of knowledge of display rules. *Social Behavior and Personality, 45*(1), 93–103.

Wu, Y., Wu, J., Chen, Y., Han, L., Han, P., Wang, P., & Gao, F. (2015). Shyness and school adjustment among Chinese preschool children: Examining the moderating effect of gender and teacher–child relationship. *Early Education and Development, 26*(2), 149–166.

Xiao, S. X., Spinrad, T. L., & Eisenberg, N. (2019). Longitudinal relations of preschoolers' dispositional and situational anger to their prosocial behavior: The moderating role of shyness. *Social Development, 28*(2), 383–397.

Yan, J. J., Feng, X., Shoppe-Sullivan, S. J., Gerhardt, M., & Wu, Q. (2021). Maternal depressive symptoms predict girls' but not boys' emotion regulation: A prospective moment-to-moment observation study. *Research on Child and Adolescent Psychopathology, 49*, 1227–1240.

Yang, W., Datu, J. A. D., Lin, X., Lau, M. M., & Li, H. (2019). Can early childhood curriculum enhance social-emotional competence in low-income children? A meta-analysis of the educational effects. *Early Education and Development, 30*(1), 36–59.

Yang, Y., Song, Q., Doan, S. N., & Wang, Q. (2020). Maternal reactions to children's negative emotions: Relations to children's socio-emotional development among European American and Chinese immigrant children. *Transcultural Psychiatry, 57*(3), 408–420.

Yelinek, J., & Grady, J. S. (2019). 'Show me your mad faces!': Preschool teachers' emotion talk in the classroom. *Early Child Development and Care, 189*(7), 1063–1071.

Yeo, K., Frydenberg, E., Northam, E., & Deans, J. (2014). Coping with stress among preschool children and associations with anxiety level and controllability of situations. *Australian Journal of Psychology, 66*, 93–101.

Yirmiya, N., Kasari, C., Sigman, M., & Mundy, P. (1989). Facial expression of affect in autistic, mentally retarded, and normal children. *Journal of Child Psychology and Psychiatry, 30*, 725–795.

Young, S. K., Fox, N. A., & Zahn-Waxler, C. (1999). The relations between temperament and empathy in 2-year-olds. *Developmental Psychology, 35*(5), 1189–1197.

Youngblade, L. M., & Dunn, J. (1995). Individual differences in young children's pretend play with mother and sibling: Links to relationships and understanding of other people's feelings and beliefs. *Child Development, 66*, 1472–1492.

Yu, T., Volling, B. L., & Niu, W. (2015). Emotion socialization and children's behavioral problems in China and the United States. *Journal of Comparative Family Studies, 46*(3), 419–434.

Yuill, N. (1984). Young children's coordination of motive and outcome in judgements of satisfaction and morality. *British Journal of Developmental Psychology, 2*, 73–81.

Yule, K., Murphy, C., & Grych, J. (2020). Adaptive functioning in high-risk preschoolers: Caregiver practices beyond parental warmth. *Journal of Child and Family Studies, 29*(1), 115–127.

Zahn-Waxler, C., Iannotti, R. J., Cummings, E. M., & Denham, S. A. (1990). Antecedents of problem behaviors in children of depressed mothers. *Development and Psychopathology, 3*, 271–292.

Zahn-Waxler, C., & Kochanska, G. (1990). The origins of guilt. In R. A. Thompson (Ed.), *Nebraska Symposium on Motivation: Vol. 36. Socioemotional development* (pp. 183–258). University of Nebraska Press.

Zahn-Waxler, C., Kochanska, G., Krupnick, J., & McKnew, D. (1990). Patterns of guilt in children of depressed and well mothers. *Developmental Psychology, 26*, 51–59.

Zahn-Waxler, C., Mayfield, A., Radke-Yarrow, M., McKnew, D., Cytryn, L., & Davenport, Y. (1988). A follow-up investigation of offspring of bipolar parents. *American Journal of Psychiatry, 145*, 506–509.

Zahn-Waxler, C., McKnew, D., Cummings, E. M., Davenport, Y., & Radke-Yarrow, M. (1984). Problem behaviors and peer interactions of young children with a manic–depressive parent. *American Journal of Psychiatry, 141*, 236–240.

Zahn-Waxler, C., & Radke-Yarrow, M. (1982). The development of altruism: Alternative research strategies. In N. Eisenberg (Ed.), *The development of prosocial behavior* (pp. 109–137). Academic Press.

Zahn-Waxler, C., & Radke-Yarrow, M. (1990). The origins of empathic concern. *Motivation and Emotion, 14*, 107–130.

Zahn-Waxler, C., Radke-Yarrow, M., & King, R. A.

(1979). Child rearing and children's prosocial initiations toward victims of distress. *Child Development, 50*, 319–330.

Zahn-Waxler, C., Radke-Yarrow, M., Wagner, E., & Chapman, M. (1992). Development of concern for others. *Developmental Psychology, 28*, 126–136.

Zahn-Waxler, C., Ridgeway, D., Denham, S. A., Usher, B., & Cole, P. (1993). Research strategies for assessing mothers' interpretations of infants' emotions. In R. Emde, J. Osofsky, & P. Butterfield (Eds.), *The IFEEL pictures: A new instrument for interpreting emotions* (pp. 217–236). International Universities Press.

Zahn-Waxler, C., Robinson, J., & Emde, R. (1992). Development of empathy in twins. *Developmental Psychology, 28*, 1038–1047.

Zahn-Waxler, C., Schiro, K., Robinson, J. L., Emde, R. N., & Schmitz, S. (2001). Empathy and prosocial patterns in young MZ and DZ twins. In R. N. Emde & J. K. Hewitt (Eds.), *Infancy to early childhood: Genetic and environmental influences on developmental change* (pp. 141–162). Oxford University Press.

Zajdel, R. T., Bloom, J. M., Fireman, G., & Larsen, J. T. (2013). Children's understanding and experience of mixed emotions: The roles of age, gender, and empathy. *Journal of Genetic Psychology, 174*(5), 582–603.

Zaman, W., & Fivush, R. (2013). Gender differences in elaborative parent–child emotion and play narratives. *Sex Roles, 68*(9–10), 591–604.

Zantinge, G., Rijn, S., Stockmann, L., & Swaab, H. (2017). Physiological arousal and emotion regulation strategies in young children with autism spectrum disorders. *Journal of Autism and Developmental Disorders, 47*(9), 2648–2657.

Zava, F., Sette, S., Baumgartner, E., & Coplan, R. J. (2020). Shyness and empathy in early childhood: Examining links between feelings of empathy and empathetic behaviours. *British Journal of Developmental Psychology, 39*(1), 54–77.

Zeman, J., & Garber, J. (1996). Display rules for anger, sadness, and pain: It depends on who is watching. *Child Development, 67*, 957–973.

Zembylas, M. (2007). Emotional ecology: The intersection of emotion knowledge and pedagogical content knowledge in teaching. *Teaching and Teacher Education, 23*, 355–367.

Zhang, L., Eggum-Wilkens, N. D., Eisenberg, N., & Spinrad, T. L. (2017). Children's shyness, peer acceptance, and academic achievement in the early school years. *Merrill–Palmer Quarterly, 63*(4), 458–484.

Zhu, J., Li, Y., Wood, K. R., Coplan, R. J., & Chen, X. (2019). Shyness and socioemotional functioning in young Chinese children: The moderating role of receptive vocabulary. *Early Education and Development, 30*(5), 590–607.

Zimmer-Gembeck, M. J., Rudolph, J., Kerin, J., & Bohadana-Brown, G. (2022). Parent emotional regulation: A meta-analytic review of its association with parenting and child adjustment. *International Journal of Behavioral Development, 46*(1), 63–82.

Zins, J. E., Bloodworth, M. R., Weissberg, R. P., & Walberg, H. J. (2007). The scientific base linking social and emotional learning to school success. *Journal of Educational and Psychological Consultation, 17*, 191–210.

Zinsser, K. M., Christensen, C. G., & Torres, L. (2016). She's supporting them; who's supporting her?: Preschool center-level social-emotional supports and teacher well-being. *Journal of School Psychology, 59*, 55–66.

Zinsser, K. M., Denham, S. A., & Curby, T. W. (2018). Being a social-emotional teacher. *Young Children, 73*(4), 77–83.

Zinsser, K. M., Denham, S. A., Curby, T. W., & Chazan-Cohen, R. (2016). Early childhood directors as socializers of emotional climate. *Learning Environments Research, 19*(2), 267–290.

Zinsser, K., Denham, S. A., Curby, T. W., & Shewark, E. (2015). "Practice what you preach": Teachers' perceptions of emotional competence and emotionally supportive classroom practices. *Early Education and Development, 26*, 899–919.

Zinsser, K. M., Gordon, R. A., & Jiang, X. (2021). Parents' socialization of preschool-aged children's emotion skills: A meta-analysis using an emotion-focused parenting practices framework. *Early Childhood Research Quarterly, 55*, 377–390.

Zinsser, K., Shewark, E., Denham, S. A., & Curby, T. W. (2014). A mixed-method examination of preschool teacher beliefs about social emotional learning and relations to observed emotional support. *Infant and Child Development, 23*(5), 471–493.

Zinsser, K. M., Weissberg, R. P., & Dusenbury, L. (2013). *Aligning preschool through high school social and emotional learning standards: A critical and doable next step.* Collaborative for Academic, Social, and Emotional Learning.

Zinsser, K. M., & Zinsser, A. (2016). Two case studies of preschool psychosocial safety climates. *Research in Human Development, 13*(1), 49–64.

Ziv, M., Smadja, M., & Aram, D. (2015). Preschool teachers' reference to theory of mind topics during different contexts of shared book reading. *Teaching and Teacher Education, 45*, 14–24.

Zsido, A. N., Arató, N., Ihasz, V., Basler, J., Matuz-Budai, T., Inhof, O., . . . Coelho, C. M. (2021). "Finding an emotional face" revisited: Differences in own-age bias and the happiness superiority effect in children and young adults. *Frontiers in Psychology, 12*.

Zumbach, J., Rademacher, A., & Koglin, U. (2021). Conceptualizing callous-unemotional traits in preschoolers: Associations with social-emotional competencies and aggressive behavior. *Child and Adolescent Psychiatry and Mental Health, 15*(1), 1–10.

# Author Index

# Subject Index

*Note. f* or *t* following a page number indicates a figure or a table.

# About the Author

**Susanne A. Denham PhD,** is an applied developmental psychologist focusing on emotional competence, especially in preschoolers: how it influences children's social and academic functioning, how it is assessed, and how parents and teachers foster it. As a University Professor at George Mason University (now Emeritus), Dr. Denham used her experience as a school psychologist in her research, which was supported by the Institute of Education Sciences, the National Institutes of Health, the W. T. Grant Foundation, the John Templeton Foundation, and the National Science Foundation. She is past coeditor of the journal *Social Development* and current editor of *Early Education and Development.*